NURSING THEORISTS *and* THEIR WORK

Ann Marriner-Tomey, Ph.D., R.N., FAAN
Professor, Indiana University School of Nursing,
Indianapolis, Indiana

SECOND EDITION

Peplau
Orem
Henderson

The C. V. Mosby Company
St. Louis • Baltimore • Philadelphia • Toronto 1989

Mosby

Editor: Allison Miller
Assistant Editor: Laurie Sparks
Production and Editing: Editing, Design & Production, Inc.

SECOND EDITION

Printed in the United States of America

The C.V. Mosby Company
11830 Westline Industrial Drive, St. Louis, Missouri 63146

Library of Congress Cataloging-in-Publication Data

Nursing theorists and their work / [edited by] Ann Marriner-Tomey.—
2nd ed.
p. cm.
Includes bibliographies and index.
ISBN 0-8016-3249-8
1. Nursing—Philosophy. I. Marriner-Tomey, Ann, 1943-
[DNLM: 1. Nurses—biography. 2. Nursing Theory. WY 86 N9738]
RT84.5.N9 1989
610.73'01—dc19
DNLM/DLC
for Library of Congress 89-3135
CIP

C/RRD/RRD 9 8 7 6 5 4 3 2

Contributors

Mary Lee Ackermann
OB/GYN Nurse Practitioner,
Louisville, Kentucky

Sr. Judith E. Alexander
Assistant Professor,
Spalding University,
Louisville, Kentucky

Jill K. Baker
Patient Care Coordinator of Plastic Surgery,
OR and Allied Areas—Long Surgery,
Indiana University Medical Center,
Indianapolis, Indiana

Carolyn J. Beagle
Clinical Charge Nurse, St. Vincent Hospital,
Indianapolis, Indiana

Sarah J. Beckman
Patient Care Coordinator, University Hospitals,
Indianapolis, Indiana

Alberta M. Bee
Major, Army Nurse Corps,
Washington, D.C.

Patricia M. Bennett
Chairperson, Department of Nursing,
Anderson University,
Anderson, Indiana

Sue Marquis Bishop
Associate Professor and Chair,
Graduate Department of Psychiatric/Mental Health Nursing,
Indiana University School of Nursing,
Indianapolis, Indiana

Carolyn L. Blue
Assistant Professor, School of Nursing,
Purdue University,
West Lafayette, Indiana

Debra A. Borchers
Head Nurse,
Children's Hospital,
Medical Center,
Cincinnati, Ohio

Sallie Anne Brink
Charge Nurse, Coronary Care Unit,
Sts. Mary and Elizabeth Hospital,
Louisville, Kentucky

Karen M. Brubaker
Staff Development Coordinator/Critical Care Nursing,
Wishard Memorial Hospital,
Indianapolis, Indiana

Pam Butler
Staff Nurse, Mental Health,
St. Vincent Stress Center,
Indianapolis, Indiana

Jane A. Caldwell-Gwin
Assistant Manager, Nursing Unit,
Adult Burn Unit,
Wishard Memorial Hospital,
Indianapolis, Indiana

Elizabeth T. Carey
Instructor, ADN Program,
Parkland College,
Champaign, Illinois

Lisa A. Carr
Graduate Student,
Indiana University,
Indianapolis, Indiana

Patricia Chapman-Boyce
Hemodialysis Home Training Coordinator,
Indiana University,
Indianapolis, Indiana

Elizabeth Chong Choi
Associate Professor,
Pediatrics, Family, and Women's Health,
Indiana University School of Nursing,
Indianapolis, Indiana

Jo Anne Clanton
LCDR, United States Navy,
Indianapolis, Indiana

Debra Trnka Cochran
PNA Student at Indiana University,
Indianapolis, Indiana

Sydney Coleman-Ehmke
Hospice Nurse,
Visiting Nurse Service,
Indianapolis, Indiana

Sharon S. Conner
Psychiatric Nurse Manager,
Caylor-Nickel Medical Center,
Bluffton, Indiana

Donna J. Crawford
Staff Nurse,
Union Hospital,
Terre Haute, Indiana

Terri Creekmur
Patient Care Coordinator, Burn Unit,
James Whitcomb Riley Hospital,
Indiana University Medical Center,
Indianapolis, Indiana

Joann Sebastian Daily
Instructor, Educational Services,
Bartholomew County Hospital,
Columbus, Indiana

Marguerite Danko
Lecturer, Indiana University School of Nursing,
Indianapolis, Indiana;
Pediatric Nurse Associate,
Marion Community Health Center,
Marion, Indiana

Janet DeFelice
Staff Nurse, Intensive Care Unit,
Winona Memorial Hospital,
Indianapolis, Indiana

Karen R. deGraaf
Nurse Educator,
Jewish Hospital,
Louisville, Kentucky

Deborah Wertman DeMeester
Cardiac Rehabilitation Instructor,
Methodist Hospital,
Indianapolis, Indiana

Marilyn Sue Doub
Long-term Care Consultant,
Bloomington, Indiana

Deborah A. Dougherty
Nursing Service Supervisor,
Johnson County Memorial Hospital,
Franklin, Indiana

Dorothy Kay Dycus
Family Nurse Practitioner,
Lake County Health Department of Lake County, Indiana,
Crown Point, Indiana

Jeanne Donohue Eben
Assistant Clinical Director,
Emergency Nursing,
Wishard Memorial Hospital,
Indianapolis, Indiana

Julia M. Fine
Staff Nurse,
Union Hospital,
Terre Haute, Indiana

Karen J. Foli
Instructor,
Lakeview College,
Danville, Illinois

Nergess N. Gashti
Head Nurse,
VA Medical Center,
Indianapolis, Indiana

Alta J.H. Gochnauer
Graduate Student,
Indiana University School of Nursing,
Indianapolis, Indiana

S. Brook Gumm
Patient Care Coordinator,
Children's Hospital,
Cincinnati, Ohio

Cheryl A. Hailway
Medical Search Specialist,
Midwest Medical Consultants,
Indianapolis, Indiana

Brenda Kay Harmon
Staff Nurse, ICU/CCU,
Indiana University Hospitals,
Indianapolis, Indiana

Susan Matthews Harris
Staff Nurse, Intensive Care Unit,
James Whitcomb Riley Hospital,
Indianapolis, Indiana

DeAnn M. Hensley
Supervisor,
University Heights Hospital,
Indianapolis, Indiana

Mary E. Hermiz
Principal Tutor,
Tenwek Hospital,
Boonet, Kenya, Africa

Deborah Hissa
Nurse Practitioner,
University of Cincinnati Medical Center,
Cincinnati, Ohio

William H. Hobble
Staff Nurse,
VA Medical Center,
Indianapolis, Indiana

Anne Hodel
Assistant Director,
Home Health Services,
Indianapolis, Indiana

Nancy E. Hunt
Clinical Head Nurse,
Lettermah Army Medical Center,
San Francisco, California

Connie Rae Jarlsberg
Manager, Nursing Unit,
Wishard Memorial Hospital,
Indianapolis, Indiana

Tamara Johnson
Assistant Manager, ICUs,
Community Hospital of Indianapolis,
Indianapolis, Indiana

Cathy Greenwell Jones
Staff Nurse II, ICU,
Sts. Mary and Elizabeth Hospital,
Louisville, Kentucky

Rhonda G. Justus
Staff Nurse,
James Whitcomb Riley Hospital,
Indianapolis, Indiana

Karla G. Kaltofen
Staff Nurse,
James Whitcomb Riley Hospital,
Indianapolis, Indiana

Juanita Fogel Keck
Assistant Professor,
Nursing of Adults with Biodissonance,
Indiana University School of Nursing,
Indianapolis, Indiana

M. Jan Keffer
Doctoral Student,
University of Illinois,
Chicago, Illinois

Kimberly A. Kilgore-Keever
Renal/Pancreas Transport Coordinator,
Methodist Hospital,
Indianapolis, Indiana

Martha J. Kirsch
Graduate Student,
Indiana University,
Indianapolis, Indiana

Jill Vass Langfitt
Graduate Student,
Indiana University School of Nursing,
Indianapolis, Indiana

Theresa Lansinger
Director Staff Development,
United Samaritans Medical Center,
Danville, Illinois

Tamara Lauer
Nurse Director of Diabetes Services,
Community Hospitals,
Indianapolis, Indiana

Rickard E. Lee
Graduate Student,
Indiana University,
Indianapolis, Indiana

Jude A. Magers
Director of Nursing,
St. Vincent Stress Center,
Indianapolis, Indiana

Judith E. Marich
Manager, Labor and Delivery,
St. Vincent Hospital,
Indianapolis, Indiana

Ann Marriner-Tomey
Professor,
Indiana University School of Nursing,
Indianapolis, Indiana

Judy Sporleder Maupin
Surgical, Emergency, Psychiatric Service,
Bartholomew County Hospital,
Columbus, Indiana

Judy McCormick
Assistant Head Nurse,
Community Hospital/North,
Indianapolis, Indiana

Cynthia A. McCreary
Chief Nurse, Children and Youth Project,
University of Texas Health Science Center at Dallas,
Dallas, Texas

Mary Meininger
Staff Nurse, Renal Intensive Care Unit,
Indiana University Hospital,
Indianapolis, Indiana

Kathleen Millican Miller
Post-Anesthesia Care Unit,
St. Elizabeth Hospital,
Lafayette, Indiana

Deborah I. Mills
Instructor,
Parkview Methodist School of Nursing,
Fort Wayne, Indiana

Sandra L. Moody
Clinical Nurse Specialist,
LaRue D. Carter Memorial Hospital,
Indianapolis, Indiana

Cynthia L. Mossman
Staff Nurse, Special Care Nursery,
Wishard Memorial Hospital,
Indianapolis, Indiana

Margaret J. Nation
Quality Assurance Coordinator,
Maxicare Indiana, Inc.,
Indianapolis, Indiana

Susan E. Neal
Public Health Nurse,
Marion County Bureau of Public Health Nursing,
Indianapolis, Indiana

John Noll
Psychiatric Nurse,
Community Hospital,
Indianapolis, Indiana

Kathryn W. Noone
Staff Nurse,
Cardiac Intensive Care,
Indiana University Hospital,
Indianapolis, Indiana

Sherry B. Nordmeyer
Instructor,
Indiana University School of Nursing,
Indianapolis, Indiana

Stephanie Oetting
Staff Nurse,
Methodist Hospital,
Indianapolis, Indiana

Nancy Orcutt
Pediatric Nurse Associate, Metro Health,
Indianapolis, Indiana

Katherine R. Papazian
Instructor, School of Nursing,
Ball State University,
Muncie, Indiana

Gwynn Lee Perlich
Nursing Supervisor,
St. Vincent Hospital and Health Care Center,
Indianapolis, Indiana

Kim Tippey Peskoe
Faculty,
Ball State University School of Nursing,
Muncie, Indiana

LaPhyllis Peterson
Student,
Indiana University School of Nursing,
Indianapolis, Indiana

Cheryl Y. Petty
Nurse Practitioner,
VA Medical Center,
Indianapolis, Indiana

Mary Carolyn Poat
Staff RN,
Indiana University Hospital,
Indianapolis, Indiana

LaDema Poppa
Clinical Nurse Specialist,
Central State Hospital,
Indianapolis, Indiana

Beverly D. Porter
Research Coordinator,
Regenstrief Health Center,
Indianapolis, Indiana

Debra L. Price
Staff Nurse,
Community Hospital,
Indianapolis, Indiana

Beth Bruns Prusinski
Staff Nurse,
St. Vincent Hospital and Health Care Center,
Indianapolis, Indiana

Rosalyn A. Pung
Graduate Student,
Indiana University School of Nursing,
Indianapolis, Indiana

LyNette Rasmussen
Staff Nurse,
Parkview Memorial Hospital,
Fort Wayne, Indiana

Cynthia M. Riester
Patient Care Coordinator,
St. Francis Hospital,
Indianapolis, Indiana

Karen D. Andrews Robards
Department Manager, CCU and Telemetry,
Johnson County Memorial Hospital,
Franklin, Indiana

Martha Carole Satterly
Manager, Outpatient Surgery,
Bartholomew County Hospital,
Columbus, Indiana

Marcia K. Sauter
Assistant Professor,
Methodist School of Nursing,
Saint Francis College,
Fort Wayne, Indiana

Donna N. Schmeiser
Co-owner and Practitioner,
Partners in Health, Inc.,
Lafayette, Indiana

Denise L. Schnell
Unit Manager,
St. Francis Hospital,
Indianapolis, Indiana

Larry P. Schumacher
Director, Critical Care Nursing,
Research Medical Center,
Kansas City, Missouri

Bryn Searcy
Staff Nurse,
St. Vincent Hospital,
Indianapolis, Indiana

Maribeth Slebodnik
Staff Nurse, Special Care Nursery,
Wishard Memorial Hospital,
Indianapolis, Indiana

Rebecca S. Sloan
Director of Research Nursing,
Kidney Disease Program,
University of Louisville,
Louisville, Kentucky

Cathy R. Smith
Staff Nurse,
Indiana University Hospitals,
Indianapolis, Indiana

Nancy L. Stark
Staff Nurse, Intensive Care Unit,
St. Vincent Hospital,
Indianapolis, Indiana

Sandra E. Steinkeler
Coordinator, Corporate Health Promotion,
Indiana Heart Insititute,
Indianapolis, Indiana

Margery Stuart
Instructor,
Lakeview Medical Center School of Nursing,
Danville, Illinois

Flossie M. Taggart
Oncology Clinical Associate,
Methodist Hospital,
Indianapolis, Indiana

Elizabeth Godfrey Terry
Health Research Editor,
The Children's Better Health Institute,
Indianapolis, Indiana

Catherine Velotta
Staff Nurse,
University of Kentucky Medical Center,
Lexington, Kentucky

Therese L. Wallace
Staff Nurse,
Indiana University Hospitals,
Indianapolis, Indiana

Judith K. Watt
Director, Community-Oriented Care,
People's Health Care,
Indianapolis, Indiana

Cynthia A. Wesolowski
Educational Nurse Specialist
Children's Hospital Medical Center,
Cincinnati, Ohio

Sandy Williams
Office Nurse,
Indianapolis, Indiana

Roberta Woeste
Staff Nurse,
St. Francis Hospital,
Indianapolis, Indiana

Roseanne Yancey
Oncology Clinical Nurse Specialist,
Riverside Methodist Hospitals,
Columbus, Ohio

Lorraine A. Yeager
Staff Nurse,
James Whitcomb Riley Hospital,
Indianapolis, Indiana

Susan T. Zoretich
Staff Nurse,
St. Vincent's Hospital,
Indianapolis, Indiana

Theorists

Faye Glenn Abdellah
Dept. Surgeon General and Chief Nurse Officer
US Public Health Service
Dept. of Health & Human Services
Room 18-67 Parklawn Building
5600 Fisher Lane
Rockville, MD 20857
(301) 443-4000

Evelyn Adam
Faculty of Nursing University of Montreal
P.O. Box 6128, Station A
Montreal, Quebec HEC-317
(514) 343-7486

Kathryn E. Barnard
University of Washington
Mail Stop WJ-10
Seattle, WA 98195
(206) 543-9200

Patricia Benner
University of California at San Francisco
School of Nursing
San Francisco, CA 94143
(415) 476-4313

Helen C. Erickson
University of Texas
Austin, TX 78701
(512) 471-7311

Joyce J. Fitzpatrick
Case Western Reserve University
Frances Payne Bolton School of Nursing
2121 Abington Road
Cleveland, OH 44106
(216) 368-2544

†Lydia E. Hall

Virginia Henderson
(retired)
164 Linden Street
New Haven, CT 06511
(203) 624-1272

Dorothy E. Johnson
(retired)
715 Grouper Lane
Key Largo, FL 33037
(305) 852-3149

Imogene King
University of Southern Florida
Medical Center
College of Nursing
Box 22
12901 North 30th Street
Tampa, FL 33612
(813) 974-2191

Madeleine Leininger
Wayne State University
5557 Cass
Detroit, MI 48202
(313) 577-4085

Myra Estrin Levine
Professor Emerita
University of Illinois
701 Forum Square, Apt. 509
Glenview, IL 60025
(312) 390-8084

Ramona T. Mercer
(retired)
1809 Ashton Avenue
Burlingame, CA 94010
(415) 697-2324

†Deceased

Betty Neuman
Box 488
Beverly, OH 45715
(614) 749-3322

Margaret A. Newman
University of Minnesota
School of Nursing
5-104 Unit F
308 Howard Street
Minneapolis, MN 55455
(612) 376-7299

†*Florence Nightingale*

Dorothea E. Orem
Orem & Shields, Inc.
55 Dear Run
Savannah, GA 31411
(912) 598-1759

Rosemarie Rizzo Parse
Nursing Science Q
320 Fort Duquesane Blvd.
Suite 25J
Pittsburgh, PA 15222
(412) 391-8471

Ida Jean Orlando (Pelletier)
80 Hawthorne
Belmont, MA 02178
(617) 489-0348

Hildegard E. Peplau
(retired)
14024 Ostego Street
Sherman Oaks, CA 91403
(818) 783-2272

Martha E. Rogers
The Division of Nursing
New York University
429 Shimkin Hall
Washington Square
New York, NY 10003
(212) 598-3921

Sister Callista Roy
Boston College
Cushing Hall
140 Commonwealth Avenue
Chestnut Hill, MA 02167
(617) 552-8811

Joan Riehl Sisca
Indiana University of Pennsylvania
Indiana, PA 15705
(412) 357-2557

Mary Ann P. Swain
Office of Academic Affairs
University of Michigan
Ann Arbor, MI 48109
(313) 764-0151

Evelyn M. Tomlin
P.O. Box 128
Big Rock, IL 60511
(312) 556-3087

†*Joyce Travelbee*

Jean Watson
University of Colorado
Health Sciences Center
School of Nursing
4200 E. Ninth Avenue
Denver, CO 80262
(303) 384-7754

Ernestine Wiedenbach
(retired)
926 Eastridge Village Drive
Miami, FL 33157
(305) 235-5931

---

†Deceased

Preface

This book is a tribute to nursing theorists. It identifies major thinkers in nursing, reviews some of their important ideas, and lists their publications, what has been written about them, and the major sources they used. The first chapter is a brief overview of the book and is appropriate for the baccalaureate level. The other chapters in Unit I define terminology and discuss history and philosophy of science, logical reasoning, the theory development process, and the evolution of nursing theory development at a graduate level.

The theorists are clustered into four categories according to major themes. The categories are not mutually exclusive. Nightingale, Henderson, Abdellah, Hall, Orem, Adam, Leininger, Watson, Parse, and Benner have written about the art and science of humanistic nursing. Peplau, Travelbee, Orlando, Wiedenbach, Riehl-Sisca, Erickson, Tomlin, Swain, Barnard, and Mercer have all dealt with interpersonal relationships. Johnson, Roy, King, and Neuman have written about systems. Levine, Rogers, Fitzpatrick, and Newman are associated with energy fields.

Credentials and background of the theorist, theoretical sources for the theory development, use of empirical data, major concepts and definitions, assumptions, theoretical assertions, logical form, acceptance by the nursing community, further development, and a critique are identified for each theorist. Baccalaureate students may be most interested in the concepts, definitions, and theoretical assertions. Graduate students will be interested in logical form, acceptance by the nursing community, the theoretical sources for theory development, and the use of empirical data. The extensive bibliographies should be particularly useful to graduate students for locating primary and secondary sources.

Many of the scholars identified in this book do not consider themselves theorists and never intended to develop theory. Is it fair to evaluate them as theorists and their work as theory? Probably not, but their thoughts are important contributions to the development of nursing theory. It is now our responsibility to analyze and synthesize their work, generate new ideas, and continue theory development.

I would like to thank the theorists for critiquing the chapters about themselves so the content could be current and accurate. So that their omission does not appear to have been an oversight, the work of Paterson and Zderad has not been included in this volume at their request. Thanks are expressed to the following graduate students for assistance with data collection: Jeanette Adam, Cynthia J. Allen, Fatmah Arafat, Judy K. Cowling, Sharon Evick, Kathy McGregor, Catherine Martin, Glenda Mitchell, Janet Pezelle, Nancy Preuss, Larry P.

Schumacher, and Anthony G. Smith. Appreciation is expressed to the following: Shirley Bastin helped obtain audiotapes for the learning laboratory. The reference librarians—Fran Brahmi, Cassandra Brooks, Janine Orr, Peggy Richwine, Sharon Schmidt, and JoAnn Switzer—helped us do computer searches to locate theorists' work. Beth Gruenwald, Marilyn Wacker, and Lorraine Brents obtained materials through interlibrary loan. Jeanne Mueller, Carole Francq, Cindy LaShorne, and Jo Chapple purchased and processed library acquisitions. Harold Shaffer, William Stoddand, and Joseph Robinson worked the circulation desk, controlled the reserved books, and searched for missing materials. Dorothy Pock did an outstanding job of typing the manuscript as she patiently worked her way through several drafts, repairing format and noting problems. Lisa Mount provided secretarial services necessary for this project. I would also like to thank my friend Art Slightom for helping my husband create a space conducive for scholarly work and my loving husband, H. Keith Tomey, for enriching my private life while supporting my professional activities.

Ann Marriner-Tomey
August 1988

Contents

UNIT IV Systems

UNIT V Energy Fields

UNIT I

Analysis of Nursing Theories

Introduction to Analysis of Nursing Theories

1

Ann Marriner-Tomey

REASONS FOR THEORY

Theory helps provide knowledge to improve practice by describing, explaining, predicting, and controlling phenomena. Nurses' power is increased through theoretical knowledge because systematically developed methods are more likely to be successful. Nurses also know why they are doing what they are doing if challenged. Theory provides professional autonomy by guiding the practice, education, and research functions of the profession. The study of theory helps develop analytical skills, challenge thinking, clarify values and assumptions, and determine purposes for nursing practice, education, and research.[10, 11, 15, 51, 56]

MAJOR CONCEPTS AND DEFINITIONS OF THEORY DEVELOPMENT

Philosophy

Philosophy is "the science comprising logic, ethics, aesthetics, metaphysics, and epistemology." It is the "investigation of causes and laws underlying reality" and is "inquiry into the nature of things based on logical reasoning rather than empirical methods."[38:985]

Science

Science is "the observation, identification, description, experimental investigation, and theoretical explanation of natural phenomena."[38:1162] It is a "body of knowledge."[10:72]

Knowledge

"Knowledge is an awareness or perception of reality acquired through learning or investigation."[10:72]

Fact

A fact is "something known with certainty."[38:469]

Model

"A model is an idea that explains by using symbolic and physical visualization."[63:62] Symbolic models may be verbal, schematic, or quantitative. They no longer have a recognizable physical form and are a higher level of abstraction than physical models. Verbal models are worded statements. Schematic models may be diagrams, drawings, graphs, or pictures. Quantitative models are mathematical symbols. Physical models may look like what they are supposed to represent, for example, body organs, or they may become more abstract while still keeping some of the physical properties, like ECG.[27] Models can be used "to facilitate thinking about concepts and relationships between them"[8] or to map out the research process.[9]

Paradigm

A paradigm is "a conceptual diagram."[63:62] It can be a large structure used to organize theory.*

Theory

A theory is "a set of concepts, definitions, and propositions that project a systematic view of phenomena by designing specific interrelationships among concepts for purposes of describing, explaining, and predicting."[10:79]

Concept

A concept is a "complex mental formulation of an object, property, or event that is derived from individual perceptual experience."[10:202] It is "an idea; a mental image; a generalization formed and developed in the mind."[1:116] Concepts label phenomena.

ABSTRACT CONCEPT. Abstract concepts are completely independent of time or place. Temperature, for example, is an abstract concept.[52:49]

CONCRETE CONCEPT. A concrete concept is specific to time and place, such as the body temperature of a specific person at a specific time on a specific day.[52:49]

Phenomenon

A phenomenon is "any occurrence or fact that is directly perceptible by the senses."[52:983] It is reality on "what exists in the real world."[24:7]

Definitions

Definitions are statements of the meaning of a word, phrase, or term.[38:346]

THEORETICAL DEFINITIONS. Theoretical definitions convey the general meaning of the concept in a manner that fits the theory.[10:207]

OPERATIONAL DEFINITIONS. Operational definitions specify "the activities or 'operations' necessary to measure a construct or a variable."[61:62]

Assumptions

Assumptions are statements supposed to be true without proof or demonstration.[34:80] They may be explicit or implicit.[10:126]

Theoretical Statements

Theoretical statements describe a relationship between two or more concepts.

LAW. A law is "a statement that describes a relationship in which scientists have so much confidence they consider it an absolute 'truth.' "[52:78]

AXIOMS. Axioms are "a basic set of statements, each independent of the others (they say different things), from which all other statements of the theory may be logically derived."[52:78] Axioms are often associated with plane geometry.

PROPOSITIONS. Propositions are theorems or statements derived from axioms. The term is often used interchangeably with hypotheses to mean "any idea or hunch that is presented in the form of a scientific statement."[52:78]

HYPOTHESIS. An hypothesis is a relationship statement to be tested.[52:78]

EMPIRICAL GENERALIZATIONS. Empirical generalizations are patterns "of events found in a number of different empirical studies."[52:79]

EXISTENCE. Existence statements establish a typology by indicating a concept exists.[52:76]

RELATIONAL STATEMENTS. Relational statements indicate that values of one concept

*References 10:76; 37:70-71; 51:21-33.

are associated or correlated with values of another. Relationships may be linear or curvilinear. Linear relationships may be either positive ("when one concept occurs, or is high, the other concept occurs, or is high, or vice versa") or negative ("when one concept occurs or is high, the other concept is low, and vice versa") or no relationship may exist (when "the occurrence of one concept gives no information about the occurrence of the other concept and vice versa").[52:70] Curvilinear relationships are characterized by curved lines (when one concept is high and low, the other concept is high or low).

CAUSAL. One concept is believed to cause the occurrence of another concept if they have a causal relationship.[52:71] Correlation is not necessarily causation.

DETERMINISTIC. Dependent variables are determined by independent variables.[52:74]

PROBABILISTIC. Probability predicts both nonoccurrence and occurrence of something.[52:75]

Research

"Research is application of systematic methods to obtain reliable and valid knowledge about empirical reality."[10:82] Research may generate theory with an inductive approach or test it by a deductive approach.

Range of Theories

"Subject matter for a theory may be very broad and all inclusive or very narrow and limited."[24:13]

GRAND THEORY. Grand theories are broad in scope and complex. "In most instances, grand theories require further specification and partitioning of theoretical statements for them to be empirically tested and theoretically verified. Grand theorists state their theoretical formulations at the most general level of abstraction, and it is often difficult to link these formulations to reality."[24:13] Grand theories contain summative concepts that incorporate smaller range theories.

MIDDLE RANGE THEORY. Middle range theory has a narrower focus than grand theory and a broader focus than micro theory. The scope is not so large as to be relatively useless for summative concepts and not so narrow that it cannot be used to explain complex life situations.[37:68]

MICRO THEORY. Micro theories are the least complex and most specific. They are "a set of theoretical statements, usually hypotheses, that deal with narrowly defined phenomena."[24:13]

DEVELOPMENT OF THEORY

Theory Development Process

Theory development is a process that primarily involves induction, deduction, and retroduction.

INDUCTION. Induction is "a form of reasoning that moves from the specific to the general. In inductive logic, a series of particulars is combined into a larger whole or set of things. In inductive research, particular events are observed and analyzed as a basis for formulating general theoretical statements, often called grounded 'theory.' "[10:204] This is a research to theory approach.

DEDUCTION. Deduction is a form of logical reasoning that progresses from general to specific. This process involves a sequence of theoretical statements derived from a few general statements or axioms. Two or more relational statements are used to draw a conclusion. Abstract theoretical relationships are used to derive specific empirical hypotheses. This is a theory to research approach.[10:202]

RETRODUCTION. Retroduction combines induction and deduction.[10:205]

Forms of Theory

Theories may be organized according to their form into three categories. These categories include set-of-laws, axiomatic, and causal process.

SET-OF-LAWS. This is an inductive approach that seeks patterns in research findings. Research findings are selected and sorted according to degree of empirical support into categories of laws, empirical generalizations, and hypotheses. It may be difficult to organize and interrelate these generalizations. Because the statements are not interrelated, support for one statement does not support another statement. Consequently, research efforts must be extensive.[52]

AXIOMATIC. The axiomatic form is an interrelated logical system of concepts, definitions, and relationship statements arranged in hierarchical order. Abstract axioms are at the top of the hierarchy with derived propositions being lower. Required research is less extensive because empirical support for one relational statement also supports the theory.[52]

CAUSAL PROCESS. The causal process increases understanding through relationship statements that specify cause between independent and dependent variables. This form also requires concepts, definitions, and relationship statements. It explains how something happens.[52,61]

CRITERIA FOR EVALUATION OF THEORY

Although many authors use different terms to describe criteria for evaluating theory, issues often discussed are clarity, simplicity, generality, empirical precision, and derivable consequences.

Clarity

Semantic and structural clarity and consistency are important. To assess this, one should identify the major concepts and subconcepts and identify definitions for them. Words should be invented only if necessary, and they should be carefully defined. Sometimes words have multiple and competing meanings within and across disciplines. Therefore, words should be borrowed cautiously and defined carefully. Diagrams and examples may provide more clarity and should be consistent. The logical development should be clear, and assumptions should be consistent with the theory's goals.[9:133-137]

Reynolds refers to intersubjectivity when he says, "there must be shared agreement of the definitions of concepts and relationships between concepts within a theory."[52:13] Hardy refers to meaning and logical adequacy when stating that "concepts and relationships between concepts must be clearly identified and valid."[19:106] Stevens also speaks of clarity and consistency.[58] Ellis refers to the criterion of terminology to evaluate theory and addresses the danger of lost meaning when terms are borrowed from other disciplines and used in a different context.[13:221] Walker and Avant say, "logical adequacy of a theory is the logical structure of the concepts and statements independent of the meaning of those concepts or statements."[62:119]

Simplicity

Chinn and Jacobs state, "In nursing, practitioners need simple theory to guide practice."[9:138] Argyris indicates that a theory "should be maximally comprehensive and concrete . . . and it should do so with the fewest concepts and the simplest relations of concepts."[4:198] In contrast, Ellis believes a theory must have complexity to be significant.[13:219] Reynolds suggests that simply counting the number of concepts is not sufficient. He says the most useful theory provides the greatest sense of understanding.[51:135] Walker and Avant refer to parsimony as ". . . elegant in its simplicity, even though it may be broad in content."[62:130]

Generality

To determine the generality of a theory, the scope of concepts and goals within the theory are examined. The more limited the concepts and goals, the less general the theory. Ada Jacox says, "There is no pressing need to develop a 'grand theory' that supposedly includes everything that nurses need to know."[58:65] Chinn and Jacobs believe situations to which the theory applies should not be limited.[9:139-140] Ellis says, "The broader the scope . . . the greater the significance of the theory."[13:219] Stevens suggests that both broad and narrow scopes are necessary and that the complexity or simplicity should be determined by the complexity of the subject matter.[58:65-66]

Empirical Precision

Empirical precision is linked to the testability and ultimate use of a theory and refers to the "extent that the defined concepts are grounded in observable reality."[9:144] Hardy states that "how well the evidence supports the theory is indicative of empirical adequacy" and agrees there "should be a match between theoretical claims and the empirical evidence."[19:105] Reynolds refers to empirical relevance and the trait that "anyone be able to examine the correspondence between a particular theory and the objective empirical data."[52:18] He notes that other scientists should be able to evaluate and verify results for themselves. Walker and Avant say, "If a theory cannot generate hypotheses, it is not useful to scientists and does not add to the body of knowledge."[62:131] In contrast, Ellis states, testability of a theory can be sacrificed in favor of scope, complexity, and clinical usefulness. Elegance and complexity of structure are preferred to precision in the meaning of concepts.[13:220] She maintains that theories should be clearly recognized as tentative and hypothetical. Chinn and Jacobs believe "if research, theory, and practice are to be meaningfully related, then theory in nursing should lend itself to research testing, and research testing should guide practice."[10:145]

Derivable Consequences

Chinn and Jacobs state, "Nursing theory ought to guide research and practice, generate new ideas, and differentiate the focus of nursing from other professions."[10:145] Ellis indicates that to be considered useful, "it is essential for theory to develop and guide practice . . . theories should reveal what knowledge nurses must, and should, spend time pursuing."[13:220] Hardy believes the nursing profession should "make use of existing theory to predict certain outcomes and control events in such a way that desired outcomes are achieved."[19:106]

NURSING THEORISTS
Art and Science of Humanistic Nursing

Nightingale, Henderson, Abdellah, Hall, Orem, Adam, Leininger, Watson, Parse, and Benner are grouped together because of their views about humanistic nursing as an art and science.

Florence Nightingale believed every woman would be responsible for someone's health at some time and consequently would be a nurse. She thought disease was a reparative process, and the nurse should manipulate the environment to facilitate the process. Her directions regarding ventilation, warmth, light, diet, cleanliness, and noise are recorded in her *Notes on Nursing.*[44]

Virginia Henderson has made enormous contributions to nursing in more than 60 years of service as a nurse, teacher, author, and researcher. She has published prolifically throughout those years. Her definition of nursing first appeared in the fifth edition of *Textbook of the Principles and Practice of Nursing* in 1955.[20] Henderson indicates, "The unique function of the nurse is to assist the individual, sick or well, in the performance of those activities contributing to health or its recovery (or to peaceful death) that he would perform unaided if he had the necessary strength, will, or knowledge and to do this in such a way as to help him gain independence as rapidly as possible."[22:7] In *The Nature of Nursing,* she also identified 14 basic needs of patients that comprise the components of nursing care: (1) breathing, (2) eating and drinking, (3) elimination, (4) movement,

(5) rest and sleep, (6) suitable clothing, (7) body temperature, (8) clean body and protected integument, (9) safe environment, (10) communication, (11) worship, (12) work, (13) play, and (14) learning.[22:16-17] She identified three levels of nurse-patient relationships: being a (1) substitute for the patient, (2) helper to the patient, and (3) partner with the patient.[22:16] She supports empathetic understanding and says the nurse needs to "get inside the skin of each of her patients in order to know what he needs."[21:63] Henderson believes many nurses' and physicians' functions overlap. She says the nurse works in interdependence with other health professionals and compares the health team to wedges on a pie graph. The sizes of pie vary depending on the patient's needs. The goal is to have the patient represented by most of the pie as he gains independence.[22:22-23]

Faye Glenn Abdellah has written prolifically about a variety of subjects since the early 1950s. She and others conceptualized 21 nursing problems based on systematic use of research data to teach and evaluate students. The typology of 21 nursing problems first appeared in the 1960 edition of *Patient-Centered Approaches to Nursing.*[2]

Lydia E. Hall used her philosophy of nursing to design and develop the Loeb Center for Nursing at Montefiore Hospital in New York. She served as Administrative Director of the Loeb Center from its opening in 1963 until her death in 1969. Most of her work was published in the 1960s. Her model for nursing was presented in "Nursing: What is it?" in *The Canadian Nurse* in 1964[17] and discussed in "The Loeb Center for Nursing and Rehabilitation" in the *International Journal of Nursing Studies* in 1969.[18] She believed nursing functions differently in the three interlocking circles that constitute aspects of the patient. She labeled the circles the body (the care), the disease (the cure), and the person (the core). Nursing functions in all three circles but share them with other providers to different degrees. She believed that more professional nursing care and teaching are needed as less medical care is needed and that professional nursing care will hasten recovery.

Dorothea E. Orem had a spontaneous insight about the concept of nursing in 1958. She has been publishing since the 1950s about nursing practice and education. She identifies her self-care deficit theory of nursing as a general theory composed of three related theories: (1) the theory of self-care, (2) the theory of self-care deficit, and (3) the theory of nursing systems. Orem identifies three types of nursing systems: (1) wholly compensatory—doing for the patient, (2) partly compensatory—helping the person do for himself, and (3) supportive-educative—helping the person learn to do for himself. The theories are discussed more fully in her book, *Nursing: Concepts of Practice.* She believes nurses share some functions with other health care providers.[45]

Evelyn Adam started publishing in the mid-1970s. Much of her work focuses on developing models and theories on the concept of nursing. She uses a model she learned from Dorothy Johnson. In her book, *To be a Nurse,*[1] she applies Virginia Henderson's definition of nursing to the model and identifies the assumptions, beliefs and values, and major units. In the latter category she includes the goal of the profession, the beneficiary of the professional service, the role of the professional, the source of the beneficiary's difficulty, the intervention of the professional, and the consequences.

Madeleine Leininger has published prolifically about a variety of topics since 1960. Although she has written several books about transcultural nursing and caring, the most complete account of transcultural care theory is found in her 1984 book, *Care: The Essence of Nursing and Health.*[28] Some of the major concepts are care, caring, culture, cultural values, and cultural variations. Leininger has generated many hypotheses and hopes to stimulate further ethnoscience research by nurses in ethnonursing.

Jean Watson started publishing in the mid-

1970s. Her book, *Nursing: The Philosophy and Science of Caring,* was published in 1979.[63] The content was further refined in *Nursing: Human Science and Health Care* in 1985.[64] In an effort to reduce the dichotomy between theory and practice, Watson proposed a philosophy and science of caring. She identified 10 carative factors: (1) the formation of a humanistic-altruistic system of values; (2) the instillation of faith-hope; (3) the cultivation of sensitivity to self and to others; (4) the development of a helping-trust relationship; (5) the promotion and acceptance of the expression of positive and negative; (6) the systematic use of the scientific problem-solving method for decision making; (7) the promotion of interpersonal teaching-learning; (8) the provision for a supportive, protective, or corrective mental, physical, sociocultural, and spiritual environment; (9) assistance with the gratification of human needs; and (10) the allowance for existential-phenomenological forces. Watson believes nurses should develop health promotion through preventive actions such as recognizing coping skills and adaptation to loss, teaching problem-solving methods, and providing situational support.

Rosemarie Rizzo Parse drew from the work of Martha Rogers and the existential-phenomenologists for the development of *Man-Living-Health: A Theory of Nursing.*[48] Major concepts include imaging, valuing, languaging, revealing-concealing, enabling-limiting, connecting-separating, powering, originating, and transforming. Parse stresses humanism.

Patrica Benner validated the Dreyfus model of skill acquisition in nursing practice by systematic description of the five stages—novice, advanced beginner, competent, proficient, and expert. In *From Novice to Expert: Excellence and Power in Clinical Nursing Practice* (1984), she provided many exemplars and described nursing practice at each stage.[6] Seven domains of nursing practice were derived from the descriptions of the cases, and a list of 31 nursing competencies was generated. From Benner's description of nursing practice, a phenomenological theory describing caring evolved and is presented in Brenner and Wrubel's 1988 book, *The Primacy of Caring: Stress and Coping in Health and Illness.*[7]

Interpersonal Relationships

Peplau; Travelbee; Orlando; Wiedenbach; Riehl-Sisca; Erickson, Tomlin, and Swain; Barnard and Mercer all address interpersonal relationships.

Hildegard E. Peplau's contributions to nursing in general and the specialty of psychiatric nursing specifically have been enormous. She has been publishing prolifically since the early 1950s, beginning with her book, *Interpersonal Relations in Nursing.*[51] She teaches psychodynamic nursing and stresses the importance of the nurse understanding his or her own behavior in order to help others identify perceived difficulties. She identifies four phases of the nurse-patient relationship: (1) orientation, (2) identification, (3) exploitation, and (4) resolution. Peplau describes six nursing roles: (1) stranger, (2) resource person, (3) teacher, (4) leader, (5) surrogate, and (6) counselor. She discusses four psychobiological experiences—needs, frustrations, conflicts, and anxieties—that compel destructive or constructive responses.

Joyce Travelbee published predominantly in the mid-1960s. She died in 1973 at a relatively young age. Travelbee promoted her Human-to-Human Relationship Model in her book, *Interpersonal Aspects of Nursing.*[59,60] She wrote about illness, suffering, pain, hope, communication, interaction, therapeutic use of self, empathy, sympathy, and rapport. She believed nursing was accomplished through human-to-human relationships that began with (1) the original encounter and then progressed through stages of (2) emerging identities, (3) developing feelings of empathy, and (4) later of sympathy, until (5) the nurse and patient attained a rapport in the final stage.

Ida Jean Orlando (Pelletier) first described her Disciplined Professional Response Theory in *The Dynamic Nurse-Patient Relationship*[46] and related research is reported in *The Discipline and Teaching of Nursing Process.*[47] Her theory stresses the reciprocal relationship between the nurse and the patient. Each is affected by what the other says and does. Orlando emphasizes the importance of exploring perceptions, thoughts, and feelings with the other party for verification. This process discipline or exploration validates the patient's need for help, which the nurse then meets directly or indirectly. Deliberative nursing actions purposefully identify and meet the patient's immediate need for help. If nursing actions are not deliberative, they are automatic and may not meet the patient's need for help.

Ernestine Wiedenbach, a maternity nurse, was stimulated by Orlando to think about the use of self and how thoughts and feelings affect a nurse's actions. She identifies and defines many concepts in her book, *Clinical Nursing: A Helping Art.*[65] Concepts and subconcepts include: patient, need-for-help, nurse, purpose, philosophy, practice (knowledge, judgment, and skills), ministration, validation, coordination (reporting, consulting, conferring), and art (stimulus, preconception, interpretation, and actions—rational, reactionary, and deliberative). Nurses need to identify the patient's need-for-help by (1) observing behaviors consistent or inconsistent with comfort, (2) exploring the meaning of patient's behavior with him, (3) determining the cause of the discomfort or incapability, and (4) determining if the person can resolve his problem or has a need-for-help. Next the nurse administers the help needed and validates that the need-for-help was met.

Joan Riehl Sisca began publishing in the mid-1970s. Her work on symbolic interactionism is presented in Riehl and Roy's book, *Conceptual Models for Nursing Practice.*[54] According to symbolic interactionism theory, people interpret each other's actions based on the meaning attached to the action before reacting. Human interaction is mediated by symbols, interpretation, and meaning, and is a process of interpretation between the stimulus and response.

Helen C. Erickson, Evelyn M. Tomlin, and *Mary Ann P. Swain's* book, *Modeling and Role-Modeling: A Theory and Paradigm for Nursing* was published in 1983.[14] Modeling is developing an understanding of the client's world. Role-modeling is the nursing intervention or nurturance that requires unconditional acceptance. Erickson, Tomlin, and Swain believe that while people are alike because of their holism, lifetime growth and development, and their affiliated individualism, they are also different because of inherent endowment, adaptation, and self-care knowledge.

Kathryn E. Barnard is an active researcher who has published prolifically about infants and children since the mid-1960s. She started by studying mentally and physically handicapped children and adults, moved into studying activities of the well child, and then expanded her work to include methods of evaluating growth and development of children and mother-infant relationships. She was also concerned about disseminating research and consequently developed the Nursing Child Satellite Training Project. While Barnard never intended to develop theory, the longitudinal nursing child assessment study provided the basis for her child health assessment interaction model. Barnard believes that the parent-infant system is influenced by individual characteristics of each member and that those characteristics are modified to meet the needs of the system by adaptive behavior.[5]

Ramona Mercer has researched and published prolifically since the 1970s. She systematically researched the field of maternal role attainment and developed a complex model about factors impacting on maternal role development over time. Mercer's work culminates in her 1986 book, *First-Time Motherhood: Experience from Teens to Forties.*[36]

Systems

Johnson's, Roy's, King's, and Neuman's works deal with systems.

Dorothy E. Johnson published from the mid-1940s to the early 1970s, with most of her work published during the 1960s. Many of her unpublished works are housed at Vanderbilt University. Johnson presented her Behavioral System Model in Riehl and Roy's book, *Conceptual Models for Nursing Practice.*[23] She identified six subsystems of the behavioral system: (1) attachment-affiliation, (2) achievement, (3) sexual, (4) ingestive-eliminative, (5) aggressive, and (6) dependency. Each subsystem can be analyzed in terms of structure and functional requirements. The four structural elements are: (1) drive or goal; (2) set, a predisposition to act; (3) choice, alternatives for action; and (4) behavior. The functional requirements are protection, nurturance, and stimulation. A need for nursing intervention exists if there is a state of instability in the behavioral system. The nurse needs to identify the source of the problem in the system and take appropriate nursing actions to maintain or restore the behavioral system balance.

Sister Callista Roy has been publishing prolifically since the late 1960s. She developed her adaptation model after being challenged by Johnson to develop a conceptual model for nursing. It is discussed at length in Roy's books, *Introduction to Nursing: An Adaptation Model*[56,57] and *Essentials of the Roy Adaptation Model.*[3] Major concepts include system, adaptation, stimuli, regulator, cognator, and adaptive modes—physiological, self-concept, role performance, and interdependence. Man's self and his environment are sources of focal, residual, and conceptual stimuli that create needs for adaptation. The four interrelated adaptive modes are physiological needs, self-concept, role function, and interdependence. The adaptation mechanisms are the regulator and the cognator. Adaptation maintains integrity. Roy believes people constantly scan the environment for stimuli so they can respond and adapt. The nurse is to help the person adapt by managing the environment.

Imogene King has been publishing since the mid-1960s. *Toward a Theory for Nursing* was published in 1971,[25] and *A Theory for Nursing* was published in 1981.[26] Many of her publications have dealt with conceptual framework, models, theory, and specifically her theory of goal attainment. Her major concepts are interaction, perception, communication, transaction, role, stress, growth and development, and time and space. She suggests that the patient's and the nurse's perceptions, judgments, and actions lead to reaction, interaction, and transaction.

Betty Neuman developed her first teaching/practice model for mental health consultation in the late 1960s. She designed the Systems Model in 1970 to help graduate students evaluate nursing problems. It was first published in *Nursing Research* in 1972[41] and further refined in the *Neuman Systems Model* in 1982 and 1989.[39,40] Major concepts include total persons approach, holism, open-system, stressors, energy resources, lines of resistance, lines of defense, degree of reaction, interventions, levels of prevention, and reconstitution. By 1989, the spiritual variable was explicitly added to the Neuman Systems Model and created-environment was added to the typology as a safety mechanism for the system. Neuman believes the nurse should use purposeful interventions and a total person approach to help individuals, families, and groups reach and maintain wellness.

Energy Fields

Levine wrote about conservation of energy during the 1960s. Fitzpatrick's, Neuman's and Parse's work has been stimulated by Rogers.

Myra Estrin Levine started publishing in the mid-1960s. She has written about numerous topics. Never intending to develop theory, she wrote *Introduction to Clinical Nursing*[34,35] as a textbook to teach medical-surgical nursing to beginning students. Journal articles containing information about holism and the four conservation principles of nursing include "Adaptation and Assessment: A Rationale for Nursing Intervention,"[29] "The Four Conservative Principles of Nursing,"[30] "For Lack of Love Alone,"[31] "The Pursuit of Wholeness,"[32] and "Holistic Nursing."[33] More recently, Levine has given presentations about the conservation principles at nurse theory conferences, some of which have been audiotaped. Wholism, holism, integrity, and conservation are major concepts. The nurse is to use the principles of conservation of (1) energy, (2) structural integrity, (3) personal integrity, and (4) social integrity to keep the holism of the individual balanced. Levine also identified four levels of organismic response—fear, inflammatory response, response to stress, and sensory response—and recommended trophicognosis, a scientific approach to determine nursing care, as an alternative to nursing diagnosis.

Levine substantially changes and clarifies her theory in her chapter, "Four Conservation Principles: Twenty Years Later" in Riehl's 1988 book, *Conceptual Models for Nursing Practice.*[53] She indicates that adaptation is the essence of conservation and elaborates on how redundancy characterizes availability of adaptive responses when stability is threatened. Adaptation processes establish a body economy to safeguard the individual's stability.

Martha E. Rogers is considered one of the most creative thinkers in nursing. She has published prolifically since the early 1960s. Her work regarding Unitary Human Beings is published in *An Introduction to the Theoretical Basis of Nursing.*[55] She characterizes life process by wholeness, openness, unidirectionality, pattern and organization, sentience, and thought. She also works with energy fields, open systems, and four-dimensionality. Her theory's principles were derived from the four concepts of energy fields, openness, pattern and organization, and four-dimensionality. The principles are: (1) complementarity, mutual and simultaneous movement of human and environmental fields; (2) resonancy, wave patterns that change from low frequency to higher frequency patterns; and (3) helicy, field changes characterized by increasing diversity of field patterns. Rogers has stimulated a number of other scholars including Fitzpatrick, Newman, and Parse.

Joyce J. Fitzpatrick derived her Life Perspective Model from Rogers' work. The major concepts are nursing, person, health, environment, temporal patterns, motion patterns, consciousness patterns, and perceptual patterns. She began publishing in 1970 and has written about aging, suicidology, temporal experience, and motor behavior.[16]

Margaret Newman started publishing in the mid-1960s. She has drawn from several fields of inquiry and was influenced by Johnson and Rogers. Her model appeared in *Theory Development in Nursing*[42] and has been explained further in subsequent chapters of various books and in her 1986 book, *Health as Expanding Consciousness.*[43] The major concepts in her model of health are movement, time, space, and consciousness. They are all interrelated. "Movement is a reflection of consciousness. Time is a function of movement. Time is a measure of consciousness. Movement is a means whereby space and time become a reality."[42:60] Health is viewed as the expansion of consciousness and can encompass pathology.

EVALUATION OF THEORY DEVELOPMENT

Early nursing scholars dealt with the philosophy, definition, and art of nursing. Interpersonal communications received considerable attention during the 1960s. By the end of the decade the focus had shifted to the science of nursing. Humanism and nursing as an art and a science gained popularity during the 1980s.

The published works share some common themes. There is also evidence that scholars use the same or similar terms differently and have divergent views of nursing, environment, health, and person. Authors have also changed their views over time as their historical perspective changed. It is appropriate to analyze the previous work for themes, similarities, and differences to generate more ideas. Several middle and micro range theories are needed to direct our nursing practice. If, in fact, we develop generalizable theories about humanism, other disciplines should be able to borrow theory from nursing as we have borrowed theories from other disciplines.

REFERENCES

1. Adam, E. (1980). *To be a nurse.* Philadelphia: W.B. Saunders.
2. Abdellah, F.G., et al. (1960). *Patient-centered approaches to nursing.* New York: Macmillan.
3. Andrews, H., & Roy, C. (1986). *Essentials of the Roy adaptation model.* Norwalk, Conn.: Appleton-Century-Crofts.
4. Argyris, C., & Schon, D. (1974). *Theory in practice.* San Francisco: Jossey-Bass.
5. Barnard, K.E. (1978). Nursing child assessment and training: Learning resource manual.
6. Benner, P. (1984). *From novice to expert: Excellence and power in clinical nursing practice.* Menlo Park, Calif.: Addison-Wesley.
7. Benner, P., & Wrubel, J. (1988). *The primacy of caring: Stress and coping in health and illness.* Menlo Park, Calif.: Addison-Wesley.
8. Bush, H.A. (1979). Models for nursing. *Advances in Nursing Science, 1*(2):13-21.
9. Chinn, P., & Jacobs, M.K. (1979). A model for theory development in nursing. *Advances in Nursing Science, 1*(1):1-11.
10. Chinn, P.L., & Jacobs, M.K. (1987). *Theory and nursing: A systematic approach.* St. Louis: C.V. Mosby.
11. DeTornyay, R. (1977, Nov.-Dec.). Nursing research: The road ahead. *Nursing Research, 26:*404-407.
12. Dickoff, J., James, P., & Wiedenbach, E. (1968). Theory in a practice discipline, Part I. Practice oriented theory. *Nursing Research, 17*(5):415-435.
13. Ellis, R. (1968). Characteristics of significant theories. *Nursing Research, 17*(5):217-222.
14. Erickson, H.D., Tomlin, E.M., & Swain, M.A. (1983). *Modeling and role-modeling: A theory and paradigm for nursing.* Englewood Cliffs, N.J.: Prentice-Hall.
15. Fawcett, J. (1980, June). A declaration of nursing independence: The relation of theory and research to nursing practice. *Journal of Nursing Administration, 10:*36-39.
16. Fitzpatrick, J., & Whall, A. (1983). *Conceptual models of nursing: Analysis and application.* Bowie, Md.: Robert J. Brady.
17. Hall, L.E. (1964, Feb.). Nursing: What is it? *The Canadian Nurse, 60:*150-154.
18. Hall, L.E. (1969). The Loeb Center for nursing and rehabilitation. *International Journal of Nursing Studies, 6:*81-95.
19. Hardy, M.E. (1978). Perspectives on nursing theory. *Advances in Nursing Science, 1:*37-48.
20. Hauner, B., & Henderson, V. (1955). *Textbook of the principles and practice of nursing.* New York: Macmillan.
21. Henderson, V. (1964, Aug.). The nature of nursing, *American Journal of Nursing, 64:* 62-68.
22. Henderson, V. (1966). *The nature of nursing: A definition and its implications for practice, research, and education.* New York: Macmillan.
23. Johnson, D.E. (1980). The behavioral system model for nursing. In J.P. Riehl & C. Roy (Eds.), *Conceptual models for nursing practice* (2d ed.). New York: Appleton-Century-Crofts.
24. Kim, H.S. (1983). *The nature of theoretical thinking in nursing.* Norwalk, Conn.: Appleton-Century-Crofts.
25. King, I. (1971). *Toward a theory for nursing: General concepts of human behavior.* New York: John Wiley & Sons.
26. King, I. (1981). *A theory for nursing: Systems, concepts, process.* New York: John Wiley & Sons.
27. Lancaster, W., & Lancaster, J. (1981). Models and model building in nursing. *Advances in Nursing Science, 3:*31-42.
28. Leininger, M. (Ed.). (1984). *Care: The essence of nursing and health.* Thorofare, N.J.: Charles B. Slack.
29. Levine, M.E. (1966). Adaptation and assessment: A rationale for nursing intervention. *American Journal of Nursing, 66*(11):2450-2453.
30. Levine, M. (1967). The four conservation principles of nursing. *Nursing Forum, 6:*45.
31. Levine, M. (1967, Dec.). For lack of love alone. *Minnesota Nursing Accent, 39:*179.
32. Levine, M.E. (1969, Jan.). The pursuit of wholeness. *American Journal of Nursing, 69:*93.

33. Levine, M.E. (1971, June). Holistic nursing. *Nursing Clinics of North America, 6*:253.
34. Levine, M.E. (1969). *Introduction to clinical nursing*. Philadelphia: F.A. Davis.
35. Levine, M.E. (1973). *Introduction to clinical nursing* (2d ed.). Philadelphia: F.A. Davis.
36. Mercer, R.T. (1986). *First-time motherhood: Experiences from teens to forties*. New York: Springer Publishers.
37. Merton, R. (1968). *Social theory and social structure*. New York: The Free Press.
38. Morris, W. (Ed.) (1978). *The American heritage dictionary of the English language*. Boston: Houghton Mifflin.
39. Neuman, B. (1982). *The Neuman systems model: Application to nursing, education, and practice*. Norwalk, Conn.: Appleton-Century-Crofts.
40. Neuman, B. (1989). The Neuman systems model: Application to nursing, education, and practice. Norwalk, Conn.: Appleton-Century-Crofts.
41. Neuman, B.M., & Young, R.J. (1972, May–June). A model for teaching total person approach to patient problems. *Nursing Research, 21*:264-269.
42. Newman, M. (1980). *Theory development in nursing*. Philadelphia: F.A. Davis.
43. Newman, M.A. (1986). *Health as expanding consciousness*. St. Louis: C.V. Mosby.
44. Nightingale, F. (1957). *Notes on nursing*. Philadelphia: Lippincott. (Originally published in 1859.)
45. Orem, D. (1985). *Nursing: Concepts of practice*. New York: McGraw-Hill.
46. Orlando, I. (1961). *The dynamic nurse-patient relationship*. New York: G.P. Putnam's Sons.
47. Orlando, I. (1972). *The discipline and teaching of nursing process*. New York: G.P. Putnam's Sons.
48. Parse, R.R. (1981). *Man-living-health: A theory of nursing*. New York: John Wiley & Sons.
49. Parse, R.R., Coyne, A.B., & Smith, M.J. (1985). *Nursing research: Qualitative methods*. Bowie, MD.: Robert J. Brady.
50. Parse, R.R. (1987). *Nursing science: Major paradigms, theories, and critiques*. Philadelphia: W.B. Saunders.
51. Peplau, H. (1952). *Interpersonal relations in nursing*. New York: G.P. Putnam & Sons.
52. Reynolds, P.D. (1971). *A primer for theory construction*. Indianapolis: Bobbs-Merrill.
53. Riehl, J.B. (Ed.). (1988). *Conceptual models for nursing practice*. New York: Appleton-Century-Crofts.
54. Riehl, J.P., & Roy, C. (Eds.). (1980). *Conceptual models for nursing practice* (2d ed.). New York: Appleton-Century-Crofts.
55. Rogers, M.E. (1970). *An introduction to the theoretical basis of nursing*. Philadelphia: F.A. Davis.
56. Roy, C. (1976). *An introduction to nursing: An adaptation model*. Englewood Cliffs, N.J.: Prentice-Hall.
57. Roy, C. (1984). *An introduction to nursing: An adaptation model* (2d ed.). Englewood Cliffs, N.J.: Prentice-Hall.
58. Stevens, B.J. (1984). *Nursing theory: Analysis, application, evaluation*. Boston: Little, Brown.
59. Travelbee, J. (1966). *Interpersonal aspects of nursing*. Philadelphia: F.A. Davis.
60. Travelbee, J. (1971). *Interpersonal aspects of nursing* (2d ed.). Philadelphia: F.A. Davis.
61. Turner, J.H. (1982). *The structure of sociological theory*. Homewood, Ill.: The Dorsey Press.
62. Walker, L., & Avant, K. (1983). *Strategies for theory construction in nursing*. Norwalk, Conn.: Appleton-Century-Crofts.
63. Watson, J. (1979). *Nursing: The philosophy and science of caring*. Boston: Little, Brown.
64. Watson, J. (1985). *Nursing: Human science and health care*. Norwalk, Conn.: Appleton-Century-Crofts.
65. Wiedenbach, E. (1964). *Clinical nursing: A helping art*. New York: Springer.

Terminology of Theory Development

2

Juanita Fogel Keck

INTRODUCTION

Terms associated with theory and theory development have been used inconsistently in the nursing literature. Establishing the meanings of terms used in this book will enable the reader to gain a better understanding of the material covered. The definitions of terms used in this chapter represent those definitions accepted by a consensus of nursing theorists and noted philosophers of science.

In the interest of professionalism nursing leaders have suggested the discipline needs an identified body of knowledge that can be used to guide nursing practice. The terms *science, philosophy, theory,* and *paradigm* all relate to the development of an identified body of knowledge that can be recognized as associated with a particular scientific discipline.

SCIENCE

Science is defined both as a unified body of knowledge concerned with specific subject matter and as the skills and methodologies necessary to provide such knowledge. Therefore, nursing science is that knowledge germane to the discipline of nursing, plus the processes and methodologies used to gain that knowledge. A goal of science is the identification of truths or facts about the subject matter of a discipline—ascertaining the what, where, when, who, and how of phenomena of interest to that discipline.

KNOWLEDGE

The term *knowledge* suggests that science is composed of what one knows about the subject matter of a discipline. A distinction is made between what is known to be (fact) and what is believed to be. Knowledge is based on factual information. One derives a fact through the use of sound logic or empirical testing. Fact is truth supported by repeated observation and replication.[1]

Science is empirically based. Feigl[3] suggested a characteristic of science is that it is replicable by scientists within a discipline using the appropriate scientific methodologies. Replication requires that the components of phenomena studied to provide knowledge be observable and measurable. One acquires knowledge about things and events comprising the subject matter of interest through experience. Experiencing things or events requires the involvement of one or more of the human senses of sight, hearing, touch, taste, and smell. An empirical entity is that which can be experienced through the human senses.

PHENOMENA

Phenomena comprise the subject matter of a discipline. A *phenomenon* is defined as an object or aspect known through the senses rather than by thought or intuition, "a fact or event of scientific interest susceptible to scientific description and explanation."[13:1696]

PHILOSOPHY

Philosophy is concerned with judgments about components of science. Philosophical concerns are not empirically based. Components of a discipline that are not amenable to empirical testing are within the realm of philosophy. The "this we believe" statements associated with nursing practice contribute to the philosophy of the discipline. Statements that reflect values, goals, or opinions contribute to philosophy. It is the philosopher who suggests the methodologies by which scientific knowledge is obtained. Philosophical statements are based on opinion. They are by their very nature untestable because there is no definitive truth about them to discover. They cannot be tested for their correctness. They are accepted in a discipline through public affirmation. The prevailing philosophy of a discipline is the one shared by the greatest number of members in terms of accepting the beliefs, values, goals, and opinions of the philosophy.

THEORY

Although it is facts about phenomena of interest to the discipline that comprise the knowledge germane to the discipline, a mass of uncollated facts provides little guidance to the members of the discipline as they attempt to use that knowledge. The facts need to be ordered in a cohesive entity that will result in an organized body of knowledge. This will allow one to explain past events, provide a sense of understanding about current events, predict future events, and provide the potential for controlling them. If one can predict events, one has the basis for control of those events. Nursing intervention is served through the ability to predict and ultimately to control phenomena associated with health and health care.

It is through the construction of theories that such ordering occurs. Theories are models of empirical real world phenomena that identify the components or elements of the phenomena and the relationships between them. The functions of theory include summarization of knowledge, explanation of phenomena of interest to the discipline employing the theory, and provision of the means to predict and ultimately to control phenomena.[8] In fact, Theobald[11] suggested that only through theory is explanation or prediction possible.

Numerous definitions of theory exist in the literature. Most reflect an understanding of theory consistent with the following: Theory is a logically consistent set of propositions that presents a systematic view of a phenomenon. A proposition is composed of the elements of the phenomenon and the relationships between them. The elements or components of a phenomenon are the concepts necessary to understand the phenomenon. The concepts are linked by specific statements identifying how two or more concepts are related to each other to provide understanding about the phenomenon. Therefore theories are composed of statements that state specific relationships between two or more concepts.

CONCEPTS

Concepts are the subject matter of theory. They are symbolic representations of the things or events of which phenomena are composed. Concepts represent some aspect of reality that can be quantified. An example of concepts necessary to explain a phenomenon is found in Hoffman's beginning theory of altruism.[5] Altruism is the phenomenon Hoffman has attempted to explain. One of the propositions of the theory is that helping behavior and empathy are related in a curvilinear manner. Both low and high levels of empathy are associated with low levels of helping behavior. Moderate empathy is associated with high level of help-

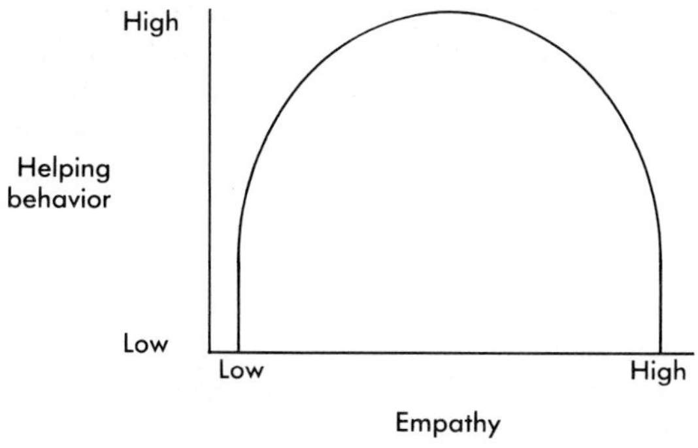

ing. *Helping behavior* and *empathy* are the concepts comprising the proposition. To be able to ultimately explain altruism by means of this theory one must include empathy and helping behavior.

Dubin[2] categorized concepts into five groups—enumerative, associative, relational, statistical, and summative.

Enumerative Concepts

Enumerative concepts are characteristics of a phenomenon that are always present. The concept of *age* is an enumerative unit. Everyone to whom a theory incorporating age is generalizable is characterized by an age. The concept is universal to all persons in the population to which the theory applies. Age is always present in the phenomenon being explained. An enumerative concept cannot have a zero value. There is no such thing as an individual with zero age. As soon as an individual exists, his or her age can be ascertained.

Associative Concepts

Associative units are those concepts that can exist in only some conditions within the phenomenon.[2] Associative concepts can have a zero value. Persons to whom a theory composed of the concepts applies can exist with none of the concepts. Examples include income, presence of disease, and anxiety. It is possible to identify persons with no income in the population to which a theory incorporating income applies. Associative and enumerative units are the simplest, least complex forms of concepts.

Relational Concepts

Relational concepts are those characteristics of a phenomenon that can be understood only through the combination or interaction of two or more enumerative or associative concepts.[2] *Elderly* is a concept that cannot be understood without an understanding of the combination of age and *longevity*. *Mother* cannot exist without the interaction of *man, woman* and *birth*. Therefore both *elderly* and *mother* are relational concepts.

Statistical Concepts

Statistical concepts are those that relate the property of the thing being represented in terms of its distribution in the population.[2] *Average blood pressure* is an example of a statistical unit.

Summative Concepts

Summative concepts are the most complex. Dubin[2] suggested summative concepts were global units that represented an entire complex entity or phenomenon. Four concepts—nursing, man, health, and environment—have been identified by numerous nurse authors and theorists as the concepts of primary concern for the discipline of nursing. They are readily identifiable as summative concepts because each represents a global and extremely complex entity.

Dubin[2] suggested many problems exist when summative concepts are used within a theory. An entire phenomenon is explained by the use of one or two words. Each summative concept is composed of numerous enumerative, associative, and relational concepts and their interactions, but none are named or defined. One can only assume which of these less complex concepts contribute to the summative unit, how they interact, and under what conditions they contribute to the phenomenon.

Dubin[2] said that summative concepts have little utility in theory development because the concepts cannot be adequately defined and the interactions between them are not readily ascertainable. For a theory to be useful in aiding the attainment of the goals of science, it must contribute to understanding, explanation, prediction, and ultimately control. Before prediction and control are possible, the theory must be testable. One can only predict future events if the proposed relationships between concepts have been repeatedly supported by empirical findings. In other words, the real world correlates of the concepts have been measured and the relationships between them verified. If such relationships have been repeatedly verified in the past, one can predict the relationship between the concepts will hold true in the future. Summative units are not measurable. How would one measure environment as a totality? One is usually interested in individual components of environment and their interactions with some specific attributes of human beings. One may be interested in a theory that states a person's recovery from illness is related to environment. However, the theory is not useful to one concerned with a specific attribute of humans, such as *recovery,* unless specific aspects of the environment that influence recovery and their interactions are stated. A useful theory then would be composed of the less complex concepts that refer to the specific environmental attributes rather than the totality of the environment. Concepts must be clearly definable and measurable to be of use to the practicing nurse in the clinical setting.

DEFINITIONS

Concepts are abstract symbols of the real world. They are mental representations constructed in language terms. The concepts of a theory reflect the theorist's own individual perception and definition of reality that the concept is supposed to represent. The concept may be open to many interpretations. Different individuals may hold differing understandings of the meanings of the words used to convey conceptual aspects of the real world. Definitions supplied by the theorist are needed so the user of theory can know what the theorist means by the concept. It is the theorist's meaning that must be used in the theory he or she developed. Therefore, the user of theory must know the meaning intended by the author.

Two classifications of definitions are associated with theory. *Conceptual definitions* relate the general meaning of the concept. *Operational definitions* identify an empirical referent for the concept. For example, *pain* may be conceptually defined as a subjective experience perceived as unpleasant initiated by potentially damaging stimuli but influenced by affective variables. It may be operationally defined as the score obtained on a 10 cm visual analogue scale in which zero represents no pain and ten represents the worst pain imaginable.

0	10
No pain	Worst pain imaginable

Scores are obtained by asking subjects to place a mark on the line to represent the severity of their pain. The resulting score is observable and is therefore an empirical referent for the subject's pain. The score is the operational definition for pain.

An additional classification of definitions may be considered. Definitions may be classified as either denotative or connotative. *Denotative definitions* define concepts in terms of what the concept is or represents. A denotative definition of father is *male parent.* Father is the male parent. A *connotative definition* suggests or implies associations one might make with the concept. A connotative definition suggests what one might think of when considering the term *father.* A connotative definition of father is *strong, provider, disciplinarian,* that is, terms that are associated with *father.*

RELATIONSHIP STATEMENTS

Concepts alone do not create theory. A theory does not exist until the specific relationships between concepts comprising the theory are expressed in relationship statements. Several labels for relationship statements may be found in the literature related to theory. Relationship statements may be classified as propositions, hypotheses, empirical generalizations, laws, axioms, or theorems. Nursing and philosophical theorists essentially agree that all relationship statements, regardless of classification, indicate specific relationships between two or more concepts. Examples of relationship statements include the following:

If one has a family history of Alzheimer's disease *then there is a specific probability that* one will develop Alzheimer's disease.

Tissue damage *is the antecedent of* pain perception.

Learning ability *varies* with anxiety *in a curvilinear relationship.*

Job satisfaction *is a function of* the fit between the job environment and the individual's personality.

Anxiety and accurate information about a diagnostic procedure *are negatively related.*

The goals of science are to aid in understanding, explaining, predicting, and controlling phenomena. These goals are achieved through the relationships proposed by theory. Meeting these goals requires that *specific* relationships between concepts be clearly stated. Simply stating that anxiety and learning ability are related is insufficient. For the theory to be useful one needs to understand how and under what conditions they are related. Stating there is a curvilinear relationship between anxiety and learning provides the practitioner with information that may allow the prediction of situations in which one is most or least able to learn. The practitioner responsible for developing and implementing a teaching program for home care following myocardial infarction would be directed to implement the program during periods of moderate anxiety for the recipients of the program rather than during periods of low or high anxiety.

Laws

Differences between classifications of relationship statements appear to reflect the abstractness of the concepts included in the statements and the amount of empirical support derived through testing the proposed relationship. Laws, empirical generalizations, and hypotheses are classifications of statements that include relatively concrete concepts.[4,9,12] The concepts incorporated in these statements represent things or events observable in the real world. Because they are observable, they can provide measures that are valid indicators of the concept. Laws and empirical generalizations are found primarily in disciplines, such as chemistry and physics, that deal with readily observable and measurable phenomena. They differ in the amount of empirical support that has been generated for the proposition. Boyle's law states that when temperature is held constant, the volume of a gas is inversely proportional to the pressure exerted on it. The statement suggests volume is influenced by the variables of temperature and pressure. To determine the influence of pressure alone, one must control for the influence of temperature. Because current technology makes temperature and pressure readily manipulatable, a researcher can control for the influence of temperature by holding temperature constant. Then by measuring volume and pressure he or she determines the influence of pressure changes on volume. If volume repeatedly and invariably decreases when pressure is increased, a law regarding the influence of pressure upon gas volume becomes tenable. A great deal of empirical support can be generated for the proposition.

Empirical Generalizations

Empirical generalizations differ from laws only in the amount of empirical support generated for the proposed relationship statements. Laws have overwhelming support; empirical generalizations have moderate support. The problem in classifying statements is deciding when moderate support becomes overwhelming support.

The decision is a philosophical one and is arrived at through agreement among scientists in a discipline.

Hypotheses

Hypotheses differ from empirical generalizations and laws again in the amount of empirical support generated. Hypotheses are the first tentative suggestions a specific relationship exists. As a hypothesis is repeatedly confirmed, it progresses to an empirical generalization and ultimately to a law. The words used in the proposition may not change. Boyle's law was Boyle's hypothesis and Boyle's empirical generalization before being accepted as a law within disciplines using the relationship.

Axioms and Theorems

Axioms and theorems are relationship statements that include abstract concepts—concepts that relate mental images of entities not readily observable. Theories emanating from the social sciences contain primarily axioms and theorems. Concepts such as anxiety, job satisfaction, learning ability, and personality are abstractions in the real world. They are neither directly observable nor measurable. Therefore they would be amenable to incorporation in either a theorem or axiom.

Axioms and theorems differ in the degree of generality incorporated in the relationship. Axioms state the most general relationship between concepts. Theorems emanate from axioms. An example of a statement that could be an axiom is "Anxiety is negatively related to accurate information about a diagnostic procedure." The statement allows for the full range of possible values associated with each concept. A theorem suggests that a specific range of values of one concept is associated with a specific range of values of the other. An example of a possible theorem would be "Low levels of anxiety are associated with a high degree of accurate information about a diagnostic procedure."

Relationship statements become an axiom or theorem through the mechanism of empirical support. A statement is not referred to as an axiom unless it has been subjected to considerable testing and repeatedly supported. However, neither axioms nor theorems are directly testable. They have no directly observable empirical referent to be measured. Hypotheses provide the mechanism for testing them. Previously it was suggested that a hypothesis is a statement of relationship between concrete measurable entities for which little empirical support has been generated. Hypotheses must also be the antecedents of axioms and theorems. The abstract concepts must be operationalized to provide an empirical referent for each. Relationships are then tested by means of the empirical referent. A previous example included a visual analogue scale to measure pain. The scale and the resulting score provide an empirical referent for the abstract concept *pain.* One cannot directly observe pain, but one can see the scale and the score used to represent it. Hypotheses are used to test propositions incorporating abstract concepts regardless of the previous empirical support for the proposed relationships among concepts.

The discussion concerning differing classifications of relationship statements is provided to explain terms often used in the literature germane to theory development. They differ primarily in degree of abstractness and amount of empirical support. The components of the statements, concepts, and specified relationships between them may not differ. One can conclude that although the classification of relationship statements may differ among scientists, there is general agreement as to the structure of the statements. Relationship statements must include appropriate concepts that have been clearly defined, and the specific relationships among those concepts must also be clearly stated.

ASSOCIATIONAL OR CAUSAL STATEMENTS

Relationship statements are generally considered to be of two types, associational and causal process.

Associational Relationship Statements

Associational relationship statements assert that values of one concept are associated with values of another. Linear and curvilinear are the two general types of associational relationships. If the relationship is linear, three possibilities exist. There may be a positive relationship, a negative relationship, or no relationship among the concepts.[9] In a linear relationship, the direction of the relationship is established in the relationship statement. If the relationship is curvilinear, such is stated in the relationship statement. An example of an associational relationship statement is "Anxiety is negatively related to the degree of accurate information one has about a diagnostic procedure." If one knows a category of values for one variable, one can infer a category of values for another. Relationship statements found in the social sciences are primarily of the associational form.

Causal Relationship Statements

Causal relationship statements state that one concept is the cause of another. Boyle's law is an example of a causal relationship statement. When temperature is held constant, a change in pressure causes an inverse change in the volume of gas. For every value of pressure there is an exact value for volume. If one knows the value for pressure, one can determine the exact value for volume.

ASSUMPTIONS

Assumptions are beliefs about phenomena one must accept as true in order to accept a theory about the phenomena as true. They are not tested but are assumed to represent reality. An example of assumptions can be found in Selye's theory of human stress.[10] Selye proposed a theory of stress based on animal studies. The theory was to operate within the realm of human stress and was to reflect the totality of the stress experience. The theory requires several assumptions before one can accept it as an explanation of the totality of human stress. One must first accept the assumption that results of animal studies are completely generalizable to humans and that the stress measured in rodents is the same as the stress experienced by humans. In addition, the theory suggests that human stress is mediated by stress energy that enables one to handle that stress. A major assumption of the theory is that everyone is born with a finite amount of stress energy and death ensues when the energy is depleted. The assumption is not testable because the amount of stress energy one might have throughout life is not measurable; it is a belief one must accept before accepting Selye's theory as an appropriate and adequate explanation of total human stress.

MODEL

The term *model* is often used in nursing literature. A model is a schematic representation of some aspects of reality. Theories are models of some phenomenon. Models fall into two broad classifications, theoretical and empirical. *Empirical models* are replicas of observable reality. A plastic model of the heart is an empirical model. *Theoretical models* are representatives of the real world expressed in language or mathematical symbols. Theories are theoretical models of reality, often a reality that is not directly observable. Models are useful in theory development because they aid in the selection of relevant concepts necessary to represent a phenomenon of interest and the determination of the relationships among the concepts. Models also allow manipulation of concepts on paper before testing in the real world. In addition, models aid theory users by providing an observable explanation of theory components. Although all theories are models, not all models are theories.

RANGE OF THEORIES

Theories differ in complexity and scope along a continuum from micro theories to grand theories. *Micro theories* are the least complex. They contain the least complex concepts and refer to specific, easily defined phenomena. They are narrow in scope because they attempt to explain a small aspect of reality. They are primarily composed of enumerative or associative concepts. *Grand theories* are the most complex and broadest in scope. They attempt to explain broad areas within a discipline. They are composed of summative concepts and incorporate numerous narrower range theories. Middle range theories fall somewhere between. They are primarily composed of relational concepts. The domain represented by mid range theory is not so large as to be useless to the user as summative concepts are useless. But neither do middle range theories represent such a narrow aspect of reality that they cannot be used in the more complex realm of real life.

Partial theories are theories in the developmental stage. In a partial theory some concepts necessary to explain a phenomenon have been identified and some relationships have been identified between them, but the theory is not complete. A criterion of a complete theory is that the concepts and proposed relationships must be exhaustive. That is, every thing or event comprising the phenomenon is represented in the theory. Theories derived from the social sciences, including nursing, are probably exclusively partial theories because there are few, if any, phenomena that have been totally and completely explained.

PARADIGM

Science, philosophy, and theory are all components of the domain of any scientific discipline. *Paradigm* is a term used to denote the prevailing network of science, philosophy, and theory accepted by a discipline. Current interest in paradigmatic issues stems from the work of Kuhn.[6] Kuhn defined a *paradigm* to reflect his belief that a paradigm was synonymous with the scientific community or community of individuals comprising discipline. The term was meant to refer to what members of the community have in common.[7] Included in the matrix shared by the scientific community are the knowledge, philosophy, theory, educational experience, practice orientation, research methodology, and literature identified with the discipline. The prevailing paradigm directs the activities of a discipline. As such, it is accepted by the majority of individuals within the discipline and suggests the areas of study of interest to the discipline and the means to study them. Nursing literature includes numerous references to conceptual models and conceptual frameworks. I believe these terms are synonymous with *paradigm.*

SUMMARY

This chapter has been concerned with the terminology associated with theory development. Science, theory, philosophy, and paradigm have been addressed. In addition, terms necessary for a clearer understanding of these terms have been included. Fact, phenomenon, concepts, definitions, categories of concepts, relationship statement, law, empirical generalization, theorem, axiom, hypothesis, associational relationship statement, causal process relationship statement, assumption, model, and range of theories have been considered. I hope this discussion will allow a clearer understanding of the theoretical work addressed on the following pages.

REFERENCES

1. Brodbeck, M. (1953). The nature and function of the philosophy of science. In H. Feigl & M. Brodbeck (Eds.), *Readings in the philosophy of science.* New York: Appleton-Century-Crofts.
2. Dubin, R. (1978). *Theory building* (Rev. ed.). New York: The Free Press.
3. Feigl, H. (1953). The scientific outlook: naturalism and humanism. In H. Feigl and M. Brodbeck (Eds.), *Readings in the philosophy of science.* New York: Appleton-Century-Crofts.
4. Hardy, M.E. (1973). The nature of theories. In M. Hardy (Ed.), *Theoretical foundation for nursing.* New York: MSS Corp.
5. Hoffman, M.L. (1981). Is altruism part of human nature? *Journal of Personality and Social Psychology, 40:*126-131.
6. Kuhn, T.S. (1970). *The structure of scientific revolutions.* Chicago: University of Chicago Press.
7. Kuhn, T.S. (1974). Second thoughts on paradigms. In F. Suppe (Ed.), *The structure of scientific theories.* Urbana: University of Illinois Press.

8. Mehlberg, H. (1962). The theoretical and empirical aspects of science. In E. Nagel, P. Suppes and A. Tarski (Eds.), *Logic, methodology and philosophy of science.* Stanford: Stanford University Press.
9. Reynolds, P.D. (1971). *A primer in theory construction.* Indianapolis: Bobbs-Merrill.
10. Selye, H. (1956). *The stress of life.* New York: McGraw-Hill.
11. Theobald, D.W. (1968). *An introduction to philosophy of science.* London: Methuen.
12. Wartofsky, M.W. (1968). *Conceptual foundations of scientific thought and introduction to the philosophy of science.* New York: Macmillan.
13. *Webster's Third New International Dictionary Unabridged* (1986). Springfield, Mass.: Merriam-Webster, Inc.

3

History and Philosophy of Science

Sue Marquis Bishop

Modern science is a relatively new intellectual activity. Established as recently as 400 years ago, it has occupied only a short span of time in the history of humankind.[2] Scientific activity has persisted because it has improved the quality of life while satisfying human needs for creative work, a sense of order, and the desire to understand the unknown.[2,8,16] If we are interested in understanding, predicting, or controlling a given phenomenon, or in describing what we know in science, we are seeking a theory.[19,29] The development of science thus requires the *formalization* of the phenomena and events with which each science is concerned.[27] The construction of nursing theories is the formalization of attempts to describe, explain, predict, or control states of affairs in nursing.

HISTORICAL VIEWS OF THE NATURE OF SCIENCE

If we are interested in formalizing the science of nursing, we must consider such basic questions as: What is science? What is to be regarded as knowledge? What is truth? What are the methods by which scientific knowledge can be produced? These are philosophical questions. The term *epistemology* is concerned with the theory of knowledge in philosophical inquiry. The particular philosophical perspective selected to answer these questions will influence how scientists choose to carry out scientific activities, how they interpret outcomes, and even what they regard as science and knowledge.[3:8] Although philosophy as an activity has been documented for 3000 years, formal science is a relatively new human pursuit.[8] Only recently has scientific activity itself become the object of investigation.[3]

Two competing theories of science have evolved (with several variations) in the era of modern science: *rationalism* and *empiricism*.[8] Gale[8] labeled these alternative epistemologies as centrally concerned with the "power of reason" and the "power of sensory experience." He noted some similarity in the divergent views of science in the time of the classical Greeks. For example, Aristotle believed advances in biological science would develop through systematic observation of objects and events in the natural world, whereas Pythagorus believed knowledge of the natural world would develop from mathematical reasoning.

Rationalism

Rationalist epistemology emphasizes the importance of a priori reasoning as the appropriate method for advancing knowledge. The scientist in this tradition approaches the task of scientific inquiry by developing a systematic explanation (theory) of a given phenomenon.[8] This conceptual system is analyzed by addressing the logical structure of the theory and the logical reasoning involved in its development. Theoretical assertions, derived by deductive reasoning, are then subjected to experimental testing to corroborate the theory. Reynolds[19] labeled this approach the "theory-then-research" strategy. If the research findings fail to correspond with the theoretical assertions, additional research is conducted or modifications are made in the theory and further tests devised, or the theory is discarded in favor of an alternative explanation.[8,29]

Popper[17] argued that science would evolve more rapidly through the process of conjectures and refutations in which new ideas are formulated and research devised to attempt to refute them.

The rationalist view is most clearly evident in the work of the theoretical physicist Einstein, who made extensive use of mathematical equations in developing his theories. The theories Einstein constructed offered an "imaginative framework," which has directed research in numerous areas.[4] As Reynolds[19] noted, if one believes that science is a process of "*inventing* descriptions of phenomena," the appropriate strategy for theory construction is the theory-then-research strategy. In Reynolds' view:[19:145]

> As the continuous interplay between theory construction (invention) and testing with empirical research progresses, the theory becomes more precise and complete as a description of nature and, therefore, more useful for the goals of science.

Empiricism

The empiricist view is based on the central idea that scientific knowledge can only be derived from sensory experience. Francis Bacon (c. 1620) is given credit for popularizing the basis for the empiricist approach to inquiry.[8] Bacon believed scientific truth was discovered by the generalization of observed facts in the natural world. This approach, which has been called the *inductive* method, is based on the idea that collection of facts precedes attempts to formulate generalizations—the "research-then-theory" approach.[19]

The strict empiricist view is reflected in the work of the behaviorists, Watson and Skinner. In a 1950 paper, Skinner[21] asserted that advances in the science of psychology could be expected if scientists would focus on the collection of empirical data. He cautioned against the drawing of premature inferences and proposed a moratorium on theory building until further facts were collected. Skinner's approach to theory construction was clearly an inductive one. His view of science and the popularity of behaviorism have been credited with influencing the shift in emphasis in psychology during the 1950s to 1970s from theory construction to fact gathering.[22] The difficulty with the inductive mode of inquiry is the world presents an infinite number of possible observations. Therefore the scientist must "bring ideas to experiences" to decide what to observe and what to exclude.[23] Although Skinner disclaimed in his early writings to be developing a theory, Bixenstine[1:465] noted:

> Skinner is startlingly creative in applying the conceptual elements of his—let's be frank—*theory* to a wide variety of issues, ranging from training pigeons in the guidance of missiles, to developing teaching machines, to constructing a model society.

During the first half of this century, philosophers focused on the analysis of the structure of theories, while scientists focused on empirical research. There was minimal interest in the history of science, the nature of scientific discovery, or the similarities between the philosophic view of science and scientific methods.[3] Positivism, a term first used by Comte, emerged as the dominant view of modern science.[8] Modern logical positivists believed empirical research and logical analysis were the two approaches that would produce scientific knowledge. The system of symbolic logic, published in 1910-1913 by Whitehead and Russell, was hailed by the logical positivists as an appropriate approach to discovering truth.[3]

The logical empiricists, offering a more lenient view of logical positivism, argued that theoretical propositions must be able to be tested through observation and experimentation.[3] This perspective is rooted in the idea that empirical facts exist independently of theories and offer the only possible basis for objectivity in science.[3] In other words, objective truth exists in the world, independent of the researcher; the task of science is to discover it. The empiricist view shares similarities with Aristotle's view of biological science and Bacon's inductive method as the true method of scientific inquiry.[8] Gale[8] argued that this view of science is often presented in methodology courses as the "single orthodox view" of the scientific enterprise. In his words, this view is taught in the following manner:

> The scientist first sets up an experiment; observes what occurs . . . ; reaches a preliminary hypothesis to describe the occurrence; runs further experiments to test the hypothesis (and) finally corrects or modifies the hypothesis in light of the results.[8:13]

The increasing use of computers permitting the analysis of large data sets may have contributed to the acceptance of the positivist approach to modern science.[22] In the 1950s, however, the literature began to reflect an increasing challenge to the positivist view, thereby ushering in a new view of science.[2]

EMERGENT VIEWS OF SCIENCE AND THEORY

In recent years, several authors have presented analyses challenging the positivist position, thus offering the basis for a new perspective of science.[7,10,13,25] In 1977, Brown[3] argued there was a new intellectual revolution in philosophy that emphasized the *history of science,* replacing formal logic as the major analytical tool in philosophy of science. One of the major perspectives in the new philosophy was the focus on science as a *process of continuing research,* as opposed to the emphasis on accepted findings. In this emergent epistemology, the emphasis was on understanding scientific discovery and the processes involved in changes in theories over time. In 1966, Foucault[7] published his analysis (in French) of the epistemology of human sciences from the seventeenth to the nineteenth centuries. His major thesis was that empirical knowledge was arranged in different patterns at a given time and in a given culture. He found changes over time in the focus of inquiry, in what was regarded as scientific knowledge, and in how knowledge was organized. Further, he concluded that humans only recently emerged as objects of study. Schutz[20] in his *Phenomenology of the Social World,* argued that scientists seeking to understand the social world cannot cognitively know an external world, independent of their own life experiences.

Empiricists argue that in order for science to maintain objectivity, data collection and analysis must be independent of theory.[3] This assertion is based on the position that objective truth exists in the world, waiting to be discovered. Brown[3] argued that the new epistemology challenged the empiricist view of perception by acknowledging that theories play a significant role in determining what the scientist will observe and how it will be interpreted. A story related to me by my grandmother illustrates Brown's thesis that observations are "concept-laden," that is, what one observes is influenced by ideas in the mind of the observer:

> A husband and wife are sitting by the fire silently watching their firstborn son asleep in the cradle. The mother looks at her infant son and imagines him learning to talk and then to walk. She continues her reverie by imagining him playing with friends, coming home from school, then going to college. She ends her daydreaming by visualizing him elected President of the United States. She smiles and glances up at her husband who also had been staring intently at their son, "What are

> you thinking, honey?" The husband replies, "I was just thinking that I can't imagine how anyone could build a fine cradle like this and sell it for $5.98 and still make a profit."

Brown[3] presented the example of a chemist and a child walking together past a steel mill. The chemist perceived the odor of sulfur dioxide, while the child smelled rotten eggs. Each of them responded to the same observable data with distinctly different cognitive interpretations. In teaching nurses to be family therapists, I frequently use videotapes of family therapy sessions for students to analyze as we progress through the study of different approaches to family therapy. Novice student therapists tend to focus on the content of family interaction (what one member says to another) or the behavior of individual family members. Following the study of the *systems view* of families, and pointing out examples of patterned transactions among family members, during the second viewing students can "see" and describe transactions among family members they did not perceive during the first viewing (the son withdrawing when his parents argue or the wife gritting her teeth when her husband talks, for example). Concepts and theories create boundaries for selecting phenomena to observe and for reasoning about specific patterns. For example, the concept *social network* may be more fruitful for studying social relations than the concept *group* because it focuses attention on a more complex set of relationships beyond the boundaries of any one setting.[12]

If, however, scientists perceive patterns in the empirical world based on their presupposed theories, how can new patterns ever be perceived or new discoveries formulated? Gale[8] answers by arguing that the scientist is able to perceive "forceful intrusions" from the environment that challenge his or her "a priori mental set," thus raising questions in regard to the current theoretical perspective. Brown[3] maintained that while a presupposed theoretical framework influences perception, theories are not the single determining factor of the scientist's perception. He identified three different views of the relationships of theories to observation:

1. Scientists are merely passive observers of occurrences in the empirical world. Observable data are objective truth, waiting to be discovered.
2. Theories structure what the scientist perceives in the empirical world.
3. Presupposed theories and observable data *interact* in the process of scientific investigation.

Brown's argument for an interactionist's perspective coincides with scientific consensus in the study of pattern recognition in human information processing. Two distinct mini theories have directed research efforts in this area: the data-driven or bottom-up theory and the conceptually driven or top-down theory. In the former, cognitive expectations (what is known or ways of organizing meaning) are used to select input and process incoming information from the environment. The second theory asserts that incoming data are perceived as unlabeled input and analyzed as raw data with increasing levels of complexity until all the data are classified. Current research evidence suggests human pattern recognition progresses by an interaction of both data-driven and conceptually driven processes, using sources of information in both currently organized cognitive categories and stimuli from the sensory environment.[15] The interactionist's perspective also is clearly reflected in Piaget's theory of human cognitive functioning:

> Piagetian man actively selects and interprets environmental information in the construction of his own knowledge rather than passively copying the information just as it is presented to his senses. While paying attention to and taking account of the structure of the environment during knowledge seeking, Piagetian man reconstrues and reinterprets that environment [according to] his own mental framework. . . . The mind neither copies the world . . . nor does it ignore the world [by] creating a private mental conception of it out of

whole cloth. . . . The mind meets the environment in an extremely active, self-directed way.[6:6]

If we are to accept the thesis that no objective truth exists, and that science is an interactive process between "invented" theories and empirical observations, how are scientists to determine truth and scientific knowledge? In the new epistemology, science is viewed as an ongoing process and much importance is given to the idea of consensus among scientists. As Brown[3] concluded, we must forgo the myth that science can establish "final truths," and accept the notion that tentative consensus based on reasoned judgments about the available evidence is the most that can be expected. In this view of science, scientific knowledge is what the community of scientists in any given historical era regard as such. The truth of a given theoretical statement is determined by current consensus among scientists as to whether it presents an "adequate description of reality."[3] This consensus is possible through the collaboration of many scientists, in making their work available for public review and debate and building on previous inquiries.[18] "The individual (scientist) *introduces* ideas, the scientific community *appraises* them" by its objective criteria.[18:59]

Science in any given era and in any given discipline is structured by an accepted set of presuppositions that define the phenomena to study and the appropriate methods for data collection and interpretation.[3] These presuppositions set the boundaries for the scientific enterprise. In Brown's view of the transactions between theory and empirical observation:

> Theory determines what observations are worth making and how they are to be understood, and observation provides challenges to accepted theoretical structures. The continuing attempt to produce a coherently organized body of theory and observation is the driving force of research, and the prolonged failure of specific research projects leads to scientific revolutions.[3:167]

The presentation and acceptance of a revolutionary theory may alter the existing presuppositions and theories, thereby creating a different set of boundaries and procedures. The result is a new set of problems or a new way to interpret observations, that is, a new picture of the world.[13] It is crucial that the emphasis in this view of science be on ongoing research rather than on established findings.

THEORY AND RESEARCH

Traditionally, theory building and research have been presented to students in separate courses. This separation has often resulted in problems for students in understanding the nature of theories and in comprehending the relevance of research efforts.[28] The acceptance of the positivist view of science may have influenced the sharp distinction between theory and research methods.[8] Although theory and research can be viewed as distinct operations, they are more appropriately regarded as interdependent components of the scientific process.[5] In constructing a theory, the theorist must be knowledgeable about available empirical findings and attempt to take these into account, since theory is, in part, concerned with the formalization of available knowledge.[29] The theory also is subject to revision if the hypotheses fail to correspond to empirical findings, or the theory may be abandoned in favor of an alternative explanation that accounts for the new information.[3,5,19]

In contemporary theories of science, the scientific enterprise has been described as a series of phases, with emphasis on the *discovery* and *verification* (or acceptance) phases.[8,9] Gale[8] described these phases as primarily concerned with the presentation and testing of new ideas. Discovery is the phase during which new ways of thinking about phenomena or new data are introduced to the scientific community. The focus during this time is on presenting a persuasive argument that the new conceptions represent an improvement over previous conceptions.[8] Verification is characterized by efforts in the scientific community to critically analyze and test the new conceptions in an attempt to refute them. During this time the new views are "put through the trial by fire."[8] Brown[3] argued, however, that discovery and verification cannot really be viewed as sharply distinct phases because a new conception is not usually accepted by the scientific community until it has "passed enough tests" to warrant acceptance as a new discovery.

At this point it should be clear that it is not appropriate in a scientific discipline to judge a theory on the basis of "authority, faith, or intuition," rather than on the basis of *scientific consensus.*[18] For example, if a specific nursing theory is to be determined acceptable, this judgment should not be made because a respected nursing leader advocates the theory. Neither should personal feelings about the theory, such as "I like this theory" or "I don't like this one," provide the basis for the judgment. The only defensible reason for judging a theory acceptable is on the basis of logical and conceptual or empirical grounds. These judgments are made by the scientific community.[2]

The advancement of science is a collaborative endeavor in which many researchers evaluate and build upon one another's work. In order for evidence to be cumulative, theories, procedures, and findings from empirical studies must be made available for critical review by scientists. In this way, the same procedures can be used to support or refute a given analysis or finding.[18] A theory is accepted when the consensus of scientists is that the theory provides an "adequate description of reality."[3] The acceptance of a scientific hypothesis depends on the appraisal of the *coherence* of theory, which involves questions of logic, and the *correspondence* of the theory, which involves efforts to relate the theory to observable phenomena through research.[24] Gale[8] labeled these criteria as epistemological and metaphysical concerns. The consensus of correspondence of the theory with reality is not based on a single study. Repeated testing is crucial, replicating the study under the same conditions and exploring the theoretical assertions under different conditions, or with different measures. Consensus is therefore based on accumulated evidence.[9] Even when the theory does not appear to be supported by research, it is not necessarily rejected by the scientific community. Rather than an automatic agreement there is a problem with the theory itself, there may be judgments made about the validity or reliability of the measures used in testing the theory or in the appropriateness of the research design. These possibilities are considered in critically evaluating attempts to test a given theory.

Dubin[5] identified three areas in which scientific consensus is necessary in regard to any given theory: (1) agreement on the boundaries of the theory (the phenomenon it addresses and the phenomena it excludes), (2) agreement on the logic used in constructing the theory so meanings can be understood from a similar perspective, and (3) agreement that the theory fits the data collected and analyzed through research. Consensus in these three areas essentially constitutes agreement among scientists to "look at the same 'things,' to do so in the same way, and to have a level of confidence certified by an empirical test."[5:13] Therefore the theory must be capable of being operationalized for testing in order to check the theory against reality. In the process of science, retroductive, deductive, and inductive forms of reasoning may be used as science progresses by building theoretical descriptions and explanations of reality, attempting to account for available findings, deriving testable hypotheses, and evaluating theories from the perspective of new empirical data.[24]

Most research can be considered to be in the category Kuhn[13] described as *normal science.* Scientific inquiry in normal science involves testing a given theory, developing new applications of theory, or extending a given theory. Occasionally a new theory with different assumptions is developed that seeks to replace previous theories. Kuhn[13] described this as *revolutionary science,* and the theory with different presuppositions as a revolutionary theory.

A change in the accepted presuppositions

creates a different set of boundaries and procedures that suggest a new set of problems or a new way to interpret observations.[13] Currently, there is some challenge in the social and behavioral sciences to the assumptions underlying accepted methods of experimental design, measurement, and statistical analysis that emphasize the search for universal laws and the use of procedures for random assignment of subjects across contexts.[14] Mishler[14] argues that scientists should develop methods and procedures for studying behavior as dependent on context for meaning, rather than eliminating context by searching for laws that hold across contexts. This critique of the methods and assumptions of research is emerging from phenomenological and ethnomethodological theorists who view the scientific process from a very different paradigm.[11,14,26]

The proper focus of research is not to attempt to prove a theory or hypothesis, but to attempt to set up research to refute a given hypothesis.[17] Failure of repeated attempts at refutation lend support to the theory and acceptance of the theory by the scientific community.[5] The emphasis, however, is always on ongoing research rather than established findings.[3] In the future, new information or a new compelling way to view the same evidence may lead to a reappraisal of the theory. One previously accepted theory may be abandoned for another theory if it fails to correspond to empirical findings or if it no longer presents clear directions for further research. The theory selected as an alternative is judged by the scientific community to account for available data and to suggest further lines of inquiry.[3]

Popper[17] observed that, unfortunately, refutations of a given theory are frequently viewed as a failure of the theorist or of the theory. In his view:

> Every refutation should be regarded as a great success; not merely as a success of the scientist who refuted the theory, but also of the scientist who created the refuted theory and who thus . . . suggested, if only indirectly, the refutation experiment.[17:243]

If a theoretical hypothesis fails to account for the observed facts in the world, one explanation is eliminated and science is thus advanced.[26]

Finally, the process of scientific inquiry may be viewed as a social enterprise.[14] In Gale's words, "Human beings *do* science."[8:290] It therefore might be anticipated that the scientific enterprise may be influenced by social, economic, or political factors.[5] For example, the popularity of certain ideologies may influence how phenomena are viewed and what problems are selected for study.[11] In addition, the availability of funds for research in a specified area may precipitate a flurry of research activity in that area. Science, however, does not depend on the "personal characteristics" or persuasions of any given scientist, or group of scientists, but is powerfully self-correcting within the community of scientists.[18] Science thus progresses by "reasoned judgments on the part of scientists and through debate within the scientific community."[3:167]

REFERENCES

1. Bixenstine, E. (1964). Empiricism in latter-day behavioral science. *Science, 145*:465.
2. Bronowski, J. (1979). *The visionary eye: Essays in the arts, literature and science.* Cambridge, Mass.: The MIT Press.
3. Brown, H. (1977). *Perception, theory and commitment: The new philosophy of science.* Chicago: The University of Chicago Press.
4. Calder, N. (1979). *Einstein's universe.* New York: Viking.
5. Dubin, R. (1978). *Theory building.* New York: The Free Press.
6. Flavell, J.H. (1977). *Cognitive development.* Englewood Cliffs, N.J.: Prentice-Hall.
7. Foucault, M. (1973). *The order of things: An archaeology of the human sciences.* New York: Vintage Books.
8. Gale, G. (1979). *Theory of science: An introduction to the history, logic and philosophy of science.* New York: McGraw-Hill.
9. Giere, R.N. (1979). *Understanding scientific rea-*

soning. New York: Holt, Rinehart & Winston.
10. Hanson, N.R. (1958). *Patterns of discovery*. Cambridge: Cambridge University Press.
11. Hudson, L. (1972). *The cult of the fact*. New York: Harper & Row.
12. Irving, H.W. (1977). Social networks in the modern city. *Social Forces, 55:*867-880.
13. Kuhn, T.S. (1962). *The structure of scientific revolutions*. Chicago: The University of Chicago Press.
14. Mishler, E.G. (1979). Meaning in context: Is there any other kind? *Harvard Educational Review, 49:*1-19.
15. Norman, D.A. (1976). *Memory and attention: An introduction to human information processing*. New York: John Wiley & Sons.
16. Piaget, J. (1970). *The place of the sciences of man in the system of sciences*. New York: Harper & Row.
17. Popper, K. (1962). *Conjectures and refutations*. New York: Basic Books.
18. Randall, J.H. (1964). *Philosophy: An introduction*. New York: Barnes & Noble.
19. Reynolds, P. (1971). *A primer in theory construction*. Indianapolis: Bobbs-Merrill.
20. Schutz, A. (1967). *The phenomenology of the social world*. Evanston, Ill.: Northwestern University Press.
21. Skinner, B.F. (1950). Are theories of learning necessary? *Psychological Review, 57:*193-216.
22. Snelbecker, G. (1974). *Learning theory, instructional theory, and psychoeducational design*. New York: McGraw-Hill.
23. Steiner, E. (1977). *Criteria for theory of art education*. Monograph presented at Seminar for Research in Art Education, Philadelphia. Unpublished.
24. Steiner, E. (1978). *Logical and conceptual analytic techniques for educational researchers*. Washington, D.C.: University Press.
25. Toulmin, S. (1961). *Foresight and understanding*. New York: Harper & Row.
26. Turner, J. (1978). *The structure of sociological theory*. Homewood, Ill.: The Dorsey Press.
27. Werkmeister, W. (1959). Theory construction and the problem of objectivity. In L. Gross (Ed.), *Symposium on sociological theory*. Evanston, Ill.: Row, Peterson, & Co.
28. Winton, C. (1974). *Theory and measurement in sociology*. New York: John Wiley & Sons.
29. Zetterberg, H.L. (1966). *On theory and verification in sociology*. Totowa, N.J.: The Bedminster Press.

4

Logical Reasoning

Sue Marquis Bishop

A theory may be evaluated by using the criterion of logical development. This requires that the development of the series of theoretical statements follow a logical form of reasoning, that is, the premises justify the conclusions. Logic is a branch of philosophy concerned with the analysis of inferences and arguments.[9] An *inference* involves the forming of a conclusion based on some evidence. Although the common meaning of argument implies a disagreement, in logic, an *argument* consists of a conclusion and its supportive evidence. The evidence supporting a conclusion may involve one or more theoretical statements, or premises. The tools of logic permit the analysis of the reasoning from the premises to the conclusion.[7]

Theories can be developed and tested through deductive, inductive, or retroductive forms of reasoning. These approaches have been explicitly presented in the literature as systematic procedures for devising theory. An in-depth discussion of these forms is beyond the scope of this chapter and the reader is referred to Geach,[1] Giere,[2] Pospesel,[7] Salmon,[8,9] and Steiner[14] for further study. It is important, however, to grasp the basic differences between these forms of reasoning in order to understand how a given theorist may choose to approach the task of theory building.

DEDUCTION

Deduction is a form of logical reasoning in which specific conclusions are inferred from more general premises or principles. Reasoning thus proceeds from the general to the particular.[13] The deductively developed theory usually involves a lengthy sequence of theoretical statements derived from a relatively few broad axioms or general statements. Conclusions thus derived may offer predictions that can be tested empirically. The deductive argument usually takes the form of a syllogism with general premises and a conclusion. In logical analysis, letters may be substituted for concepts, since emphasis on the analysis of the argument is focused on the *form of the argument*. Example A presents a valid deductive argument with letter notation.

EXAMPLE A

Premise: All victims of abuse have low self-esteem. (All S are M)
Premise: Martha and Tom are victims of abuse. (All P are S)
Conclusion: Therefore, Martha and Tom have low self-esteem. (*Ergo,* All P are M)

In Example A, the conclusion follows from, or was deduced from the general premises. There may be a lengthy number of premises in a given argument preceding the conclusion. Note in the above example there is no new information presented in the conclusion that is not at least implied in the premises. The deductive form of reasoning is defined as:

1. If A were true, then B would be true.
2. A is true.
3. Hence, B is true.[14:9]

As you study the nursing literature, you will not often find arguments presented in the form in Example A with the premises and conclusions placed in order and clearly labeled. But with practice you can sharpen your skills in identifying arguments and labeling the premises and conclusions from your reading of narrative text. You may find the conclusion may be presented at the beginning or end, or even in the middle of an argument.[9] Salmon[9] suggests that certain words or phrases are clues that specific statements are offered as premises or conclusions. Examples of terms that often precede a premise include *since, for,* and *because*. Examples of terms that often precede a conclusion are *therefore, consequently, hence, so,* and *it follows that*.[9]

Arguments may be evaluated in two different ways: (1) the validity of the argument may be assessed as to whether the conclusion logically follows from the premises, and (2) the content of the premises may be assessed in terms of the truth or falsity of the statements.[7] The validity of a deductive argument refers to the logic involved in reasoning from the premises to the conclusion in such a way that if the premises are true, the conclusion must necessarily be true.[7,9,14] A deductive argument may contain all true statements or one or more false statements and be considered either valid or invalid. This judgment is made on the basis of whether the conclusion is supported by the premises. For example:

EXAMPLE B
Premise: All victims of abuse have low self-esteem.
Premise: Martha has low self-esteem.
Conclusion: Therefore, Martha is a victim of abuse.

Although Martha may very well be the victim of abuse, the truth or falsity of the conclusion (or any of the statements) is not an issue when evaluating the validity of an argument. In Example B, the conclusion that Martha is a victim of abuse is not established by the supporting evidence in the premises. The conclusion goes beyond the explicit and implicit information in the premises. This is not a valid argument. (Compare the reasoning in Examples A and B.)

Whereas *validity* refers to the form of the deductive argument, *truth* refers to the content of a given theoretical statement. It is therefore inappropriate to label a single theoretical statement valid or an argument true.[9]

In a valid deductive argument, if the premises are true, it necessarily follows that the conclusion must be true. (This combination is marked [R] in Figure 4-1.) It is therefore impossible for the conclusion to be false. (This combination is marked [S] in Figure 4-1.) If, however, one or more of the premises are false, two outcomes are possible: the conclusion may be either true or false.

Example C presents a deductively valid argument that leads from false premises to a false

		The conclusion is:	
		True	False
If the premises are:	All true	Necessary (R)	Impossible (S)
	Not all true	Possible (Y)	Possible (X)

(R) If the premises are true, it *necessarily follows* that the conclusion be true.

(S) If the premises are true, it is therefore *impossible* for the conclusion to be false.

(Y), (X) If one or more of the premises are false, it is *possible* the conclusion may be *either* true or false.

Figure 4-1. Potential outcomes of a valid deductive argument.

Adapted from Giere, R.N. (1979). *Understanding scientific reasoning*. New York: Holt, Rinehart & Winston.

conclusion. (This combination is marked [X] in Figure 4-1.)

EXAMPLE C

Premise: The dime is larger than the nickel. (FALSE)
Premise: The nickel is larger than the Susan B. Anthony dollar. (FALSE)
Conclusion: Thus, the dime is larger than the Susan B. Anthony dollar. (FALSE)

As Figure 4-1 suggests, and Example D illustrates, it is also possible that a valid argument can lead from one or more false premises to a true conclusion. (This combination is marked [Y] in Figure 4-1.)

EXAMPLE D

Premise: The nickel is larger than the Susan B. Anthony dollar. (FALSE)
Premise: The Susan B. Anthony dollar is larger than the dime. (TRUE)
Conclusion: Thus, the nickel is larger than the dime. (TRUE)

It may be helpful to study Examples C and D to understand how the conclusions are derived from the information given in the premises. (Note in these examples that "larger than" refers to physical size, not the value of the coins.) In science, deductive arguments can be a powerful form of reasoning for deriving new conclusions by making explicit the implied information contained in what is known. These derived conclusions can then be subjected to empirical test.

INDUCTION

Induction is a form of logical reasoning in which a generalization is induced from a number of specific observed instances. Inductive reasoning has been less well developed than deductive reasoning.[7] The form of the inductive argument is:

1. A is true of $b_1, b_2 \ldots b_n$.
2. $b_1, b_2 \ldots b_n$ are some members of class B.
3. Hence, A is true of all members of class B.[14:9]

The inductive form is based on the assumption that members of any given class share common characteristics. Therefore what is true of any randomly selected members of the class is accepted as true for all members of the class.[14] Suppose a sample of the population of victims of abuse has been selected for study. Example E presents an argument in the inductive form that may be developed based on this hypothetical study:

EXAMPLE E

Premise: Every victim of abuse that has been observed has low self-esteem.
Conclusion: All victims of abuse have low self-esteem.

The premise in Example E states observations from a number of instances, that is, a limited number of subjects. The conclusion states a generalization extending beyond the observations to the whole class of victims of abuse.

The inductive generalization also may be stated in terms of a mathematical quantity.[9] For example, assume a researcher decides to survey a sample of 400 nurses to determine their opinions as to whether nurses should establish independent private practices. Results indicate sixty-five percent of nurses in the sample support independent private practice activities in nursing. The inductive statement may be stated as:

EXAMPLE F

Premise: Sixty-five percent of nurses in the sample support independent private practice activities in nursing.
Conclusion: Sixty-five percent of all nurses support independent private practice in nursing.

Whereas, in a deductive argument, if the premises are true, the conclusion must necessarily be true, the inductive argument can have true premises and yet produce a false conclusion.

An inductive conclusion based on limited or biased evidence can clearly lead to a fallacious argument and perhaps a false conclusion.[9] Suppose the argument in Example E was developed by one nurse's experience with observing five victims of abuse. The conclusion that victims of abuse have low self-esteem may or may not be true. However, this conclusion is not warranted based on the number of observed instances. There is too little evidence in this case to justify the conclusion about all victims of abuse.

Even if the sample size is appropriately sufficient (or based on several studies), the sample may be biased. Assume in Example F that the sample of nurses was drawn from faculty in schools of nursing. The opinions of this select group of nurses may be expected to be different in some respects and may not reflect the opinions of all nurses. It may be that a greater proportion of nursing faculty members are engaged in private practice activities than the proportion of all nurses. Considering a number of factors in selecting representative samples can help avoid introducing bias into observations. This reasoning is the basis for the random selection of subjects in research projects. Descriptive and inferential statistics are used to characterize the sample and population and help with decisions about the strength of the evidence.[2] The inductive inference thus has been termed the statistical inference.[14,17]

A distinguishing characteristic of inductive arguments is that the inferred conclusion goes beyond the implicit and explicit information in the premises. In Example E not all victims of abuse have been observed. This conclusion is inferred on the basis of selected instances. In a deductive argument, the conclusion can be considered true if the argument is structured so that implicit information in the premises is made explicit.[9] The inductive argument, on the other hand, goes beyond the information in the premises. The inductive argument thus expands on the information presented. Giere[2] has argued this characteristic permits the justification of scientific conclusions that may not be justifiable by deductive reasoning, since they contain information beyond the premises. An example would be a scientific hypothesis about the future based on observations in the present.

Whereas deductive arguments are considered to be either valid or invalid, the concept of validity does not apply to inductive arguments. The correctness of inductive arguments is not viewed in either/or terms, but on degrees of strength, measured in terms of the *probability* with which the premises lead to a given conclusion. The inferred conclusion then can be determined to have low, medium, or high probability.[9] Statistical procedures can be used for making these judgments.

In Example A, the only possibility for the conclusion being false is if one or more of the premises are false, that is, if all victims of abuse do not have low self-esteem, or if Martha and Tom are not victims of abuse. If these are true, the conclusion must necessarily be true. However, in Example E the reasoning suggests that all victims of abuse have low self-esteem. But the premises state only selected victims of abuse have been observed. The premises may lend some support for the conclusion. The fact that no victims of absue without low self-esteem have been observed may be considered some evidence, but not conclusive evidence that a victim with high self-esteem will not be observed in the future.[9]

Deductive arguments are considered "truth preservers," while inductive arguments can be a source of new information.[2,9] Scientific generalizations about instances not observed in the present or projections about the future are examples. Although this form of reasoning is useful in advancing science, the very nature of induction may introduce error into the scientific process.[3] Even if we could be sure the premises were accurate, we could not be absolutely certain of the accuracy of the conclusion. In Giere's view, if we assume the premises are true:

> The difference between a *good inductive argument* and a *valid deductive argument* is that the deduc-

tive argument guarantees the *truth* of its conclusion while the inductive argument guarantees only an *appropriately high probability* of its conclusion.[2:37-38]

RETRODUCTION*

Whereas deduction and induction may explicate and evaluate ideas, retroduction originates ideas.[13] The retroductive form of reasoning is an approach to inquiry using analogy as a method for devising theory. In 1878 Pierce described three kinds of reasoning as comprising the major steps of inquiry: retroduction, deduction and induction.[14] Pierce viewed retroductive reasoning as the first stage in the search for understanding some "surprising phenomenon" in which a viewpoint offering a possible explanation is identified. Pierce stated that once a viewpoint was identified that held the promise of explanation for the observed phenomenon, deductive reasoning was used to develop the explanation. Pierce considered the final stage of inquiry in terms of induction with the focus on checking out the devised hy-

*The following discussion of retroduction has been adapted from the work of Elizabeth Steiner (see references 11, 12, and 13).

Table 4-1. Deduction, induction, and retroduction summary table

Type	Question	Techniques
Deduction	Given the premises are true, what other propositions may be inferred as necessary conclusions from the premises?[12:67]	Logical and conceptual analysis[12]
Induction	Given the premises are true, what is the strength of the link between them and the conclusion?[12:87]	Logical and conceptual analysis based on statistical analysis[11,15]
Retroduction	Given a surprising observation, what explanation would result in the expectation that the observation would be a matter of course?[12]	Logical and conceptual analysis[11]

potheses in experience.[14] The theory models approach using retroductive inference was further developed by Steiner* as a method for devising theory. The form of the retroductive inference follows:

1. The surprising fact C, is observed.
2. But if A were true, C would be a matter of course.
3. Hence, there is reason to suspect that A is true.[14:9]

An analysis of the above form reveals that the theory models (or retroductive) approach does not establish truth. Its function is to originate ideas about selected phenomena that can be developed further and tested. The theory models approach is most useful as a strategy for devising theory in a field in which there are few available theories and innovation is indicated to advance knowledge in describing and understanding selected observations.[14,16]

The retroductive theorist approaches the development of a wanted theory by identifying a source theory in another field that may have potential for developing the wanted theory. The theory models approach is based on the use of analogy and metaphor between two sets of phenomena, which requires considerable creativity

*References 3, 4, 11, 12. Elizabeth Steiner-Maccia's earlier published work on theory models was under her married name of Maccia.

Definition	Example	Function
1. If A were true, then B would be true. 2. A is true. 3. Hence, B is true.[14:9]	*Premises* All victims of abuse have low self-esteem. Marty & Tom are victims of abuse. *Conclusion* Marty & Tom have low self-esteem.	*Explicates and derives further truths*[11:9] If premises are true, establishes truth of something else by derivation.[11:9]
1. A is true of $b_1, b_2 \ldots b_n$. 2. $b_1, b_2 \ldots b_n$ are members of some class B. 3. Hence, A is true of all members of class B.[14:9]	*Premise* $b_1, b_2 \ldots b_n$ victims of abuse that have been observed have low self-esteem. *Conclusion* All victims of abuse have low self-esteem.	*Evaluates and expands information*[2] Based on probability of observed cases. Does not establish truth. Establishes probability of certainty. New data may change conclusion.[2,8,11]
1. The surprising fact C is observed. 2. But if A were true, C would be a matter of course. 3. Hence, there is reason to suspect that A is true.[14:9]	*Proposition 1* The role of expecting *reward* determines a relation between *student* and *teacher* that establishes a path for influence of the *teacher* on the *student*.[4:121] *Proposition 2* The role of expecting *care and comfort* determines a relation between *patient* and *nurse* that establishes a path for influence of *nurse* on the *patient*.	*Originates ideas*[11:9] Does not establish truth. Suggests lines of thought worthy of exploration and testing.[11:9]

on the part of the theorist and an intuitive knowledge of the phenomena of interest.[12] The theory models approach is represented as:[13,14]

THEORY$_1$ ------→ THEORY MODEL ----→ THEORY$_2$

(Source theory) (Wanted theory)

Thus theory models are not "models-of," but are "models-for" devising representations of selected phenomena.[12] The theory model is essentially a meta-model which serves as a model to develop theory.[13]

To devise theory using retroductive inference, the theorist seeks out a source theory to form a theory model from which the wanted theory will be devised. The source theory is selected on the basis of a "suspected similarity in the structure of form or pattern of relations" between the two sets of phenomena.[14] The selected source theory is perceived to present ideas that may be useful for developing a theory about the observations of interest. These ideas are selected from theory$_1$ and formed into a point of view or theory model that will serve as the framework for developing theory$_2$. This approach is based on the assumption that new conjectures, or ideas, in a given field may be devised from other conjectures in theories in other fields.[3,4,14] The ideas selected from theory$_1$ for the theory model may involve any combination of concepts, hypothesized relationships or theory structures. The viewpoint presented by the theory model is used to develop theory$_2$ by adding content to the theory model and by altering concepts and relationships to fit with the phenomenon of interest for theory$_2$. It should be clear that this process of theory building is not simply borrowing a theory from one field and applying it unchanged to another. The deliberate selection of aspects of theory$_1$ to form the theory model, the addition of new information, and the alteration of concepts and relationships for congruence with different phenomena in a new context, result in a new theory. Of course a theory devised by this method must meet the criteria for adequacy of a theory (see Chapter 1). As Steiner[4,13,14] argued, the theory models approach cannot be considered reductive since theory$_1$ is not equivalent to theory$_2$. To be reductive, the theorist would simply borrow concepts and hypotheses and use them as formulated in a new context. Neither can this approach be considered deductive, since theory$_2$ was not developed by deduction from theory$_1$. The hypotheses in theory$_2$ cannot be derived from theory$_1$.[13,14]

The use of analogy to develop theory has been a common occurrence in the development of a number of scientific fields. In Sigmund Freud's day, the machine model was a popular advanced model of the times. Freud used the notion of machine operations to develop his theoretical assertions about psychological tension-reduction relationships in his theory of psychosexual development. Three or more decades ago basic texts in human anatomy and physiology used the telephone switchboard as an analogy for explaining the functioning of the brain. Currently, the computer is often used as a model for thinking about the brain and in developing theories of human information processing.[5,10] In nursing, General Systems Theory has been used as a model for developing nursing theory.[6] Steiner's development of the theory models approach provides guidelines for using this strategy in theory building.

Stevens[15] has argued that one of the reasons much of nursing research has so little impact on nursing practice is that nursing research is often based on the "categories and characteristics" of borrowed theories. A borrowed theory tends to be used unchanged in the new context. Although theories in other fields may suggest a possible framework for addressing phenomena in the field of nursing, this framework may need to be contextualized within nursing. That is, aspects of the "borrowed theory" may need to be altered to reflect the appropriate categories and characteristics within nursing. Walker and Avant's "derivation strategy" for theory construction[16] draws from the theory models approach developed by Steiner. Walker and Avant[16] present a number of examples of using the derivation strategy to "shift and reformulate" concepts, theoretical statements, and theories from other fields to nursing. The theory models approach permits the translation and expansion of ideas within the milieu of nursing and may result in the development of a new nursing theory. A nursing theory devised by this method can be further developed through the use of deductive and inductive strategies.

A summary of deductive, inductive, and retroductive forms of reasoning is presented in Table 4-1.

REFERENCES

1. Geach, P.T. (1979). *Reason and argument.* Los Angeles: University of California Press.
2. Giere, R.N. (1979). *Understanding scientific reasoning.* New York: Holt, Rinehart & Winston.
3. Maccia, E.S., & Maccia, G. (1966). *Construction of educational theory derived from three educational theory models* (Project No. 5-0638). Washington, D.C.: U.S. Department of Health, Education, and Welfare.
4. Maccia, E.S., Maccia, G., & Jewett, R. (1963). *Construction of educational theory models* (Cooperative Research Project No. 1632). Washington, D.C.: Office of Education, U.S. Department of Health, Education, and Welfare.
5. Norman, D.A. (1976). *Memory and attention: An introduction to human information processing.* New York: John Wiley & Sons.
6. Nursing Theories Conference Group (1980). *Nursing theories: The base for professional nursing practice.* Englewood Cliffs, N.J.: Prentice-Hall.
7. Pospesel, H. (1974). *Propositional logic.* Englewood Cliffs, N.J.: Prentice-Hall.
8. Salmon, W.C. (1967). *The foundations of scientific inference.* Pittsburgh: University of Pittsburgh Press.
9. Salmon, W.C. (1973). Logic. Englewood Cliffs, N.J.: Prentice-Hall.
10. Shepherd, G.M. (1974). *The synaptic organization of the brain.* New York: Oxford University Press.
11. Steiner, E. (1976). *Logical and conceptual analytic techniques for educational researchers.* Paper presented at the American Educational Research Association, San Francisco. © Copyright Elizabeth Steiner. All rights reserved.
12. Steiner, E. (1976). *The complete act of educational inquiry.* © Copyright Elizabeth Steiner. All rights reserved.
13. Steiner, E. (1977). *Criteria for theory of art education.* Paper presented at the Seminar for Research in Art Education, Philadelphia. © Copyright Elizabeth Steiner. All rights reserved.
14. Steiner, E. (1978). *Logical and conceptual analytic techniques for educational researchers.* Washington, D.C.: University Press.
15. Stevens, B. (1979). *Nursing theory: Analysis, application, evaluation.* Boston: Little, Brown.
16. Walker, L., & Avant, K. (1983). *Strategies for theory construction in nursing.* Norwalk, Conn.: Appleton-Century-Crofts.
17. Weiner, P. (1958). *Values in a universe of chance.* New York: Doubleday.

5

Theory Development Process

Sue Marquis Bishop

Nursing theory development is not a mysterious, magical activity. Many nurses have been developing their own private ideas of nursing since their first day in nursing (or perhaps before) and have continued to develop private assumptions based on their readings and experiences. These private notions may include such generalizations as "A clean, smooth bed allows greater rest and less need for pain medication for a patient," or "Encouraging the patient to have some say in his or her care leads to greater cooperation with treatment procedures." Nurses usually don't talk explicitly about their private theories, although these theories may influence the nursing activities they choose to implement and the manner in which they practice nursing.

If, in fact, all nurses are evolving private theories of nursing, why all the fuss about studying published theories? The major reason is that nurses' private conceptions of nursing may be "incomplete, inconsistent, or muddled."* This leads to considerable problems in using the private theory as a sound basis for practice. Further, an incomplete, inconsistent, or muddled theory may be difficult to use in studying clinical nursing situations to advance our knowledge of nursing. If we agree that the availability of more systematic theories would provide a clearer understanding and enable us to explore whether this understanding corresponds with activities in the nursing environment, then we also must agree with Hardy[7] and others that rigorous development of nursing theory is a priority. The systematic development of nursing theory has a better chance of advancing nursing and may lead to the basis for nursing science.

It is important to grasp the concept of *systematic development*. Approaches to the construction of theory differ. But one aspect they have in common is the agreement among scientists to approach this task in a systematic fashion and to make the stages in development explicit so others can review the logical processes and test the hypotheses presented. The nurse who devises a theory of nursing and presents it for public review by the nursing community is engaging in the process essential to advancing theory development.

THEORY COMPONENTS

Hage[6] identified six components of a complete theory and specified the contribution each

*I wish to acknowledge my indebtedness to Nicholas Mullins, one of my former teachers, for his discussion of private and public theories, and for communicating both the complexity and creative playfulness in theoretical work.

makes to the whole theory (Table 5-1). He argued that the failure to include one or more of the components resulted in the elimination of that particular contribution to the total theory. These six aspects of a theory are discussed as a basis for understanding the function of each element in the theory building process.

Concepts

Concepts, the building blocks of theories, classify the phenomena with which we are concerned.[8] It is crucial in any separate discussion of concepts to recognize that concepts must not be considered separately from the theoretical system in which they are embedded and from which they derive their meaning.[2] Concepts may have completely different meanings in different theoretical systems. Because scientific progress is based on the critical review and testing of a researcher's work by others in the scientific community, consensus regarding the meaning of scientific concepts is important.[2,6]

Table 5-1. Theory components and their contributions to the theory

Theory Components	Contributions
Concepts	Description and classification
Theoretical statements	Analysis
Definitions	
Theoretical	Meaning
Operational	Measurement
Linkages	
Theoretical	Plausability
Operational	Testability
Ordering of concepts and definitions into primitive and derived terms	Elimination of overlap (tautology)
Ordering of statements and linkages into premises and equations	Elimination of inconsistency

Modified from Hage, J. (1972). *Techniques and problems in theory construction in sociology.* New York: John Wiley & Sons.

Concepts may be abstract or concrete. Abstract concepts are independent of a specific time or place, while concrete concepts relate to a particular time and place.[6,13]

Abstract concepts	*Concrete concepts*
Social System	The Vaughn Family Indiana University School of Nursing
Debate	Bush-Dukakis Debate

In the above example, the Vaughn family is an instance of the more general abstract concept of social system.

Concepts may label discrete categories (or classes) of phenomena (such as patient, nurse, or environment), or dimensions of phenomena (the amount of self-care or degree of marital conflict, for example).[3,6,11,13] Theories may be developed by using nonvariable discrete concepts to build typologies.[6,13,16]

The nonvariable concept is devised to capture a number of different aspects.[6] Phenomena are then identified as belonging or *not* belonging to a given class. The sorting of phenomena into nonvariable, discrete categories carries the assumption that the reality associated with the given phenomena is captured by the classification.[6] The nonvariable concept of bureaucracy was devised by Max Weber as an ideal type to characterize organizations.[9] Organizations can thus be classified as bureaucratic or nonbureaucratic.

On the other hand, the use of variable concepts based on a range or continuum tend to be focused on one dimension without the assumption that a single dimension "captures all the reality" connected with the phenomenon.[6] Additional dimensions may be devised to measure further aspects of the phenomenon. In contrast to the nonvariable term *bureaucracy,* variable concepts such as rate of conflict, ratio of professional to nonprofessional staff, and communication flow may be used to characterize organizations. Although nonvariable concepts are useful in classifying phenomena in theory development, it has been argued that major breakthroughs occurred in several fields when the focus shifted from nonvariable to variable concepts.[6] Variable concepts permit scoring the full range of the phenomenon on a continuum.

The development of theoretical concepts permits the *description* and *classification* of phenomena.[6] The labeled concept suggests boundaries for selecting phenomena to observe and for reasoning about the phenomena of interest. New concepts may focus attention on new phenomena or may facilitate thinking about and classifying phenomena in a different way.[6]

Theoretical Statements

Although concepts are considered the building blocks of theory, they must be connected in some way with a set of theoretical statements to devise theory.* The development of theoretical statements asserting a connection between two or more concepts introduces the possibility of *analysis*.[6]

Statements in a theory can be classified into three general categories: existence statements, definitions, and relational statements.[13,18] Existence statements and definitions relate to specific concepts. Whereas definitions provide descriptions of the concept, existence statements simply assert that a given concept exists and is labeled with the concept name. Relational statements assert relationships between the properties of two or more concepts (or variables). Various types of relational statements have been described in the literature.[11,13,18] Discussion in this chapter is limited to an introduction to probabilistic statements and necessary and sufficient conditional statements. These types of statements are important in understanding scientific reasoning.[5]

In the connections between variables, one variable may be assumed to influence a second variable. In this instance, the first variable may be labeled a determinant (or antecedent) and the second variable a resultant (or consequent).[5,16,20] The first variable may be viewed as the independent variable and the second as the dependent variable.[5] Because of its complexity, nursing presents a situation in which multiple antecedents and consequents may be involved in studying a selected phenomenon. Zetterberg[20] concluded, however, that the development of two-variate theoretical statements may be an important intermediate step in the development of a theory. These statements later can be reformulated as the theory evolves or new information is known.

An example of a relational statement expressed as a sufficient condition is, "If nurses react with approval of patients' independent behaviors, patients increase their efforts in self-care activities." This is a type of compound statement linking antecedent and consequent. The statement does not assert the truth of the antecedent. Rather, the assertion is made that *if* the antecedent is true, then the consequent also is true.[5] In addition, there is no assertion in the statement explaining *why* the antecedent is related to the consequent.[6] In symbolic notation form, the above statements can be expressed as:

NA --------►	PSC
(Nurse Approval)	(Patient Self-Care)

This statement asserts that nurse approval of a patient's independent behaviors is sufficient for the occurrence of the patient's self-care activities. However, patient assumption of self-care activities resulting from other factors such as the patient's health status and personality variables is not ruled out. In other words, there could be other antecedents that are sufficient conditions for the patient's assumption of self-care activities.

A statement in the form of a necessary condition asserts that one variable is required for the occurrence of another variable.[5,12,15] For example:

*References 2, 3, 6, 13, 20.

Without the motivation to get well (MGW), patients will not assume strict adherence to following their prescribed treatment regimen (PTR).

MGW ---------▶ PTR

This means PTR never occurs when MGW does not occur.[5,12] No assertion is made that patients' strict adherence to the prescribed treatment regimen follows from their motivation to get well. It is asserted, however, that if motivation to get well is absent, patients will not assume strict adherence to their treatment regimen. The motivation to get well is thus a necessary, but not a sufficient, condition for the occurrence of this consequent.

The term *if* is most generally used to introduce a sufficient condition, whereas, *only if* and *if . . . then* are used to introduce necessary conditions.[5] In most instances conditional statements are not both necessary and sufficient.[5] It is possible, however, for a statement to express both conditions. In such instances the term, *if and only if* is used to imply the conditions are both necessary and sufficient for one another.[5] In this case: (1) the consequent never occurs in the absence of the antecedent, and (2) the consequent always occurs when the antecedent occurs.[5,12]

Although causal statements (one variable causes another) may be expressed as a conditional statement, not all conditional statements are causal.[5] For example, the statement "If this month is March, then the next month is April," does not assert that March causes April to occur. Rather the sequence of months suggests that April follows March.[5] (For an extensive discussion of conditional and unconditional causal statements see Nowak.[12])

Probabilistic statements are generally derived from statistical data and express connections that do not always occur but are likely to occur based on some estimate of probability.[18] Walker and Avant[18] used as an example the statement "Cigarette smoking will most likely lead to cancer of the lung." It is clear that cigarette smoking does not always lead to lung cancer since some persons who smoke do not develop this disease. However, the probability of developing cancer of the lung is enhanced for cigarette smokers. In symbolic notation:[18]

If CS ---------▶ P LC.

The development of relational statements asserting connections between variables provides for *analysis* and establishes the basis for explanation and prediction.[6]

Definition

The development of science is a collaborative endeavor in which the community of scientists critique, test, and build upon one another's work.[2] It is therefore crucial that concepts be as clearly defined as possible to reduce ambiguity in understanding a given concept or a set of concepts. While it is not possible to entirely eliminate perceived differences in meaning, these differences can be minimized by setting forth explicit definitions. In the development of a complete theory, both theoretical and operational definitions provide meaning for the concept and a basis for searching for empirical indicators.[6] *Theoretical definitions* also permit consideration of the relationships of a given concept to other theoretical ideas.

But a clear meaning for concepts is not sufficient. If theories are to be tested against reality, concepts also must be measurable.[6] *Operational definitions* relate the concepts to observable phenomena by specifying empirical indicators.[6] Hage[6] asserted that the concept name and the theoretical and operational definitions establish reference points for "locating the concept," that is, viewing the concept as related to both theoretical systems and the observable environment.

Linkages

The specification of linkages is an important part of the development of theory.[6] Although the theoretical statements assert connections between concepts, the rationale for the stated connections need to be developed. The development of *theoretical linkages* offers a reasoned explanation of why the variables may be connected in some manner, that is, the theoretical reasons for asserting particular interrelationships.[6] This rationale contributes *plausibility* to the theory.[6]

Operational linkages, on the other hand, contribute the element of *testability* to the theory by specifying how variables are connected.[6] Whereas operational definitions provide for measurability of the concepts, operational linkages provide for testability of the assertions. The operational linkage contributes a perspective for understanding the nature of the relationship between concepts, such as whether the relationship between concepts is negative or positive and linear or curvilinear.[6]

Ordering

Finally, Hage,[6] concluded that a theory may be considered to be "fairly complete" if it presents the elements of *concepts, definitions, statements,* and *linkages.* Complete development of the theory, however, requires the organization of concepts and definitions into primitive and derived terms and the organization of statements and linkages into premises and equations.[6] As the theory evolves, concepts and theoretical statements multiply, and the need arises to establish some logical arrangement or ordering of the theoretical components to bring conceptual order to the theory.[6] Hage stated the concepts should be ordered if the theory contains more than ten variables. He also recommended the concepts and definitions be ordered into primitive and derived terms. Primitive terms are terms not defined within the theory. Derived terms are defined with primitive terms or other terms already defined. Derived terms are thus defined within the theory. This process of ordering may point up any existing overlap between concepts and definitions.[6] The conceptual arrangement of statements and linkages into premises and equations may reveal areas of inconsistency.[6] Premises (or axioms) are regarded as the more general assertions from which the hypotheses are derived in the form of equations. Hage suggested that the ordering of statements and linkages is indicated when the theory contains a large number of theoretical statements.

FORMS OF THEORY ORGANIZATION*

A formal theory is a systematically developed conceptual system that addresses a given set of phenomena. There are different ideas of how this conceptual system should be organized so as to constitute a theory. Three forms for organizing theory include: set-of-laws, axiomatic, and causal process.

Set-of-Laws Form

The set-of-laws approach attempts to organize findings from empirical research.[13] The theorist first reviews the research literature in an area of particular interest. Empirical findings from available research are identified and selected from the literature for evaluation. Findings are evaluated and sorted into categories based on the degree of empirical evidence supporting each assertion.[13] The available categories are *laws, empirical generalizations* and *hypotheses.*[13]

Since construction of the set-of-laws theory requires the selection and evaluation of research findings in terms of degree of empirical support, several limitations emerge as a result of this approach to constructing theory. Reynolds[13] discussed these limitations as disadvantages to the set-of-laws approach to theory building. First, the nature of research requires focusing on relationships between a limited set of variables, often two variables. Therefore attempts to develop a set-of-laws theory from statements of findings may result in a lengthy number of statements that assert relationships between two or more variables. This lengthy set

*The section on forms of theory organization is largely based on Reynolds' discussion[13] of these forms.

SET-OF-LAWS FORM

Laws (Overwhelming empirical support)
1.
2.
3.
Empirical Generalizations (Some empirical support)
1.
2.
3.
4.
Hypotheses (No empirical support)
1.
2.
3.
4.
5.

From Reynolds, P. (1971). *A primer in theory construction*. Indianapolis: Bobbs-Merrill.

of generalizations may be difficult to organize and interrelate. Second, in order for research to be conducted, concepts must be operationally defined so as to be measurable. Concepts in the statements of empirical findings are therefore most likely to be measurable and operational concepts. This procedure eliminates other more highly abstract or theoretical concepts that might be useful in developing an understanding of the phenomenon of interest. Reynolds[13] concluded that although the set-of-laws form may provide for classification of phenomena or predictions of relationships between selected variables, it does not permit a "sense of understanding" crucial for the advancement of science. Finally, Reynolds[13] noted that each statement in the set-of-laws form is considered to be independent in that the various statements have not been interrelated into a system of description and explanation (see box above). Therefore each statement must be tested. Because the statements are not interrelated, research support for one statement does not provide support for any other statement. Research efforts must therefore be more extensive.

The set-of-laws approach to theory building is consistent with the view that scientific knowledge consists of the body of empirical findings and that science is advanced by conducting research and then looking for patterns in the data.[13] This strategy is clearly an inductive one and may be based on the positivist belief that knowledge exists independent of theories and is waiting for discovery.[2,13] Patterns do not, of their own accord, arise from empirical data.[16] The theorist must bring "ideas to experience" to conceptualize and order theoretical relationships.[16] Reynolds[13] stated this may be difficult to do with a "lengthy catalogue" of empirical findings in the set-of-laws form.

Axiomatic Form

In contrast to the set-of-laws form, the axiomatic form of theory organization is an interrelated logical system. Specifically, an axiomatic theory consists of a set of concepts, explicit definitions, a set of existence statements, and a set of relationship statements arranged in hierarchical order.[13,17,20] The concepts include highly abstract concepts, intermediate concepts, and more concrete concepts. The set of existence statements describes situations in which the theory is applicable.[13,17,18] Statements helping delineate the boundaries of the theory are referred to as describing the scope conditions of the theory.[3,6,13] The relational statements consist of axioms and propositions. The highly abstract theoretical statements, called axioms, are organized at the top of the hierarchy.[17] All other propositions are developed through logical deduction from the axioms or from other more abstract propositions[17] (see box on p. 46).

The axiomatic theory is determined to be integrated when there are no propositions in Set B that cannot be logically derived from Set A.[19] This results in a highly interrelated explanatory

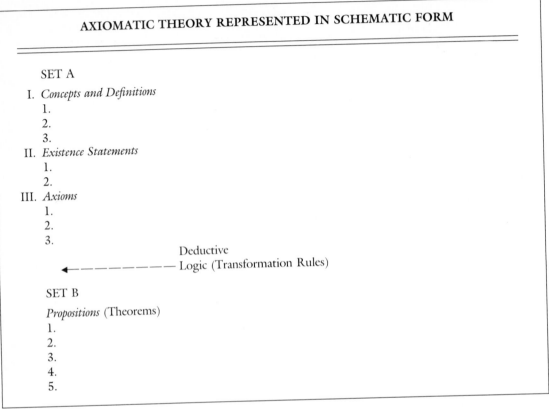

AXIOMATIC THEORY REPRESENTED IN SCHEMATIC FORM

SET A

I. *Concepts and Definitions*
   1.
   2.
   3.

II. *Existence Statements*
   1.
   2.

III. *Axioms*
   1.
   2.
   3.

Deductive
←——————— Logic (Transformation Rules)

SET B

Propositions (Theorems)
1.
2.
3.
4.
5.

This schemata on axiomatic theory is a modified version of Werkmeister's schemata[19] using Reynolds' terms[13] for the theory comments.

system. An essential criterion for the axiomatic form is that the theoretical statements may not be contradictory.[19] A basic principle of logic asserts that when two statements are contradictory, one or both of the statements must be false.[15,19] Thus, axiomatic theorists seek to avoid this problem by developing a conceptual system with a few broad axioms from which a set of propositions can be derived.[19] As science progresses and new empirical data become known, the general axioms may be modified or extended. If, however, these additions to the logical system produce contradictions in the theory, the theory must be rejected for one without contradictions.[19] New theories often subsume portions of previous theories as special cases.[2,19] For example, Einstein's theory of relativity incorporated Newton's law of gravitation as a special case within the theory.

Axiomatic theories are not common in the social and behavioral sciences, but are clearly evident in the fields of physics and mathematics. For example, Euclidean geometry is an axiomatic theory.[19,20]

Developing theories in axiomatic form has several advantages.[13,20] First, since theory is a highly interrelated set of statements, some of which are derived from others, all concepts do not need to be operationally defined.[13] This allows the theorist to incorporate some highly abstract concepts that may be unmeasurable but provide for explanation. The interrelated axiomatic system may also be more efficient for explanation than the lengthy number of theoreti-

ELEMENTS OF CAUSAL THEORY

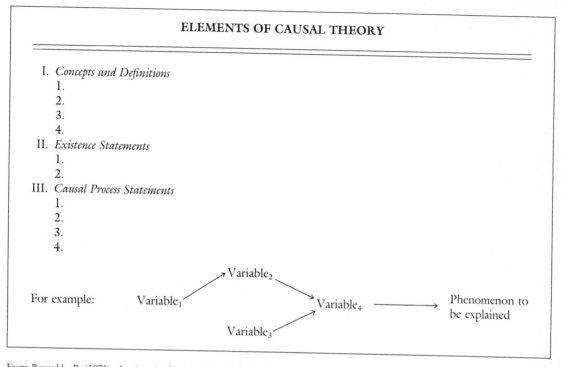

I. *Concepts and Definitions*
   1.
   2.
   3.
   4.

II. *Existence Statements*
   1.
   2.

III. *Causal Process Statements*
   1.
   2.
   3.
   4.

For example:

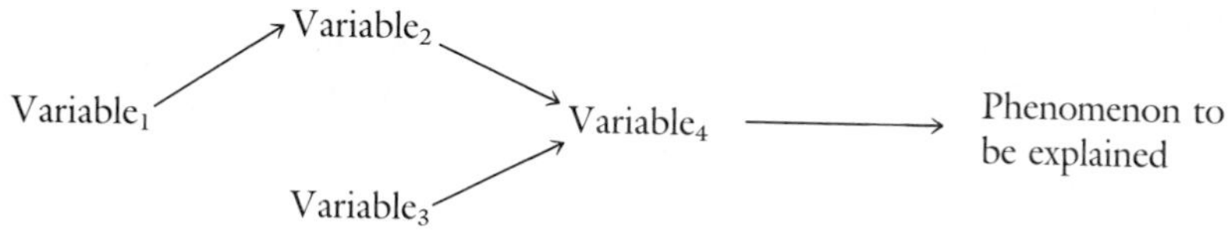

From Reynolds, P. (1971). *A primer in theory construction.* Indianapolis: Bobbs-Merrill Educational Publishing; and Turner, J. (1978). *The structure of sociological theory.* Homewood, Ill.: The Dorsey Press.

cal statements in the set-of-laws form. In addition, empirical support for one theoretical statement may be judged to provide support for the theory, thus permitting less extensive research than the requirement to test each statement in the set-of-laws form. Finally, Reynolds[13] concluded that in certain instances the axiomatic theory may be organized in a causal process form to increase a sense of understanding.

Causal Process Form

The distinguishing feature of the causal process form of theory is the development of theoretical statements specifying causal mechanisms between independent and dependent variables.[12,13] This form of theory organization consists of a set of concepts, a set of definitions, a set of existence statements, and a set of theoretical statements specifying causal process.[13] Concepts include abstract as well as concrete concepts. Existence statements function as in axiomatic theories to describe the scope conditions of the theory—the situations to which the theory applies.[3,6,13] In contrast to the hierarchical arrangement in the axiomatic theory, causal process theories contain a set of statements describing the causal mechanisms or effects of one variable on one or more other variables.[11,13] Causal process theories may be limited to a few variables or may be quite complex with several variables (see box above).

The causal statements specify the hypothesized effects of one variable on one or more variables. In complex causal process theories, feedback loops and paths of influence through several variables may be hypothesized in the set of interrelated causal statements.[11,12] Reynolds concluded that the causal process form of theory provides for an explanation of "how something happens." He identified several advantages of the causal process form of organization. First, it provides for highly abstract theoretical concepts, as does axiomatic theory. Second, also like axiomatic theory, this form with its interrelated theoretical statements permits more efficient research testing. Finally, the causal process statements provide a sense of understanding about the phenomenon of interest not possible with other forms. However Turner[17] observed that causal process theories may not necessarily include highly abstract concepts, since a number of available theories contain simply "descriptions of causal connections among events." This approach does permit the development of a causal explanation of the sequence of events that may effect the phenomenon of interest.[17]

CREATIVITY IN THEORY BUILDING

Although a number of strategies for developing theory have been presented in the literature, the theorist who attempts to approach theory construction in a mechanical way by applying structured procedures may have limited success. Theory building involves discovery and creativity. A scientific theory is clearly "a creation of the human mind."[1] Bronowski[1] has written about the similarities in the processes of constructing theories and works of art, with each requiring a high level of imagination. In his view, "There is no difference in the use of such words as 'beauty' and 'truth' in the poem, and such symbols as 'energy' and 'mass' in the equation."[1:21]

While it is possible to teach specific techniques and content, we don't really know how to facilitate creativity and originality in students. In Rosenberg's words,[14:2] "You can teach someone how to look, but not how to see; how to search, but not how to find." Bronowski[1] suggests a sense of imagination, playfulness, and participation is essential not only for the theorist but for the reader who seeks to understand theories:

> If science is a form of imagination, if all experiment is a form of play, then science cannot be dry-as-dust. . . . Science, or art, every creative activity is fun. . . . If a theorem in science seems dull to you, that is because you are not reading it with the same active sense of participation (and imagination) which you bring to the reading of a poem.[1:22-23]

In addition to imagination, developing and presenting theories requires personal discipline. Novel ideas tend to occur in a vague, disconnected, and tenuous form.[10] Self-discipline is required to work with the idea, develop it, and express it in written form for others to review. Rosenberg[14] stated that although "critical acumen" and creativity cannot be taught, they can be "nourished, enhanced, and matured." The individual's role is to attain familiarity with the phenomenon of interest and "practice, practice, practice."[14]

DO WE HAVE NURSING THEORIES?

It has been argued that there has been a preoccupation in nursing with the question of whether current nursing formulations are really theories. Flaskerud and Halloran[4] noted that although nurses identify formulations in nursing as "simply models or conceptual frameworks," they are not reluctant to label frameworks from other fields, such as psychology and sociology, as "theories." They argued that this has resulted in a depreciation of available efforts to systematize nursing. I recently encountered a nursing colleague who informed me she had returned to graduate school for doctoral work and had just completed a graduate course on nursing theories. When I inquired about what she had learned from the course, she responded, "Well, I didn't learn anything. You know there *really* aren't any nursing theories anyway." The application of rigorous criteria for a scientific theory will surely result in nursing theories being found deficient since theory construction in nursing is currently in the early stages of development. However, is the conclusion of negation of theory work in nursing (that there are no theories) the desired outcome from the study of nursing formulations?

The debate about whether nursing formulations are theories is often based on the conceptual sorting of theories into two categories: theories (T) and not-theories ($\not{T}$).

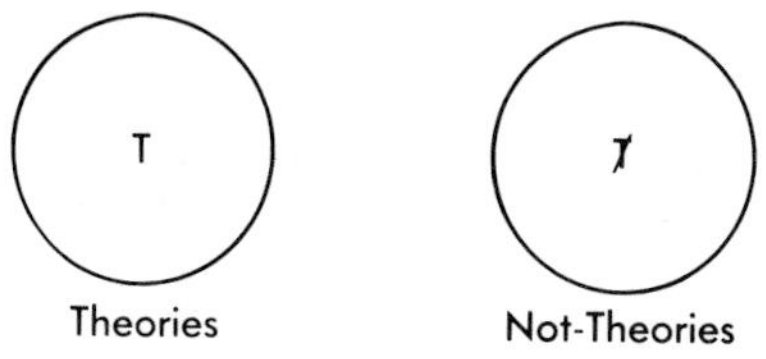

In using these conceptual classes for analysis, there are two categories for placing nursing formulations. If the T category (theory) is defined on the basis of rigorous criteria for a scientific theory, most and perhaps all nursing formulations would fall into the $\not{T}$ category. The result may be that all nursing formulations would occupy only one category. What has been gained, in terms of advancing knowledge of nursing, by the time spent on the analysis of whether nursing formulations are or are not *theories,* especially if analysis ends at this point? Turner[17] labeled this approach the "game" of "criticize-the-discipline."

Suppose, hypothetically, we have two distinct sets of nursing formulations, *X* and *Y*. Let's assume we determine *X* meets the rigorous criteria for the theory class, while *Y* is incompletely developed and does not. However, let's further suppose that the formulations in *X* do not address the phenomenon we are interested in describing, understanding, or predicting. It is also possible that *X* does not even address anything we find particularly interesting. On the other hand, *Y*, which is now labeled *not-theory,* addresses a domain of interest that fits our particular concerns in our practice area. What do we do? Develop *Y* further!

In our efforts to prepare a new generation of nurse scholars to advance theory building in nursing, it may be more fruitful to give less attention to whether a given nursing formulation is a theory or not, and concentrate on analyzing how much of a theory it is.[6] In this perspective the category of theory is defined so a range of theoretical formulations can be considered (see Mullins[11]; Hage[6]). We have therefore expanded the conceptual categories from two, in which all nursing formulations tend to fall into the $\not{T}$ category, to the notion of a continuum in the theory category. In this sorting system, sets of nursing formulations can be evaluated in terms of their relative completeness, according to where they fall in the following schematic:

T		$\not{T}$
Complete theories	Incomplete theories High Medium Low	Not-theory

Once a set of nursing formulations that fits our area of interest has been identified, several questions arise: How complete is it? What components or relationships are missing? Is it internally consistent? What is its correspondence with available empirical findings? Is it operationally defined for testing? Analyses of this nature logically lead to the question: What are the next steps in the further development of this theory? In Turner's view[17:12-13]:

> As soon as the question becomes one of *potential* for theory building, critical analysis must move beyond the mechanical comparisons of a particular theoretical perspective with the canons of scientific theory. While such comparisons . . . are an important and appropriate concern . . . , their polemic intent often gets in the way of the productive analysis of a particular conceptual perspective.

Turner recommended for his own discipline of sociology that any analysis of theory should begin with the "blunt admission" that theory construction in sociology "has a long way to go" and progress to the more important questions of beginning to identify and address current inadequacies in available theories. Hage's similar conclusions about sociological knowledge are quoted below, substituting nursing for sociology to illustrate relevance for states of affairs in nursing.

> The major difficulty in discussing whether there is any [nursing] knowledge is that many individuals think about this issue in either-or terms. . . . We do not want an either-or conception of knowledge. Because we are used to reasoning in this way, we are prevented from perceiving that perhaps there is some knowledge in [nursing], albeit it is incomplete.[6:182]

I recommend that at this point in the development of nursing, we acknowledge the following:

1. Widespread interest in the development of nursing theory is only a recent phenomenon in the history of the discipline.
2. The systematic development of nursing theories is currently in its infancy.
3. The application of rigorous criteria for a scientific theory to nursing formulations will most likely result in nursing theories being found to be far from the ideal scientific theory.
4. There is an increasing priority in nursing for the development of nursing science.

If we can accept there is a reasonable consensus in the community of nurse scholars on these assertions, perhaps we can direct our attention and energies to the critical analysis of existing incomplete theories in terms of their potential for further development.

REFERENCES

1. Bronowski, J. (1979). *The visionary age: Essays with arts, literature, and science.* Cambridge, Mass.: The MIT Press.
2. Brown, H. (1977). *Perception, theory and commitment: The new philosophy of science.* Chicago: The University of Chicago Press.
3. Dubin, R. (1978). *Theory building.* New York: The Free Press.
4. Flaskerud, J., & Halloran, E. (1980). Area of agreement in nursing theory development. *Advances in Nursing Science, 3*:1-7.
5. Giere, R.N. (1979). *Understanding scientific reasoning.* New York: Holt, Rinehart, & Winston.
6. Hage, J. (1972). *Techniques and problems in theory construction in sociology.* New York: John Wiley & Sons.
7. Hardy, N. (1983). Metaparadigms and theory development. In N. Chaska (Ed.), *The nursing profession: A time to speak.* New York: McGraw-Hill.
8. Kaplan, A. (1964). *The conduct of inquiry: Methodology for behavioral science.* New York: Chandler.
9. Merton, R., et al. (Eds.). (1952). *Reader in Bureaucracy.* New York: The Free Press.
10. Mills, C.W. (1959). On intellectual craftmanship. In L. Gross (Ed.), *Symposium on sociological theory.* Evanston, Ill.: Row, Peterson, & Co.
11. Mullins, N. (1971). *The art of theory: Construction and use.* New York: Harper & Row.
12. Nowak, S. (1975). Causal interpretations of statistical relationships in social research. In H. Blalock, et al. (Eds.), *Quantitative sociology: International perspectives on mathematical and statistical modeling.* New York: Academic Press.
13. Reynolds, P. (1971). *A primer in theory construction.* Indianapolis: Bobbs-Merrill.
14. Rosenberg, J. (1978). *The practice of philosophy.* Englewood Cliffs, N.J.: Prentice-Hall.
15. Salmon, W.D. (1973). *Logic.* Englewood Cliffs, N.J.: Prentice-Hall.
16. Steiner, E. (1978). *Logical and conceptual analytic techniques for educational researchers.* Washington, D.C.: University Press.
17. Turner, J. (1978). *The structure of sociological theory.* Homewood, Ill.: The Dorsey Press.
18. Walker, L., & Avant, K. (1983). *Strategies for theory construction in nursing.* Norwalk, Conn.: Appleton-Century-Crofts.
19. Werkmeister, W. (1959). Theory construction and the problem of objectivity. In L. Gross (Ed.), *Symposium on sociological theory.* Evanston, Ill.: Row, Peterson, & Co.
20. Zetterberg, H.L. (1966). *On theory and verification in sociology.* New York: John Wiley & Sons.

Evolution of Nursing Theory Development

6

Elizabeth Chong Choi

Nursing as a profession has been practiced for more than a century, but theory development in nursing has evolved most rapidly in the past three decades. In the mid-1800s, Nightingale[40] expressed her firm conviction that nursing required knowledge distinct from medical knowledge. She described what she believed was a nurse's proper function—to put the patient in the best condition for nature to act upon him. However, as Chinn and Jacobs noted,[7] not until the 1950s did members of the profession begin serious efforts to develop, articulate, and test nursing theory. Until the emergence of nursing as a science in the 1950s, nursing practice was based on rules, principles, and traditions passed on through an apprenticeship form of education and common wisdom that came from years of experience. Meleis[34] states that progress in nursing theory is a most significant aspect of scholarly evolution and the cornerstone of the nursing discipline.

Today there are many debates about theory in nursing that characterize the preparadigm period.[28] It is marked by frequent and deep debates over legitimate methods, problems, and standards of solutions, though these serve to define schools of thought rather than to produce agreement.[28] Kuhn[28] states that science progresses only when groups that now doubt their own status achieve consensus about their past and present accomplishments.

Kim[24] identified that interest in nursing theory development emerged for two reasons. First, nursing leaders saw theory development as a means of clearly establishing nursing as a profession. Theory development was inherent in the long-standing interest in defining nursing's unique body of knowledge. Second, the theorists were motivated by the intrinsic value of theory for nursing and the importance of the growth and enrichment of theory for nursing in itself. "Today's theories represent the individual and collective efforts of nurses to define and direct the profession and, as such, provide the basis for continued theoretical development."[7:5]

Furthermore, two kinds of efforts are formed in the works of nursing scientists, both dealing with the definitional ambiguities in nursing. The first type is the grand theorist in nursing. Related models are used to describe the aspects of human conditions the discipline is concerned with and what the members of the discipline do as practitioners in a scientific field. On the other hand, middle range theorists have focused on developing elementary theoretical statements that deal with a few selected concepts relative to nursing.[24] This chapter examines both the grand theorists and middle range theorists in their theory development and traces the origin of their influence and their orientation to paradigms such as philosophy, interpersonal relationship, energy field, and system, that have influenced nursing.

FLORENCE NIGHTINGALE

The first author to be examined is Florence Nightingale. Her theory of nursing is closely related to her philosophical orientation of the client-environment interaction, and the principles and rules on which nursing practice was founded. Nightingale's emphasis on environment reflected a predominant concern of the late 1800s when sanitation was a major health problem.[61] Nightingale believed that disease was a reparative process. The manipulation of the external environment such as ventilation, warmth, light, diet, cleanliness, and noise would contribute to the reparative process and the patient's well being. She did not believe in the germ theory that was being postulated during her lifetime.[44] Nightingale's beliefs about nursing, what it is and what it is not, form the foundation upon which her notes on nursing were written. Her contribution to theory development is in explicating nursing's domain as the patient environment relationship and in pioneering statistical analysis for health and professional nursing. Nightingale's writings represent philosophy of nursing.[63]

HILDEGARD PEPLAU

Hildegard Peplau[46] referred to a partial theory for the practice of nursing. Her work was heavily influenced by Sullivan's interpersonal relationship model and reflects the view of the contemporaneous psychoanalytical model. Peplau is the first author to borrow from other scientific fields and relate this to nursing theory. Her influence in nursing through her theory development is praised as the second order of change in nursing.[58] Blake[4] calls Peplau's model developmental. However, it has strong emphasis on interaction too. Thus it can be categorized as an interpersonal relationship.

IDA JEAN ORLANDO

Ida Jean Orlando[42,43] uses the interpersonal relationship as the basis for her work. She focuses on the patient's verbal and nonverbal expressions of needs. The nurse reacts to the patient's behavior by discerning both the meaning of the distress and what would alleviate the distress. Three elements—patient behavior, nurse reaction, and nursing actions—comprise a nursing situation. Orlando delineated automatic actions and deliberate actions. The deliberate actions are those that may yield solutions to problems and also prevent problems. She used the nursing process to meet the patient's need and thus alleviate distress. Her contribution as a theorist has advanced nursing, from personal and automatic responses to disciplined and professional practice responses.[57] Orlando's model can be categorized as interpersonal relationship.

ERNESTINE WIEDENBACH

Ernestine Wiedenbach[68] concentrated on the art or practice aspect of nursing. She focused on the need of the patient. Wiedenbach's model grew from 40 years of experience, primarily in maternity nursing, and her definition of nursing reflects that background. She said, "People may differ in their concept of nursing, but few would disagree that nursing is nurturing or caring for someone in a motherly fashion."[68:1] Wiedenbach's orientation[68] is a philosophy of nursing. It tells the nurse what to do or is a prescriptive level of theory.[8] According to Wiedenbach, clinical nursing has four elements: (1) philosophy, (2) purpose, (3) practice, and (4) art. Clinical nursing is directed toward the fulfillment of a specific purpose. The nurse's goal is to meet the perceived need-for-help the patient is experiencing.[68:15] Wiedenbach's theory of practice is influenced by her conception of nursing as an art. Her vision of nursing reflects the period of nursing theory development during which emphasis was on the art of nursing. She also follows Orlando's tradition of automatic versus deliberate nursing and incorporates the steps of the nursing process. Wiedenbach's model can be called philosophy of nursing.

JOYCE TRAVELBEE

Joyce Travelbee's model[62] is an extension of Peplau and Orlando's Interpersonal Relationship Model, but her unique synthesis of their ideas has strengthened her model in terms of the therapeutic relationship between nurse and patient. Her emphasis on caring, which stresses empathy, sympathy, and rapport, focuses on the emotional aspect and can be used as a philosophy for nursing. The model is categorized as interpersonal relationship.

JOAN RIEHL SISCA

Joan Riehl Sisca's interaction model[50] is a synthesis of works by Mead, Rose, and Erickson and uses symbolic interaction as the focus of nurse-client interaction. Her symbolic interaction was developed primarily to explain a philosophy of meaning. Communication is a major ingredient of symbolic interaction. Her work is borrowed from sociology and is categorized as interpersonal relationship.

HELEN ERICKSON, EVELYN TOMLIN, MARY ANN SWAIN

Erickson, Tomlin, and Swain's[11] modeling and role-modeling theory is a synthesis of the works of Erickson, Maslow, Selye, Engel, and Piaget. From the synthesis of multiple concepts related to basic needs, developmental tasks, object attachment, and adaptive coping potential, they developed their role-modeling theory, which is highly abstract. Role-modeling provides a framework for understanding the way clients structure their world. Erickson, Tomlin, and Swain view nursing as a self-care model based on the client's perception of the world and adaptations to stressors. This is a holistic model that promotes the client's growth and development while recognizing individual differences according to the client's world view and inherent endowment. Erickson, Tomlin, and Swain's work can be categorized as an interpersonal relationship model.

RAMONA MERCER

Mercer's[35] model is focused on parenting and maternal role attainment in diverse populations. The maternal role attainment theory is a middle range theory with close linkages between theory, research, and practice. This model follows the more traditional social science approach to theory development. Mercer's early research was based on Goffman's systems theory. She has sytstematically researched the field of maternal role attainment and has developed a complex model to understand the factors impacting the development of the maternal role over time. The application of Mercer's theory has derivable consequences for nursing practice in women's health and maternal child health. Mercer's model can be categorized with the interpersonal relationship theories.

KATHERINE BARNARD

Katherine Barnard's middle range theory[3] borrows from psychology and human development and focuses on the mother-infant interaction with the environment. Her model is based on empirical evidence accumulated through scales developed to measure feeding, teaching, and environment. Barnard's theory is at a descriptive level that follows traditional science. Her contribution to theory development is the limitation of her concepts to mother-infant interaction and environment during the first 3 years of life, allowing the development of conceptual and operational definitions. Continuous research refined the model by providing a closer link between the available data and the model. Barnard further extended scientific knowledge across disciplines, since knowledge is not unique to nursing. She has provided a role model for future scholars who would engage in theory development for furthering the science of nursing. Barnard's model is interpersonal relationship.

VIRGINIA HENDERSON

Virginia Henderson[18] views the patient as an individual who requires help toward independence. She envisions the practice of nursing as independent from physicians. Henderson acknowledges her interpretation of the nurse's function as a synthesis of many influences. Her conceptual model is based on Thorndike's work, her experience in rehabilitation nursing, and Orlando's work regarding the continuation of deliberate nursing action.[2] Henderson emphasizes the art of nursing. She has identified 14 problems. Her contributions include delineating autonomous nursing functions, stressing goals of interdependence for the patient, and creating self-help concepts that influenced Abdellah and Adam. Henderson's model is philosophy of nursing.

FAYE ABDELLAH

Faye Abdellah's model is based on the problem solving method, which had a great impact on nursing curriculum development.[1,59:165] Problem solving is the vehicle for delineating the nursing problems as the client is moved toward a healthy outcome. According to Abdellah,[1] nursing is both an art and a science that mold the attitude, intellectual competencies, and technical skills of the individual nurse into the desire and ability to help people, whether ill or not, cope with their health needs. She believes nursing actions are carried out under general or specific medical direction. Abdellah has formulated 21 nursing problems based on research studies. Her work seems to be based somewhat on Henderson's 14 principles and on research studies to establish the classification of nursing problems.[12] Abdellah may have been influenced by Maslow's hierarchy of needs, which encompasses both physical and psychological needs of a client.[12] The major difference between Henderson and Abdellah is that Abdellah's problems are formulated in terms of nursing-centered services, which can be incorporated to determine the client's needs. Abdellah's contribution to nursing theory development is the systematic use of research data in formulating and validating 21 nursing problems. Abdellah's model is philosophy of nursing.

LYDIA HALL

Lydia Hall[17] stressed the autonomous function of nursing. She identified three overlapping parts that comprise nursing: (1) the therapeutic use of self (the core aspect), (2) treatment within the health team (the cure aspect), and (3) the nurturing component (the care aspect). Her model is a philosophy of nursing influenced by Carl Rogers and other psychologists.[51,52] Her conceptualization encompasses adult patients who have passed the acute stage of illness. The goal for the client is rehabilitation and feelings of success in self-actualization and self-love. Her contribution to theory development is the actual implementation of her philosophy of care in Loeb Center and encouragement of professional nursing's contribution to client outcome. Hall's model is philosophy of nursing.

DOROTHEA OREM

Dorothea Orem[41] explicated self-care as a human need. Orem defines nursing as a human service and indicates that nursing's special concern is a person's need for the provision and management of self-care actions on a continuous basis in order to sustain life and health or to recover from disease or injury.[41] Fawcett[13] stated that the components of Orem's model, which focuses primarily on the individual, are capable of generating theories. Orem's contribution to theory development is further delineating nursing function in self-care needs and continuing to work for empirical support through research and previous work. Orem's model is a philosophy of nursing.

MADELEINE LEININGER

Madeleine Leininger[29,30] espouses caring as the central theme in nursing care, nursing knowledge, and practice. Caring includes assistive, supportive, or facilitative acts toward an individual or a group with evident or anticipated needs. Caring serves to ameliorate or improve human conditions and life ways. Her methodology is borrowed from anthropology, but the concept of caring is an essential characteristic of nursing practice. She is credited with the foundation of transcultural nursing, and the resultant nursing research, education, and practice in this subfield of nursing. Leininger's model is a philosophy of nursing.

JEAN WATSON

Jean Watson's theory[66,67] could be an extension of the Leininger model and borrows from an existential phenomenologist's view of psychology, and humanities. Nursing concerns itself with promoting health, preventing illness, caring for the sick, and restoring health. Clients require holistic care that promotes humanism, health, and quality living. Caring is a universal social phenomenon that is only effectively practiced interpersonally. The 10 caring factors represent both feelings and actions pertaining to the nurse, the patient, and the professional and include things to be felt, experienced, communicated, expressed, and promoted by every nurse.

Her theory contribution is in sensitizing individual practitioners to humanistic aspects and caring. Further work is needed for testability, but her work may currently be classified as a philosophy of nursing.

ROSEMARIE RIZZO PARSE

Rosemarie Rizzo Parse[45] derives her theory from Rogers' principles and concepts, and synthesizes this with the existential-phenomenological views, such as those of Heidegger, Ponty, and Sartre. Parse's view of nursing is based on humanism as opposed to positivism.[33] Even though Parse developed her model largely from Rogers, whose model is highly abstract and lacking in testability, further work is needed in explicating each concept to form an operational definition and in linking existentialist relevancy to nursing phenomena. The strength of Parse's model may be a more humanistic approach as a philosophy of nursing. In addition, more emphasis on the relationship of man, environment, and health is addressed. Parse's model can be categorized as a philosophy of nursing.

PATRICIA BENNER

Benner's[4] contribution to nursing theory development has been to describe caring in the context of nursing practice with rich meaning and a broader understanding of personhood. She validated the Dreyfus model of skill acquisition in nursing practice by systematic descriptions of the five stages. Benner has provided many exemplars describing nursing practice at each stage: novice, advanced beginner, competent, proficient, and expert. Seven domains of nursing practice were derived from the descriptions of "paradigm cases" with a list of 31 nursing competencies. From her description of nursing practice Benner and Wrubel's (1988) theory of *The primacy of caring: Stress and coping in health and illness* has evolved.[5] This phenomenological theory describes caring as a common bond of persons situated in meaning, a state of being that is essential to nursing.

MYRA LEVINE

Myra Levine borrowed from sciences such as psychology, sociology, and physiology, used this knowledge to analyze varied nursing practice suggestions, and described detailed nursing skills and activities.[31,32,47] Levine's Nursing Activity Analysis resulted in the formulation of four conservation principles in helping clients adapt to environment. She presented the person in a holistic manner and as the center of nursing activities. Her emphasis on the ill person in the health care setting is also reflective of the history of health care in the 1960s and the fact that she was writing a textbook to teach medical-surgical nursing to beginning students. Levine's model building has been influenced by the use of borrowed theory as well as nursing practice theory development.[47] She, in turn, influenced Roy. Levine's model can be categorized as energy field.

MARTHA ROGERS

Martha Rogers was influenced by general systems theory as well as electromagnetic theory. She clearly emphasizes the science of nursing versus the art of nursing in her delineation of the unitary human being as central to the discipline of nursing.[53,54] Quillen and Runk have stated that Rogers' model had a significant influence on current scientific inquiry and professional nursing practice.[48] In addition, the model has served as a basis for the explication of other nursing conceptualizations, including those of Newman, Parse, and Fitzpatrick. It has also promoted research that has influenced the scientific community of nursing scholars who are investigating this model. Rogers' model can be categorized as energy field.

JOYCE FITZPATRICK

Joyce Fitzpatrick's rhythm model[14] is based on research which extends and refines Rogers' theory. Fitzpatrick uses Rogers' conceptualization of unitary man as a building block for her life perspective rhythm model.[53,54] She proposes that human development occurs within the context of continuous person-environment interaction.[14:300] Fitzpatrick's major concept relates to the development of persons as indices of temporal patterns, motion patterns, and consciousness patterns. She believes the meaning attached to life as the basic understanding of human existence is a central concern of nursing science and the nursing profession.[14:301] The model's contribution to theory development is that one of the indices—the temporal pattern—was developed by previous researchers. Other indices are largely untested, and research is needed to explicate the interrelation of indices in the future. Fitzpatrick's model can be called energy field.

MARGARET NEWMAN

Margaret Newman's model[39] of health is a direct expansion of Rogers' theory. The goal of nursing is not to make well or to prevent illness, but to help people use the power within them as they evolve toward a higher level of consciousness.[39:37] Her contribution to theory development is the replication of earlier works and further expansion on the interaction of time, movement, space, and consciousness in maintaining life processes. She had also defined health differently, as a fusion of disease and nondisease. Further research and testing are needed to clarify relationships among variables. Newman's model, like Rogers', is highly abstract in its present form and further linking of concept to operational definition is needed for validation or refutation. The model can be categorized as an energy field.

SISTER CALLISTA ROY

Sister Callista Roy[56] has based her work on Helson's adaptation model. Her model is a good example of how borrowed knowledge becomes unique in nursing.[56] It combines divergent thinking, such as systems, stress, and adaptation, into convergent views for explication of a person interacting with the environment. According to Roy, humans are biopsychosocial beings who exist within an environment. Environment and self provide three classes of stimuli: focal, residual, and contextual. Stimuli impact on humans and create needs in one or more interrelated adaptation modes, that is, physiological needs, self-concept, role function, and interdependence. Through two adaptative mechanisms, a regulator and a cognator, an individual can demonstrate adaptive responses (some successful, some not) or ineffective responses that require nursing intervention. The strength of Roy's model[55] is continued work related to the model, linking it to education, practice, and research and continued changes in the model to fit the growing empirical evidences. Roy's model is a system.

IMOGENE KING

Imogene King[26,27] believes the patient is a personal system within an environment, coexisting with other personal systems. The nurse and the patient perceive one another and the situation, act and react, interact, and transact. King[26:144] defined nursing as a process of human interactions between nurse and clients, who communicate to set goals, explore means for achieving the goals, and then agree on the means to be used. King speaks of nursing as a discipline and an applied science, with emphasis on the derivation of nursing knowledge from other disciplines. King's work can be categorized as a systems model. Fawcett[12] commented that King's conceptual framework is capable of generating a theory. Her contribution in theory development can be characterized as specifying outcome for nurse-client interactions, which are the end state of transaction for mutual satisfaction.

BETTY NEUMAN

Betty Neuman's model[37,38] is influenced by Gestalt theory, stress, and levels of prevention and can be characterized a systems model. Her conceptualization of the total person approach to client care is to help individuals, families, and groups attain and maintain a maximum level of total wellness by purposeful interventions.[38:119] Nursing intervention is aimed at the reduction of stress factors and adverse conditions that potentially or actually impact on optimal client functions. Her model represents the grand level theory focusing on the problem of summative concepts that are difficult at best to delineate for empirical testing.[10] At present, these are highly abstract and lack consistent operational definitions.[64] Her contribution to theory development is differentiating the level of prevention in nursing intervention as it relates to stress reduction. Neuman's model can be called a system.

DOROTHY JOHNSON

Dorothy Johnson[20,23] developed the behavioral system and labeled it a model for nursing practice, education, and research. Her model is influenced by ethological theorist and general systems theory. Johnson[23:212] considered attachment, or the affiliative subsystem, the cornerstone and critical for all social organizations. Her behavioral system also includes the dependency, achievement, aggressive, ingestive, eliminative, and sexual subsystems. "Nursing problems arise because there are disturbances in the structure or function of the subsystems or the system, or because the level of behavioral functioning is at less than a desirable optimal level."[23:214] Johnson's contributions to nursing theory development are her actual model development, her writings related to philosophical issues on theory development, and her influence on students, such as Roy and Adams, who have subsequently contributed to nursing theory development.[21,22] Her model employs the system theory orientation.

EVELYN ADAM

Evelyn Adam[2] is a Canadian nurse who uses the structure of a conceptual model to present Henderson's writings as the basis of nursing practice, research, and education. Adam's work is a good example of using a unique basis of nursing for further expansion or addition. Adam has contributed to theory development by clarification of the earlier theorists' models. Adam's model is a philosophy of nursing.

Through this overview, one can sense complete evolution of theory development in nursing (see box p. 58). First evolved a philosophy for nursing (Nightingale), then an emphasis on interpersonal relationships (Peplau, Orlando, Travelbee, Mercer), the art of nursing (Henderson, Wiedenbach, Hall), and the beginning emphasis on the scientific aspects of nursing (Abdellah). These are followed by the systems approach and the emphasis of science (Johnson, Neuman, Roger, King, Orem, Roy, Barnard), with the philosophy for a humanistic nursing approach resurfacing (Watson, Leininger,

THE EVOLUTION OF NURSING THEORY DEVELOPMENT

PHILOSOPHY

Nightingale (1860)
Abdellah (1960s-70s)
Wiedenbach (1960s)
Hall (1960s)
Henderson (1960s)
Leininger (1970s-80s)
Orem (1970s-80s)
Watson (1979-80s)
Adam (1980s)
Parse (1980s)
Benner (1980s)

INTERPERSONAL RELATIONSHIP

Peplau (1950s)
Orlando (1960s)
Travelbee (1970s)
Barnard (1970s-80s)
Mercer (1970s-1980s)
Riehl (1980s)
Erickson, Swain, Tomlin (1980s)

ENERGY FIELD

Levine (1960s-70s)
Fitzpatrick (1970s-80s)
Rogers (1970s-80s)
Newman (1979-80s)

SYSTEMS

Roy (1970s-80s)
King (1970s-80s)
Neuman (1970s-80s)
Johnson (1980s)

Parse, Benner). Finally, there is further elaboration of earlier models (Parse, Newman, Fitzpatrick, Adam).

Before we look to the future, a prospective critical reexamination of where we are may help clarify our goals for the future of theory development. After reading all the theorists, it seems as if we are in the midst of a coined word explosion. Every theorist has defined nursing, environment, health, and person differently along with other terms such as adaptation, system, and stress. This profusion of definitions only creates further confusion.

A think tank should be created where all theorists could work together to eliminate the redundancies and inconsistencies among the theories when defining identical phenomena, such as Roy and Riehl attempted in suggesting a unified nursing model.[55] In this regard, Wartofsky[65:5] may have referred to the present status of nursing theory development by noting:

> Philosophy is nothing if not a dedicated search for coherence, for the synthesis of what we know in one field with what we know in others. Sometimes this enthusiasm for synthesis leads to excess, to fanciful systems and wishful unities of everything-all-at-once which evaporate under critical examination, and are often no more than expressions of scientifically illiterate goodwill and pious hopes for coherence.

As Naisbitt[36] said in *Megatrends,* we are living in the time of the parenthesis, the time between eras. "It is as though we have bracketed off the present from both the past and the future, for we are neither here nor there."[36:279] This is a period of change, when anything can take place, and perhaps the rapid changes in nursing that are resulting from the theory development occurring now reflect the time.

The future of nursing is bright and full of hope. The theorists' different conceptualizations of nursing will enrich the discipline and its search for truth about persons, health, environment, and nursing. Our task for the future is to use further testing and collaboration to refute or support the truth about the nature of human beings from conceptual models. Kuhn[28:42] eloquently stated that a "paradigm can guide research in the absence of rules"; however, normal science cannot progress without the paradigm. These contributions represent the status of nursing as a discipline, and further development needs to occur for the explication of nursing phenomena. A great debate has occurred over what is nursing phenomena, whether nursing is an applied or a basic science, and whether it has a borrowed or unique body of knowledge.* What is more important is that models can predict or account for the phenomena of nursing, and are becoming more and more accepted by the nursing community of scholars. The debate should not be what each model represents, but rather how does it represent the truth we are seeking. The future direction should be toward the further clarification of each testable conceptual model so that each theorist's efforts should be replicating and refining her original model. Some theorists have already been working in this regard. The development of nursing theory has come a long way, but there is still much to be done, for the future of nursing as a discipline depends on theory development.

The ultimate goal in theory development for nursing could be a multiple model, or a paradigm, that could guide scientists, and those who learn from them, closer and closer to the truth.[28] In addition, we should not insist on including all four concepts of person, health, environment, and nursing within a conceptual framework. Working at micro or middle range theory development would facilitate testability and establish further a scientific knowledge base. A philosophy of nursing should address the issues related to nursing practice or nursing as a discipline. Theory development should be directed toward explicating person, health, and environment interactions (although not simultaneously) by learning more about each relationship through theory and through research strategy.[49]

REFERENCES

1. Abdellah, F., et al. (1973). *New direction in patient-centered nursing.* New York: Macmillan.
2. Adam, E. (1980). *To be a nurse.* Toronto: W.B. Saunders.
3. Barnard, K.E., et al. (1977). *The nursing child assessment satellite training study guide.* Unpublished program learning manual. Seattle: University of Washington.
4. Benner, P. (1984). *From novice to expert: Excellence and power in clinical nursing practice.* Menlo Park, Calif.: Addison-Wesley.
5. Benner, P., & Wrubel, J. (1988). *The primacy of caring: Stress and coping in health and illness.* Menlo Park, Calif.: Addison-Wesley.
6. Blake, M. (1980). The Peplau development model. In J. Riehl & C. Roy (Eds.), *Conceptual models for nursing practice* (2d ed.). New York: Appleton-Century-Crofts.
7. Chinn, P., & Jacobs, M. (1983). *Theory and nursing.* St. Louis: C.V. Mosby.
8. Dickoff, J., & James, P. (1968). A theory of theories: A position paper. *Nursing Research, 17:*197-203.
9. Donaldson, S.K., & Crowley, D.M. (1978). The discipline of nursing. *Nursing Outlook, 26:*113-120.
10. Dubin, R. (1978). *Theory building.* New York: The Free Press.
11. Erickson, H., Tomlin, E., & Swain, M. (1983). *Modeling and role-modeling: A theory and paradigm for nursing.* Englewood Cliffs, N.J.: Prentice-Hall.
12. Falco, S.M. (1980). Faye G. Abdellah. In Nursing Theories Conference Group, J.B. George (Ed.), *Nursing theories: The base for professional practice.* Englewood Cliffs, N.J.: Prentice Hall.
13. Fawcett, J. (1983). Hallmarks of success in nursing theory development. In P. Chinn (Ed.), *Advances in nursing theory development.* Rockville, Md.: Aspen Systems.
14. Fitzpatrick, J. (1983). A life perspective rhythm model. In J. Fitzpatrick & A. Whall (Eds.), *Conceptual models of nursing: Analysis and application.* Bowie, Md.: Robert J. Brady.
15. Gale, G. (1979). *Theory of science: An introduction to the history, logic and philosophy of science.* New York: McGraw-Hill.
16. Giere, R.N. (1979). *Understanding scientific reasoning.* New York: Holt, Rinehart & Winston.
17. Hall, L. (1969). The Loeb Center for Nursing

*References 9, 13, 19, 20, 63.

and Rehabilitation. *International Journal of Nursing Studies, 6*:81-95.
18. Henderson, V. (1966). *The nature of nursing: A definition and its implications, practice, research, and education.* New York: Macmillan.
19. Jacox, A. (1974). Theory construction in nursing: An overview. *Nursing Research, 23*:4-13.
20. Johnson, D.E. (1968). State of the art of theory development in nursing. In *Theory development: What, why, how?* New York: National League for Nursing.
21. Johnson, D.E. (1968). *One conceptual model of nursing.* Unpublished paper presented April 25 at Vanderbilt University, Nashville, Tenn.
22. Johnson, D.E. (1974). Development of a theory: A requisite for nursing at a primary health profession. *Nursing Research, 23*(5):372-377.
23. Johnson, D.E. (1980). The behavioral system model for nursing. In J.P. Riehl & S.C. Roy (Eds.), *Conceptual models for nursing practice* (2d ed.). New York: Appleton-Century-Crofts.
24. Kim, H.S. (1983). *The nature of theoretical thinking in nursing.* Norwalk, Conn.: Appleton-Century-Crofts.
25. King, I. (1968). A conceptual frame of references for nursing. *Nursing Research, 17*:27-31.
26. King, I. (1971). *Towards a theory of nursing.* New York: John Wiley & Sons.
27. King, I. (1981). *A theory of nursing: systems, concepts, process.* New York: John Wiley & Sons.
28. Kuhn, T.S. (1970). *The structure of scientific revolutions.* Chicago: University of Chicago Press.
29. Leininger, M. (1981). *Caring: An essential human need. Proceedings of the Three National Caring Conferences.* Thorofare, N.J.: Charles B. Slack.
30. Leininger, M. (1978). *Transcultural nursing concepts, theories, and practice.* New York: John Wiley & Sons.
31. Levine, M.E. (1967). The four conservation principles of nursing. *Nursing Forum, 6*:45-59.
32. Levine, M.E. (1973). *Introduction to clinical nursing.* Philadelphia: F.A. Davis.
33. Limandri, B. (1982). Review of Man-living-health: A theory of nursing by Rosemarie Rizzo Parse. *Western Journal of Nursing Research,* 4(1):105.
34. Meleis, A. (1983). The evolving nursing scholars. In P. Chinn (Ed.), *Advances in nursing theory development.* Rockville, Md.: Aspen Systems.
35. Mercer, R. (1986). *First-time motherhood: Experience from teens to forties.* New York: Springer.
36. Naisbitt, J.C. (1984). *Megatrends: Ten new directions transforming our lives.* New York: Warner.
37. Neuman, B. (1980). The Betty Neuman health-care systems model: A total person approach to patient problems. In J. Riehl & C. Roy (Eds.), *Conceptual models for nursing practice* (2d ed.). New York: Appleton-Century-Crofts.
38. Neuman, B. (Ed.) (1982). *The Neuman systems model.* New York: Appleton-Century-Crofts.
39. Newman, M. (1979). *Theory development in nursing.* Philadelphia: F.A. Davis.
40. Nightingale, F. (1969). *Notes on nursing: What it is and what it is not.* New York: Dover. (Originally published, 1859.)
41. Orem, D.E. (1985). *Nursing: Concepts of practice* (3d ed). New York: McGraw-Hill.
42. Orlando, I.J. (1961). *The dynamic nurse-patient relationship.* New York: G.P. Putnam's Sons.
43. Orlando, I.J. (1972). *The discipline and teaching of nursing process.* New York: G.P. Putnam's Sons.
44. Palmer, I.S. (1977). Florence Nightingale: Reformer, reactionary, researcher. *Nursing Research, 26*(2):84-89.
45. Parse, R.R. (1981). *Man-living-health: A theory of nursing.* New York: John Wiley & Sons.
46. Peplau, H.E. (1952). *Interpersonal relations in nursing.* New York: G.P. Putnam's Sons.
47. Pieper, B.C. (1983). Levine's nursing model. In J. Fitzpatrick & A. Whall (Eds.), *Conceptual models of nursing: Analysis and application.* Bowie, Md.: Robert J. Brady.
48. Quillen, S., & Runk, J. (1983). Martha Rogers' model. In J. Fitzpatrick & A. Whall (Eds.), *Conceptual models of nursing: Analysis and application.* Bowie, Md.: Robert J. Brady.
49. Reynolds, P. (1971). *A primer in theory construction.* Indianapolis: Bobbs-Merrill.
50. Riehl, J. (1980). The Riehl interaction model. In J. Riehl & C. Roy (Eds.), *Conceptual models for nursing practice* (2d ed.). New York: Appleton-Century-Crofts.
51. Rogers, C. (1951). *Client-centered therapy.* Boston: Houghton Mifflin.
52. Rogers, C. (1961). *On becoming a person.* Boston: Houghton Mifflin.

53. Rogers, M.E. (1970). *The theoretical basis of nursing*. Philadelphia: F.A. Davis.
54. Rogers, M.E. (1980). A science of unitary man. In J.P. Riehl & C. Roy (Eds.). *Conceptual models for nursing practice* (2d ed.). New York: Appleton-Century-Crofts.
55. Roy, C. (1984). *An introduction to nursing: An adaptation model* (2d ed.). Englewood Cliffs, N.J.: Prentice-Hall.
56. Roy, C.S. (1976). *Introduction to nursing: An adaptation model*. Englewood Cliffs, N.J.: Prentice-Hall.
57. Schmieding, N.C. (1983). An analysis of Orlando's nursing theory based on Kuhn's Theory of science. In P. Chinn (Ed.), *Advances in nursing theory development*. Rockville, Md.: Aspen Systems.
58. Sills, G. (1978). Leader, practitioner, academician, scholar, theorist. *Perspectives in Psychiatric Care, 16*(3):122-128.
59. Stevens, B.J. (1984). *Nursing Theory: Analysis, Application, Evaluation* (2d ed.). Boston: Little, Brown.
60. Sullivan, H.S. (1952). *The interpersonal theory of psychiatry*. New York: W.W. Norton.
61. Torres, G. (1980). Florence Nightingale. In Nursing Theories Conference Group, J.B. George, Chairperson, *Nursing theories: The base for professional nursing practice*. Englewood Cliffs, N.J.: Prentice-Hall.
62. Travelbee, J. (1971). *Interpersonal aspects of nursing*. Philadelphia: F.A. Davis.
63. Walker, L.O. (1971). Toward a clearer understanding of the concept of nursing theory. *Nursing Research, 20*:428-435.
64. Walker, L.O., & Avant, K.C. (1983). *Strategies for theory construction in nursing*. Norwalk, Conn.: Appleton-Century-Crofts.
65. Wartofsky, M. (1968). *Conceptual foundations of scientific thought*. New York: Macmillan.
66. Watson, J. (1979). *Nursing: The philosophy and science of caring*. Boston: Little, Brown.
67. Watson, J. (1985). *Nursing: Human science and health care*. Norwalk, Conn.: Appleton-Century-Crofts.
68. Wiedenbach, E. (1964). *Clinical nursing: A helping art*. New York: Springer.

UNIT II

Art and Science of Humanistic Nursing

Florence Nightingale

7

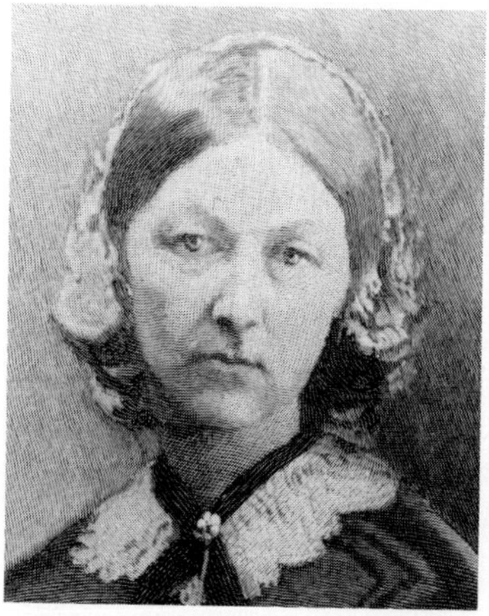

Modern Nursing

Karen R. deGraaf, Ann Marriner-Tomey, Cynthia L. Mossman, Maribeth Slebodnik

CREDENTIALS AND BACKGROUND OF THE THEORIST

Florence Nightingale, the matriarch of modern nursing, was born May 12, 1820, while her British parents were on an extended European tour. Her parents, Edward and Frances Nightingale, named their daughter for her birthplace, Florence, Italy.

The Nightingales were affluent and well-educated members of a Victorian family. So as Nightingale grew older her father tutored her in mathematics, languages, religion, and philosophy. In her teens Nightingale was active in aristocratic society, but she felt her life should be more useful. In 1837 she confided in her diary that "God spoke to me and called me to his service."[6:8;7:41]

In 1851, Nightingale went to Kaiserswerth, Germany, for her early nursing training. After leaving Kaiserswerth, she continued to examine the facilities at hospitals, reformatories, and charitable institutions. In 1853 she became Superintendent of the Hospital for Invalid Gentlewomen in London.

During the Crimean War Nightingale volunteered to go to Scutari, Turkey. There she organized a nursing department and devoted her efforts to eliminating sanitation problems in the wards. At that time women working in hospitals were not respectable, reliable, or educated. There were no trained nurses and no British Red Cross. Consequently, Nightingale solicited and received help from the Sisters of Mercy.

Conditions in the army wards were poor. In addition to their wounds, the soldiers suffered from exposure, frostbite, lice infestations, and disease. There were few chamber pots; latrines were blocked; cess pools overflowed; and the water was contaminated. Patients who couldn't feed themselves starved. There were no surgery tables or anesthesia.

Nightingale's work made her popular with the men. They called her "the Lady of the Lamp" in recognition of her Turkish candle lantern she carried through the corridors packed with wounded soldiers. While at Scutari Nightingale became critically ill with Crimean fever, which might have been typhus.

Nightingale returned to England following the war and established a teaching institution for nurses at St. Thomas Hospital and at King's College Hospital in London. These were established from funds received in recognition of her war service. Nightingale kept close contact with her graduates through encouraging letters. Within a few years after its foundation, the Nightingale School began receiving requests for nurses to found new schools at hospitals worldwide and Florence Nightingale's reputation as the founder of modern nursing was assured.

During her carreer Nightingale concentrated on army sanitation reform, army hospitals, and sanitation in India and among the poorer classes in England. She wrote *Notes on Matters Affecting the Health, Efficiency, and Hospital Administration of the British Army* (1858), *Notes on Hospitals* (1858), *Notes on the Sanitary State of the Army in India* (1871), and *Life or Death in India* (1874). For her efforts, Nightingale received numerous awards, including the Order of Merit from King Edward VII, Germany's Cross of Merit, and France's Secours aux Blesses Militaires.

Nightingale wrote between 15,000 and 20,000 letters to friends and distinguished acquaintances. These often displayed her beliefs, observations, and desire for change in health care. She worked into her eighties gathering data and writing about nursing and health care. She enjoyed a robust old age before suffering a gradual loss of vision, which made reading and writing difficult. She was widely recognized for her knowledge, drive, and compassion.

Nightingale died in her sleep at the age of 90 on August 13, 1910, in London. But many of her revolutionary ideas continue to inspire contemporary nursing.

THEORETICAL SOURCES FOR THEORY DEVELOPMENT

Many factors influenced the development of Nightingale's theory for nursing. Individual, societal, and professional values were all integral in the development of her work. She combined her individual resources with societal and professional resources to produce change.

Nightingale, who considered nursing a religious calling to be answered only by women, believed she should strive to change the things she saw as unacceptable. Chinn and Jacobs[2:46] note that "When individual or professional values are in conflict with and challenge societal values, there is potential for creating change in society." Nightingale lived up to that potential. The health care system of her era used the uneducated and incompetent to care for the ill. But Nightingale transformed it into the system of professional nursing practices we value today.

Nightingale knew that contact with the professionals of her time was important. She expanded her philosophy of nursing through association with numerous prominent physicians and other influential members of society.

The strongest influences on the development

of her practice were her education, experience, and observation. She gained these through years of charitable and hospital work and military nursing. They established the logical base for her nursing philosophy.

USE OF EMPIRICAL EVIDENCE

Nightingale was a devoted statistician. She used her carefully collected information to prove the efficacy of her system of hospital nursing and organization during the Crimean War. The report of her data and experiences, entitled *Notes on Matters Affecting the Health, Efficiency, and Hospital Administration of the British Army,* was given to the British Royal Sanitary Commission, which had been organized in response to Nightingale's charges of poor sanitary conditions. "It showed that for every man killed in battle in the Crimea, seven died from disease. Even in peacetime the mortality rate in the barracks was twice that of the general population."[3:396]

Palmer[12:88] identified Nightingale's research skills as recording, communicating, ordering, coding, conceptualizing, inferring, analyzing, and synthesizing. Nightingale viewed observation and practice as concurrent activities.

MAJOR CONCEPTS AND DEFINITIONS

Nightingale's grand theory focused on the environment. Murray and Zentner[8:149] state that the environment, which is capable of preventing, suppressing or contributing to disease, accidents, or death, is all the external conditions and influences affecting the life and development of an organism. While the term environment does not itself appear in Miss Nightingale's writings, her major concepts of ventilation, warmth, light, diet, cleanliness, and noise comprise the components of environment as defined above.

Although Nightingale usually defined concepts precisely, she did not clearly separate the patient's environment into physical, emotional, or social aspects. She assumed these aspects were encompassed by the environment, but made no clear distinction of how to differentiate them. "Although she tends to emphasize the physical more than the psychological or social environment, this needs to be viewed in the context of her time and her activities as a nurse leader in a war-torn environment."[11:28]

Nightingale emphasized several aspects of the environment in her work. She believed healthy surroundings were necessary for proper nursing care. Although she specifically addressed the issue of health in homes with this passage, it may be assumed she was referring to hospitals as well when she said:

> There are five essential points in securing the health of houses: (1) pure air, (2) pure water, (3) efficient drainage, (4) cleanliness, [and] (5) light. Without these, no house can be healthy. And it will be unhealthy just in proportion as they (sic) are deficient.[10:24]

Nightingale felt the public needed to believe and practice these procedures in order to have healthy homes. She wanted people to use common sense, but only after they were educated to essential facts regarding health.

The aspect of the environment that concerned Nightingale most was providing proper ventilation for a patient. This meant the nurse was "to keep the air he breathes as pure as the external air, without chilling him."[10:12] Nightingale believed a steady supply of fresh air was the most important principle in nursing. She said pure air was "the very first canon of nursing, the first and the last thing upon which a nurse's attention must be fixed, the first essential to a patient, without which all the rest you can do for him is nothing."[10:12]

Light was another element of nursing care that Nightingale believed could not be ignored.

> It is the unqualified result of all my experience with the sick, that second only to their need of fresh air is their need of light. . . . And that it is not only light, but direct sun-light they want. . . . Without going into any scientific exposition we must admit that light has quite as real

> and tangible effects upon the human body. . . . Who has not observed the purifying effect of light, and especially of direct sunlight, upon the air of a room?[10:84-85]

Nightingale firmly believed in the beneficial aspects of direct sunlight. She even suggested that a nurse might have to carry the patient "about after the sun, according to the aspects of the rooms, if circumstances permit."[10:84]

The need for cleanliness extended to the patient, the nurse, and the environment, Nightingale believed. She stated that dirty carpets and walls contained large quantities of organic matter and provided a ready source of infection, just as dirty sheets and beds did. A well-ventilated dirty room and a clean unventilated room were both deemed dirty areas. Nightingale also believed that unwashed skin interfered with the healing process and that washing removed noxious matter from the system quickly. Therefore nurses should wash their hands frequently and keep their patients very clean.[10:94]

In addition to her five main points of emphasis, Nightingale also believed a nurse should attend to a patient's warmth, quiet, and diet.[10:8] She advised nurses to constantly monitor patients' body temperatures by palpatating the extremities to prevent the effects of vital heat loss.[10:17] Nightingale delineated specific instructions for providing fresh air while avoiding a chilly climate. She castigated medical and nursing personnel who neglected ventilation for the sake of warmth and thereby exposed their patients to the dangers of foul, infected air.[10:15] "The safest atmosphere of all for a patient is a good fire and open window, excepting in extremes of temperature."[10:19]

Noise was another environmental element Nightingale believed the nurse should manipulate. "Unnecessary noise, or noise that creates an expectation in the mind, is that which hurts a patient. . . . Any sacrifice to secure silence . . . is worthwhile, because no air, however good, no attendance however careful, will do anything . . . without quiet."[10:45,47] By maintaining that noise could impede the progress of the patient's recovery, even if there were fresh air and good attendance by nurses, she clarified the interrelatedness of her major concepts.

Nightingale was also concerned with a patient's diet. She believed a nurse should not only assess the dietary intake, but also assess the timeliness of the food and its effect on the patient. Observation, ingenuity, and perserverance were the qualities Nightingale felt should distinguish a good nurse so that patients were not starved to death because of chronic illnesses.[10:65] She said "If the nurse is an intelligent being, and not a mere carrier of diets to and from the patient, let her exercise her intelligence in these things."[10:67]

MAJOR ASSUMPTIONS

Nightingale believed that every woman, at one time or another, would be a nurse in the sense that nursing was to have the responsibility for someone's health. Thus, she provided women with guidelines for nursing care and advice on how to "think how to nurse."[10:3-4]

Nightingale refers to the person as a patient in most of her writings. However, the patient is regarded as being acted upon by the nurse or affected by the environment. The patient is passive and does not seem to influence the nurse or the environment.

Nightingale defined health as being well and using to the fullest extent every power we have.[10:334-5] Additionally, she saw disease as a reparative process nature instituted because of some want of attention.[10:7] Nightingale envisioned health as being maintained through the prevention of disease via environmental health factors. She called this health nursing and distinguished it from nursing proper, which was nursing of the diseased patient so he could survive or at least live better until his death.[10:199]

The environment, Nightingale asserted, was one of the chief sources of infection. Fitzpatrick and Whall[4:16-7] state that Nightingale's concept of the environment was "those elements external to and which affect the health of the sick and healthy person" and included "everything from the patient's food and flowers to the nurse's verbal and nonverbal interactions with the patient."

THEORETICAL ASSERTIONS

Nightingale believed disease was a reparative process. Disease, she felt, was nature's effort to remedy a process of poisoning or decay, or a reaction against the conditions in which a person was placed. Nightingale directed that nursing's role was to prevent the reparative process from being interrupted and to provide optimal conditions for its enhancement. Nurses encouraged this process by providing proper environmental conditions such as fresh air, light, pure water, efficient drainage, cleanliness, warmth, quiet, and appropriate diet. Nightingale also felt nurses had to use common sense to achieve these conditions, but that it had to be coupled with perserverance, observation, and ingenuity. Nightingale assumed the person was desirous of health, so that the nurse, nature, and the person would cooperate to allow the reparative process to occur.

LOGICAL FORM

Nightingale used inductive reasoning to extract laws of health and nursing from her observations and experiences. For example, she noticed that disease flourished in confined, dark, damp areas and concluded it was generated in such environments. She also derived from this observation her belief that disease could be prevented, or its cure hastened, by providing an environment antithetical to the one in which disease originated. Many of these observations and derived principles originated during her wartime experiences.

ACCEPTANCE BY NURSING COMMUNITY

Practice

Nightingale's nursing principles remain applicable to nursing practice today. Ventilation, warmth, quiet, diet, and cleanliness are integral parts of nursing care. Pure water and efficient drainage are controlled by public health regulations. In her book, *Notes on Nursing,* Nightingale suggested concepts that are relatively simple to apply in practice, yet many of them are overlooked in the highly technical areas of nursing. Contemporary practitioners would find value in examination and use of her concepts.

Much of Nightingale's rationale has been modified or disproved because of advances in medicine and nursing. However, it is important to remember Nightingale's background and the advances she made in her era. Her inclusion of both health teaching and sick nursing within nursing's domain was a then-revolutionary concept that still defines nursing practice, and her insistence upon proper education and social support systems for nursing remains pertinent today. The numerous articles and books written regarding Nightingale's attitudes and contributions demonstrate her continued acceptance by nursing in the area of practice.

Education

The Nightingale system was the basis for the origination of many early nurse training schools, including St. Thomas Hospital and King's College Hospital in London. This system is no longer in general use, but its influence lingers on in the combination of practical and didactic training found in today's nursing programs. Nightingale advocated the nursing school's independence from hospitals so that students were not involved in the hospital's labor pool as part of their training. Nightingale felt the "art of nursing" could not be standardized and therefore licensing examinations were inappropriate, but her opinion was overridden shortly after her death. Scholarships and grants in her honor continue to allow students to pursue advanced studies in nursing.

Research

Nightingale's interest in statistics and their importance to nursing continues to influence nursing research. She was exceptionally efficient and resourceful in her ability to gather and analyze data. Much of these data may be found in her numerous letters. She was one of the first to use graphic illustrations in statistics.[1:665] Many of these illustrations continue to be used by statisticians today. Nightingale recognized the importance of data collection in nursing care. While her methods have had a continued effect on research in nursing, her theory lacks complexity and testability.[4:23] Therefore, it has not generated nursing research.

FURTHER DEVELOPMENT

Nightingale's theory for nursing is stated clearly and concisely. *Notes on Nursing* was Nightingale's most widely known work and one that seems most amenable to theory analysis. The organization of chapters treating various aspects of nursing care suggests that perhaps the main goal is definition and elaboration of concepts rather than organization of a theory. Fitzpatrick and Whall[4:18] state that this theory can be described as a "set of laws" theory. Laws are theoretical statements with overwhelming empirical support.

It might also be proposed that Nightingale formulated a grand theory, as described by Margaret Hardy:[5:42]

> A theory in the early stage of development is characterized by discursive presentation and descriptive accounts of anecdotal reports to illustrate and support its claims. The theoretical terms are usually vague and ill defined, and their meaning may be close to everyday language. A paradigm at this embryonic stage is very readable and provides a perspective rather than a set of interrelated theoretical statements. . . . This type of formulation, the "grand theory" or "general orientation," is aimed at explaining the totality of behavior. Grand theories tend to use vague terminology, leave the relationships between terms unclear and provide formulations that cannot be tested.

Nightingale's intention to provide a first step for the formalization and development of nursing seems to have been accomplished. Her achievements spawned the beginning of nursing as we know it today. Nightingale's theory was a lower level theory, but it sets the stage for further work in the development of nursing theories.

CRITIQUE

Simplicity

Nightingale's theory contains three major relationships: environment to patient, nurse to environment, and nurse to patient. She viewed environment as the main factor acting upon the patient to produce an illness state, and regarded disease as "the reactions of kindly nature against the conditions in which we have placed ourselves."[10:32] The nurse as manipulator of environment and actor on the patient is described when Nightingale said nursing "ought to signify the proper use of fresh air, light, warmth, cleanliness, quiet, and the proper selection and administration of diet—all at the least expense of vital power to the patient."[10:8] These relationships are expanded on in the text of *Notes on Nursing*. The book is organized into chapters dealing with the components of environment, such as ventilation, warmth, light, noise, and cleanliness. Relationships between these environmental components are also described, as when Nightingale states, "Without cleanliness, within and without your house, ventilation is comparatively useless."[10:27]

The concepts and their relationships cannot be combined in order to increase simplicity; they are in economical form as Nightingale stated them. Various diagrams for the theory have been proposed, suggesting that it is simple and logical enough to allow such visual representation. This theory tends toward description and explanation rather than prediction. Nightingale did not intend to develop theory, but to define nursing and set forth general rules for its practice and development. Simplicity of the theory was therefore necessary and is present.

Generality

Nightingale's theory attempts to provide general guidelines for all nurses in all times. Although many of her specific directives are no longer applicable, the general concepts, such as the relationships between nurse, patient, and environment, are still pertinent. The theory is specifically directed toward the nurse, defined as a woman who at some time has charge of somebody's health, and is thus not restricted to the professional nurse. In order to address her audience, the proposed theory is of necessity very broad. Generality is a criterion met by Nightingale's theory.

Empirical Precision

Concepts and relationships within Florence Nightingale's theory are frequently stated implicitly and are presented as established truths rather than tentative, testable statements. Little or no provision is made for empirical examination. Indeed, Nightingale suggested that the practice of nursing should be built upon individual observation rather than systematic research when she advised, "Let experience, not theory, decide upon this as upon all other things."[10:76]

Derivable Consequences

Nightingale's writings, to an extraordinary degree, direct the nurse to action in the behalf of her patient and herself. These directives encompass the areas of practice, research, and education. Most specific are her principles attempting to shape nursing practice. She urges nurses to provide doctors with "not your opinion, however respectfully given, but your facts."[10:113] She goes on to say, "If you cannot get the habit of observation one way or other, you had better give up the being a nurse, for it is not your calling, however kind and anxious you may be."[10:122] Her encouragement of a measure of independence and precision previously unknown in nursing may still guide and motivate us today as nursing continues to evolve.

Nightingale's view of humanity was consistent with her theories of nursing. She believed in creative, universal humanity with the potential and ability for growth and change.[12:85] Deeply religious, she viewed nursing as a means of doing the will of her God. Perhaps it is because of this concept of nursing as a divine calling that she relegated the patient to a passive role, essentially infantile, with every want and need provided by the nurse. The excessive zeal and self-rightousness of a religious reformer might partially account for this behavior. Although the lack of patient involvement in health seems to be a gap in Nightingale's views, it may be accounted for by the historical period in which she lived and wrote.

Basic principles of environmental manipulation and psychological care of the patient can be applied with modification in many contemporary nursing settings. Of course, many technological and societal changes have occurred since Nightingale's day, which reduce some of her fondest assertions to the ludicrous. Her unshakable disdain for the germ theory of disease and adherence to the belief that dirt and dampness are pathogenic now seems less than progressive.[12:87] Likewise, her emphasis on personal observation rather than formation of a unified body of nursing knowledge has fallen into disuse.

Lack of specificity has hindered use of Nightingale's ideas for the generation of nursing research. However, her writings continue to stimulate productive thinking for the individual nurse and the nursing profession. Nightingale was brilliant and creative. She gave nursing much food for thought—food that continues to nourish us 130 years later.

REFERENCES

1. Agnew, L.R. (1958, May). Florence Nightingale, statistician. *American Journal of Nursing, 58:*644.
2. Chinn, P., & Jacobs, M. (1983). *Theory and nursing: A systematic approach.* St. Louis: C.V. Mosby.
3. Cruse, P. (1980, Sept.). Florence Nightingale. *Surgery 88*(3):394-9.
4. Fitzpatrick, J., & Whall, A. (1983). *Conceptual models of nursing.* Bowie, Md.: Prentice-Hall.
5. Hardy, M. (1978). Perspectives on nursing theory. *Advances In Nursing Science, 1:*37-48.

6. Isler, C. (1970). *Florence Nightingale: Rebel with a cause.* Oradell, N.Y.: Medical Economics.
7. Isler, C. (1970, May). Florence Nightingale: Rebel with a cause, *RN, 33:*39-55.
8. Murray, R., & Zenter, J. (1975). *Nursing concepts in health promotion.* Englewood Cliffs, N.J.: Prentice Hall.
9. Nightingale, F. (1954). *Selected writings.* Compiled by Lucy R. Seymer. New York: Macmillan.
10. Nightingale, F. (1969). *Notes on nursing: What it is and what it is not.* New York: Dover.
11. Nursing Theories Conference Group, J.B. George, Chairperson. (1980). *Nursing theories: The base for professional practice.* Englewood Cliffs, N.J.: Prentice-Hall.
12. Palmer, I.S. (1977, March-April). Florence Nightingale: Reformer, reactionary, researcher. *Nursing Research,* 26:84-9.
13. *World Who's Who in Science.* (1968). Florence Nightingale. Chicago: A.N. Marquis.

BIBLIOGRAPHY

Primary Sources

Books

Nightingale, F. (1911). *Letters from Miss Florence Nightingale on health visiting in rural districts.* London: King.

Nightingale, F. (1954). *Selected writings.* Compiled by Lucy R. Seymer. New York: Macmillan.

Nightingale, F. (1956). *The institution of Kaiserswerth on the Rhine, Dusseldorf, Germany.* Anna Sticker.

Nightingale, F. (1957). *Notes on nursing.* Philadelphia: Lippincott. (Originally published, 1859).

Nightingale, F. (1969). *Notes on nursing: What it is and what it is not.* New York: Dover.

Nightingale, F. (1974). *Letters of Florence Nightingale in the history of nursing archive.* Boston: Boston University.

Nightingale, F. (1976). *Notes on hospitals.* New York: Gordon.

Nightingale, F. (1978). Notes on nursing. London: Duckworth.

Nightingale, F. (1979). *Cassandra, an essay.* Old Westbury, N.Y.: Feminist Press.

Journal Articles

Nightingale, F. (1930, July). Trained nursing for the sick poor, *International Nursing Review, 5:*426-433.

Nightingale, F. (1954, May 7). Maternity hospital and midwifery school. *Nursing Mirror, 99:*ix-xi, 369.

Nightingale, F. (1954). The training of nurses, *Nursing Mirror, 99:*iv-xi.

Secondary Sources

Book Reviews

Nightingale, F. (1954). Selected writings.
*Nursing Mirror 100:*846, Dec. 24, 1954.
Roy San Inst. J. *75:*275-276, April 1955.
*American Journal of Nursing, 55:*162, May 1955.
*Nursing Times, 51:*502-503, 507, May 6, 1955.

Nightingale, F. (1969). *Notes on Nursing: What it is and what it is not.*
*Nursing Times, 66:*828, June 25, 1970.
*Nursing Mirror, 131:*47, Oct. 9, 1970.

Nightingale, F.: *Notes on nursing: What it is and what it is not, the science and art.*
*Nursing Times, 76:*187, Oct. 23, 1980.
*Nursing Mirror, 151:*41, Dec. 11, 1980.
*Australian Nurses Journal, 10:*29, Feb. 1981.

Nightingale, F. (1979). *Cassandra, an essay. American Journal of Nursing, 81:*1059–1061, May 1981.

Seymer, L.R.: *Florence Nightingale.* (1950).
*Nursing Mirror, 92:*31, Nov. 17, 1950.
*Nursing Times, 46:*1285, Dec. 16, 1950.
*Journal of the American Medical Association, 146:*605, June 9, 1951.
Public Health Nursing, 43: 459, Aug. 1951.

Books

Aiken, C.A. (1915). *Lessons from the life of Florence Nightingale.* New York: Lakeside.

Aldis, M. (1914). *Florence Nightingale.* New York: NOPHN.

Andrews, M.R. (1929). *A lost commander.* Garden City, N.J.: Doubleday.

Baly, M.E. (1986). *Florence Nightingale & the nursing legacy.* New York: Methuen.

Barth, R.J. (1945). *Fiery angel: The story of Florence Nightingale.* Coral Gables, Fla.: Glade House.

Bishop, W.J. (1962). *A bio-bibliography of Florence Nightingale.* London: Dawson's of Pall Mall.

Boyd, N. (1982). *Three Victorian women who changed their world.* New York: Oxford.

Bull, A. (1985). *Florence Nightingale.* North Pomfret, Vt: David and Charles.

Collins, D. (1985). *Florence Nightingale.* Milford, Mi: Mott Media.

Columbia University Faculty of Medicine and Department of Nursing. (1937). *Catalogue of the Florence Nightingale collection* New York: the Department.

Cook, E.T. (1913). *The life of Florence Nightingale.* London: Macmillan.

Cook, E.T. (1941). *A short life of Florence Nightingale,* New York: Macmillan.

Cope, Z. (1958). *Florence Nightingale and the doctors.* Philadelphia: Lippincott.

Cope, Z. (1961). *Six disciples of Florence Nightingale.* New York: Pitman.

Editors of *RN.* (1970). *Florence Nightingale: Rebel with a cause.* Oradell, N.J.: Medical Economics.

French, Y. (1953). *Six great Englishwomen.* London: H. Hamilton.

Goldsmith, M.L. (1937). *Florence Nightingale: The woman and the legend.* London: Hodder and Stoughtons.

Goldwater, S.S. (1947). *On hospitals.* New York: Macmillan.

Gordon, R. (1979). *The private life of Florence Nightingale.* New York: Atheneum.

Haldale, E. (1931). *Mrs. Gaskell and her friends.* New York: Appleton.

Hall, E.F. (1920). *Florence Nightingale.* New York: Macmillan.

Hallock, G.T., & Turner, C.E. (1928). *Florence Nightingale.* New York: Metropolitan Life Insurance Co.

Herbert, R.G. (1981). *Florence Nightingale: Saint, reformer, or rebel?* Melbourne, Fla.: Krieger.

Holmes, M. (n.d.) *Florence Nightingale—A cameo life-sketch.* London: Woman's Freedom League.

Huxley, E.J. (1975). *Florence Nightingale.* London: Putnam.

Hyndman, J.A. (1969). *Florence Nightingale: Nurse to the world.* Cleveland, Ohio: World Publishing.

Keele, J. (Ed.). (1981). *Florence Nightingale in Rome.* Philadelphia: American Philosophical Society.

Lammond, D. (1935). *Florence Nightingale.* London: Duckworth.

Miller, B.W. (1947). *Florence Nightingale: The lady with the lamp.* Grand Rapids, Mich.: Zondervan.

Miller, M. (1987). *Florence Nightingale.* Minneapolis, Minn: Bethany House.

Mosby, C.V. (1938). Little journey to the home of Florence Nightingale. New York: C.V. Mosby.

Muir, D.E. (1946). *Florence Nightingale.* Glasgow: Blackie and Son.

Nash, R. (1937). *A sketch for the life of Florence Nightingale.* London: Society for Promoting Christian Knowledge.

Newton, M.E. (1949). *Florence Nightingale's philosophy of life and education.* Ed.D. dissertation. Stanford, Calif.: Stanford University.

O'Malley, I.B. (1931). *Life of Florence Nightingale, 1820-1856.* London: Butterworth.

Pollard, E. (1902). *Florence Nightingale: The wounded soldiers' friend.* London: Partridge.

Presbyterian Hospital, School of Nursing. (1937). *Catalogue of the Florence Nightingale collection.* New York: the School.

Quiller-Couch, A.T. (1927) *Victors of peace.* New York: Nelson.

Rappe, E.C. (1977). *God bless you, my dear Miss Nightingale.* Stockholm: Almqvist and Wiksell.

Sabatini, R. (1934). *Heroic lives.* Boston: Houghton.

St. Thomas's Hospital. (1960). *The Nightingale Training School: St. Thomas's Hospital, 1860-1960.* London: St. Thomas's Hospital.

Saleeby, C.W. (1912). *Surgery and society: A tribute to Listerism.* New York: Moffat, Yard & Co.

Schmidt, M.M. (1933). *400 outstanding women of the world and costumology of their time.* Chicago: the author.

Shor, D. (1987). *Florence Nightingale.* Lexington, N.H.: Silver.

Seymer, L.R. (1951). *Florence Nightingale.* New York: Macmillan.

Smith, F.B. (1982). *Florence Nightingale: Reputation and power.* New York: St. Martin.

Stephenson, G.E. (comp.) (1924). *Some pioneers in the medical and nursing world.* Shanghai.: Nurses' Association of China.

Strachey, L. (1918). *Eminent Victorians.* London: Chatto & Windus.

Tabor, M.E. (1925). *Pioneer Women.* London: Sheldon.

Todey, S.A. (1905). *The life of Florence Nightingale.* New York: Macmillan.

Turner, D. (1986). *Florence Nightingale.* New York: Watts.

Wilson, W.G. (1940). *Soldier's heroine.* Edinburgh: Missionary Education Movement.

Woodham-Smith, C. (1983). *Florence Nightingale.* New York: Atheneum.

Woodham-Smith, C.B. (1951). *Florence Nightingale, 1820-1910.* New York: McGraw-Hill.

Woodham-Smith, C.B. (1951). *Lonely crusader: The*

life of Florence Nightingale, 1820-1910. New York: Whittlesey House.

Woodham-Smith, C.B. (1956). *Lady-in-chief.* London: Methven.

Woodham-Smith, C.B. (1977). *Florence Nightingale, 1820-1910*. London: Collins.

Woodsey, A.H. (1950). *A century of nursing*. New York: Putnam.

World Who's Who in Science: Florence Nightingale (entry). (1968). Chicago: A.N. Marquis.

Wren, D. (1949). *They enriched humanity: Adventurers of the 19th century*. London: Skilton.

Book Chapters

Reed, P.G., & Zurakowski, T.L. (1983). Nightingale: A visionary model for nursing. In J. Fitzpatric & A. Whall, *Conceptual models of nursing: Analysis and application*. Bowie, Md.: Robert J. Brady.

Torres, G.C. (1980). Florence Nightingale. In Nursing Theories Conference Group, J.B. George, Chairperson, *Nursing theories: The base for professional nursing practice*. Englewood Cliffs, N.J.: Prentice-Hall.

Journal Articles

Abbott, M.E. (1916, Sept. 14). Portraits of Florence Nightingale. *Boston Medical and Surgical Journal 1975:*361-367.

Abbott, M.E. (1916, Sept. 21), Portraits of Florence Nightingale. *Boston Medical Surgery Journal, 175:*413-422.

Abbott, M.E. (1916, Sept. 28). Portraits of Florence Nightingale, *Boston Medical Surgery, 175:*453-457.

Address by the Archbishop of York. (1970, May 21). Florence Nightingale *Nursing Times, 66:*670,

Address given at fiftieth anniversary of founding by Florence Nightingale of first training school for nurses at St. Thomas's Hospital, London, England. (1911, Feb.). *American Journal of Nursing 11:*331–361.

Agnew, L.R.C. (1958, May). Florence Nightingale: Statistician. *American Journal of Nursing, 58:*644+.

At Embley Park and East Wellow. (1937, July 24). *Nursing Times, 33:*730-731.

Ball, O.F. (1952, May). Florence Nightingale. *Modern Hospital, 78:*88-90, 144.

Baly, M. (1986, June 11–18). Shattering the Nightingale myth. *Nursing Times, 82*(24):16-18.

Baly, M.E.: (1969, Jan. 2). Florence Nightingale's influence on nursing today. *Nursing Times, 65(suppl.):*1-4.

Barber E.M. (1935, July). A culinary compaign. *Journal of the American Dietetic Association, 11:*89-98.

Barritt, E.R. (1973). Florence Nightingale's values and modern nursing education. *Nursing Forum, 12:*7-47.

Boylen, J.O. (1974, April). The Florence Nightingale–Mary Stanley controvery: Some unpublished letters. *Medical History, 18(2):*186-193.

Berentson, L. (1982, April-May), Florence Nightingale: Change agent. *RN, Idaho, 6(2):*3, 7.

Berman J.K. (1974, Aug.). Florentia and the Clarabellas—A tribute to nurses. *Journal of the Indiana State Medical Association, 67:*717-719.

Bishop, W.J. (1957, Jan.). Florence Nightingale bibliography. *International Nursing Review, 4:*64+.

Bishop W.J. (1957, May). Florence Nightingale's letters. *American Journal of Nursing, 57:*607+.

Bishop, W.J. (1960, May). Florence Nightingale's message for today. *Nursing Outlook, 8:*246+.

Black, B.W. (1939, July). A tribute to Florence Nightingale. *Pacific Coast Journal of Nursing, 35:*408-409.

Blanc, E. (1980, May). Nightingale remembered: Reflections on times past. *California Nurse, 75(10):7*.

Blanchard, J.R. (1939, June). Florence Nightingale: A study in vocation. *New Zealand Nursing Journal, 32:*193-197.

Book reviews and digests. (1920, May). *Public Health Nursing, 12:*442-448.

Bridges, D.C. (1954, April). Florence Nightingale centenary. *International Nurses Review 1:*3.

Brow, E.J. (1954, April). Florence Nightingale and her international influence. *International Nursing Review, (ns) 1:*17-19.

The call to war. (1970, May). *RN, 33:*42+.

Cartwright, F.F. (1976, March). President's address: Miss Nightingale's dearest friend. *Proceedings of the Royal Society of Medicine, 69(3):*169-175.

Centenary celebrations [Florence Nightingale]. (1954, Nov.). *Nursing Times, 50:*1213-1214.

Centenary (Editorial). (1960, May). *Nursing Times,* 56:587.

Cherescavich, G.: (1971, June). *Nursing clinics of North America, 6:*217-223.

Choa, G.H. (1971, May). Speech by Dr. the Hon.

G.H. Choa at the Florence Nightingale Day Celebration on Wednesday, 12th May, 1971, at City Hall, Hong Kong. *Nursing Journal, 10:*33-34.

Clayton, R.E. (1974, April). How men may live and not die in India: Florence Nightingale. *Australasian Nurses Journal, 2:*10-11 passim.

Collins, W.J. (1945, May 12). Florence Nightingale and district nursing. *Nursing Mirror 81:*74.

Cope, Z. (1960, May 13). Florence Nightingale and her nurses. *Nursing Times, 56:*597.

Coxhead, E. (1973, May 10). Miss Nightingale's country hospital. *Nursing Times, 65:*615-617.

A criticism of Miss Florence Nightingale. (1907, Feb. 2). *Nursing Times, 3:*89.

Crowder, E.L.: (1978, May). Florence Nightingale. *Texas Nursing, 52(5):*6-7.

Cruse, P. (1980, Sept.). Florence Nightingale. *Surgery, 88(3):*394-399.

Davidson, C. (1937, March). Jeanne Mance and Florence Nightingale. *Hospital Progress, 18:*83-85.

de Guzman, G. (1935, July). [Florence Nightingale]. *Filipino Nurse, 10:*10-14.

de Tornayay, R. (1976, Nov.-Dec.). Past is prologue: Florence Nightingale. *Pulse, 12(6):*9-11.

The death of Florence Nightingale. (1910, Sept.). *American Journal of Nursing, 10:*919-920. (Editorial).

Dennis, K.E. & Prescott, P.A. (1985, Jan.). Florence Nightingale: Yesterday, today, and tomorrow. *Advances in Nursing Science, 7(2):*66-81.

Draper, J.M. (1907, Jan.). A brief sketch of the life of Florence Nightingale. *Trained Nurse, 38:*1-4.

Duggan, R. (1981, June). Florence Nightingale memorial service. *Australasian Nurses Journal 10(6):*30.

Dunbar, V.M. (1954, Oct.). Florence Nightingale's influence on nursing education. *International Nursing Review, (ns) 1:*17-23.

Dwyer, B.A. (1937, Jan.). The mother of our modern nursing system. *Filipino Nurse, 12:*8-10.

Echoes of the past. (1907, Nov. 16). *British Journal of Nursing, 39:*396-397.

Echoes of the past. (1907, Dec. 21). *British Journal of Nursing, 39:*497-498.

Ellett, E.C. (1904, May). Florence Nightingale. *Trained Nurse, 32:*305-310.

Extracts from letters from the Crimea. (1932, May). *American Journal of Nursing, 32:*537-538.

Fink, L.G. (1934, Dec.). Catholic influences in the life of Florence Nightingale. *Hospital Progress, 15:*482-489.

Florence Nightingale. (1903, July). *Medical Dial, 5:*122-124. (Editorial).

Florence Nightingale. (1964, May 15.). *Nursing Mirror, 118:*131. (Editorial).

Florence Nightingale as a leader in the religious and civic thought of her time. (1936, July). *Hospitals, 10:*78-84.

The Florence Nightingale bibliography. (1956, April). *South African Nursing Journal, 22:*16.

Florence Nightingale bibliography. (1956, Oct.). *Nursing Research, 5:*87.

Florence Nightingale bibliography is compiled. (1931, May). *Modern Hospital, 36:*126.

Florence Nightingale: Looking back . . . notes on hospitals. (1979, Sept.). *Lamp, 36:*39-43.

Florence Nightingale O.M. (1910, Aug. 20). *British Journal of Nursing, 45:*141-147.

Florence Nightingale: The original geriatric nurse. (1980, May). *Oklahoma Nurse, 25(4):*6.

Florence Nightingale: Rebel with a cause. (1970, May). *RN, 33:*39-55.

Florence Nightingale's influence on nursing today. (1969, Jan. 3). *Nursing Times, 65:*1+.

Florence Nightingale's letter. (1932, July 2). *Nursing Times, 28:*699.

Florence Nightingale's letter of advice to Bellevue. (1911, Feb.). *American Journal of Nursing 11:*361-364.

Florence Nightingale's tomb. (1957, June). *Canadian Nurse, 53:*529.

Florence Nightingale's work for public health. (1914, June). *American Journal of Public Health 4:*510-511. (Editorial).

Food for thought. (1958, Aug.). *Nursing Outlook, 6:*437. (Editorial).

Footnote to a dedicated life. (1958, Aug.). *RN, 21:*53+.

Fraga, M., & Tanenbaum, L. (1980, May). Florence Nightingale: Model for today's nurse. *Florida Nurse, 29(5):*11.

Frankenstein, L. The lady with a lamp. *Red Cross Courier, 16:*15-17.

Gordon, J.E. (1972, Oct.). Nurses and nursing in Britain. 21. The work of Florence Nightingale. I. For the health of the army, *Midwife Health Visitor and Community Nurse, 8:*351-359.

Gordon, J.E. (1972, Nov.). Nurses and nursing in Britain. 22. The work of Florence Nightingale. II.

The establishment of nurse training in Britain, *Midwife Health Visitor and Community Nurse, 8*:391-396.

Gordon, J.E. (1973, Jan.). Nurses and nursing in Britain. 23. The work of Florence Nightingale. III. Her influence throughout the world. *Midwife Health Visitor and Community Nurse, 9*:17-22.

Gottstein, W.K. (1956, May). Miss Nightingale's personality. *RN, 19*:58-60, 80, 82.

Gould, M.E. (1970, May 7). A woman of parts. *Nursing Times, 66*:606+.

Graham, S. (1980, Oct. 23). Notes on nursing, 1860-1980: Angels of plain speech. *Nursing Times, 76(43)*:1874.

Greatness in little things. (1954, May 8). *Nursing Times, 50*:508-510.

Grier, B., & Grier, M. (1978, Oct.). Contributions of the passionate statistician (Florence Nightingale). *Research in Nursing and Health, 1(3)*:103-109.

Grier, M.R. (1978, Oct.). Florence Nightingale: Saint or scientist? *Research in Nursing and Health, 1(3)*:91. (Editorial).

Hallowes, R. (1957, Sept. 27). Florence Nightingale. In Distinguished British nurses. *Nursing Mirror, 105*:viii-x.

Hamash Dash, D.M. (1971, June). Florence Nightingale's writings. *Nursing Journal of India, 62*:179.

Headberry, J. (1966, Feb.). Florence Nightingale and modern nursing. *Australian Nurses Journal, 64*:32-36.

Headberry, J.E. (1966, Jan.). Florence Nightingale and modern nursing. *Journal of the West Australian Nurses, 32*:7-16.

Headberry, J.E. (1966, March-April). Florence Nightingale and modern nursing. *UNA Nursing Journal, 64*:80-87.

Headberry, J.E. (1966, Sept. 2). Florence Nightingale and modern nursing. *Nursing Mirror, 122*:xiii.

Health as a personal and community asset. (1926, Dec. 13). *Journal of Education 104*:566.

Hearn, M.J. (1920, April). Florence Nightingale. *Quart. J. Chinese Nurses, 1*:12-14.

Her letters [Florence Nightingale]. (1955, June). *Nursing Journal of India,* 46:210.

Her letters [Florence Nightingale]. (1955, July). *Nursing Journal of India,* 46:236.

Her letters [Florence Nightingale]. (1955, Aug.). *Nursing Journal of India,* 46:268.

Her letters [Florence Nightingale]. (1955, Oct.). *Nursing Journal of India,* 46:326.

Holly, H. (1967, Winter). Wanted: A day's work for a day's pay. *Nevada Nurses Association Newsletter.* 1 passim.

Hurd, H.M. (1910, June). Florence Nightingale: A force in medicine. *Johns Hopkins Nurses Alumnae Magazine, 9*:68-81.

Ifemesia, C.C. (1976, July-Sept.). Florence Nightingale (1820-1910). *Nigerian Nurse, 8(3)*:26-34.

In her memory. (1957, May). *RN, 20*:53.

Isler, C. (1970, May). Florence Nightingale. *RN, 33*:35-55.

Iu, S. (1971, May). President's address at Florence Nightingale Day Celebration 12th May 1971, City Hall Theatre. *Hong Kong Nursing Journal, 10*:27-32.

Iveson-Iveson, J. (1983, May 11). Nurses in society: A legend in the breaking (Florence Nightingale). *Nursing Mirror 156(19)*:26-27.

Jake, D.G. (1975, Nov.). Florence Nightingale: Mission impossible. *Arizona Medicine 32(11)*:894-895.

Jamme, A.C. (1920, May). Florence Nightingale, the great teacher of nurses. *Pacific Coast Journal of Nursing, 16*:282-285.

Jones, H.W. (1940, Nov.). Some unpublished letters of Florence Nightingale. *Bulletin of the History of Medicine, 8*:1389-1396.

Jones, O.C. (1972, Aug.). A useful memorial (Florence Nightingale). *Canadian Nurse, 68*:38-39.

Journey among women: Responsibility at the top. Part 2. (1970, June 4). *Nursing Times,* 66:77+.

Kalisch, B.J., & Kalisch, P.A. (1983, April). Heroine out of focus: Media images of Florence Nightingale. *Nursing and Health Care, 4*:181-187.

Kalisch, B.J. & Kalisch, P.A. (1983, May). Heroine out of focus: Media images of Florence Nightingale. *Nursing and Health Care, 4*:270-278.

Kelly, L.Y. (1976, Oct.). Our nursing heritage: Have we renounced it? (Florence Nightingale). *Image* (NY) 8(3):43-48.

Kerling, N.J. (1976, July 1). Letters from Florence Nightingale. *Nursing Mirror, 143(1)*:68.

Kiereini, E.M. (1981, June). The way ahead: On the occasion of Florence Nightingale oration at the Perth Concert Hall, Australia, 24th October, 1979. *Kenya Nursing Journal, 10(1)*:5-8.

King, A.G. (1964, June). The changing role of the nurse. *Hospital Topics 42*:89+.

King, F.A. (1954, Oct. 22). Miss Nightingale and her ladies in the Crimea. *Nursing Mirror, 100*:xi-xii.

King, F.A. (1954, Oct. 29). Miss Nightingale and her ladies in the Crimea. *Nursing Mirror, 100*:viii-ix.

King, F.A. (1954, Nov. 5). Miss Nightingale and her ladies in the Crimea. *Nursing Mirror, 100*:v-vi.

King, F.A. (1954, Nov. 12). Miss Nightingale and her ladies in the Crimea. *Nursing Mirror, 100*: x-xi.

Konderska, Z. (1971, Oct.). [The birthday of nursing, (Florence Nightingale)]. *Pielig Polozna, 8*:12-13.

Konstantinova, M. (1923, Oct.). In the cradle of nursing. *American Journal of Nursing, 24*:47-49.

Kopf, E.W. (1978, Oct.). Florence Nightingale as statistician. *Research in Nursing & Health, 1(3)*:93-102.

Kovacs, A.F. (1973, May-June). The personality of Florence Nightingale. *International Nursing Review, 20*:78-79+.

The lady with a lamp. (1929, Feb. 9). *Nursing Times, 25*:154.

Large, J.T. (1985, May). Florence Nightingale: A multifaceted personality. *Nursing Journal of India, 76(5)*:110, 114.

Lee, C.A. (1987, Feb.). Thrusts of Florence Nightingale in the social context of the 19th century. *62(2)*: 3–4.

Lee, C.A. (1987, May). Discussion/life of Florence Nightingale. *Kansas Nurse, 62(5)*:12-13.

Levine, M.E. (1963, April). Florence Nightingale: The legend that lives. *Nursing Forum, 2*:24+.

Literature of Florence Nightingale. (1931, April). *Hospital Progress, 12*:188.

Loane, S.F. (1911, Feb.). Florence Nightingale and district nursing. *American Journal of Nursing, 11*:383-384.

McKee, E.S. (1909, Sept.). Florence Nightingale and her followers. *Nashville Journal of Medicine and Surgery, 103*:385-392.

Mackie, T.T. (1942, Jan.). Florence Nightingale and tropical and military medicine. *American Journal of Tropical Medicine, 22*:1-8.

Materials for the study of Florence Nightingale. (1931, May). *Trained Nurse and Hospital Review* 86:656-657.

The meaning of the lamp. (1956, May). *RN, 19*:61+.

Menon, M. (1980, Aug.). The lamp she lit [Florence Nightingale]. *Nursing Journal of India, 81(8)*:214-215.

Miss Nightingale's book of the Crimea. (1954, May 7). *Nursing Journal of India, 99*:ii-iii.

Monteiro, L. (1972, Nov.-Dec.). Research into things past: Tracking down one of Miss Nightingale's correspondents. *Nursing Research, 21*:526-529.

Monteiro. L. (1973, Nov. 8). Letters to a friend. *Nursing Times, 69*:1474-1476.

Monteiro, L.A. (1985, Feb.). Florence Nightingale on public health nursing. *American Journal of Public Health, 75(2)*:181-186.

Monteiro, L.A. (1985, Nov.). Response in anger: Florence Nightingale on the importance of training for nurses. *Journal of Nursing History, 1(1)*:11-18

The most beautiful old lady. (1951, May 11). *Nursing Journal of India, 93*:101.

Nelson, J. (1976, May 13). Florence: The legend [Florence Nightingale]. *Nursing Mirror, 142(20)*: 40-41.

Newton, M.E. (1952, May). Florence Nightingale's concept of clinical teaching. *Nursing World, 126*:220-221.

Newton, M.E. (1951, Sept.). The power of statistics. *Public Health Nursing, 43*:502-505.

Nightingale bibliography. (1957, May). *American Journal of Nursing, 57*:585.

Nightingale letter to Alice Fisher in Philadelphia. (1976, Jan.). *American Nurse, 8(2)*:2.

The Nightingale Saga (Vol. 1). (1962, Aug. 13). *Nursing Mirror 114*:425.

Ninan, R. (1982, June). The lady with the lamp: A profile. *Nursing Journal of India, 73(6)*:154-155.

No other earth. (1962, Nov.). *Today's Health, 40*:63.

Noguchi, M. (1969, Oct.). [Nightingale's philosophy and its limitations: My theory on Nightingale]. *Japanese Journal of Nursing, Art 10*:65-75.

Noyes, C.D. (1931, Jan.). Florence Nightingale: sanitarian and hygienist. *Red Cross Courier, 10*:41-42.

Notting, M.A. (1927, May). Florence Nightingale as a statistician. *Public Health Nursing, 19*:207-209.

O'Malley, I.B. (1935, May). Florence Nightingale after the Crimean War (1856-1861). *Trained Nurse, 94*:401-407.

Oman C. (1950, Nov. 17). Florence Nightingale as seen by two biographers, *Nursing Mirror, 92*:30-31.

The other side of the coin. (1967, May). *New Zealand Nursing Journal, 60*:40. (Editorial).

Palmer I.S. (1976, Sept.-Oct.). Florence Nightingale and the Salisbury incident. *Nursing Research 25(5)*:370-377.

Palmer, I.S. (1977, March-April). Florence Nightingale: Reformer, reactionary, researcher. *Nursing Research, 26*:84-89.

Palmer, I.S. (1981, June). Florence Nightingale and international origins of modern nursing. *Image, 13*:28-31.

Palmer, I.S. (1983, July-Aug.). Nightingale revisited. *Nursing Outlook, 31(4)*:229-233.

Palmer, I.S. (1983, Aug. 3). Florence Nightingale: The myth and the reality. *Nursing Times, 79*:40-42.

Parker, P. (1977, March). Florence Nightingale: First lady of administrative nursing. *Supervisor Nurse, 8*:24-25.

The passing of Florence Nightingale. (1910, Nov.). *Pacific Coast Journal of Nursing, 6*:481-519.

A passionate statistician. (1931, May). *American Journal of Nursing, 31*:566.

Penner, S.J. (1987, May). The remarkable Miss Nightingale. *Kansas Nurse, 62(5)*:11.

Pearce, E.C. (1954, April). The influence of Florence Nightingale on the spirit of nursing. *International Nursing Review, (ns)1*:20-22.

Peter, M. (1936, May). A personal interview with Florence Nightingale. *Pacific Coast Journal of Nursing, 32*:270-271.

Phillips, E.C. (1920, May). Florence Nightingale: A study. *Pacific Coast Journal of Nursing, 16*:272-274.

Pickering, G. (1974, Dec. 14). Florence Nightingale's illness. *British Medical Journal, 4(5945)*:656. (Letter).

Public health nursing: Florence Nightingale as a consultant. (1920, May). *Pacific Coast Journal of Nursing, 16*:299-300.

Rains, A.J. (1982, Feb.). Mitchiner memorial lecture: "The Nightingale touch." *Journal of the Royal Army Medical Corps, 128(1)*:4-17.

Rao, G.A. (1971, June). Florence Nightingale's writings. *Nursing Journal of India, 62*:179.

The real Florence Nightingale. (1912, April 6). *British Journal of Nursing, 48*:267.

Remembering Florence Nightingale. (1979, Sept.). *Nursing Focus, 1(1)*:34.

The revolting revisionist historian perspective. (1979, Jan.). *Arizona Medicine, 36(1)*:65-66.

Rhynas, M. (1931, May). Intimate sketch of the life of Florence Nightingale. *Canadian Nurse 27*:229-233.

Richards, L. (1920, May). Recollections of Florence Nightingale. *American Journal of Nursing, 20*:649.

Richards, L. (Ed.).(1934). Letters of Florence Nightingale, *Yale Review, 24*:326-347.

Roberts, M.M. (1937, July). Florence Nightingale as a nurse educator. *American Journal of Nursing, 37*:773-778.

Rogers, P. (1982, July). Florence Nightingale: The myth and the reality. *Nursing Focus, 3(11)*:10.

The romantic Florence Nightingale. (1968, May). *Canadian Nurse, 64*:57+.

Ross, M. (1954, May). Miss Nightingale's letters. *American Journal of Nursing, 53*:593-594.

Scovil, E.R. (1911, Feb.). Personal recollections of Florence Nightingale. *American Journal of Nursing, 11*:365-368.

Scovil, E.R. (1913, Oct.). Florence Nightingale. *American Journal of Nursing, 14*:28-33.

Scovil, E.R. (1914, Oct.). Florence Nightingale and her nurses. *American Journal of Nursing, 15*:13-18.

Scovil, E.R. (1916, Dec.). The love story of Florence Nightingale. *American Journal of Nursing, 17*:209-212.

Scovil, E.R. (1920, May). The later activities of Florence Nightingale. *American Journal of Nursing, 20*:609-612.

Scovil, E.R. (1927, May). Florence Nightingale's notes on nursing. *American Journal of Nursing, 27*:355-357.

Seden, F. (1947, July). Florence Nightingale and Turkish education. *Public Health Nursing, 39*:349.

Seymer, L.R. (1947, Sept.). Florence Nightingale oration. *International Nursing Bulletin, 3*:12-17.

Seymer, L.R. (1951, July). Florence Nightingale at Kaiserswerth. *American Journal of Nursing, 51*:424-426.

Seymer, L.R. (1954, April 2). Florence Nightingale. *Nursing Mirror, 99*:34-36.

Seymer, L.R. (1960, May). Nightingale Nursing School: 100 years ago. *American Journal of Nursing, 60*:658+.

Seymer, S. (1979, May). The writings of Florence Nightingale. *Nursing Journal of India, 70(5)*:121-128.

Skeet, M. (1980, Oct. 23). Nightingale's notes on nursing, 1860-1980 [interview by Alison Dunn]. *Nursing Times, 76(43)*:1871-1873.

Smith, F.T. (1981, May). Florence Nightingale:

Early feminist. *American Journal of Nursing, 81*:1059-1061.

Some letters from Florence Nightingale. (1935, Feb.). *Hospital (London), 31*:50.

Sotejo, J.V. (1970, April-June). Florence Nightingale: Nurse for all seasons. *ANPHI Papers, 5*:4.

Stewart, I.M. (1939, Dec.). Florence Nightingale: Educator. *Teacher's College Record*, 41: 208-223.

Swain V. (1983, March 16-22). No plaster saint! *Nursing Times, 79(11)*:62-63.

That lamp. (1966, May 13). *Nursing Times, 62*:631.

Thompson, J.D. (1980, May). The passionate humanist: From Nightingale to the new nurse. *Nursing Outlook, 28(5)*:290-295.

Tinkler, L.F. (1973, Aug. 2). The barracks at Scutari: Start of a nursing legend. *Nursing Times, 69*:1006-1007.

Tobin, J. (1969, March). Observations on Florence Nightingale. *Tar Heel Nurse, 31*:52-55 passim.

Tracy, M.A. (1940, July). Florence Nightingale and her influence on hospitals. *Pacific Coast Journal of Nursing, 36*:406-407.

Trautman, M.J. (1971, April). Nurses as poets. *American Journal of Nursing, 71*:725-728.

Two unpublished letters. (1937, May). *Public Health Nursing, 29*:307.

Verney, H. (1980, Spring). The perfect aunt: FN 1820-1910. *News Letter of the Florence Nightingale International Nurses Association, 70*:13-16.

Walton, P. (1972, Jan.-March). The lady with the lamp: Florence Nightingale. *Phillipine Journal of Nursing, 41*:11-12.

Walton, P. (1986, May). The lady with the lamp (Florence Nightingale). *Nursing Journal of India, 77(5)*:115-116.

Watkin, B. (1976, May 6). Notes on Nightingale. *Nursing Mirror, 142(19)*:42.

Welch, M. (1986, April). Nineteenth-century philosophic influences on Nightingale's concept of the person. *Journal of Nursing History, 1(2)*:3-11

Westminster Abbey Florence Nightingale Commemoration Service, May 12th, 1970: The 150th anniversary of her birth. (1970, Autumn). *News Letter of the Florence Nightingale International Nurses Association,* pp. 21-24.

White, F.S. (1923, June). At the gate of the temple. *Public Health Nursing, 15*:279-283.

Whittaker, E. & Olesen, V.L. (1967, Nov.). Why Florence Nightingale? *American Journal of Nursing, 67*:2338+.

The wider education of the nurse. (1951, Sept. 14). *Nursing Journal of India, 93*:438.

Williams, C.B. (1961, May). Stories from Scutari. *American Journal of Nursing, 61*:88.

Winchester, J.H. (1967, May). Tough angel of the battlefield. *Today's Health, 45*:30+.

Winslow, C.E.A. (1946, July). Florence Nightingale and public health nursing, *Public Health Nursing, 38*:330-332.

Wolstenholme, G.E. (1980, Dec.). Florence Nightingale: New lamps for old. *Proceedings of the Royal Society of Medicine, 63*:1282-1288.

Woodham-Smith, Mrs. C. (1947, May 10). Florence Nightingale as a child. *Nursing Mirror, 85*:91-92.

Woodham-Smith, Mrs. C. (1952, May). Florence Nightingale revealed. *American Journal of Nursing, 52*:570-572.

Woodham-Smith, Mrs. C. (1954, July 10). The greatest Victorian. *Nursing Times, 50*:737, 738-741.

The works of mercy window (1956, May). *American Journal of Nursing, 56*:574.

Yeates, E.L. (1962, May 11). The prince consort and Florence Nightingale. *Nursing Mirror, 114*:iii-iv.

8

Virginia Henderson

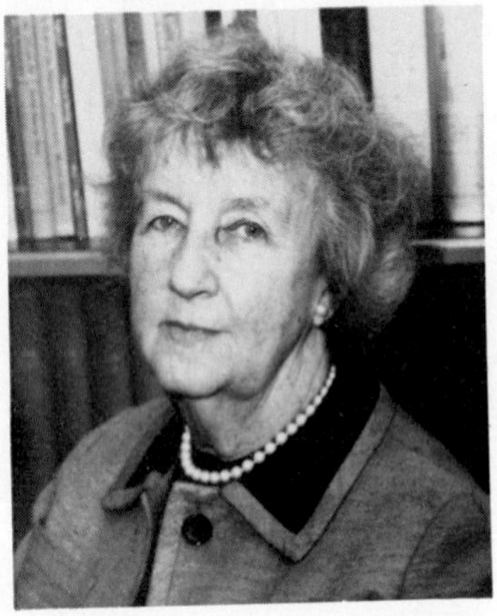

Definition of Nursing

Deborah Wertman DeMeester, Tamara Lauer, Susan E. Neal, Sandy Williams

CREDENTIALS AND BACKGROUND OF THE THEORIST

Virginia Henderson was born in 1897, the fifth of eight children in her family. A native of Kansas City, Mo., Henderson spent her developmental years in Virginia because her father practiced law in Washington, D.C.

During World War I Henderson developed an interest in nursing. So in 1918 she entered the Army School of Nursing in Washington, D.C. Henderson graduated in 1921 and accepted a position as a staff nurse with the Henry Street Visiting Nurse Service in New York. In 1922 Henderson began teaching nursing in the Norfolk Protestant Hospital in Virginia. Five years later she entered Teacher's College at Columbia University, where she subsequently earned her B.S. and M.A. degrees in nursing education. In 1929 Henderson served as a teaching supervisor in the clinics of Strong Memorial Hospital in Rochester, New York. She returned to Teacher's College in 1930 as a faculty member, teaching courses in the nursing analytical process and clinical practice until 1948.*

The authors wish to express appreciation to Virginia Henderson for critiquing the chapter.

*References 3:49; 23:87; 24:116-117.

Henderson has enjoyed a long career as an author and researcher. While on the Teacher's College faculty she rewrote the fourth edition of Bertha Harmer's *Textbook of the Principles and Practice of Nursing* following the author's death. This edition was published in 1939. The fifth edition of the textbook was published in 1955 and contained Henderson's own definition of nursing. Henderson has been associated with Yale University since the early 1950s, and has done much to further nursing research through this association. From 1959 to 1971 Henderson directed the Nursing Studies Index Project sponsored by Yale. The *Nursing Studies Index* was developed into a four-volume annotated index to nursing's biographical, analytical, and historical literature from 1900 to 1959. Concurrently, Henderson authored or coauthored several other important works. Her pamphlet, *Basic Principles of Nursing Care,* was published for the International Council of Nurses in 1960 and translated into more than 20 languages. Henderson's 5-year collaboration with Leo Simmons produced a national survey of nursing research that was published in 1964. Her book, *The Nature of Nursing,* was published in 1966 and described her concept of nursing's primary, unique function. The sixth edition of *The Principles and Practice of Nursing,* published in 1978, was coauthored by Henderson and Gladys Nite and edited by Henderson. This textbook has been widely used in the curriculums of various nursing schools. In the 1980s, Henderson remains active as a Research Associate Emeritus at Yale. Henderson's achievements and influence in the nursing profession have brought her more than seven honorary doctoral degrees and the first Christiane Reimann Award. At the 1988 American Nurses' Association Convention, she received a special citation of honor for her lifelong contributions to nursing research, education, and professionalism.*

*References 23:87; 24:117-130; 25:58.

THEORETICAL SOURCES FOR THEORY DEVELOPMENT

Henderson first published her definition of nursing in the 1955 revision of Harmer and Henderson's, *The Principles and Practice of Nursing*. There were three major influences upon Henderson's decision to synthesize her own definition of nursing. First, she revised the *Textbook of Principles and Practice of Nursing* in 1939. Henderson identifies her work for this text as the source that made her realize "the necessity of being clear about the function of nurses."[24:119] A second source was her involvement as a committee member in a regional conference of the National Nursing Council in 1946. Her committee work was incorporated into Ester Lucile Brown's 1948 report, *Nursing for the Future*. Henderson[7:62] says this report represented "my point of view modified by the thinking of others in the group." Finally, the American Nurses' Association's 5-year investigation of the function of the nurse interested Henderson, who was not fully satisfied with the definition adopted by the ANA in 1955.

Henderson labels her work a definition rather than a theory because theory was not in vogue at that time. She describes her interpretation as the "synthesis of many influences, some positive and some negative."[7:64] In *The Nature of Nursing* she identifies sources of influence during her early years of nursing. These include the following.

ANNIE W. GOODRICH. Goodrich was the Dean of the Army School of Nursing, where Henderson achieved her basic nursing education, and served as an inspiration to Henderson. Henderson[8:7] recalls, "Whenever she visited our unit, she lifted our sights above techniques and routine." She also attributes Goodrich with "my early discontent with the regimentalized patient care in which I participated and the concept of nursing as merely ancillary to medicine."[8:7]

CAROLINE STACKPOLE. Stackpole was a physiology professor at Teacher's College, Columbia University when Henderson was a graduate student. She impressed upon Henderson the importance of maintaining physiological balance.[8:10-11]

JEAN BROADHURST. Broadhurst was a microbiology professor at Teacher's College. The importance of hygiene and asepsis made an impact on Henderson.[8:10-11]

DR. EDWARD THORNDIKE. Thorndike worked in psychology at Teacher's College. He conducted investigational studies on the fundamental needs of humans. Henderson[8:11] realized that illness is "more than a state of disease" and that most fundamental needs are not met in hospitals.

DR. GEORGE DEAVER. Deaver was a physicist at the Institute for the Crippled and Disabled and, later, at Bellevue Hospital, Henderson observed that the goal of the rehabilitative efforts at the Institute was rebuilding the patient's independence.[8:12]

BERTHA HARMER. Harmer, a Canadian nurse, was the original author of *Textbook of the Principles and Practice of Nursing,* which Henderson revised. Henderson never met Harmer, but similarities of their respective definitions of nursing are obvious. Harmer's 1922 definition begins, "Nursing is rooted in the needs of the humanity."[3:54]

IDA ORLANDO. Henderson identifies Orlando as an influence upon her concept of the nurse-patient relationship. She says, "Ida Orlando (Pelletier), [has] made me realize how easily the nurse can act on misconceptions of the patient's needs if she does not check her interpretation of them with him."[8:14]

USE OF EMPIRICAL EVIDENCE

Henderson incorporated physiological and psychological principles into her personal concept of nursing. Her background in these areas stems from her association with Stackpole and Thorndike during her graduate studies at Teacher's College.

Stackpole based her physiology course on Claude Bernard's dictum that health depends on keeping lymph constant around the cell.[8:10] From this, Henderson surmised that "A definition of nursing should imply an appreciation of the principle of physiological balance."[8:11] From Bernard's theory, she also gained an appreciation for psychosomatic medicine and its implications for nursing. She states, "It was obvious that emotional balance is inseparable from physiological balance once I realized that an emotion is actually our interpretation of cellular response to fluctuations in the chemical composition of the intercellular fluids."[8:11]

Henderson does not identify the precise theories supported by Thorndike, only that they involved the fundamental needs of man. A correlation with Abraham Maslow's Hierarchy of Needs is seen in Henderson's 14 components of nursing care, which begin with physical needs and progress to the psychosocial components. Although she doesn't cite Maslow as an influence, she describes his theory of human motivation in the sixth edition of *Principles and Practice of Nursing Care* in 1978.

MAJOR CONCEPTS AND DEFINITIONS

NURSING. Henderson[8:15] defines nursing in functional terms:

> The unique function of the nurse is to assist the individual, sick or well, in the performance of those activities contributing to health or its recovery (or to peaceful death) that he would perform unaided if he had the necessary strength, will, or knowledge. And to do this in such a way as to help him gain independence as rapidly as possible.

HEALTH. Henderson does not state her own definition of health. But in her writing she equates health with independence. In the sixth edition of *Textbook of Principles and Practice of*

Nursing she cites several definitions of health from various sources, including the one from the charter of the World Health Organization. She views health in terms of the patient's ability to perform the 14 components of nursing care unaided. She says it is "the quality of health rather than life itself, that margin of mental and physical vigor that allows a person to work most effectively and to reach his highest potential level of satisfaction in life."[15:122]

ENVIRONMENT. Again, Henderson does not give her own definition of environment. She uses *Webster's New Collegiate Dictionary,* 1961, which defines environment as "the aggregate of all the external conditions and influences affecting the life and development of an organism."[15:829]

PERSON (PATIENT). Henderson[7:65] views the patient as an individual who requires assistance to achieve health and independence or peaceful death. The mind and body are inseparable. The patient and his family are viewed as a unit.

NEEDS. No specific definition of need is found, but Henderson identifies 14 basic needs of the patient, which comprise the components of nursing care.* These include the need to:

1. Breathe normally.
2. Eat and drink adequately.
3. Eliminate body wastes.
4. Move and maintain desirable position.
5. Sleep and rest.
6. Select suitable clothes—dress and undress.
7. Maintain body temperature within normal range by adjusting clothing and modifying the environment.
8. Keep the body clean and well groomed and protect the integument.
9. Avoid dangers in the environment and avoid injuring others.
10. Communicate with others in expressing emotions, needs, fears, or opinions.
11. Worship according to one's faith.
12. Work in such a way that there is a sense of accomplishment.
13. Play or participate in various forms of recreation.
14. Learn, discover, or satisfy the curiosity that leads to normal development and health and use the available health facilities.

*Reprinted with the permission of Macmillan Publishing Company *The Nature of Nursing* by Virginia Henderson. Copyright © 1966 by Virginia Henderson.

MAJOR ASSUMPTIONS

Virginia Henderson does not directly cite what she feels her underlying assumptions include. We have adapted the following assumptions from Henderson's publications.

Nursing

The nurse has a unique function to help well or sick individuals.

The nurse functions as a member of a medical team.

The nurse functions independently of the physician, but promotes his or her plan, if there is a physician in attendance. Henderson stressed that the nurse (for example, the nurse-midwife) can function independently and *must* if he or she is the best-prepared health worker in the situation. The nurse can and *must* diagnose and treat if the situation demands it. (Henderson is especially emphatic on this in the sixth edition of *Principles and Practice of Nursing*).

The nurse is knowledgeable in both biological and social sciences.

The nurse can assess basic human needs.

The 14 components of nursing care encompass all possible functions of nursing.[7:63;8:16-17;15]

Person (Patient)

The person must maintain physiological and emotional balance.

The mind and body of the person are inseparable.

The patient requires help toward independence.
The patient and his family are a unit.
The patient's needs are encompassed by the 14 components of nursing.[8:11]

Health

Health is a quality of life.
Health is basic to human functioning.
Health requires independence and interdependence.
Promotion of health is more important than care of the sick.[11:33]
Individuals will achieve or maintain health if they have the necessary strength, will, or knowledge.[8:15]

Environment

Healthy individuals may be able to control their environment, but illness may interfere with that ability.
Nurses should have safety education.
Nurses should protect patients from mechanical injury.
Nurses should minimize the chances of injury through recommendations regarding construction of buildings, purchase of equipment, and maintenance.
Doctors use nurses' observations and judgments upon which to base prescriptions for protective devices.
Nurses must know about social customs and religious practices to assess dangers.[6:652]

THEORETICAL ASSERTIONS

The Nurse-Patient Relationship

Three levels comprising the nurse-patient relationship can be identified, ranging from a very dependent to a quite independent relationship: (1) the nurse as a *substitute* for the patient; (2) the nurse as a *helper* to the patient; and (3) the nurse as a *partner* with the patient. In times of grave illness, the nurse is seen as a "substitute for what the patient lacks to make him 'complete,' 'whole,' or 'independent,' by the lack of physical strength, will, or knowledge."[7:63] Henderson[8:16] portrays this view when she says the nurse "is temporarily the consciousness of the unconscious, the love life for the suicidal, the leg of the amputee, the eyes of the newly blind, a means of locomotion for the infant, knowledge and confidence for the young mother, the 'mouthpiece' for those too weak or withdrawn to speak, and so on."

During conditions of convalescence, the nurse helps the patient acquire or regain his independence. Henderson[21:120] states, "Independence is a relative term. None of us is independent of others, but we strive for a healthy interdependence, not a sick dependence."

As partners, the nurse and patient together formulate the care plan. Basic needs exist regardless of diagnosis but are modified by pathology and other conditions such as age, temperament, emotional state, social or cultural status, and physical and intellectual capacities.[6:415]

The nurse must be able not only to assess the patient's needs, but also those conditions and pathologic states that alter them. Henderson[7:63] says the nurse must "get 'inside the skin' of each of her patients in order to know what he needs." The needs must then be validated with the patient.

The nurse can alter the environment where she deems necessary. Henderson[15:831] believes, "In every situation nurses who know physiologic and psychologic reactions to temperature and humidity, light and color, gas pressures, odors, noise, chemical impurities, and microorganisms can organize and make the best use of the facilities available."

The nurse and patient are always working toward a goal, whether it be independence or peaceful death. One goal of the nurse must be to keep the patient's day as "normal as possible."[7:67] Promotion of health is another important goal of the nurse. Henderson[11:33] states, "There is more to be gained by helping every man learn how to be healthy than by preparing the most skilled therapists for service to those in crises."

The Nurse-Physician Relationship

Henderson insists the nurse has a unique function from that of physicians. The care plan, formulated by the nurse and patient together, must be implemented in such a way as to promote the physician's prescribed therapeutic plan. Henderson[11:34] stresses that nurses do *not* follow doctor's orders, for she "questions a philosophy that allows a physician to give orders to patients or other health workers." Recently she has extended this to emphasize that the nurse helps patients with health management when physicians are unavailable.[15:121] She also indicates that many nurse and physician's functions overlap.[19]

The Nurse as a Member of the Health Team

The nurse works in interdependence with other health professionals. The nurse and other team members help each other carry out the total program of care, but they should not do each others' jobs. Henderson[7:63] reminds us that "No one of the team should make such heavy demands on another member that anyone of them is unable to perform his or her unique function."

Henderson compares the entire medical team, including the patient and his family, to wedges on a pie graph (Figure 8-1). The size of each member's section depends on the patient's current needs, and therefore changes as the patient progresses toward independence. In some situations, certain team members are not included in the pie at all. The goal is for the patient to have the largest wedge possible or to take the whole pie.

Just as the patient's needs change, so may the definition of nursing. Henderson[24:121] admits, "This does not say that it is a definition that will stand for all time. I believe nursing is modified by the era in which it is practiced, and depends to a great extent on what other health workers do."

Henderson believes her sixth edition of *Principles and Practice of Nursing,* coauthored with Gladys Nite, expands her definition to include nurse practitioners. She says, "Nursing must not exist in a vacuum. Nursing must grow and learn to meet the new health needs of the public as we encounter them."[18]

LOGICAL FORM

Henderson appears to have used the deductive form of logical reasoning to develop her definition of nursing. She deduced her definition of nursing and 14 needs from physiological and psychological principles. One must study the assumptions of Henderson's definition to assess logical adequacy. Many of the assumptions have validity because of their high level of agreement with the literature and research conclusions of scientists in other fields. For example, her 14 basic needs correspond closely to Maslow's widely accepted human needs hierarchy, even though they were listed before she read Maslow's work.

In her book, *To be a Nurse,* Evelyn Adam analyzes Henderson's work using a framework she learned from Dorothy Johnson. Adam[1] identifies Henderson's assumptions, values, the goal of nursing, the client, the role of the nurse, the source of difficulty, the intervention, and the desired consequences.

ACCEPTANCE BY THE NURSING COMMUNITY

Practice

Henderson's definition of nursing as it relates to nursing practice points out that the nurse who sees her primary function as the direct care-giver to the patient will find an immediate reward in the patient's progress from dependence to independence. The nurse must make every effort to understand the patient when he lacks will, knowledge, or strength. As Henderson[8:24] states, the nurse will "get inside his skin." The nurse can help the patient move to an independent state by assessing, planning, implementing, and evaluating each of the 14 components of basic nursing care.

Henderson's approach to patient care is de-

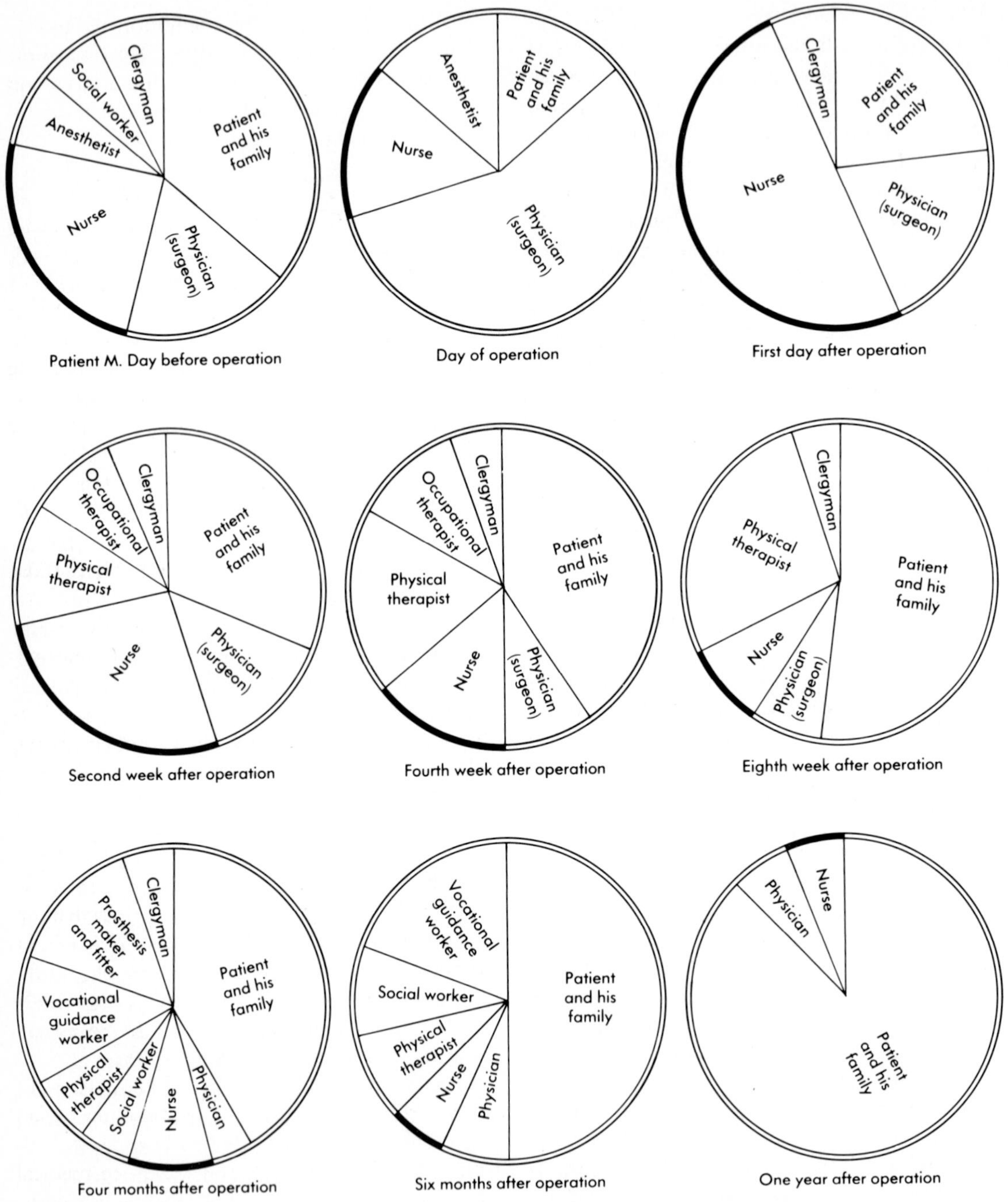

Figure 8-1. Showing how nurse's role diminishes as rehabilitation progresses in case of young man having leg amputated, for example.

liberative and involves decision-making. Although she does not specifically mention the steps in the nursing process, one can see how the concepts are interrelated. Henderson[17,18,20] believes the nursing process is the problem-solving process and is not peculiar to nursing.

In the assessment phase, the nurse would assess the patient in all 14 components of basic nursing care. After the first component was completely assessed, the nurse would move on to the next component until all 14 areas were assessed. In gathering data, the nurse uses observation, smell, feeling, and hearing. To complete the assessment phase, the nurse must analyze the data she has collected. This requires knowledge of what is normal in health and disease.

Henderson states, "As long as nursing is the only service available on a 24-hour, 7-day-a-week basis, the ability of nurses to differentiate the normal from the abnormal in patient health, . . . the assessment function of nurses is indisputable."[21]

According to Henderson,[15:416] the planning phase involves making the plan fit the individual's needs, updating the plan as necessary based on the changes, using the plan as a record and ensuring it fits with the physician's prescribed plan. A good plan, in her opinion, integrates the work of all those on the health team.[18]

In the implementation phase, the nurse helps the patient perform activities to maintain health, to recover from illness, or to aid in peaceful death. Interventions are individualized, depending on physiological principles, age, cultural background, emotional balance, and physical and intellectual capacities. Henderson[8:24-31;12] would evaluate the patient according to the degree to which he performs independently. However, the infant cannot be independent, nor can the unconscious. In some phases of illness, we should accept the patient's desire to depend on others.

Education

Henderson[8:69] states, "In order for a nurse to practice as an expert in her own right and to use the scientific approach to the improvement of practice, the nurse needs the kind of education available only in colleges and universities." The nurse's education demands universal understanding of diverse human beings. The statement supports the position taken in 1965 by the American Nurses' Association.

In addition, Henderson believes "the value of education comes not only with the added knowledge that is gained but also from the added confidence the individual develops in the institute of higher education environment." She says "nursing is a universal occupation and higher education allows you to do it better."[22]

In her book, *The Nature of Nursing: A Definition and Its Implications for Practice, Research, and Education,* Henderson has designed three phases of curriculum development students should progress through in their learning. The focus in all three phases remains the same—assisting the patient when he needs strength, will, or knowledge in performing his daily activities or in carrying out prescribed therapy with the ultimate goal of independence.

In the first phase, emphasis is placed on the fundamental needs of the patient, planning nursing care, and the unique function of the nurse in helping the patient carry out his activities of daily living. In this phase the curriculum plan does not emphasize pathological states or specific illnesses, but takes into account conditions always present that affect basic needs.[8:51] In the second phase, emphasis is placed on helping patients meet their needs during marked body disturbances or pathological states that demand modifications in the nurse's plan of care. The patient presents the student with problems of greater complexity. More medical science is involved, and the student begins to understand the rationale of symptomatic treatment.[8:51] In the third phase, instruction is patient- and family-centered. The student becomes involved in the complete study of the patient and all his needs.[8:55]

Henderson[16] has stressed the importance of having nursing students develop a habit of inquiry; take courses in biological, physical, and social sciences, and in the humanities; study with students in other fields; observe effective care; and give effective care in a variety of settings.

The textbook in which Henderson's definition of nursing is found, *Principles and Practices of Nursing,* is an excellent source that can be used by nursing students and by practicing nurses. It provides depth usually lacking in such texts. Kelly states, "If only one nursing book can be saved when the bomb falls, *PPN* is that book. In it are the breadth and depth of nursing, framed within the accumulated wisdom of law, medicine, and religion, documented from the world literature, fascinatingly footnoted—and eminently practical."[25:59]

Research

Henderson recommends library research and has done a vast amount of it herself. She has surveyed library resources and nursing research.[5] She supports developing nurses in a research atmosphere, introducing research at the baccalaureate level, and believes research is needed to evaluate and improve practice.[4]

"Nurses need to acquire the habit of looking for research upon which to base their practice," Henderson says.[22] She recommends that nurses make greater use of library resources and hopes nurses will conduct research to improve practice rather than merely for academic respectability.[9;10;13;14:164]

In a survey and assessment of nursing research reported by Henderson and Leo W. Simmons in 1964 several reasons for lack of research in clinical nursing were identified. These reasons included:

1. Major energies of the profession have gone into improving the preparation for nursing.
2. Learning how to recruit and to hold sufficient numbers of nurses to meet the growing demand has taken considerable energy.
3. The need for administrators and educators has almost exhausted the supply of degree nurses.
4. A lack of support from administrators, nursing service administrators, and physicians has discouraged researchers.[8:34]

Research questions arise from each of the 14 components for basic nursing care, and it is the nurse's function to assume responsibility for identifying problems, for continually validating her function, for improving the methods she uses, and for reassuring the effectiveness of nursing care.

Henderson[8:39] concludes, "No profession, occupation, or industry in this age can evaluate adequately or improve its practice without research." Research is the most reliable type of analysis.

She believes that until practicing nurses learn how to use library resources, such as indexes from the National Library of Medicine, "nurses will not have taken the most elementary step to becoming part of a research-based profession—a claim nurses now like to make."[19]

FURTHER DEVELOPMENT

Henderson has no plans to further develop her definition of nursing.[18] Neither does she anticipate any further revisions of the text, *Principles and Practices of Nursing.* She stresses continued assessment of the patient's needs and continued revision of the patient's needs as his condition and goals change. Henderson[17] encourages the nurse to identify new needs beyond the 14 she enumerated.

CRITIQUE

Before one attempts to evaluate Virginia Henderson's theory of nursing with respect to the generally accepted criteria of simplicity, generality, empirical precision, and derivable consequences, one must understand that she did not intend to develop a definitive nursing *theory.* Instead, she developed a personal concept or definition in an attempt to clarify what she considers to be the unique function of nursing. She states, "My interpretation of the nurse's function is the synthesis of many influences, some positive and some negative. . . . I should first make clear that I do not expect everyone to agree with me. Rather, I would urge every nurse to develop her own concept."[7:64]

Henderson's definition can be considered a grand theory or philosophy within the preparadigm stage of theory development in nursing. Her concept is descriptive and easy to read. It is defined in common language terms. Her definitions of nursing and enumeration of the 14 basic nursing functions presents a perspective aimed at explaining a totality of nursing behavior. Because she had no intention of developing a theory, Henderson does not develop the interrelated theoretical statements or operational definitions necessary to provide the theory testability. However, that can be done.

Simplicity

Henderson's concept of nursing is complex rather than simplistic. It contains many variables and several different descriptive and explanatory relationships. It is not associated with structural organizations within a framework or model form to enhance simplicity, although some work has been done in this area. Diagrams of Henderson's and Orem's concepts of nursing from the Nursing Developmental Conference Group's book, *Concepts Formation in Nursing,* have been reproduced in the Henderson and Nite book.[15:23] In addition, the 14 basic needs appear simple as stated, but they become complex when an alteration of a need occurs and all the parameters relating to that need are considered. The sixth edition of *Principles and Practices of Nursing* is extremely comprehensive and well illustrated to add clarity.

Generality

Generality is present in Henderson's definition since it is broad in scope. It attempts to include the function of all nurses and all patients in their various interrelationships and interdependencies.

Derivable Consequences

Henderson's perspective has been useful in promoting new ideas and in furthering conceptual development of emerging theorists. In her many published works she has discussed the importance of nursing's independence from, and interdependence with, other branches of the health care field. She has also influenced curriculum development and made a great contribution in promoting the importance of research in the clinical practice of nursing. She has made extensive use of other theorists' research in her own work. Evans[2] states that *Principles and Practice of Nursing* has made "a revolutionary change in one's thinking about nursing research." He states that the revolutionary thesis of the book is:

> The habits of minds which inform the everyday tasks of a nurse are exactly the same as those which undergird the very finest published research; in this way, every nurse ought not just to *do* simple research tasks as part of her work, but she ought also *always* to *be* a researcher, whether or not she writes or speaks a word in print or public.[2:338-339]

Since Henderson's definition of the unique function of nursing has been widely read, it has functioned as a major stepping-stone in the emergence of nursing as a professional scientific discipline.

She continues to be cited in current nursing literature and publications in all areas of nursing practice from holistic nursing to the nursing process.

REFERENCES

1. Adam, E. (1980). *To Be a Nurse.* New York: W.B. Saunders.
2. Evans, D.L. (1980). Everynurse as researcher: An argumentative critique of Principles and Practice of Nursing, *Nursing Forum, xix:*335-349.

3. Furukawa, C.Y., & Howe, J.K. (1980). Virginia Henderson. In Nursing Theories Practice Group, J.B. George, Chairperson, *Nursing theories: The base for professional nursing practice*. Englewood Cliffs, N.J. Prentice-Hall.
4. Henderson, V. (1956, Feb.). Research in nursing practice—When? *Nursing Research, 4:*99.
5. Henderson, V. (1957, Oct.). An overview of nursing research. *Nursing Research, 6:*61-71.
6. Henderson, V. (1958, May 9). The basic principles of nursing care. *Nursing Mirror, 107:* 337-338, 415-416, 497-498, 583-584, 651-652, 733-734, 803-804.
7. Henderson, V. (1964, Aug.). The nature of nursing. *American Journal of Nursing, 64:*62-68.
8. Henderson, V. (1966). *The nature of nursing: A definition and its implications for practice, research, and education*. New York: Macmillan.
9. Henderson, V. (1968). Library resources in nursing: Their development and use. *International Nursing Review, 15:*164-174, 236-246.
10. Henderson, V. (1971, Jan.). Implications for nursing in the library activities of the regional medical programs. *Bulletin of the Medical Library Association, 59:*53-64.
11. Henderson, V. (1971, March). Health is everybody's business. *Canadian Nurse, 67:*31-34.
12. Henderson, V. (1973, June). On nursing care plans and their history. *Nursing Outlook, 21:*378-379.
13. Henderson, V. (1977). Awareness of library resources: A characteristic of professional workers; an essential in research and continuing education. *Reference resources for research and continuing education in nursing*. Kansas City, Mo.: American Nurses' Association.
14. Henderson, V. (1977, May-June). We've "come a long way," but what of the direction? *Nursing Research, 26:*163-164.
15. Henderson, V., & Nite, G.A. (1978). *The principles and practice of nursing*. New York: Macmillan.
16. Henderson, V. (1978, March). The concepts of nursing, *Journal of Advanced Nursing, 3*:13-30.
17. Henderson, V. (1982, March). The nursing process—is the title right? *Journal of Advanced Nursing, 7:*103-109.
18. Henderson, V. (1984-1985). Telephone interviews.
19. Henderson, V. (1985, Summer). The essence of nursing in high technology. *Nursing Administration Quarterly, 9(4):*1-9.
20. Henderson, V. (1985). Personal correspondence.
21. Henderson, V. (1987, May). Nursing process—a critique. *Holistic Nursing Practice, 1(3):*7-18.
22. Holmes, P. (1985, Aug.). Who's afraid of Virginia Henderson? *Nursing Times, 81(32):*16-17.
23. Runk, J.A., & Muth, Quillin, S.I. (1983). Henderson's definition of nursing. In J.J. Fitzpatrick & A.L. Whall, *Conceptual models of nursing: An analysis and application*. Bowie, Md.: Robert J. Brady.
24. Safier, G. (1977). Virginia Henderson: Practitioner. In G. Safier, *Contemporary American leaders in nursing: An oral history*. New York: McGraw-Hill.
25. 70 Plus and going strong: Virginia Henderson, a nurse for all ages. (1983). *Geriatric Nursing, 4:*58-59.

BIBLIOGRAPHY

Primary Sources

Books

Harmer, B., & Henderson, V. (1939). *Textbook of the principles and practice of nursing* (4th ed.). New York: Macmillan.

Harmer, B., & Henderson, V. (1955). *Textbook of the principles and practice of nursing* (5th ed.). New York: Macmillan.

Henderson, V. (1966). *The nature of nursing: A definition and its implications for practice, research, and education*. New York: Macmillan.

Henderson, V. (1969). *ICN Basic principles of nursing care*. Geneva: International Council of Nursing.

Henderson, V. (1970). *Basic principles of nursing care*. Basel, N.Y.: Karger. (Pamphlet prepared for International Council of Nurses.)

Henderson, V., & Nite, G. (1978). *The principles and practice of nursing* (6th ed.). New York: Macmillan.

Henderson, V., & Simons, L.W. (1957). *The yearbook of modern nursing: 1956*. New York: G.P. Putnam's Sons.

Simmons, L.W., & Henderson, V. (1964). *Nursing research: A survey and assessment*. New York: Appleton-Century-Crofts.

Yale University School of Nursing Index Staff under the direction of Virginia Henderson. (1963-1972). *Nursing Studies Index* (4 vols.). Philadelphia: J.B. Lippincott.

Book Chapters

Henderson, V. (1974). On nursing care plans and their history. In American Journal of Nursing, *The nursing process in practice.* Kansas City, Mo.: American Nurses' Association.

Henderson, V. (1977). Annie Warburton Goodrich. In *Dictionary of American Biography: Supplement Five, 1951-1955.* New York: Charles Scribners' Sons.

Henderson, V. (1977). Awareness of library resources: A characteristic of professional workers. In American Nurses' Association, *Reference resources for research and continuing education.* Kansas City, Mo.: American Nurses' Association.

Articles

Henderson, V. (1937, Jan.). Paper and other substitutes for woven fabric. *American Journal of Nursing, 37:*23-32.

Henderson, V., et al. (1938, Nov.). Oxygen therapy: A study of some aspects of the operation of an oxygen tent. *American Journal of Nursing, 38:*1203-1216.

Henderson, V. (1955, Dec.). Annie Warburton Goodrich. *American Journal of Nursing, 55:*1488-1492.

Henderson, V. (1956, Feb.). Research in nursing practice—when? *Nursing Research, 4:*99.

Henderson, V. (1957, Oct.). An overview of nursing research. *Nursing Research, 6:*61-71.

Henderson, V. (1958, May 2). The basic principles of nursing care. *Nursing Mirror, 107:*337-338.

Henderson, V. (1958, May 9). The basic principles of nursing care, *Nursing Mirror, 107:*415-416.

Henderson, V. (1958, May 16). The basic principles of nursing care. *Nursing Mirror, 107:*497-498.

Henderson, V. (1958, May 23). The basic principles of nursing care. *Nursing Mirror, 107:*583-584.

Henderson, V. (1958, May 30). The basic principles of nursing care. *Nursing Mirror, 107:*651-652.

Henderson, V. (1958, June 6). The basic principles of nursing care. *Nursing Mirror, 107:*733-734.

Henderson, V. (1958, June 13). The basic principles of nursing care. *Nursing Mirror, 107:*803-804.

Henderson, V. (1964, Aug.). The nature of nursing. *American Journal of Nursing, 64:*63-68.

Henderson, V. (1965, Jan.-Feb.). The nature of nursing. *International Nursing Review, 12(1):*23-30.

Henderson, V. (1968, Spring). Some comments for nurses today. *The Alumnae Magazine* (Columbia University–Presbyterian Hospital School of Nursing Alumnae Association), pp. 5-15.

Henderson, V. (1968, April). Library resources in nursing: Their development and use (Part I). *International Nursing Review, 15(2):*164-182.

Henderson, V. (1968, July). Library resources in nursing: Their development and use (Part II). *International Nursing Review, 15(3):*236-247.

Henderson, V. (1968, Oct.). Library resources in nursing: Their development and use (Part III). *International Nursing Review, 15(4):*348-358.

Henderson, V. (1968, Oct.). Is the role of the nurse changing? *Weather Vane,* pp. 12-43.

Henderson, V. (1969, Oct.). Excellence in nursing. *American Journal of Nursing, 69:*2133-2137.

Henderson, V. (1971, Jan.). Implications for nursing in the library activities in regional medical programs. *Bulletin of the Medical Library Association, 59(1):*53-61.

Henderson, V. (1971, March). Health is everybody's business. *Canadian Nurse, 67:*31-34.

Henderson, V. (1973, June). On nursing care plans and their history. *Nursing Outlook, 21:*378-379.

Henderson, V. (1977, Jan.-Feb.). We've "come a long way," but what of the direction? *Nursing Research, 26:*163-164. (Guest editorial).

Henderson, V. (1977). The essence of nursing. *Virginia Nurse.*

Henderson, V. (1978, May 1). Professional writing. *Nursing Mirror and Midwives Journal,* pp. 5-18.

Henderson, V. (1978). The concept of nursing. *Journal of Advances in Nursing, 3:*113-130.

Henderson, V. (1979, Nov. 22-23). Preserving the essence of nursing in a technological age. *Nursing Times, 75:*2012.

Henderson, V. (1980, May). Preserving the essence of nursing in a technological age. *Journal of Advanced Nursing, 5:*245-260.

Henderson, V. (1980, May 22). Nursing—yesterday and tomorrow. *Nursing Times, 76:*905-907.

Henderson, V. (1982, March). The nursing process—is the title right? *Journal of Advanced Nursing, 7:*103-109.

Book Reviews

Henderson, V. (1969, January). Review of *Edith Cavell: Pioneer and patriot* by A.E. Clark-Kennedy. *Journal of the History of Medicine and Allied Sciences, 24(1):*100-101.

Henderson, V. (1973). Review of *Mary Adelaide Nutting: Pioneer of modern nursing* by Helen F. Marshall. *Journal of the History of Medicine and Allied Sciences.*

Henderson, V. (1976, Aug.). Review of *Equity in health services: Empirical analysis in social policy* by Ronald Anderson et al. *American Journal of Nursing, 76(1)*:1339-1340.

Henderson, V. (1979, Aug.). Review of *The advance of American nursing* by Philip A. Kalish and Beatrice J. Kalish. *Nursing Outlook, 27(8)*:554.

Henderson, V. (1969, March-April). Review of *A bibliography of nursing literature: 1859-1960* edited by Alice M.C. Thompson. *Nursing Research, 18(2)*:174-176.

Thesis

Henderson, V. (1935, June). *Medical and surgical asepsis: The development of asepsis and a study of current practice with recommendations in relation to certain aseptic nursing methods in hospitals.* (Department of Nursing Education, Teacher's College, Columbia University).

Correspondence

Henderson, V. (1984-1985). Telephone interviews.

Henderson, V. (1985). Personal correspondence.

Interviews

Community Health Nursing Revisited: A conversation with Virginia Henderson. By S.L. Shamansky. *Public Health Nursing, 1(4).*

70 plus and going strong: Virginia Henderson, a nurse for all ages. (1983). *Geriatric Nursing, 4:*58-59.

Virginia Henderson: A nursing's treasure. (1984). *Focus on Critical Care 11(3)*:60-61.

Who's afraid of Virginia Henderson? (1977, May 11). By C. Darby. *Nursing Mirror and Midwives Journal, 146:*15-18.

Videotapes

A Distinguished Leader in Nursing: Virginia Henderson. (1979). Capitol Heights, MD.: The National Advisory Center. Videotapes available from National Institute of Health, National Library of Medicine, and Sigma Theta Tau International, 1200 Waterway Blvd. Indianapolis, Ind. 46202

Nursing Theory: A Circle of Knowledge. (1987). New York: National League for Nursing. Available from the author, 10 Columbus Circle, New York, New York 10019.

The Nurse Theorists: Portraits of Excellence: Virginia Henderson. (1988). Oakland: Studio III, from Fuld Video Project, 370 Hawthorne Avenue, Oakland, Calif. 94609.

Secondary Sources

Books

Adam, E. (1980). *To be a nurse.* New York: W.B. Saunders.

Chinn, P.L., & Jacobs, M.K. (1983). *Theory and nursing: A systematic approach.* St. Louis: C.V. Mosby.

Walker, L.O., & Avant, K.C. (1983). *Strategies for theory construction in nursing.* Norwalk, Conn.: Appleton-Century-Crofts.

Book Chapters

Furukawa, C.Y., & Howe, J.K. (1980). Virginia Henderson. In Nursing Theories Practice Group, J.B. George, Chairperson, *Nursing theories: The base for professional nursing practice.* Englewood Cliffs, N.J.: Prentice-Hall.

Runk, J.A., & Muth Quillin, S.I., (1983). Henderson's definition of nursing. In J.J. Fitzpatrick, & A.L. Whall, *Conceptual models of nursing: Analysis and application.* Bowie, Md.: Robert J. Brady.

Safier, G. (1977). Virginia Henderson: Practitioner. In G. Safier, *Contemporary American leaders in nursing: An oral history.* New York: McGraw-Hill.

Articles

Ellis, R. (1968, May-June). Characteristics of significant theories. *Nursing Research, 17:*217-222.

Hardy, M.E. (1978). Perspectives on nursing theory. *Advances in Nursing Science, 1:*37-48.

9

Faye Glenn Abdellah

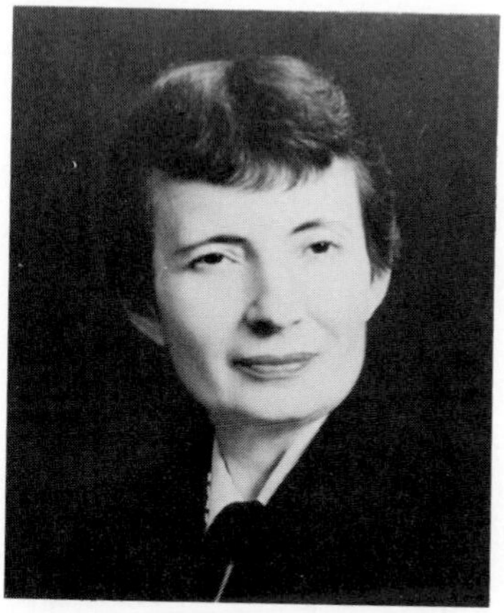

Twenty-one Nursing Problems

Dorothy Kay Dycus, Donna N. Schmeiser, Flossie M. Taggart, Roseanne Yancey

CREDENTIALS AND BACKGROUND OF THE THEORIST

Faye Glenn Abdellah was born in New York City. A 1942 Magna Cum Laude graduate of Fitkin Memorial Hospital School of Nursing (now Ann May School of Nursing), she received her B.S., M.A., and Ed.D. from Teacher's College at Columbia University. She completed her doctoral work in 1955.

Abdellah has practiced in many settings. She has been a staff nurse, a head nurse, a faculty member at Yale University and at Columbia University, a public health nurse, a researcher, and an author of more than 132 articles and books. Since 1949, Abdellah has held various positions in the U.S. Public Health Service, including nurse consultant to the states, chief of the nurse education branch, senior consultant of nursing research, principle investigator in the progressive patient care project, chief of the research grants branch, director of nursing home affairs, and director of long-term care.

Abdellah was appointed Chief Nurse Officer of the USPHS in 1970, and served in that position for 17 years. Concurrently, in 1982 she

The authors wish to express their appreciation to Dr. Faye G. Abdellah for critiquing the chapter.

was selected as Deputy Surgeon General, the first nurse and first woman to hold the post. Her office makes her the focal point for nursing and a chief adviser on long-term care policy within the Office of the Surgeon General. Abdellah represents the interests of health professionals in all categories in the PHS. She acts as advisor on matters related to nursing, long-term care policy, mental retardation, developmentally disabled, home health services, aging, and hospice. Because her efforts are directed toward improvement of the quality of health care for all Americans, she supervises the activities in both health and nonhealth agencies.

She is the recipient of over 40 academic awards and professional honors. These include selection as a Charter Fellow of the American Academy of Nursing; eight honorary degrees, including an honorary Doctor of Laws degree from Case Western Reserve University for pioneering nursing research and being responsible for the advent of the nurse-scientist scholar; an honorary degree from the University of Bridgeport for devoting her career to advancing the quality of health care through research and being an innovative and inspirational leader for nursing professionals; the Federal Nursing Service Award for the advancement of professional nursing; and the Distinguished Service Honor Award of the U.S. Department of Health, Education, and Welfare for exceptional leadership and professional commitment and the first presidential award of Sigma Theta Tau International.

Abdellah realized that for nursing to gain full professional status and autonomy, a strong knowledge base was imperative. Nursing also needed to move away from the control of medicine and toward a philosophy of comprehensive patient-centered care. Abdellah and her colleagues conceptualized 21 nursing problems to teach and evaluate students. The typology of 21 nursing problems first appeared in the 1960 edition of *Patient-centered Approaches to Nursing* and had a far-reaching impact on the profession and on the development of nursing theories.[9:34]

THEORETICAL SOURCES

A critique of Abdellah's work cannot be isolated from the background in which her typology of nursing problems was developed. Nursing practice and education in the 1950s were facing major problems resulting from technological advancement and social change. Old methods of educational preparation and practice based on functions and medical services were inadequate to meet the demands of the rapid change. The definition of nursing was becoming clouded. In Abdellah's opinion, one of the greatest barriers keeping nursing from a professional status was lack of a scientific body of knowledge unique to nursing. The educational system was not providing students and practitioners a means to cope with changing technology. Evaluation of students' clinical experiences based on a services approach provided no measure of quality of that experience. The delivery of care to patients was organized around meeting the needs of the institution rather than those of the patient.

The problem-solving method is the basis for Abdellah's model. It was formulated as a remedy to the problems facing nursing. The typology of 21 nursing problems and skills was developed to constitute the unique body of knowledge that is nursing.

Abdellah states that "nursing is both an art and a science that mold the attitude, intellectual competencies, and technical skills of the individual nurse into the desire and ability to help people, whether ill or not, cope with their health needs."[12]

"Her work is related to Henderson's fourteen principles and to her own research studies to establish the classification of nursing problems."[5] Knowledge of the problem-solving approach to nursing problems would provide a method of change with advancing technology. A qualititative assessment of student experiences could be made based on the nursing problems encountered and alleviated, while providing patients with patient-centered nursing care.

ABDELLAH'S TYPOLOGY OF 21 NURSING PROBLEMS

1. To maintain good hygiene and physical comfort.
2. To promote optimal activity: exercise, rest, and sleep.
3. To promote safety through prevention of accident, injury, or other trauma and through the prevention of the spread of infection.
4. To maintain good body mechanics and prevent and correct deformity.
5. To facilitate the maintenance of a supply of oxygen to all body cells.
6. To facilitate the maintenance of nutrition of all body cells.
7. To facilitate the maintenance of elimination.
8. To facilitate the maintenance of fluid and electrolyte balance.
9. To recognize the physiological responses of the body to disease conditions—pathological, physiological, and compensatory.
10. To facilitate the maintenance of regulatory mechanisms and functions.
11. To facilitate the maintenance of sensory function.
12. To identify and accept positive and negative expressions, feelings, and reactions.
13. To identify and accept interrelatedness of emotions and organic illness.
14. To facilitate the maintenance of effective verbal and nonverbal communication.
15. To promote the development of productive interpersonal relationships.
16. To facilitate awareness of self as an individual with varying physical, emotional, and developmental needs.
17. To create and/or maintain a therapeutic environment.
18. To facilitate awareness of self as an individual with varying physical, emotional, and developmental needs.
19. To accept the optimum possible goals in the light of limitations, physical, and emotional.
20. To use community resources as an aid in resolving problems arising from illness.
21. To understand the role of social problems as influencing factors in the cause of illness.

USE OF EMPIRICAL EVIDENCE

The typology was developed from several studies conducted during the 1950s. In the study, *Appraising the Clinical Resources in Small Hospitals,* Abdellah and Levine[6] classified medical diagnoses of more than 1700 patients into 58 categories thought to represent common nursing problems. Abdellah's dissertation,[1] *Methods of Determining Covert Aspects of Nursing Problems as a Basis for Improved Clinical Teaching,* reported findings from her study designed to identify what interview technique provided the most complete list of patients' problems. The study revealed that a free-answer method was the most productive for identifying nursing problems. When used with patients, this method elicited many more covert (emotional-social) problems than a pictorial interview technique or direct questioning approach.[2] Also in 1955, the National League for Nursing (NLN) Committee on Records formed a subcommittee to develop a meaningful clinical evaluation tool. The subcommittee members, with the assistance of faculties from 40 NLN-accredited collegiate schools of nursing, compressed the 58 patient categories into 21 common nursing problems, and reported their development and use in *Patient-centered Approaches to Nursing* in 1960.

MAJOR CONCEPTS AND DEFINITIONS

NURSING. In writing the typology of 21 nursing problems, which served as a basis of her nursing theory,[5] Abdellah was also creating a guide for nurses to use in identifying and solving patient problems. The concept of nursing was therefore a primary component of her writing. Abdellah[11:24] defined nursing as:

> service to individuals and families; therefore, to society. It is based upon an art and science which mold the attitudes, intellectual competencies, and technical skills of the individual nurse into the desire and ability to help people sick or well cope with their health needs, and may be carried out under general or specific medical direction.

Abdellah was clearly promoting the image of the nurse who was not only kind and caring, but also intelligent, competent, and technically well prepared to provide service to the patient.

NURSING PROBLEM. A second major concept in Abdellah's work was the nursing problem. The "nursing problem presented by the patient is a condition faced by the patient or family which the nurse can assist him or them to meet through the performance of her professional functions."[11:7] The problem can be either an overt or covert nursing problem.

Abdellah states that her present perception would be to change nursing problem to patient/client problem. An "overt nursing problem is an apparent condition faced by the patient or family which the nurse can assist him or them to meet through the performance of her professional functions."[2:4] The "covert nursing problem is a concealed or hidden condition faced by the patient or family which the nurse can assist him or them to meet through the performance of her professional functions."[2:4]

Although Abdellah spoke of the patient-centered approaches, she wrote of nurses identifying and solving specific problems. This identification and classification of problems was called the typology of 21 nursing problems (see box on p. 95). Abdellah's typology[11:11] was divided into three areas: (1) the physical, sociological, and emotional needs of the patient; (2) the types of interpersonal relationships between the nurse and the patient; and (3) the common elements of patient care. Abdellah and her colleagues thought the typology would provide a method to evaluate a student's experiences and also a method to evaluate a nurse's competency.

PROBLEM SOLVING. "The process of identifying overt and covert nursing problems and interpreting, analyzing, and selecting appropriate courses of action to solve these problems" is problem solving, the final building block of Abdellah's writing.[11:26] Abdellah wrote that the nurse must be able to solve problems in order to give the best professional nursing care. This process, which closely resembles the steps of the nursing process, involves identifying the problem, selecting data, and formulating, testing, and revising hypotheses. According to Abdellah, the patient will not receive quality nursing care if the steps to problem solving are done incorrectly.

Abdellah identifies nursing diagnosis as a subconcept of the problem-solving process. It is defined as the "determination of the nature and extent of nursing problems presented by individual patients or families receiving care."[11:9]

MAJOR ASSUMPTIONS

Nursing

Nursing is a helping profession. In Abdellah's model, nursing care is doing something to or for the person or providing information to the person with the goal of meeting needs, increasing or restoring self-help ability, or alleviating an impairment.

Determination of nursing care strategies to

be administered is based on the problem-solving approach. The nursing process is viewed as problem solving and the correct identification of nursing problems is a paramount concern. Direct observation of overt needs may be possible, but determination of covert needs requires mastery of communication skills and patient interaction. Deciding how patient needs can best be met is considered the responsibility of hospital and public health personnel.

"As long as self-help ability is developed and maintained at a level at which need satisfaction can take place without assistance, nursing care will not be required."[11:56] The role of the nurse in health promotion is limited to circumstances of anticipated impairment. In 1960 Abdellah[11:23] stated that physicians need more knowledge about prevention and rehabilitation than do nurses. But in correspondence with the authors in 1984, Abdellah indicated it is important that nurses also know about prevention and rehabilitation.

Also in 1984 she stated, "It is hoped that preoccupation with illness-oriented assessment methods will not diminish concern with the promotion of wellness."[16:111] No consideration is given to achievement of a higher level of wellness than is present when personal needs are met or when actual and anticipated impairments are absent.

Person

Abdellah describes people as having physical, emotional, and sociological needs. These needs may be overt, consisting of largely physical needs, or covert, such as emotional and social needs. The typology of nursing problems is said to evolve from the recognition of a need for patient-centered approaches to nursing. The patient is described as the only justification for the existence of nursing. But as previously discussed, the patient is not the central focus of Abdellah's work.

People are helped by the identification and alleviation of problems they are experiencing. The model implies that by resolving each problem the person returns to a healthy state or one with which he can cope; therefore, the idea of holism is absent in this model. The whole, which is the patient, is not greater than the sum of its parts, which are his problems.

In Abdellah's model all persons have self-help ability and the capacity to learn, both of which vary from one individual to another. Because identifying these qualities in a comatose patient or an infant without family resources may be difficult, omissions could result when organizing such patients' care with this model.

Environment

The environment is the least-discussed concept in Abdellah's model. Nursing problem number 17, from the typology, is "to create and/or maintain a therapeutic environment."[11:17] Abdellah also states that if the nurse's reaction to the patient is hostile or negative, the atmosphere in the room may be hostile or negative. This suggests that patients interact with and respond to their environment and that the nurse is part of that environment.

The environment is also the home and community from which the patient comes. Although fleetingly discussed, Abdellah urges that nurses not limit the identification of nursing problems to those existing only in the hospital. She predicts a future community center that will extend beyond the four walls of the hospital into the community.

Abdellah states that in 1988 she would "give greater emphasis to environment and health promotion."[5]

Health

Health, as Abdellah discusses in *Patient-centered Approaches to Nursing,* is a state mutually exclusive of illness. Health is defined implicitly as a state when the individual has no unmet needs and no anticipated or actual impairments. Much of nursing practice in the 1950s focused on remedial or illness care, so it is not surprising that health was not clearly defined. But 30 years have passed since the book was published and Abdellah[4] now says she "would certainly place greater emphasis today on health status as an important part of the wellness-sickness continuum." She also fully supports the holistic approach to patient-centered care and the need for greater attention on environmental factors.

THEORETICAL ASSERTIONS

Several assertions were repeatedly stated by Abdellah although they were not labeled as such. These assertions are:

1. "The nursing problem and nursing treatment typologies are the principles of nursing practice and constitute the unique body of knowledge that is nursing."[11:12]
2. "Correct identification of the nursing problem influences the nurse's judgment in selecting steps in solving the patient's problem."[9:492]
3. The core of nursing is patient/client problems that focus on the patient and his/her problems.[5]

According to Reynolds,[17:68] statements of assertion can be either existence or relational statements. Assertions 1 and 3 are of the existence type, while assertion 2 is relational.

Neither the major components of the nursing paradigm nor the central concepts are clearly linked with relational statements. Such structure cannot be diagrammed without imposing the critic's conclusions regarding the existence of relationships. Because the components of person, health, and environment were only implicitly defined, no attempt will be made to propose relationships between them. The major concepts that are more clearly defined by Abdellah are thought to be associated in this manner. Nursing, through the identification of nursing problems and usage of the problem-solving process, helps the client meet his needs. As late as 1972 Abdellah[3:234] stated, "The patient, his needs, and the nurse meeting his needs through nursing service is the only raison d'être for the nursing profession." Abdellah's statement exemplifies her major concerns and implied relationships.

LOGICAL FORM

The logical form can best be described as an inductive approach that generalizes from particulars. Abdellah used her multiple observations from the studies mentioned previously as the basis for her typology. Thus the typology developed from research toward theory.

ACCEPTANCE BY THE NURSING COMMUNITY

In discussing the acceptance by the nursing community, one must be aware of two distinct times within the history of nursing—the mid-1950s through early 1960s and the present. When *Patient-centered Approaches to Nursing* was published in 1960, the profession of nursing was striving to clarify its practice area and to identify rationale for its actions based on scientific knowledge. The introduction of the 21 nursing problems had profound effects on the areas of practice, education, and research. Now they are associated with nursing diagnosis.

Practice

Abdellah's typology of 21 nursing problems helps nurses practice in an organized, systematic way. The use of this scientific base enabled the nurse to understand the reasons for her actions. The clinical practitioner, using the 21 nursing problems, could assess the patient, make a nursing diagnosis, and plan interventions. Through the problem-solving process the nurse attempted to make the patient, rather than his medical condition, the central figure. By using the typology and the problem-solving process in the clinical setting, nurses gave their practice a scientific basis.

When asked to contrast the 21 nursing problems with the nursing diagnoses being promoted today, Dr. Abdellah says that it would have been heresy to use the term diagnosis in relation to nursing 25 years ago. Today she would describe them as being problems presented by patients or clients rather than nursing problems. But, she adds, there is a lot of similarity between the 21 nursing problems and the recently established diagnostic related groupings (DRGs). Both involve classification systems. The former could be used to provide the basis for determining acuity of illness, nursing outcomes, and costs of nursing services. This is particularly important as DRGs move into home care and ambulatory settings.[13:32]

Education

Abdellah's 21 nursing problems had their most dramatic effect on the educational system within nursing. Nursing educators were aware that curricula changes were needed if nurses were to become autonomous. They recognized that the greatest weakness in the profession was the lack of a scientific body of knowledge unique to nursing. The typology provided such a body of knowledge and an opportunity to move away from the medical model of educating nurses. The typology of 21 problems was widely accepted in the nursing community in all types of programs—2-, 3-, and 4-year.

Research

Because the typology of 21 nursing problems was created through research, it is not surprising that more research followed its introduction. Was this typology really necessary from an administrative point of view? Had not hospitals been doing well without it? The amount of time the nurse spent with the patient was examined in the form of function studies. How could the patient receive comprehensive patient care in 18 minutes per 8-hour shift? Does the hospital administration serve the patient or does it serve someone else? To answer these questions Abdellah and Strachan[10] extended the research and used the typology as the basis for developing the nursing care model used for planning staffing patterns in clinical settings. These staffing patterns were based on patients' identified needs and as Abdellah envisioned, consisted of intensive care, intermediate care, long-term care, self-care, and home-care units. By grouping patients with similar needs instead of diagnoses, nursing service could provide the best staffing patterns to meet patients' needs.

FURTHER DEVELOPMENT

According to Dickoff and James' categories,[14] Abdellah's typology may be recognized as a level one theory—categories or classifications. Currently, the nursing community's use of the 21 nursing problems has moved into a second generation of development, which includes patient problems and patient outcomes rather than nursing problems and outcomes.

Abdellah[4] is pleased with the shift of emphasis from nursing problems to patient outcomes. She believes that 30 years ago the concept of nursing problems was used to identify a strong nursing role in patient care. If the initial emphasis had been on patient problems instead, the concept would *not* have been accepted and the medical model would have been perpetuated.

The concepts of problem-solving and nursing diagnosis continue to be used in the settings of practice, education, and research. Critical thinking and validating of theory in the practice area is needed within the profession. More sophisticated research tools might be designed to thoroughly study problem solving and how nurses apply this concept. The nursing diagnosis classification system may be considered an outgrowth of the typology. Currently nursing diagnosis is a classification system describing patient signs and symptoms. Expanding this system to explain outcomes may be possible through additional research.

CRITIQUE

Simplicity

The typology is very simple and is descriptive of nursing problems thought to be common among patients. The concepts of nursing, nursing problems, and the problem-solving process, which are central to this work, are defined explicitly. The concepts of person, health, and environment, which are associated with the nursing paradigm today, are implied. There are no stated relationships between Abdellah's major concepts or those of the nursing paradigm in her writing. This model has a limited number of concepts, and its only structure is a list. A somewhat mixed approach to concept definition is present in this work. Nursing and nursing problems are connotatively defined, while the problem-solving process is defined denotatively. These approaches to definitions do not seem to detract from the clarity of definitions. The typology does not yet constitute a theory because it lacks sufficient relationship statements.

Generality

The 21 nursing problems are general and linked to neither time nor environment. "She acknowledges that her list is neither exhaustive nor listed according to priorities."[13:32] Assuming that persons experience similar needs, the nursing goals stated in the list of 21 problems could be used by nurses in any time frame to meet patients' needs. However, according to this model, some persons do not need nursing.

Other service professions could use the typology of 21 nursing problems to focus on the psychosocial and emotional needs presented by patients. The goals of this model vary in generality. The broadest goal is to positively affect nursing education, while subgoals are to provide a scientific basis on which to practice and to provide a method of qualitative evaluation of educational experiences for students. The goals are appropriate for nursing.

Empirical Precision

The concepts are very specific with empirical referents easily identifiable. The concepts are within the domain of nursing. Ready linkage of the concepts and the typology to reality is secondary to an inductive approach to theory development. Validation of the typology was done by the faculty of 40 collegiate schools of nursing. Chapters 4, 5, and 6 of *Patient-centered Approaches to Nursing* describe different approaches to implementation and use of the typology in three programs of nursing.

Derivable Consequences

The typology provided a general framework in which to act, but continued neither specific nursing actions nor patient-centered outcomes, despite the title of the book. However, two subsequent publications did address outcome measures (effect variables) and suggested models for organizing curricula to emphasize patient-centered outcomes.[6,10] Except for stating the importance of nursing the whole patient, today's idea of holism is not apparent in this work. The skills list includes skills thought necessary for nurses to meet patients' needs but is not prescriptive. Abdellah suggests nursing research as a method for validating treatments toward resolution of patients' needs.

The emphasis on problem-solving is not limited by time or space and therefore provides a means for continued growth and change in the provision of nursing care. The problem-solving process and the typology of 21 nursing problems can be respectively considered precursors of the nursing care process and classification of nursing diagnoses in evidence today.

In *Patient-centered Approaches to Nursing Care,* Abdellah addressed nursing education problems linked to the use of the medical model. Her typology provided a new way to qualitatively evaluate experiences and emphasized a practice based on sound rationales rather than rote.

"She proposes that nurses could take a leadership role in making the public aware that quality nursing health care is available. Quality is defined as the care that the patient needs. Need is determined by a classification system that identifies the medical treatment and nursing care essential for that individual."[13:33]

Abdellah has made significant contributions to patient care, education, and research in nursing and health care in this country and throughout the world.[13:33]

REFERENCES

1. Abdellah, F.G. (1955). *Methods of determining covert aspects of nursing problems as basis for improved clinical teaching.* Doctoral dissertation, New York Teacher's College, Columbia University.
2. Abdellah, F.G. (1957, June). Methods of identifying covert aspects of nursing problems. *Nursing Research, 6:*4.
3. Abdellah, F.G. (1972). Evolution of nursing as a profession: Perspective on manpower development. *International Nursing Review, 19:*3.
4. Abdellah, F.G. (1984, March 7). Personal Correspondence.
5. Abdellah, F.G. (1988, April 28). Personal Correspondence.
6. Abdellah, F.G., & Levine, E. (1954). *Appraising the clinical resources in small hospitals* (U.S. Public Health Service. Pub. No. 389). Washington, D.C.: U.S. Government Printing Office.
7. Abdellah, F.G., & Levine, E. (1958). Effect of nurse staffing on satisfactions with nursing care. In *Hospital Monograph Series No. 4.* Chicago: American Hospital Association.
8. Abdellah, F.G., & Levine, E. (1965). *Better patient care through nursing research.* New York: Macmillan.
9. Abdellah, F.G., Levine, E., & Levine, B.S. (1986). *Better patient care through nursing research* (3d ed.). New York: Macmillan.
10. Abdellah, F.G., & Strachan, E.J. (1959, May). Progressive patient care, *American Journal of Nursing, 59:*5.
11. Abdellah, F.G., et al. (1960). *Patient-centered approaches to nursing.* New York: Macmillan.
12. Abdellah, F.G., et al. (1973). *New directions in patient-centered nursing: Guidelines for systems of service, education, and research.* New York: Macmillan.
13. Abdellah, F.G. (1986. Oct.). Faye G. Abdellah—working to enrich the profession (interview). *Focus on Critical Care. 13(5):*32-33.
14. Dickoff, J., & James, P. (1968, March). A theory of theories: A position paper. *Nursing Research, 17:*3.
15. Falco, S.M. (1980). Faye G. Abdellah. In Nursing Theories Conference Group & J.B. George Chairperson, *Nursing Theories: The base for professional practice.* Englewood Cliffs, N.J.: Prentice-Hall.
16. Levine, E., & Abdellah, F.G. (1984, Summer). DRGs: Nursing has been using them for a long time. *Inquiry.*
17. Reynolds, P.D. (1971). A primer in theory construction. Indianapolis: Bobbs-Merrill.

BIBLIOGRAPHY

Primary Sources

Books

Abdellah, F.G. (1968). *An overview of nurse-scientist programs in the country.* National League for Nursing No. 15-1342.

Abdellah, F.G. (1972). *A career in nursing.* B'nai B'rith Career and Counseling Services Occupational Brief Series. Washington, D.C.: B'nai B'rith.

Abdellah, F.G. (1972). *Extending the scope of nursing practice.* National League for Nursing Pub. No. 15-1473.

Abdellah, F.G., & Levine, E. (1954). *Appraising the clinical resources in small hospitals* (U.S. Public Health Service Pub. No. 389). Washington, D.C.: U.S. Government Printing Office.

Abdellah, F.G., & Levine, E. (1957). *Patients and personnel speak: A method of studying patient care in hospitals* (U.S. Public Health Service Pub. No. 527). Washington, D.C.: U.S. Government Printing Office.

Abdellah, F.G., & Levine, E. (1958). *Effect of nurse staffing on satisfactions with nursing care: A study of how omissions in nursing services, as perceived by patients and personnel, are influenced by the number of nursing hours available.* Chicago: American Hospital Association.

Abdellah, F.G., & Levine, E. (1965). *Better patient care through nursing research.* New York: Macmillan.

Abdellah, F.G., & Levine, E. (1979). *Better patient care through nursing research* (2d ed). New York: Macmillan.

Abdellah, F.G., Levine, E., & Levine, B.S. (1986). *Better patient care through nursing research.* (3d ed.). New York: Macmillan.

Abdellah, F.G., Meltzer, L.E., & Kitchell, J.R. (Eds.). (1969). *Concepts and practices of intensive care for nurse specialists*. Philadelphia: Charles Press.

Abdellah, F.G., Meltzer, L.E., & Kitchell, J.R. (Eds.). (1976). *Concepts and practices of intensive care for nurse specialists* (2d ed). Bowie, Md.: Charles Press.

Abdellah, F.G., Schwartz, D.R., & Smoyak, S.A. (1975). *Models for health care delivery: Now and for the future* (American Nurses Association No. G 119). American Academy of Nursing.

Abdellah, F.G., Walsh, M.E., & Brown, E.L. (1979). *Health care in the 1980's: Who provides? Who plans? Who pays?* National League for Nursing Pub. No. 52-1755.

Abdellah, F.G., et al. (1960). *Patient-centered approaches to nursing*. New York: Macmillan.

Abdellah, F.G., et al. (1968). *Patient-centered approaches to nursing* (2nd ed.). New York: Macmillan.

Abdellah, F.G., et al. (1973). *New directions in patient-centered nursing*. New York: Macmillan.

Dissertation

Abdellah, F.G. (1955). *Methods of determining covert aspects of nursing problems as basis for improved clinical teaching*. New York Teacher's College, Columbia University.

Book Chapters

Abdellah, F.G. (1985). The aging woman and the future of health care delivery. In M.R. Haug, A.B. Ford, & M. Scheafor (Eds.). *The physical and mental health of aged women*. New York: Springer Publishing Co.

Abdellah, F.G. (1986). The nature of nursing science. In L.H. Nicoll (Ed.). *Perspectives on nursing theory*. Boston: Little, Brown.

Abdellah, F.G. (1986). Nurses as primary health care providers in USA. In [*The accountability of nurses in a changing society*.] International Nurses' Foundation of Japan (INFI).

McCormick, K.A., & Abdellah, F.G. (1984). Respiratory failure: Technological care in the home and hospital. In S.J. Reiser & M. Anbar (Eds.). *The machine at the bedside*. Mass.: Cambridge University Press.

Articles

Abdellah, F.G. (1952, June). State nursing surveys and community action. *Public Health Reports, 67*:554-560.

Abdellah, F.G. (1953, July) Some trends in nursing education. *American Journal of Nursing, 53*:841-843.

Abdellah, F.G. (1954, May). Surveys stimulate community action. *Nursing Outlook, 2*:268-270.

Abdellah, F.G. (1957, June). Methods of identifying covert aspects of nursing problems. *Nursing Research, 6*:4.

Abdellah, F.G. (1959, May). How we look at ourselves. *Nursing Outlook, 7*:273.

Abdellah, F.G. (1960, June). Progressive patient care: A challenge for nursing. *Hospital Management, 89*:102.

Abdellah, F.G. (1960, Aug.). Nursing patterns vary in progressive care. *Modern Hospital, 95*:85.

Abdellah, F.G. (1961, April). The decision is yours. *Nursing Outlook, 9*:223.

Abdellah, F.G. (1961, Winter). Criterion measures in nursing. *Nursing Research, 10*:21.

Abdellah, F.G. (1965, Oct.). Search or research? An experiment to stimulate research. *Nursing Outlook, 13*:65-67.

Abdellah, F.G. (1966). Frontiers in nursing research. *Nursing Forum, 5*:28-38.

Abdellah, F.G. (1967, Fall). Approaches to protecting the rights of human subjects. *Nursing Research, 16*:315-320.

Abdellah, F.G. (1969, Sept.-Oct.). The nature of nursing science. *Nursing Research, 18*:390-393.

Abdellah, F.G. (1969, Dec.). Nursing research in the health services, *Nursing Research Reports, 4*:2. (Editorial).

Abdellah, F.G. (1970, Jan.-Feb.). Overview of nursing research: 1955-1968 (Part I). *Nursing Research, 19*:6-17.

Abdellah, F.G. (1970, March-April). Overview of nursing research: 1955-1968 (Part II). *Nursing Research, 19*:151-162.

Abdellah, F.G. (1970, May-June). Overview of nursing research: 1955-1968 (Part III). *Nursing Research, 19*:239-252.

Abdellah, F.G. (1970, May). Training and development of the health care team. *AORN Journal, 11*:86-91.

Abdellah, F.G. (1970, Summer). Conference on the nature of science in nursing. The nature of nursing science. *Japanese Journal of Nursing Research, 3*:248-252.

Abdellah, F.G. (1971, May). Problems, issues, challenges of nursing research. *Canadian Nurse, 67*:44-46.

Abdellah, F.G. (1972, Oct.). No legal bars to expanded nursing practice. *Stat, 41:*4.
Abdellah, F.G. (1972, Sept.). The physician-nurse team approach to coronary care. *Nursing Clinics of North America, 7:*423-430.
Abdellah, F.G. (1972). Evolution of nursing as a profession: Perspective on manpower development. *International Nursing Review, 19:*219-238.
Abdellah, F.G. (1973, Jan.-Feb.). Criterios de avaliac as em enfermagen. *Revista Brasileira de Enfermagem, 26:*17-32. (Portugal).
Abdellah, F.G. (1973, May). Research on career development in the health professions: Nursing. *Occupational Health Nursing, 21:*12-16.
Abdellah, F.G. (1973, June). School nurse practitioner: An expanded role for nurses. *Journal of the American College Health Association, 21:*423-432.
Abdellah, F.G. (1973, Dec.). Nursing and health care in the USSR. *American Journal of Nursing, 73:*2096-2099.
Abdellah, F.G. (1974, Spring). Long-term care: A top health priority. *Journal of Long-Term Care Administration, 2(2):*1-3. (Guest editorial).
Abdellah, F.G. (1974, Fall). Health care issues: Overview of emerging health services delivery projects. *Health Care Dimensions,* pp. 125-139.
Abdellah, F.G. (1974). A national health strategy for the delivery of long-term health care: Implications for nursing. *Journal of New York State Nurses' Association, 5(4):*7-13.
Abdellah, F.G. (1975, Jan.-Feb.). National library of medicine is official nursing archives. *Nursing Research, 24(1):*64. (Letter).
Abdellah, F.G. (1975, Sept.-Oct.). The nursing archives at the national library of medicine. *Nursing Research, 24(5):*389. (Letter).
Abdellah, F.G. (1975, Nov.). Three views. Patient assessment: Its potential and use (Part 1). *American Health Care Association Journal, 1:*69.
Abdellah, F.G. (1976, March). Nurse practitioners and nursing practice. *American Journal of Public Health, 66(3):*245-246. (Editorial).
Abdellah, F.G. (1976, Aug.). Nursing's role in future health care. *AORN Journal, 24(2):*236-240.
Abdellah, F.G. (1977, July-Aug.). U.S. Public Health Service's contribution to nursing research—past, present, future. *Nursing Research, 26(4):*244-249.
Abdellah, F.G. (1978, July). Long-term care policy issues: Alternatives to institutional care. *American Academy of Political and Social Science Annals, 438:*28-29.
Abdellah, F.G. (1981, Nov.). Nursing care of the aged in the United States of America. *Journal of Gerontological Nursing, 7(11):*657-663.
Abdellah, F.G. (1982, Summer). The nurse practitioner 17 years later: Present and emerging issues. *Inquiry, 19(2):*105-116.
Abdellah, F.G. (1982, Dec.). Keynote address, 75th anniversary of the West Virginia State Nurse's Association. *Weather Vane, 51(6):*10-13, 15.
Abdellah, F.G. (1983, Feb.-March). Future directions: Impact on NSNA 1982 and 2012. *Imprint, 30(1):*66-74.
Abdellah, F.G. (1983, April-May). Future directions of the profession: Impact on NSNA 1982 and 2012 (Part II). *Imprint, 30(2):*91-97.
Abdellah, F.G. (1983, March-April 6-7). 1983-2008: Nursing practice. *Arizona Nurse.*
Abdellah, F.G. (1984, Feb.). New roles in the Federal Nursing Services. *Today's OR Nurse. 6(2):*6.
Abdellah, F.G. (1984, July). Nursing in the world: 35 years of development after World War II. Changes affecting nursing in the United States 1949-1984. *Kango Tenbo, 36(8):*2-10. (Japanese Journal of Nursing Science).
Abdellah, F.G. (1985, June 5-11). Standards of care: Hospitals mean business. *Nursing Times, 81(23):*36-37.
Abdellah, F.G. (1987, Feb.), Practice model of nursing for "Health for All." *Kango Tenbo, 12(2):*164–169. (Japanese Journal of Nursing Science).
Abdellah, F.G. (1987, Sept.-Oct.). The federal role in nursing education. *Nursing Outlook, 35(5):*224-225.
Abdellah, F.G., Chamberlain, J.G., & Levine, I.S. (1986, Sept.-Oct.). Role of nurses in meeting needs of the homeless: Summary of a workshop for providers, researchers, and educators. *Public Health Reports, 101(5):*494–498.
Abdellah, F.G., & Chow, R.K. (1976, Nov.-Dec.). The long-term care facility improvement campaign: The PACE project. *Association of Rehabilitation Nurses' Journal, 1(7):*3-4.
Abdellah, F.G., & Chow, R.K. (1976, Winter). Long-term care facility improvement—a nationwide research effort. *Journal of Long-Term Care Administration, 4(1):*5-19.
Abdellah, F.G., Foerst, H.V., & Chow, R.K. (1979, June). PACE: An approach to improving the care

of the elderly. *American Journal of Nursing, 79(6)*:1109-1110.

Abdellah, F.G., & Levine, E. (1954, June). Why nurses leave home. *Hospitals, 28*:80-81.

Abdellah, F.G., & Levine, E. (1957, Feb.). Developing a measure of patient and personnel satisfaction with nursing care. *American Journal of Nursing, 5*:100.

Abdellah, F.G., & Levine, E. (1957, Nov. 1). Polling patients and personnel: What patients say about their nursing care (Part I). *Hospitals, 31*:44.

Abdellah, F.G., & Levine, E. (1957, Nov. 16). What factors affect patients' opinions of their nursing care? (Part 2). *Hospitals, 31*:61.

Abdellah, F.G., & Levine, E. (1957, Dec. 1). What personnel say about nursing care (Part 3). *Hospitals, 31*:53.

Abdellah, F.G., & Levine, E. (1957, Dec. 16). What hospitals have done to improve patient care (Part 4). *Hospitals*, 31:43.

Abdellah, F.G., & Levine, E. (1965, April). Better patient care through nursing research. *International Journal of Nursing Studies, 2*:1.

Abdellah, F.G., & Levine, E. (1965, Winter). The aims of nursing research. *Nursing Research, 14*:27.

Abdellah, F.G., & Levine, E. (1966, Jan.). Future directions of research in nursing. *American Journal of Nursing, 66*:112-116.

Abdellah, F.G., & Levine, E. (1968, Summer). The aims of nursing research. *Comprehensive Nursing Monthly, 3*:12-31. (Japan).

Abdellah, F.G., & Levine, E. (1982, Aug.). Better patient care through nursing research (Part 1). *Kango Tenbo, 7(8)*:714-719. (Japanese Journal of Nursing Science).

Abdellah, F.G., & Strachan, E.J. (1959, May). Progressive patient care. *American Journal of Nursing, 59*:649.

Levine, E., & Abdellah, F.G. (1984, Summer). DRGs: A recent refinement to an old method. *Inquiry, 21(2)*:105–112.

Matarazzo, J.D., Abdellah, F.G. (1971, Sept.-Oct.). Doctoral education for nurses in the U.S. *Nursing Research, 20*:404-414.

Muller, J.E., et al. (1972, March). The Soviet health system: Aspects of relevance for medicine in the U.S. *New England Journal of Medicine, 286*:693-702.

Conferences

Hogness, J.R., Atkinson, H., Abdellah, F.G., Foster, J., Haley, R.W., & Patterson, R.A. (1984, March 29-30). International Conference on the Reuse of Disposable Medical Devices in the 1980's. Final Report of the Conference Panel, Washington, D.C.: Institute for Health Policy Analysis, Georgetown University Medical Center. (Conference proceedings also published by the Institute for Health Policy Analysis.)

Correspondence

Abdellah, F.G. (1984, March 7). Personal letter.

Abdellah, F.G. (1988, April 28). Personal letter.

Secondary Sources

Book Reviews

Abdellah, F.G., & Levine, E. (1957). *Patients and personnel speak: A method of studying patient care in hospitals.*
American Journal of Nursing, 59:634-635, May 1959.

Abdellah, F.G., & Levine, E. (1965). *Better patient care through nursing research* (1st ed.).
Hospitals, 39:115, November 1965.
Nursing Outlook, 13:18, December 1965.
Catholic Nurse, 14:63, March 1966.
American Journal of Nursing, 66:828, April 1966.
Nursing Research, 15:217, Summer 1966.
Nursing Research Reports, 2:6, June 1967.

Abdellah, F.G., & Levine, E. (1979). *Better patient care through nursing research* (2d ed.).
American Journal of Nursing, 80:67-68, January 1980.

Abdellah, F.G., et al. (1963). *Patient-centered approaches to nursing.*
Hospital Administration, 8:48, Spring 1963.

Abdellah, F.G., et al. (1973). *New directions in patient-centered nursing.*
American Journal of Nursing, 73:1439, August 1973.
Nursing Outlook, 22:555, September 1974.

Interviews

Abdellah, F.G. (1984, Jan.). Interview with Faye Abdellah (interview by Judith Rodin). *American Psychologist, 39(1)*:67-70.

Abdellah, F.G. (1986, May). An interview with Faye G. Abdellah (interview by S. Senno). *Kango*

Tenbo, 11(6):592-593. (Japanese Journal of Nursing Science).

News Releases

Two Named to Top Nurse Rank in P.H.S. (1970, Nov.). *Nursing Outlook,* 18:10.

Public Health Service Now Has Two Lady Admirals: Jessie Scott and Faye Abdellah. (1970, Nov.). *American Journal of Nursing, 70:*2281.

Appointments. (1971, Jan.). *H.S.M.H.A. Health Report, 36:*27-38.

Department of Health, Education, and Welfare (1971, Jan.-Feb.). Faye C. Abdellah: A New Appointment. *Journal of Continuing Education in Nursing, 2:*9.

Biographic Sources

Directory of Nurses with Doctoral Degrees. (1980, Aug.). American Nurses Association. (ANA Publication No. G-143).

Faye Abdellah Sees Bright Future for Nurses. (1980, September). *American Journal of Nursing, 80:*1671-1672.

The National Nursing Directory. (1982). Rockville, Md.: Aspen Systems.

Who's Who in America: 1982-1983. (42nd ed.). (1982). Chicago, Marquis.

Books

Dolan, J.A., Fitzpatrick, M.L., & Herrmann, E.K. (1983). *Nursing in society: A historical perspective* (15th ed.). Philadelphia: W.B. Saunders.

Griffin, J.G., & Griffin, J.K. (1973). *History and trends of professional nursing.* St. Louis: C.V. Mosby.

Nursing Theories Conference Group, J.B., George, Chairperson. (1980). *Nursing theories: The base for professional practice.* Englewood Cliffs, N.J.: Prentice-Hall.

Orem, D.E. (ed.) (1979). *Concept formalization in nursing, process and product.* Boston: Little, Brown, & Co.

Book Chapters

Falco, S.M. (1980). Faye Abdellah. In Nursing Theories Conference Group, J.B. George, Chairperson, *Nursing theories: The base for professional nursing practice.* Englewood Cliffs, N.J.: Prentice Hall.

Articles

Adebo, E.O. (1974). Identifying problems for nursing research. *International Nursing Review, 21(2):*53.

Alward, R.R. (1983). Patient classification system: The ideal vs. reality. *Journal of Nursing Administration, 13(2):*14-19.

Armiger, B. (1977). Ethics of nursing research: Profile, principles perspective. *Nursing Research, 26(5):*330-336.

Auger, J.A., & Dee, V. (1983). A patient classification system based on the behavioral system model of nursing. *Journal of Nursing Administration, 13(4):*38-43.

Auster, D. (1978). Occupational values of male and female nursing students. *Sociology of Work and Occupations, 5(2):*209-233.

Ballard, S., & McNamara, R. (1983). Qualifying nursing needs in home health care. *Nursing Research, 32(4):*236-241.

Bergman, R., et al. (1981). Role, selection and preparation of unit head nurses (Part I). *International Journal of Nursing Studies, 18(2):*123-152.

Bergman, R., et al. (1981). Role, selection and preparation of unit head nurses (Part II). *International Journal of Nursing Studies, 18(3):*191-211.

Bergman, R., et al. (1981). Role, selection and preparation of unit head nurses (Part III). *International Journal of Nursing Studies, 18(4):*237-250.

Carnegie, M.E. (1975). Financial assistance for nursing research: Past and present. *Nursing Research, 24(3):*163.

Carter, M.D. (1973). Identification of behaviors displayed by children experiencing prolonged hospitalization. *International Journal of Nursing Studies, 10(2):*125-135.

Caterinicchо, R.P., & Davies, R.H. (1983). Developing a client focused allocation statistic of inpatient nursing resource use: An alternative to the patient day. *Social Science and Medicine, 17(5):*259-272.

Chamorro, I.L., et al. (1973). Development of an instrument to measure premature infant behavior and caretaker activities: Time-sampling methodology. *Nursing Research, 22(4):*300-309.

Chamorro, T. (1981). The role of a nurse clinician in joint practice with gynecologic oncologists. *Cancer, 48(2):*622-631.

Chow, R.K. (1974). Significant research and future

needs for improving patient care. *Military Medicine, 139(4)*:302-306.
Colaizzi, J. (1975). Proper object of nursing science. *International Journal of Nursing Studies, 12(4)*:197-200.
Conine, T.A., & Hopper, D.L. (1978). Work sampling: Tool in management. *American Journal of Occupational Therapy, 32(5)*:301-304.
Copp, L.A. (1973). Professional change: Which trends do nurses endorse? *International Journal of Nursing Studies, 10(1)*:55-63.
Copp, L.A. (1974). Critical concerns and commitments of a new department of nursing. *International Journal of Nursing Studies, 11(4)*:203-210.
Cornell, S.A. (1974). Development of an instrument for measuring quality of nursing care. *Nursing Research, 23(1)*:103-117.
Craig, S.L. (1980). Theory development and its relevance for nursing. *Journal of Advanced Nursing, 5(4)*:349-355.
Crow, R.A. (1981). Research and the standards of nursing care: What is the relationship? *Journal of Advanced Nursing, 6(6)*:491-496.
Daeffler, R.J. (1977). Outcomes of primary nursing for the patient. *Military Medicine, 142(3)*:204-208.
Delacuestra, C. (1983). The nursing process: From development to implementation. *Journal of Advanced Nursing, 9(5)*:365-371.
Denton, J.A., & Wisenbaker, V.B. (1977). Death experience and death anxiety among nurses and nursing students. *Nursing Research, 26(1)*:61-64.
Dickoff, J., James, P., & Semradek, J. (1975). Stance for nursing research: Tenacity or inquiry? *Nursing Research, 24(2)*:84-88.
Dickoff, J., James, P., & Semradek, J. (1975). Designing nursing research: Eight points to encounter. *Nursing Research, 24(3)*:164-176.
Dickson, W.M. (1978). Measuring pharmacist time use: Note on use of fixed interval work sampling. *American Journal of Hospital Pharmacy, 35(10)*:1241-1243.
DiMarco, N., et al. (1976). Nursing resources on nursing unit and quality of patient care. *International Journal of Nursing Studies, 13(3)*:134-152.
Doerr, B.C., & Jones, J.W. (1979). Effect of family preparation on the state anxiety level of the C.C.U. patient. *Nursing Research, 28(5)*:315-316.
Duhart, J., & Chartonb, J. (1973). Hospital reform and health care in medical ordinance. *Revue Francaise De Sociologic, 14*:77-101.
Dungy, C.I., & Mullins, R.G. (1981). School nurse practitioner: Analysis of questionnaire and time-motion data. *Journal of School Health, 51(7)*:475-478.
Ellis, R. (1977). Fallibilities, fragments, and frames: Contemplation on 25 years of research in medical-surgical nursing. *Nursing Research, 26(3)*:177-182.
Elms, R.R. (1972). Recovery room behavior and postoperative convalescence. *Nursing Research, 21(5)*:390-397.
Eriksen, L.R. (1987, July). Patient satisfaction: An indicator of nursing care quality? *Nursing management, 18(7)*:31-35.
Falcone, A.R. (1983). Comprehensive functional assessment as an administrative tool. *Journal of the American Geriatrics Society, 31(11)*:642-650.
Fielder, J.L. (1981). A review of the literature on access and utilization of medical care with special emphasis on rural primary care, social science and medical (Part C). *Medical Economics, 15(3c)*:129-142.
Flook, E. (1973). Health services research and R and D in perspective. *American Journal of Public Health and the Nations Health, 63(8)*:681-686.
Fortinsky, R.H., Granger, C.V., & Seltzer, G.B. (1981). The use of functional assessment in understanding home care needs. *Medical Care, 19(5)*:489-497.
Foster, S.B. (1974). Adrenal measure for evaluating nursing effectiveness. *Nursing Research, 23(2)*:118-124.
Fox, R.N., & Ventura, M.R. (1983). Small scale administration of instruments procedures. *Nursing Research, 32(2)*:122-125.
Frelick, R.W., & Frelick, J.H. (1976). Coming to grips with main issues. *American Journal of Public Health, 66(8)*:795.
French, K. (1981). Methodological considerations in hospital patient opinion surveys. *International Journal of Nursing Studies, 18(1)*:7-32.
Golden, A.S. (1975). Task analysis in health manpower development and utilization. *Medical Care, 13(8)*:704-710.
Goodwin, J.D., & Edwards, B.S. (1975). Developing a computer program to assist nursing process: Phase 1: From systems analysis to an expandable program. *Nursing Research, 24(4)*:299-305.

Gordon, M. (1980). Determining study topics. *Nursing Research, 2*:83-87.

Gordon, M., Sweeney, M.A., & McKeehan, K. (1980). Development of nursing diagnoses. *American Journal of Nursing, 4*:669.

Gortner, S.R., & Nahm, H. (1977). Overview of nursing research in the United States. *Nursing Research, 26(1)*:10-33.

Greaves, F. (1980). Objectively toward curriculum improvement in nursing: Education in England and Wales. *Journal of Advanced Nursing, 5(6)*:591-599.

Grier, M.R., & Schnitzler, C.P. (1979). Nurses' propensity to risk. *Nursing Research, 28(3)*:186-191.

Gunter, L.M., & Miller, J.C. (1977). Toward a nursing gerontology. *Nursing Research, 26(3)*:208-221.

Hardy, L.K. (1982). Nursing models and nursing: A restrictive view. *Journal of Advanced Nursing. 7(5)*:447-451.

Hayesbautista, D.E. (1976). Classification of practitioners by urban Chicano patients: Aspects of sociology of lay knowledge. *American Journal of Ostometry and Physiological Optics, 53(3)*: 156-163.

Heagarty, M.C., et al. (1973). Evaluation of activities of nurses and pediatricians in a university outpatient department. *Journal of Pediatrics, 83(5)*: 875-879.

Hodgman, E.L. (1979). Closing the gap between research and practice: Changing the answer to the who, the where and the how of nursing research. *International Journal of Nursing Studies, 16(1)*:105-110.

Hooker, B.B. (1977). Diploma school of nursing: Option in post secondary education. *Journal of Nursing Education, 16(3)*:36-42.

Hubbard, S.M., & Donehower, M.G. (1980). The nurse in a cancer research setting. *Seminars in Oncology, 1*:9-17.

Jackson, B.S., & Kinney, M.R. (1978). Energy-expenditure, heart rate, rhythm and blood pressure in normal female subjects engaged in common hospitalized patient positions and modes of patient transfer. *International Journal of Nursing Studies, 15(3)*:115-128.

Jennings, C.P., & Jennings, T.F. (1977). Containing costs through perspective reimbursement. *American Journal of Nursing, 77(7)*:1155-1159.

Ketefian, S. (1975). Application of selected nursing research findings into nursing practice: Pilot study. *Nursing Research, 24(2)*:89-92.

Ketefien, S. (1976). Curriculum change in nursing education: Sources of knowledge utilized. *International Nursing Review, 23(4)*:107-115.

Krueger, J.C. (1980). Establishing priorities for evaluation and evaluation research: Nursing perspective. *Nursing Research, 2*:115-118.

Kuhn, B.G. (1980). Prediction of nursing requirements from patient characteristics. *International Journal of Nursing Studies, 1*:5-15.

Lanara, V.A. (1976). Philosophy of nursing and current nursing problems. *International Nursing Review, 23(2)*:48-54.

Lebow, J.L. (1974). Consumer assessments of quality of medical care. *Medical Care, 12(4)*:328-337.

Leininger, M. (1976). Doctoral trends for nurses: Trends, questions, and projected plans. Part I: Trends, questions and issues on doctoral programs. *Nursing Research, 25(3)*:201-210.

Lewandowski, L.A., & Kositsky, A.M. (1983). Research priorities for critical care nursing: A study by the American Association of Critical Care Nurses. *Heart and Lung, 12(1)*:35-44.

Leyden, D.R. (1983). Measuring patients attitudes in a comprehensive health care setting. *Computers in Biology and Medicine, 13(2)*:99-124.

Lindeman, C.A. (1975). Delphi survey of priorities in clinical nursing research. *Nursing Research, 24(6)*:434-441.

Majesky, S.J., Brester, M.H., & Nishio, K.T. (1978). Development of a research tool: Patient indications of nursing care. *Nursing Research. 27*(6):365-371.

McGilloway, F.A. (1980). The nursing process: A problem-solving approach to patient care. *International Journal of Nursing Studies, 2*:79-90.

McKinnon, E.L. (1978). Circulation research: Exploring its potential in clinical nursing. *Nursing Research, 21(6)*:494-498.

McLane, A.M. (1978). Core competencies of masters-prepared nurses. *Nursing Research, 27(1)*:48-53.

Meleis, A.I. (1979). Development of a conceptually based nursing curriculum: International experiment. *Journal of Advanced Nursing, 6*:659-671.

Mickley, B.B. (1974). Physiologic and psychologic responses of elective surgical patients: Early definite or late indefinite scheduling of surgical procedures. *Nursing Research, 23(5)*:392-401.

Nunnally, D.M. (1974). Patients' evaluation of their

prenatal and delivery care. *Nursing Research, 23(6)*:469-474.

Orr, J.A. (1979). Nursing and the process of scientific injury. *Journal of Advanced Nursing, 6*:603-610.

Penchansky, R., & Thomas, J.W. (1981). The concept of access: Definitions and relationship to consumer satisfaction. *Medical Care, 19(2)*:127-140.

Rankin, M.A. (1974). Pienschke's theoretical framework for guardedness or openness on cancer unit. *Nursing Research, 23(5)*:434.

Risser, N.L. (1975). Development of an instrument to measure patient satisfaction with nurses and nursing care in primary care settings. *Nursing Research, 24(1)*:45-52.

Schlotfeldt, R.M. (1975). Research in nursing and research training for nurses: Retrospect and prospect. *Nursing Research*, 24(3):177-183.

Seither, F.G. (1974). Predictive validity study of screening measures used to select practical nursing students: *Nursing Research, 23(1)*:60-63.

Sheahan, J. (1980). Some aspects of the teaching and learning of nursing. *Journal of Advanced Nursing, 5(5)*:491-511.

Shopa, M.A. (1975). Historical materials in nursing. *Nursing Research, 24(4)*:308.

Smoyak, S.A. (1976). Is practice responding to research? *American Journal of Nursing, 76(7)*:1146-1150.

Spiegel, A.D., Hyman, H.H., & Gary, L.R. (1980). Issues and opportunities in the regulation of home health care. *Health Policy and Education, 1(3)*:237-253.

Taylor, S.D. (1974). Development of a classification system for current nursing research. *Nursing Research, 23(1)*:63-68.

Taylor, S.D. (1975). Bibliography on nursing research: 1950-1974. *24(3)*:207-225.

Temkingreener, H. (1983). Interprofessional perspectives on teamwork in health care: A case study. *Milbank Memorial Fund Quarterly: Health and Society, 61(4)*:641-658.

Tornary, R.D. (1977). Nursing research: Road ahead. *Nursing Research, 26(6)*:404-407.

Trivedi, V.M., & Hancock, W.M. (1975). Measurement of nursing workload using head nurses' perceptions. *Nursing Research, 24(5)*:371-376.

Trivedi, V.M., & Warner, D.M. (1976). Branch and bound algorithm for optimum allocation of float nurses. *Management Science, 22(9)*:972-981.

Turnbull, E.M. (1978). Effect of basic preventive health practices and mass-media on practice of breast self-examination. *Nursing Research, 27(2)*: 98-102.

Ventura, M.R., & Waligoraserofur, B. (1981). Study priorities identified by nurses in mental health setting. *International Journal of Nursing Studies, 19(1)*:41-46.

Vredevoe, D.L. (1972). Nursing research involving physiological mechanisms: Definitions of variables. *Nursing Research, 21(1)*:68-72.

Warner, D.M. (1976). Nurse staffing, scheduling, reallocation in hospital. *Hospital and Health Services Administration, 21(3)*:77-90.

White, M.B. (1972). Importance of selected nursing activities. *Nursing Research, 21(1)*:4-14.

Wolfer, J.A. (1973). Definition and assessment of surgical patients' welfare and recovery. *Nursing Research, 22(5)*:394-401.

10

Lydia E. Hall

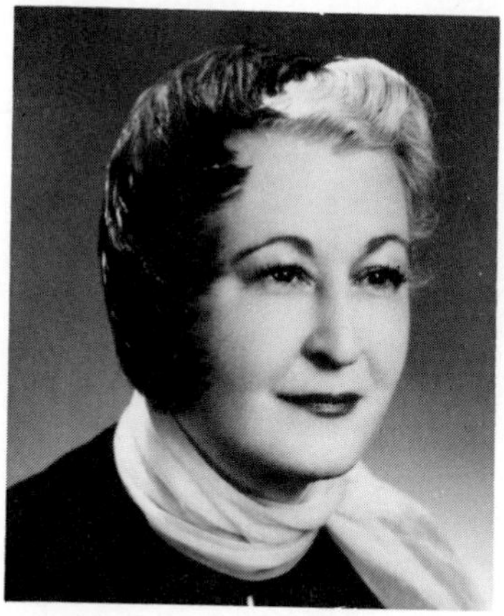

Core, Care, and Cure Model

Ann Marriner-Tomey, Kim Tippey Peskoe, S. Brook Gumm

CREDENTIALS AND BACKGROUND OF THE THEORIST

Lydia Hall began her prestigious career in nursing as a graduate of the York Hospital School of Nursing in York, Pa. She then earned her B.S. and M.A. degrees from Teacher's College, Columbia University in New York, like many other contemporary nursing theorists.

Hall had faculty positions at the York Hospital School of Nursing and the Fordham Hospital School of Nursing, and was a consultant in Nursing Education to the nursing faculty at State University of New York, Upstate Medical Center. She also was an instructor of Nursing Education at Teacher's College, Columbia University.

Hall's career interests revolved around public health nursing, cardiovascular nursing, pediatric cardiology, and nursing of long-term illnesses. She authored 21 publications, with the bulk of articles and addresses regarding her nursing theories published in the early to middle 1960s. In 1967 she received the Award for Distinguished Achievement in Nursing Practice from Columbia University.

Perhaps Hall's greatest achievement in nursing was her design and development of the Loeb Center for Nursing at Montefiore Hospital in New York. Established to apply her theory to nursing practice, the center opened in January 1963. It demonstrated extreme success and provided empirical evidence to support the major concepts in Hall's theory. Hall served as Administrative Director of the Loeb Center for Nursing from its opening until her death in February 1969.

THEORETICAL SOURCES

Hall drew extensively from the schools of psychiatry and psychology in theorizing about the nurse-patient relationship. She was a proponent of Carl Rogers' philosophy of "client-centered therapy." This method of therapy entails establishing a relationship of warmth and safety, conveying a sensitive empathy with the client's feelings and communications as expressed.[8:34] A major premise Hall borrowed from Rogers[8:280] is that patients achieve their maximal potential through a learning process. Rogers[8:47] states that psychotherapy facilitates significant learning by (1) pointing out and labeling unsatisfying behaviors, (2) exploring objectively with the client the reasons for the behaviors, and (3) establishing through reeducation more effective problem-solving habits. In client-centered therapy, changes occur when:

1. The person accepts himself and his feelings more fully
2. He becomes more self-confident and self-directing
3. He changes maladaptive behaviors, even chronic ones
4. He becomes more open to evidence of what is going on both inside and outside of himself[8:280-281]

Extensive documentation indicates the result of this treatment is that physiological and psychological tensions are reduced and that the change lasts.[8:65]

The major therapeutic approach advocated by Hall is also Rogerian. This is the use of reflection, a nondirective method of helping the patient clarify, explore, and validate what he says. Rogers[8:43] states, "The therapist procedure which [clients] had found most helpful was that the therapist clarified and openly stated feelings which the client had been approaching hazily and hesitantly."[8:73]

Hall derived her postulates regarding the nature of feeling-based behavior from Rogers, who repeatedly speaks to the interaction of known feelings and feelings out-of-awareness. Rogers[8:36] hypothesizes that in a client-centered relationship the patient

> will re-organize himself at both the conscious and deeper levels of his personality in such a manner as to cope with life more constructively. . . . He shows . . . more of the characteristics of the healthy, well-functioning person. . . . He is less frustrated by stress, and recovers from stress more quickly.

Hall also adopted Rogers' theory on motivation for change. In this theory Rogers asserts that although the therapist does not motivate the client, neither is the motivation supplied by the client. Alternatively, motivation for change "springs from the self-actualizing tendency of life itself."[8:285] In the proper psychological climate, this tendency is released.

USE OF EMPIRICAL EVIDENCE

Rogers' theories have received wide acclaim in the fields of psychiatry, psychology, and social work. His methods of therapy have been used in caring for clients, and in the area of education, where a nondirective approach is less than common. In *On Becoming a Person,* one of Rogers' students, Samuel Tenenbaum, discussed learning through a nondirective approach and then teaching that way.[8:285]

The application of client-centered therapy in play therapy for children is addressed by Elaine Dorfman in Rogers' book, *Client-Centered Therapy*. In this specialized area, the therapist must work at the child's level of communication. Even with small children, reflection and clarification techniques are instrumental in helping children examine their feelings.[8:299]

Client-centered therapy concepts are also

used in leadership and administration situations. Thomas Gordon has addressed Rogers' concepts as they relate to group dynamics and group-centered leadership.[8:338] Gordon believes a leader can strive to create a nonthreatening psychological climate by conveying warmth and acceptance; clarification statements can be used to link chains of thought.

The multiplicity of applications of Rogerian theory in everyday life is almost endless. Rogers deserves his venerable title of the "founder of nondirective client-centered therapy."[6] His writings would have constituted the most current literature on this topic in the 1960s, when Hall was building her theory of nursing.

While Hall did not actually research her theory, Blue Cross Insurance studies indicated patients at Loeb recovered in half the time, at less than half the cost, and with fewer readmissions than patients who stayed in Montefiore Hospital. Twenty-two home-care programs in the New York area had a readmission rate five times higher than Loeb.[5:91-92] On a follow-up questionnaire, 40 physicians indicated the hospital stay of patients at the Loeb Center ranged from 3 to 43 days shorter than at other hospitals, but the difference was more usually 1 to 3 weeks. Patients and physicians were both pleased with the care.[5:82]

MAJOR CONCEPTS AND DEFINITIONS

BEHAVIOR. Hall broadly defines behavior as everything that is said or done. Behavior is dictated by feelings, both conscious and unconscious.

REFLECTION. Reflection is a Rogerian method of communication in which selected verbalizations of the patient are repeated back to him using different phraseology, to invite him to explore his feelings further.[4:88]

SELF-AWARENESS. Self-awareness refers to the state of being that nurses endeavor to help their patients achieve. The more self-awareness a person has of his feelings, the more control he has over his behavior.

SECOND STAGE ILLNESS. Hall[4:84] defines second stage illness as the nonacute recovery phase of illness. This stage is conducive to learning and rehabilitation.[4:84] The need for medical care here is minimal although the need for nurturing and learning is great. Therefore this is the ideal time for wholly professional nursing care.

WHOLLY PROFESSIONAL NURSING. Wholly professional nursing implies nursing care given exclusively by RNs educated in the behavioral sciences who take the responsibility and opportunity to coordinate and deliver the total care of their patients.[4:91] This concept includes the roles of nurturing, teaching, and advocacy in the fostering of healing.

Nursing circles of Care, Core, and Cure are the central concepts of Hall's theory (Figure 10-1). Care alludes to the "hands-on," intimate bodily care of the patient and implies a comforting, nurturing relationship.[4:85] Core involves the therapeutic use of self in communicating with the patient. The nurse reflects questions appropriately and helps the patient clarify motives and goals, facilitating the process of increasing the patient's self-awareness. Cure is the aspect of nursing involved with administration of medications and treatments. The nurse functions in this role as an investigator and potential "painer."[3:152]

MAJOR ASSUMPTIONS

The following assumptions are basic to Hall's theory of nursing. They are explicit and for the most part are adequately defined in her writings.

Nursing

Nursing can and should be professional.[4:81] Hall stipulated patients should be cared for

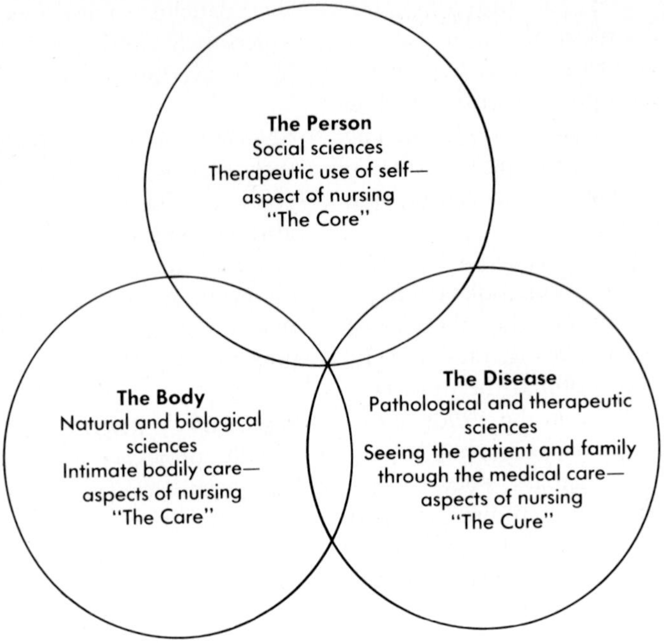

Figure 10-1. Core, Care, and Cure model.
From Hall, L. (1964, Feb.). Nursing: What is it? *The Canadian Nurse, 60(2)*:151. Reproduced with permission from *The Canadian Nurse.*

only by professional RNs who can take total responsibility for the care and teaching of their patients. This interesting after-note appears in one of her articles on the Loeb Center:[4:95]

> We hire from 3-year schools, community colleges, baccalaureate, and even master's degree programmes. . . . Although all learn to master satisfactorily, those from the 2 and 3-year programmes reach a plateau. The baccalaureate graduates keep on learning and being and don't seem to stop growing in their ability to gain skills in the nurturing process.

The professional nurse functions most therapeutically when patients have entered the second stage of their hospital stay.[4:84] The second stage is the recuperating or nonacute phase of illness. The first stage of illness is a time of biological crisis, with nursing being ancillary to medicine. After the crisis period the patient is more able to benefit and learn from the teaching that nurses can offer.

Nursing is all complex.[4:84] The patient is certainly complex. Not only is he a human being, bringing with him the influences of his culture and environment, but he may be suffering from an illness that medicine is still struggling to understand and treat. The nurse giving the care is also a unique human being, interacting with the patient in a complex process of teaching and learning.

Nursing expertise centers around the body.[4:85] This refers to Hall's theoretical model because she viewed the patient as composed of Body, Pathology, and Personality. The uniqueness of nursing lies not only in knowing bodily care, but also in knowing how to modify these processes in line with the pathology and treatment, and amend them in line with the personality of the patient.

Person

Patients achieve their maximal potential through a learning process; therefore the chief therapy they need is teaching.[4:82] Rehabilitation is a process of learning to live within limitations. Physical and mental skills must be learned, but a prerequisite to these is learning about oneself as a person, becoming aware of feelings and behaviors, and clarifying motivations. Hall believed this process could best be facilitated by the professional nurse educated in communication skills.

People strive for their own goals, not goals others set for them.[4:82] Hall declared that in the usual medical setting the doctor defines the goals for the patient, but too often these goals do not coincide with the patient's goals for himself. In this situation, effective teaching and learning cannot occur.

A patient is composed of three aspects: Body, Pathology, and Person.[4:84] (These elements are discussed later.) This particular assumption is crucial to Hall's theory of nursing.

People behave on the basis of their feelings, not on the basis of knowledge.[4:89] The evidence that learning has occurred is a resultant change in some behavior. This does not usually happen strictly as a result of knowing information. Actions occur in conjunction with feelings, and feelings are not influenced by rationality.

There are two types of feelings: known feelings and feelings-out-of-awareness.[4:90] When people act on the basis of known feelings, they are *free* and in control of their behavior. When they act on feelings-out-of-awareness, they have no choice as to their behavior and the feelings make them act.

Health

Becoming ill is behavior,[4:90] according to Hall's definition of behavior. Illness is directed by one's feelings-out-of-awareness, which are the root of adjustment difficulties.

Healing may be hastened by helping people move in the direction of self-awareness.[4:90] Once people are brought to grips with their true feelings and motivations, they become free to release their own powers of healing.

Through the process of reflection, "the patient has a chance to move from the unlabeled threat of anxiety . . . through a mislabeled threat of 'phobia' or 'dis-ease' . . . to a properly labeled threat (fear) with which he can deal constructively."[4:91]

Environment

Hospital nursing services are organized to accomplish tasks efficiently.[4:83] Hall viewed these organizations as being an end unto themselves. She did not believe they have patient care and teaching as their goal, but rather that their goal is helping the physicians and administrators get their work done.

Hall was not pleased with the concept of team nursing. She said, "any career that is defined around the work that has to be done, and how it is divided to get it done, is a trade."[4:83] She vehemently opposed the idea of anyone other than educated, professional nurses taking direct care of patients and decried the fact that nursing has trained nonprofessionals to function as practical nurses so that professional nurses can function as practical doctors.

There are two phases of medical care practiced in medical centers: biological crisis and evaluative medicine.[4:84] The biological crisis phase involves intensive medical and diagnostic treatment of the patient. The evaluative medicine phase follows and generally is the time when the patient is observed in order to appraise whether he is meeting the doctor's goals.

THEORETICAL ASSERTIONS

Hall's theory consists of three major tenets. The first is that nursing functions differently in the three interlocking circles which constitute aspects of the patient.[4:81] These three circles are interrelated and are influenced by each other. They are: the patient's *Body,* the *Disease* affecting the body, and the *Person* of the patient, which is being affected by both of the other circles. Nursing operates in all three circles, but shares them with other professions to different degrees. Because pathologic conditions are treated with medical care (Cure), nursing shares this circle with physicians. The Person aspect (Core) is cared for by therapeutic use of the self. Therefore this arena is shared with psychiatry, psychology, social work, and religious ministry. The body of the patient is cared for exclusively by nursing (Care). This circle includes all intimate bodily care such as feeding, bathing, and toileting the patient.

Hall's second assertion[2:806] is the Core postulate of her theory: As the patient needs less medical care, he needs more professional nursing care and teaching. This inversely proportional relationship alters the ratio of nursing care in the three circles. Patients in the second stage of illness (nonacute phase) are primarily in need of rehabilitation through learning: thus, the Care and Core circles predominate the Cure circle. The Loeb Center was designed for the care of nonacute patients in need of teaching and rehabilitation; the fact that it is staffed and run by nurses with physicians functioning as ancillaries is no surprise.

The third assertion of this theory is that wholly professional nursing care will hasten recovery. Hall decried the concept of team nursing, which gives the care of less complicated cases to caregivers with less training. Nurses are complex people using a complex process of teaching and learning in caring for complex patients with complex diseases. Only professional nurses are inherently qualified to provide the teaching, counseling, and nurturing needed in the second stage of illness.[3:150;4:83-84] At the Loeb Center, secretaries and messenger-attendants are employed for the indirect patient care. But they are not permitted to do anything directly related to the patient. The professional nurse is the coordinator for all her patients' therapies, and all disciplines act in a consulting capacity to nursing.[4:82]

LOGICAL FORM

Hall's theory is formulated using inductive logic, moving from specific observations to a generalized concept. For example:

- Nursing care shortens patient recovery time;
- Nursing care facilitates patient recovery;
- Professional nursing improves patient care;
- Therefore "wholly professional nursing will hasten recovery."[5:82]

ACCEPTANCE BY THE NURSING COMMUNITY

Practice

Hall's theory closely resembles the modern nursing model of primary care. Her emphasis on the professional nurse as the primary caregiver parallels primary care nursing to the extent that continuity and coordination of patient care are provided. In addition, Hall's concepts of nurses being accountable and responsible for their own practice are ideas that are pertinent and applicable today. Concern for these concepts demonstrates support for her theory.

Education

Hall's theory delineates definite ideas regarding nursing care being provided for by a professional nursing staff. The acceptance of this philosophy can be seen in the current shift toward professional staffing in many health care facilities, and in the growing trend toward the BSN as the minimum entry level requirement for professional practice. Hall[2:806] also emphasized the concept of nurses practicing nursing while completing their educational programs, instead of practicing as practical doctors. Today's issues of narrowing the divide between nursing education and service, and of using nursing diagnoses as a guide for patient care instead of medical diagnoses support Hall's concepts from her theory.

Research

Currently available literature suggests that only at the Loeb Center for nursing is further research on Hall's theories being conducted.

FURTHER DEVELOPMENT

Much research and testing of Hall's theory is needed before it can be applicable and useful to areas of nursing other than long-term illnesses and rehabilitative nursing. In particular, the theory needs to be adapted to health care facilities that differ from the Loeb Center for Nursing before its true impact and contribution to nursing can be judged. This step would require flexibility and change in several of Hall's main concepts and relationships, particularly those relating to the age and illness orientation of the client. It would be interesting to further develop in a variety of settings the concept of increased nursing care as a means to hasten patient recovery. This tenet has been highly successful at the Loeb Center in reducing both patient days and health care costs. However, other research relating nursing care to patient outcomes has not been based on Hall's model.

CRITIQUE

Simplicity

Hall's theory is simple and easily understood. The major concepts and relationships are limited and clear. The three aspects of professional nursing are identified both individually and as they relate to each other in the total process of patient care. Hall designed basic models to represent the major concepts and relationships of her theory, using individual and interlocking circles to define the three aspects of the patient, and their relationships to the three aspects of nursing. The language used to define and describe the theory is easily understood and is indigenous to nursing.

Generality

Perhaps the most serious flaw in Hall's theory of nursing is its limited generality. Hall's primary target[5:80] in nursing theory is the adult patient who has passed the acute phase of his or her illness and has a relatively good chance at rehabilitation. This concept severely limits application of the theory to a small population of patients of specific age and stage of illness. Although the ideas of Care, Cure, and Core can possibly be applied to patients in the acute phase of their illness, the theory would be most difficult to apply to infants, small children, and comatose patients. In addition, Hall[5:80,82] devotes her theory to adult individuals who are ill. The function of the nurse in preventive health care and health maintenance is not addressed, nor is the nurse's role in community health, even though the model could be adapted.

Hall viewed the role of the nurse as heavily involved in the Care and Core aspects of patient care. Unfortunately, this concept provides for little family interaction with the nurse, as her theory delineates the family aspect of patient care only in the Cure circle.[3:151;4:87]

The use of therapeutic communication to help the patient look at and explore his feelings regarding his illness and the potential changes the illness might cause is discussed in the Core aspect of nursing care. Therapeutic communication is also thought to motivate the patient by making him aware of his true feelings. However, the only communication technique Hall[4:91] described in her theory as a means to assist the patient toward self-awareness was reflection. This is a very limited approach to therapeutic communication, because not all nurses can effectively use the technique of reflection, and it is not always the most effective and successful communication tool in dealing with patients.[1:47]

Empirical Precision

Hall's concept of professional nursing hastening patient recovery with increased care as the patient improves has been subjected to a great amount of testing at the Loeb Center for Nursing.[5:80] The fact that the theory is identified with empirical reality cannot be disputed. Evidence obtained through research at the Loeb Center demonstrates that Hall's theory[4:92] does in fact obtain its goal of shortening patient recovery time through concentrated, professional nursing efforts. Currently, the available literature supports the results obtained at the Loeb Center in testing the theory. Although research support has been demonstrated by the success of the Center, a wider range of testing in various settings is necessary to allow for increased empirical precision of the theory.

Derivable Consequences

The theory provides a general framework for nursing, and the concepts are within the domain of nursing although the aspects of Cure and Core are shared with other health professionals and family members. Although the theory does not provide for the resolution of specific issues and problems, it does address itself to the pertinent and contemporary issues of accountability, responsibility, and professionalism. Application of the theory in practice has produced valued outcomes in all three areas. In addition, the theory demonstrates a great impact on the educational preparation of nursing students. Hall[2:806] stated, "With early field experience in a center where nursing rather than medicine is emphasized, the student may emerge a nurse first." Hall believed that in nursing centers the student would benefit from experiencing nursing as it is taught to them in the classroom.

Despite the shortcomings of Hall's theory of nursing, her contribution to nursing practice is tremendous. Her insight into the problems of nursing in the 1960s has provided a base for professional practice in the multidimensional modern domain of nursing in the 1980s.

REFERENCES

1. Hale, K., & George, J. (1980). Lydia E. Hall. In Nursing Theories Conference Group, J.B. George, Chairperson, *Nursing theories: The base for professional practice.* Englewood Cliffs, N.J.: Prentice-Hall.
2. Hall, L.E. (1963, Nov). Center for nursing. *Nursing Outlook, 11*:805-806.
3. Hall, L.E. (1964, Feb.). Nursing: What is it? *Canadian Nurse, 60*:150-154.
4. Hall, L.E. (1969). The Loeb Center for Nursing and Rehabilitation. *International Journal of Nursing Studies, 6*:81-95.
5. Henderson, C. (1964, June). Can nursing care hasten recovery? *American Journal of Nursing, 64*:80-83.
6. Knech, D., et al. (1976). *Psychology: A basic course.* New York: Alfred Knopf.
7. Rogers, C. (1951). *Client-centered therapy.* Boston: Houghton Mifflin.
8. Rogers, C. (1961). *On becoming a person.* Boston: Houghton Mifflin.

BIBLIOGRAPHY

Primary Sources

Book Chapters

Hall, L. (1965). Nursing—what is it? In H. Baumgarten, Jr., *Concepts of nursing home administration.* New York: Macmillan.

Hall, L. (1966). Another view of nursing care and quality. In M.K. Straub, *Continuity of patient care: The role of nursing.* Washington, D.C.: Catholic University of America Press.

Articles

Hall, L. (1955, June). Quality of nursing care. *Public Health News.* (New Jersey State Department of Health.) *36(6)*:212-215.

Hall, L. (1963, Nov.). Center for nursing. *Nursing Outlook, 11*:805-806.

Hall, L. (1964, Feb.). Nursing: What is it? *Canadian Nurse, 60*:150-154.

Hall, L. (1969). The Loeb Center for nursing and rehabilitation. *International Journal of Nursing Studies, 6*:81-95.

Hall, L., Hauck, M., & Rosenson, L. (1949, March). The cardiac child in school and community. *New York Heart Association Publication.*

Pamphlets

Hall, L. (1951). *What the classroom teacher should know and do about children with heart disease.* American Heart Association.

Reports

Hall, L. (1960). *Report of a work conference on nursing in long-term chronic disease and aging.* National League for Nursing as a League Exchange #50. New York: National League for Nursing.

Hall, L. (1963, June). *Report of Loeb Center for nursing and rehabilitation project report.* Congressional Record Hearings before the Special Subcommittee on Intermediate Care of the Committee on Veterans' Affairs. Washington, D.C., pp. 1515-1562.

Secondary Sources
Book Chapters

Alfano, G.J. (1987). The Loeb Center for Nursing and Rehabilitation: A model for extended care. In B.C. Vladeck & G.J. Alfano (Eds.). *Medicare and extended care: Issues, problems and prospects.* Owings Mills, Md.: Rynd Comm.

Chinn, P.L., & Jacobs, M.K. (1987). Theory in nursing: A current overview. In P.L. Chinn & M.K. Jacobs, *Theory and nursing*. St. Louis: C.V. Mosby.

Griffith, J. (1982). Other frameworks and models. In J. Griffith & P. Christenson, *Nursing Process: Application of theories, frameworks, and models.* St. Louis: C.V. Mosby.

Hale, K., & George, J. (1980). Lydia E. Hall. In Nursing Theories Group Conference, J.B. George, Chairperson, *Nursing theories: The base for professional practice.* Englewood Cliffs, N.J.: Prentice-Hall.

Articles

Alfano, G.J. (1988, Jan.-Feb.). A different kind of nursing. *Nursing Outlook, 36:*34-37.

Alfano, G. (1964, June). Administration means working with nurses. *American Journal of Nursing, 64*:83-85.

Bernardin, E. (1964, June). Loeb Center: As the staff nurse sees it. *American Journal of Nursing, 64*:85-86.

Bowar-Ferres, S. (1975, May). Loeb Center and its philosophy of nursing. *American Journal of Nursing, 65*:810.

Henderson, C. (1964, June). Can nursing care hasten recovery? *American Journal of Nursing, 64*:80-83.

Isler, C. (1964, June). New concepts in nursing therapy: More care as the patient improves. *RN, 27*:58-70.

Correspondence

Alfano, G.J. (1984, Jan. 26). Personal correspondence.

Alfano, G.J. (1984, Feb. 15). Personal correspondence.

Wender, B. (1984, Jan. 25). (Secretary of the Loeb Center) Telephone interview.

Other Sources

Chinn, P.L., & Jacobs, M.K., (1983). *Theory and nursing*. St. Louis: C.V. Mosby.

Rogers, C. (1951). *Client-centered therapy*. Boston: Houghton Mifflin.

Rogers, C. (1961). *On becoming a person*. Boston: Houghton Mifflin.

11

Dorothea E. Orem

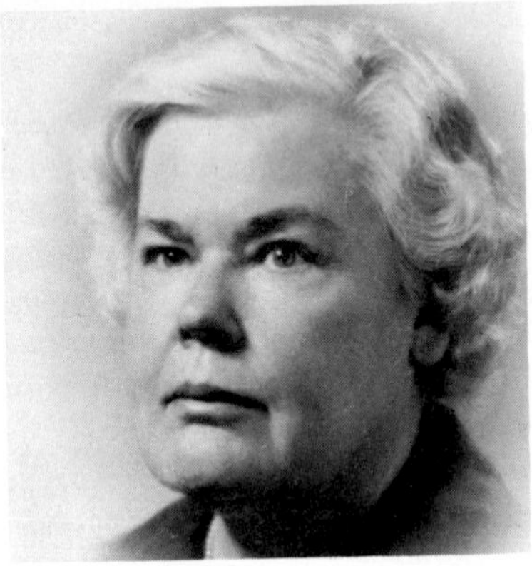

Self-Care Deficit Theory of Nursing

Jeanne Donohue Eben, Nergess N. Gashti, Margaret J. Nation, Ann Marriner-Tomey, Sherry B. Nordmeyer

CREDENTIALS AND BACKGROUND OF THE THEORIST

Dorothea Elizabeth Orem, one of America's foremost nursing theorists, was born in Baltimore, Maryland. Her father was a construction worker who liked fishing, and her mother was a homemaker who liked reading. She was the second of two daughters. She began her nursing career at Providence Hospital School of Nursing in Washington, D.C., where she received her diploma certificate of nursing in the early 1930s. Orem continued her education and received a B.S.N. from Catholic University of America in 1939 and an M.S. in nursing education in 1945 from the same university.

Her nursing experience included private duty nursing, hospital staff nursing, and teach-

The authors wish to express appreciation to Dorothea E. Orem for critiquing the first edition.

ing. Orem held directorship of both the nursing school and the department of nursing at Providence Hospital, Detroit, during 1940 to 1949. After leaving Detroit, Orem spent seven years (1949 to 1957) in Indiana working in the Division of Hospital and Institutional Services of the Indiana State Board of Health. Her goal while in Indiana was to upgrade the quality of nursing in general hospitals throughout the state. During this time, Orem developed her definition of nursing practice.

In 1957 Orem moved to Washington, D.C., where she was employed by the Office of Education, U.S. Department of Health, Education, and Welfare, as a curriculum consultant from 1958 to 1960. During this time she began to see deficits in the training of practical nurses. While at HEW she worked on a project to upgrade practical nursing training that stimulated a need to address the question, What is the subject matter of nursing? As a result, she published *Guidelines for Developing Curricula for the Education of Practical Nurses.*

In 1959, Orem became an assistant professor of Nursing Education at Catholic University of America. She subsequently served as acting dean of the School of Nursing and as associate professor of Nursing Education. She continued to develop her concept of nursing and self-care while at Catholic University. While there, she wrote "The Hope of Nursing" (1962), which was published in the *Journal of Nursing Education.* In 1970 Orem left Catholic University and started her own consulting firm of Orem and Shields, Inc., of Chevy Chase, Maryland. Orem's first book, published in 1971, was *Nursing: Concepts of Practice.* Georgetown University conferred Orem with the honorary degree of Doctor of Science in 1976. "Levels of Nursing Education and Practice" was published in the alumnae magazine of Johns Hopkins School of Nursing in 1979. She received the Catholic University of America Alumni Association Award for Nursing Theory in 1980. The second edition of *Nursing: Concepts of Practice* was published in 1980, and the third edition followed in 1985. Since 1984, Dorothea Orem is retired in Savannah, Georgia, where she enjoys reading, traveling, consulting, attending nursing conferences regarding her theory, and working on her fourth edition of *Nursing: Concepts of Practice.* Orem has been working alone and with colleagues on the continued conceptual development of S.C.D.N.T. She participates in conferences and prepares papers about various conceptual elements of the theory. She continues to contribute to the work of her colleagues through discussions about the structure of the theory and its use in nursing.[45]

THEORETICAL SOURCES

Although Orem cites Eugenia K. Spaulding as a great friend and teacher, she indicates that no particular nursing leader was a direct influence on her work. She believes association with many nurses over the years provided many learning experiences, and she views her work with graduate students and collaborative works with colleagues as valuable endeavors.[41] While crediting no one as a major influence, she does cite many other nurses' works in terms of their contributions to nursing including, but not limited to, Abdellah, Henderson, Johnson, King, Levine, Nightingale, Orlando, Peplau, Riehl, Rogers, Roy, Travelbee, and Wiedenbach.* She also cites numerous authors in other disciplines including, but not limited to, Gordon Allport, Chester Barnard, René Dubos, Erich Fromm, Gartly Jaco, Robert Katz, Kurt Lewin, Ernest Nagel, Talcott Parsons, Hans Selye, and Ludwig von Bertalanffy.[42:222-225]

USE OF EMPIRICAL EVIDENCE

In 1958, Orem had a spontaneous insight about why individuals required and could be helped through nursing that enabled her to formulate and express her concept of nursing. Her knowledge of the features of nursing practice situations was acquired over many years.[41]

---

*References 9:38, 39, 61, 100-103.

MAJOR CONCEPTS AND DEFINITIONS

Orem labels her self-care deficit theory of nursing as a general theory. This general theory is composed of three related theories: (1) the theory of self-care (describes and explains self-care); (2) the theory of self-care deficit (describes and explains why people can be helped through nursing); and (3) the theory of nursing systems (describes and explains relationships that must be brought about and maintained for nursing to be produced).[38:209;39:214] The major concepts of these theories are identified here and discussed more fully in Orem's book *Nursing: Concepts of Practice* (Figure 11-1).

SELF-CARE. "The production of actions directed to self or to the environment in order to regulate one's functioning in the interests of one's life, integrated functioning, and well-being."[44:31]

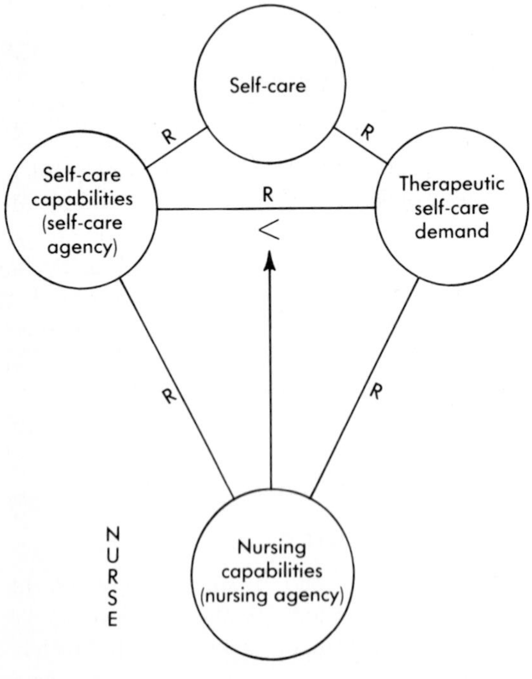

Figure 11-1. Conceptual framework for nursing. *R*, relationship; <, deficit relationship, current or projected.

Used with permission from Orem, D.E. (1980). *Nursing: Concepts of practice*. New York: McGraw-Hill.

Self-care requisites. Self-care requisites are "the purposes to be attained through the kinds of actions termed self-care."[40:37;44:85] They may be broken down into three categories.

Universal self-care requisites. Universal self-care requisites are common to all human beings and include the maintenance of air, water, food, elimination, activity and rest, and solitude and social interaction, prevention of hazards, and promotion of human functioning.[40:42;44:90-91]

> These eight requisites represent the kinds of human actions that bring about the internal and external conditions that maintain human structure and functioning, which in turn support human development and maturation. When it is effectively provided, self-care or dependent care organized around universal self-care requisites fosters positive health and well being.[44:91]

Developmental self-care requisites. Developmental self-care requisites were separated from universal self-care requisites in the second edition of *Nursing: Concepts of Practice*. They promote processes for life and maturation and prevent conditions deleterious to maturation or mitigate those effects.[38:47]

Health deviation self-care requisites. Orem[40:48-50;44:98-99] defined health deviation self-care requisites in the following way.

> Disease or injury affects not only specific structures and physiological or psychological mechanisms but also integrated human functioning. When integrated functioning is seriously affected . . . the individual's power of agency are seriously impaired either permanently or temporarily. . . . When a change in health state brings about total or almost total dependence on others for the needs to sustain life or well-being, the person moves from the position of self-care agent to

that of patient or receiver of care. . . . Evidence of health deviations leads to demands for determining what should be done to restore normalcy. . . . Seeking and participating in medical care for health deviations are self-care actions. . . . Pain, discomfort, and frustration resulting from medical care also create requisites for self-care to bring relief. . . . If persons with health deviations are to become competent in managing a system of health-deviation self-care, they must also be able to apply relevant medical knowledge to their own care.

THERAPEUTIC SELF-CARE DEMAND. "The measures of care required at moments in time in order to meet existent requisites for regulatory action to maintain life and to maintain or promote health and development and general well-being."[44:31]

SELF-CARE AGENCY. "The complex capability for action that is activated in the performance of the actions or operations of self-care."[43:31]

Agent. An agent is the "person taking action."[40:35;44:84]

Self-care agent. A self-care agent is "the provider of self-care."[40:35;44:84]

Dependent-care agent. A dependent-care agent is "the provider of infant care, child care, or dependent adult care."[40:35;44:84]

SELF-CARE DEFICIT. "A relationship between self-care agency and therapeutic self-care demand in which self-care agency is not adequate to meet the known therapeutic self-care demand."[44:31]

NURSING AGENCY. "The complex capability for action that is activated by nurses in their determination of needs for, design of, and production of nursing for persons with a range of types of self-care deficits."[44:31]

NURSING SYSTEM. "A continuing series of actions produced when nurses link one way or a number of ways of helping to their own actions or the actions of persons under care that are directed to meet these person's therapeutic self-care demands or to regulate their self-care agency."[44:31]

Types of nursing systems. Three types of nursing systems are identified (Figure 11-2). Whether the nursing system is wholly compensatory, partly compensatory, or supportive-educative depends on "who can or should perform those self-care actions."[38:96-97;44:152]

Wholly compensatory nursing systems. Wholly compensatory nursing systems are needed when the "nurse should be compensating for a patient's total inability for (or prescriptions against) engaging in self-care activities that require ambulation and manipulation movements."[38:97-98;44:154]

Partly compensatory systems. Partly compensatory systems exist when "both nurse and patient perform care measures or other actions involving manipulative tasks or ambulation."[38:101;44:156]

Supportive-educative systems. Supportive-educative systems are "for situations where the patient is able to perform or can and should learn to perform required measures of externally or internally oriented therapeutic self-care but cannot do so without assistance."[38:101;44:156]

Methods of assistance. Methods of assistance include: "(1) acting or doing for; (2) guiding; (3) teaching; (4) supporting; and (5) providing a developmental environment."[38:61]

MAJOR ASSUMPTIONS

Assumptions basic to the general theory were formalized in the early 1970s and were presented at Marquette University School of Nursing in 1973.[42] Orem[38:33-34] lists the five as-

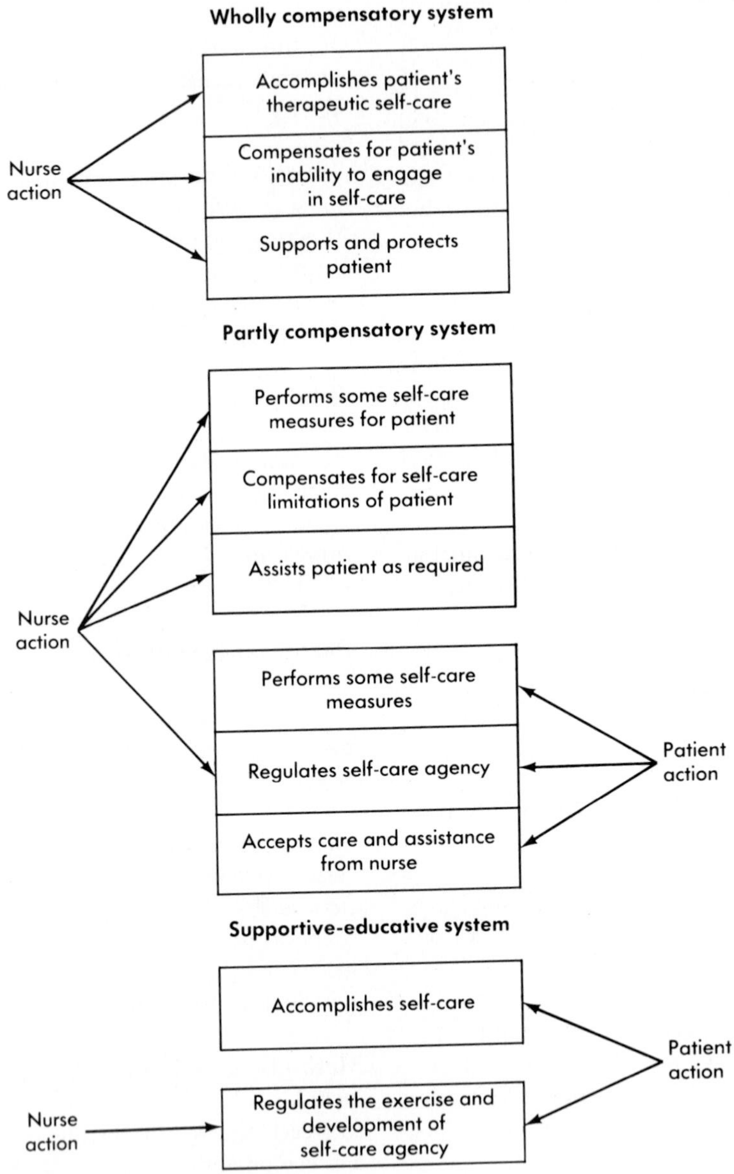

Figure 11-2. Basic nursing systems.
Used with permission from Orem, D.E. (1980). *Nursing: Concepts of practice.* New York: McGraw-Hill.

sumptions underlying the general theory of nursing as:

1. Human beings require continuous deliberate inputs to themselves and their environments in order to remain alive and function in accord with natural human endowments.
2. Human agency, the power to act deliberately, is exercised in the form of care of self and others in identifying needs for and in making needed inputs.
3. Mature human beings experience privations in the form of limitations for action in care of self and others involving the making of life-sustaining and function-regulating inputs.
4. Human agency is exercised in discovering, developing, and transmitting to other ways and means to identify needs for and make inputs to self and others.
5. Groups of human beings with structured relationships cluster tasks and allocate responsibilities for providing care to group members who experience privations for making required deliberate input to self and others.

Orem lists presuppositions for the theory of Self-Care, the theory of Self-Care Deficit, and the theory of Nursing Systems in *Nursing: Concepts of Practice.*[43:33-38]

THEORETICAL ASSERTIONS

The model shows that when an individual's self-care capabilities are less than the therapeutic self-care demand, the nurse compensates for the self-care or dependent-care deficits. The relational structure is discussed in Orem's book, *Nursing: Concepts of Practice,* as central ideas and propositions of the three related theories of self-care, self-care deficits, and nursing systems.[38:26-30;44:33-38]

Self-Care

> Self-care and care of dependent family members are learned behaviors that purposely regulate human structural integrity, functioning, and human development. The theory of self-care denotes the relationship between the deliberate self-care actions of mature and maturing members of social groups and their own development and functioning as well as the relationship of the continuing care of dependent members to their functioning and development.[38:28;44:36]

Self-Care Deficit

Individuals experience a self-care deficit when they are unable to care for themselves.

> People can benefit from nursing because they are subject to health-related or health-derived limitations that render them incapable of continuous self-care or dependent care or that result in ineffective or incomplete care.[38:27;44:34-36]

Nursing Systems

> Nursing systems are formed when nurses use their abilities to prescribe, design, and provide nursing for legitimate patients (as individuals or groups) by performing discrete actions and systems of action. These actions or systems regulate the value of or the exercise of individuals' capabilities to engage in self-care and meet the self-care requisites of the individual therapeutically.[38:29;44:37-38]

LOGICAL FORM

Orem's spontaneous insight led to her initial formalization and subsequent expression of a general concept of nursing. That generalization then made possible deductive thinking about nursing.[41]

Susan and Thomas Taylor from the University of Missouri at Columbia have worked with Orem's general theory of nursing using a mathematical logic approach to explicate its syntactical structure or internal logic as a step toward identifying rules and modes of inquiry.[42,45]

ACCEPTANCE BY THE NURSING COMMUNITY

Orem's self-care theory has achieved a greater level of acceptance by the nursing community than the works of the majority of other theorists.

Practice

Many articles document the use of the self-care theory as a basis for clinical practice. In 1971

Lucille Kinlein established an independent nurse practice in College Park, Md. Although Kinlein's concepts differ from Orem's, her practice was stimulated by Orem's self-care theory. In 1977 Kinlein[26,27] published *Independent Nursing Practice with Clients* in which she documented her experience in setting up an independent practice and her use of self-care.

At Johns Hopkins Hospital in Baltimore the self-care theory was used in several outpatient clinics. Nurse specialists managed three of those units—two cardiac clinics and a diabetic clinic. These clinics were managed separately from the standard medically managed clinics. Although there was a mechanism for referral to a medical doctor, the nurse specialists controlled the clinics and used Orem's self-care theory in their daily practice.[1]

A group of graduate students at the University of Texas School of Nursing, as part of their course work, applied Orem's theory in a nursing home to specific patients. Their conclusions were "that through the employment of the self-care conceptual framework the nurses developed a greater respect for the patient, the patient realized his right of choice as a consumer of health care and participated in care geared to re-establishing his self-sufficiency."[2:11]

An article by Virginia Mullin states that implementation of Orem's self-care theory faces many constraints within the acute care setting. Mullin[31:183] wrote that "these constraints can be dealt with effectively in nursing by each individual nurse internalizing the beliefs about self-care and translating those beliefs into practice."

Orem's self-care concept has been used in work with adolescent alcohol abusers,[33] employees with rheumatoid arthritis,[9] women recovering from radical mastectomies,[31] families and children with cystic fibrosis,[28] patients with congestive heart failure,[7] pretransfer teaching for cardiac patients,[51] diabetic patients,[1,3,16] persons receiving enterostomal therapy,[5] renal transplant recipients,[22] and patients receiving peritoneal dialysis.[47] It has been related to family-centered maternity care,[20] hospitalized children,[14] and hospice care.[54] Orem's self-care deficit theory has been used in the context of the nursing process to teach patients to increase their self-care agency,[24] to evaluate nursing practice,[51] and to differentiate nursing from medical practice.[32]

The general theory was applied to practical settings in many states in the United States. Beth Israel Medical Center in Newark, New Jersey, has become the first acute-care hospital in the northeastern United States to have its nursing care philosophy on Dorothea Orem's Self-Care Deficit Model. The hospital has a national information center in their reading room with collections of Orem's own work and what others have written or done about her theory. The hospital has been providing information and news letters to those nurses who are interested.[35]

Orem's general theory of nursing has been translated into different languages and has been used worldwide in Sweden, France, Australia, and Canada.[45] Maagard and Nordstrom (1984) examined the extent to which Orem's theory is applicable to the nursing of colostomy patients in Sweden. The postoperative care was described according to Orem's nursing system as wholly compensatory, partly compensatory, and supportive educative. Patient education started immediately after operation, depending on the amount of the assistance they need.[29,30]

Education

Orem's self-care deficit theory has been used as a basis for the focus of the curriculum in nursing education at many schools of nursing, such as Thornton Community College, South Holland, Illinois[15]; Georgetown University, Washington, D.C.; University of Southern Mississippi at Hattiesburg[21]; and Southern Missouri State at Springfield.[51]

At Georgetown University School of Nursing, Orem's self-care deficit theory was introduced as early as the freshman year. This establishes the theory early in the educational process, which allows the student to have a broader perspective on nursing.[48]

The curriculum for the Southwest Missouri State School of Nursing RNBSN program uses the self-care theory extensively. Students are taught to incorporate the theory in nursing care plans, patient teaching, and everyday nursing practice.[51] Goodwin[18] proposed a model of the nursing process for faculty to use to have students apply models incorporating theories to clinical practice.

University of Missouri at Columbia School of Nursing offers conferences on Orem's theory each fall and winter semesters for nursing students. The university is also offering annual self-care deficit theory conferences, nursing research conferences, and annual institutes on self-care theory. Most of these conferences are national and international.[43]

Research

Orem's self-care concept provided the conceptual framework for Dickerson and Lee-Villasenor's[16] research[11] and for Gallant and McLane's outcome criteria.[17] Denyes[10] developed a Likert scale questionnaire for clinical nursing assessment and studies with adolescents, and Crockett[8] described the self-reported development of coping beliefs and practices of adult psychiatric and nonpsychiatric subjects.

Kearney and Fleischer developed an instrument to measure a person's excercise of self-care agency and administered it to nursing students in an associate degree program and to students in two psychology courses. Findings concluded that people who exercise a high degree of self-care agency describe themselves as self-controlled, dependable, assertive, intelligent, confident, responsible, helpful, and adaptable. Kearney and Fleischer recommended that the scale be administered to other populations to further validate the results of the study.[24]

Barbara J. Horn, Mary Ann Swain, and their associates have developed criteria measures of nursing care around the universal self-care requisites and health-deviation self-care requisites along with instruments and procedures to measure the quality of nursing care provided.[22]

In a study done at the University of Michigan, the authors, who were research assistants on the Horn and Swain study, developed eight categories of patient outcomes related to health-deviation self-care actions. The study had not been concluded when the article was published because a method of data collection still needed to be determined. The ultimate goal of the study was to establish an instrument that could be used to measure the health status of hospitalized patients along dimensions related to their requirements for universal and health-deviations self-care.[6]

Rothlis (1984) reviewed reactive depression as a health-deviation self-care deficit in Orem's framework.[50] Dodd (1984) studied the self-care behaviors of cancer patients in chemotherapy. She stated that because there is little information about how patients manage their illnesses, study of self-care is necessary. The research was conducted in three groups of cancer patients and found that the patients who were informed about the side effects of medications performed more self-care than those who had not received the information.[12,48]

FURTHER DEVELOPMENT

Orem's work has been used most with ill adults. However, Orem defined dependent care agent as the provider of infant or child care and identified early on developmental as one of the three types of self-care requisites. She added a section on "age-specific factors in nursing children" in the 1980 edition of her book *Nursing: Concepts of Practice*[38:155-159;44:259-262] and a section on multiperson units in the 1985 edition.[38:251-256] She had addressed the multiperson unit in a table in the 1980 edition.[38] Orem[40] discussed her conceptual model and community health nursing at the eighth annual community health nursing conference at the University of North Carolina at Chapel Hill, and has addressed the relationship of her model to rehabilitation in Cincinnati.[45]

CRITIQUE

Simplicity

Orem identified six major concepts in the self-care deficit theory of nursing. They are self-care, therapeutic self-care demand, self-care agency, self-care deficit, nursing agency, and nursing system. She uses these six concepts to express the three constituent theories of the general theory of nursing.[43,44] The conceptual framework appears simple. Subconcepts are identified to express the substantive structure of the six broad conceptual elements of the theory.

Generality

> The self-care deficit theory of nursing as expressed is universal. It is a theory of nursing as nursing regardless of time or place. Its use as a guide to practice was initially and at present most commonly applied in the care of ill adults. From the beginning, it has been applied in the care of both well and sick children. The universality of the theory should be differentiated from its application in terms of time, place, and individuals.[43]

Empirical Precision

This theory identifies concepts, provides definitions, describes relationships, and states assumptions. It can be, and has been, used for research.

Derivable Consequences

Orem's self-care deficit theory of nursing provides a general framework to direct nursing action. Orem[36:92-103] views nursing within the framework of the theory as related to patients' therapeutic self-care demands, their self-care agency, and the relationships between them. She sees three types of nursing systems: doing self-care for the individual (wholly compensatory), assisting the individual with self-care (partially compensatory), and educating and supporting the individual to help him or her better perform self-care.

Orem believes her self-care theory applies to other groups in addition to nurses.

> The self-care theory component of the general theory of nursing is common to the health professions and to all members of social groups. Physicians as well as paramedical groups help people with aspects of self-care and with development of capabilities to engage in self-care. Persons helped may or may not be in need of nursing or may or may not be under nursing care.[43]

The assumptions used in this theory are logically sound and accepted by the nursing community. The concepts are relevant for nursing. The relationships explained and implied are useful in explaining patiency and the nurse-patient relationship.

Orem's theory does direct nursing practice, the stated goal. Her nursing systems provide a framework for nursing practice, based on the amount and kind of nursing agency needed. In her books Orem also addresses educational needs for nurses to be able to practice as well as the use of various levels of nursing practice. Additional research is desirable.

REFERENCES

1. Allison, S. (1973). A framework for nursing action in a nurse-conducted diabetic managed clinic. *Journal of Nursing Administration, 3(4)*:53-60.
2. Anna, D., et al. (1978, Nov.). Implementing Orem's conceptual framework, *Journal of Nursing Administration, 8:*8-11.
3. Bachschieder, J. (1974). Self-care requirements, self-care capabilities and nursing systems in the diabetic nurse managed clinic. *American Journal of Public Health, 64(12)*:1138-1146.
4. Bennett, J.G. (Ed.) (1980). Symposium on the self-care concept of nursing. *Nursing Clinics of North America, 15:*129-217.
5. Bromley, B. (1980, Feb.). Applying Orem's self-care theory in enterostomal therapy. *American Journal of Nursing, 80:*245-249.
6. Clinton, J.E., et al. (1977, Sept.). Developing criterion measures of nursing care: Case study of

a process. *Journal of Nursing Administration, 7(7):*41-45.
7. Crews, J. (1972). Nurse-managed cardiac clinics. *Cardiovascular Nursing, 8:*15-18.
8. Crockett, M.S. (1982). Self reported coping histories of adult psychiatric and nonpsychiatric subjects and controls. *Nursing Research,* 31:122. (Abstract).
9. Dear, M.R., & Keen, M.F. (1982). Promotion of self-care in the employee with rheumatoid arthritis. *Occupational Health Nursing, 30(1):*32-34.
10. Denyes, M.J. (1982). Measurement of self-care agency in adolescents. *Nursing Research, 31:*63. (Abstract).
11. Dickson, G.L., & Lee-Villasenor, H. (1982). Nursing theory and practice: A self-care approach. *Advances in Nursing Science, 5(1):*29-40.
12. Dodd, M.J. (1984). Measuring informational intervention for chemotherapy: Knowledge and self-care behavior. *Research in Nursing and Health, 7:*43-50.
13. Eichelberger, K.M., et al. (1980). Self-care nursing plan: Helping children to help themselves. *Pediatric Nursing 6(3):*9-13.
14. Facteau, L.M. (1980). Self-care concepts and the care of the hospitalized child. *Nursing Clinics of North America, 15:*145-155.
15. Fenner, K. (1979). Developing a conceptual framework. *Nursing Outlook, 27:*122-126.
16. Fitzgerald, S. (1980). Utilizing Orem's self-care nursing model in designing an educational program for the diabetic. *Topics in Clinical Nursing, 2(2):*57-65.
17. Gallant, B.W., & McLane, A.M. (1979). Outcome criteria: A process for validation at the unit level. *Journal of Nursing Administration, 9(1):*14-21.
18. Garavan, P., et al. (1980). Self-care applied to the aged. *New Jersey Nurse, 10(1):*3-5.
19. Goodwin, J.O. (1980, Nov.-Dec.). A cross-cultural approach to integrating nursing theory and practice. *Nurse Educator, 5(6):*15-20.
20. Harris, J.K. (1980). Self-care is possible after Cesarean delivery. *Nursing Clinics of North America. 15:*191-204.
21. Herrington, J.V., & Houston, S. (1984, Jan.). Using Orem's theory: A plan for all seasons. *Nursing and Health Care, 5(1):*45-47.
22. Hoffart, N. (1982, June). Self-care decision making by renal transplant recipients. *AANNT Journal, 9(3):*43-47.
23. Horn, B.J., & Swain, M.A. (1977). *Development of Criterion Measures of Nursing Care* (Vols. 1 and 2). Springfield, Va.: University of Michigan and National Center for Health Services Research, U.S. Department of Commerce. (NTIS Nos. 267-004 and 267-005).
24. Joseph, L.S. (1980). Self-care and the nursing process. *Nursing Clinics of North America, 15:*131-143.
25. Kearney, B., & Fleischer, B.L. (1979). Development of an instrument to measure exercise of self-care agency. *Research in Nursing and Health, 2(1):*25-34.
26. Kinlein, M. (1977). *Independent nursing practice with clients.* Philadelphia: J.B. Lippincott.
27. Kinlein, M.L. (1977, April). The self-care concept, *American Journal of Nursing, 77:*598-601.
28. Kruger, S., Shawver, M., & Jones, L. (1980). Reactions of families to the child with cystic fibrosis. *Image, 12:*67-72.
29. Lundh, U., Soder, M., & Warness, K. (1988, Spring). Nursing theories: A critical view, *Image, 20 (1):*36-40.
30. Maagard, B., & Nordström, G. (1984). Orems vårdteori [The Nursing Theory of Orem]. *Omvårdaren, 1:*16-20.
31. Martin, L. (1980). Self-care nursing model for patients experiencing radical change in body image. *Journal of Obstetric, Gynecologic, and Neonatal Nursing, 7(6):*9-13.
32. McIntyre, K. (1980). The Perry model as a framework for self-care. *Nurse Practitioner, 5(6):*34-38.
33. Michael, M.M., & Sewall, K.S. (1980). Use of adolescent peer group to increase the self-care agency of adolescent alcohol abusers. *Nursing Clinics of North America, 15:*157-176.
34. Mullin, V.I. (1980, March). Implementing the self-care concept in the acute care setting. *Nursing Clinics of North America, 15(1):*183.
35. NLN Editorial Review Board News. (1987, Dec.). Newark Beth Israel Medical Center adopts Orem's Self-Care Model. *Nursing and Health Care. 8(10):*593-594.
36. Orem, D.E. (1956). *Hospital nursing service: An analysis and report of a study of administrative positions in one hospital nursing service.* Indianapolis: Indiana State Board of Health.

37. Orem, D.E. (1979). *Concept formalization in nursing: Process and product*. Boston: Little, Brown.
38. Orem, D.E. (1980). *Nursing: Concepts of practice*. New York: McGraw-Hill.
39. Orem, D.E. (1983). The self-care deficit theory of nursing: A general theory. In I. Clements & F. Roberts (Eds.), *Family health: A theoretical approach to nursing care*. New York: Wiley.
40. Orem, D.E. (1984, May). Orem's conceptual model and community health nursing. In M.K. Asay & C.C. Ossler (Eds.), *Proceedings of the Eighth Annual Community Health Nursing Conference: Conceptual Models of Nursing Applications in Community Health Nursing*. Chapel Hill: University of North Carolina Press.
41. Orem, D. (1984). Vitae.
42. Orem, D. (1984). Personal correspondence.
43. Orem, D. (1988). Personal correspondence.
44. Orem, D. (1985). *Nursing: Concepts of practice*. New York: McGraw-Hill.
45. Orem, D. (1985). Telephone interviews.
46. Orem, D. (1988). Telephone interviews.
47. Perras, S.T., & Zappacosta, A.R. (1982, June). The application of Orem's theory in promoting self-care in a peritoneal dialysis facility. *AANNT Journal, 9(3)*:37-40.
48. Piemme, J.A., & Trainor, M.A. (1977). A first-year nursing course in a baccalaureate program. *Nursing Outlook, 25(3)*:185-186.
49. Polit, D.F., & Hungler, B.P. (1987). *Nursing research principles and methods* (3d ed.). Philadelphia: J.B. Lippincott.
50. Rothlis, J. (1984). The effect of a self-help group on feelings of hopelessness and helplessness. *Western Journal of Nursing Research, 6*:157-168.
51. Runtz, S.E., & Urtal, J.G. (1983, March). Evaluating your practice via a nursing model. *Nurse Practitioner, 8(3)*:30-40.
52. Schumacher, L. (1984, April). Interview.
53. Toth, J.C. (1980). Effects of structured preparation for transfer on patient anxiety on leaving coronary care unit. *Nursing Research, 29*:28-34.
54. Walborn, K.A. (1980). A nursing model for the hospice: Primary and self-care nursing. *Nursing Clinics of North America, 15*:205-217.

BIBLIOGRAPHY

Primary Sources

Books

Orem, D.E. (Ed.) (1959). *Guides for developing curricula for the education of practical nurses*. Vocational Division #274, Trade and Industrial Education #68. Washington, D.C., U.S. Department of Health, Education, and Welfare.

Orem, D.E. (1971). *Nursing: Concepts of practice*. Scarborough, Ontario: McGraw-Hill.

Orem, D.E. (Ed.) (1973). *Concept formalization in nursing: Process and product*. Boston: Little, Brown.

Orem, D.E. (Ed.) (1979). *Concept formalization in nursing: Process and product* (2d ed.). Boston: Little, Brown.

Orem, D.E. (1980). *Nursing: Concepts of practice*. (2d ed.). New York: McGraw-Hill.

Orem, D.E. (1985). *Nursing: Concepts of practice* (3d ed.). New York: McGraw-Hill.

Orem, D.E., & Parker, K.S. (Eds.). (1963). *Nurse education workshop proceedings*. Washington, D.C.: Catholic University of America.

Orem, D.E., & Parker, K.S. (Eds.). (1964). *Nursing content in preservice nursing curriculum*. Washington, D.C.: The Catholic University of America Press.

Book Chapters

Orem, D.E. (1966). Discussion of paper—Another view of nursing care and quality. In K.M. Straub, & K.S. Parker *Continuity of patient care: The role of nursing*. Washington, D.C.: The Catholic University of America Press.

Orem, D.E. (1969). Inservice education and nursing practice forces affecting nursing practice. In D.K. Petrowski & K.M. Staub (Eds.), *School of Nursing Education*. Washington, D.C.: The Catholic University of America Press.

Orem, D.E. (1981). Nursing: A triad of action systems. In G.E. Lasker (Ed.), *Applied systems and cybernetics* (Vol. IV). Systems research in health care, biocybernetics and ecology. New York: Pergamon Press.

Orem, D.E. (1982). Nursing: A dilemma for higher education. In Sister A. Power (ed.), *Words commemorated: Essays celebrating the centennial of Incarnate Word College*. San Antonio, Tex.: Incarnate Word College.

Orem, D.E. (1983). The self-care deficit theory of

nursing: A general theory. In I. Clements & F. Roberts (Eds.), *Family health: A theoretical approach to nursing care.* New York: Wiley Medical Publications.

Orem, D.E. (1984). Orem's conceptual model and community health nursing. In M.K. Asay & C.C. Ossler, *Proceedings of the Eighth Annual Community Health Nursing Conference: Conceptual models of nursing applications in Community Health Nursing.* Chapel Hill: University of North Carolina, Dept. of Public Health Nursing, School of Public Health.

Orem, D.E., & Taylor, S. (1986). Orem's general theory of nursing. In P. Winstead-Fry (Ed.), *Case Studies in Nursing Theory* (pp. 37-71). Pub. No. 15-2152. New York: National League for Nursing.

Orem, D.E. (1988). Nursing administration: A theoretical approach. In B. Henry, C. Arndt, M. DiVincenti, & A. Marriner-Tomey (Eds.), *Dimensions of Nursing Administration.* Boston: Blackwell Scientific.

Articles

Orem, D.E., & O'Malley, M. (1952, Aug.). Diagnosis of hospital nursing problems. *Hospitals, 26:*63.

Orem, D.E. (1962, Jan.). The hope of nursing. *Journal of Nursing Education, 1:*5+.

Orem, D.E. (1979, March). Levels of nursing education and practice. *Alumnae Magazine, The Johns Hopkins School of Nursing, 68:*2-6.

Orem, D.E. (1985, May-June). Concepts of self-care for the rehabilitation client. *Rehabilitation Nursing, 10(3):*33-36.

Orem, D.E. (1988, May). The forum of nursing science. *Nursing Science Quarterly 1(2):*75-79.

Reports

Orem, D.E. (1955). *Indiana hospitals: a report.* Author of three sections of ten-year report of status and problems of Indiana hospitals. The Indiana State Board of Health.

Orem, D.E. (1956). *Hospital nursing service: An analysis and report of a study of administrative positions in one hospital nursing service.* The Indiana State Board of Health.

Orem, D.E., Dear, M., & Greenbaum, J. (1976). *Organization of nursing faculty responsibilities.* (Project Report, Public Health Service Grant No. 03D-005-3666). Washington, D.C.: Georgetown University School of Nursing.

Audiotape

Orem, D.E. (1978, Dec.). Paper presented at the Second Annual Nurse Educator Conference, New York. Audio tapes available from Teach 'em, Inc., 160 E. Illinois Street, Chicago, Ill. 60611.

Videocassette

National League for Nurses. (1987). *Nursing Theory: A Circle of Knowledge.* Available from the author, 10 Columbus Circle, New York, N.Y. 10019.

The Nurse Theorists. Portraits of excellence: Dorothea Orem. (1988). Oakland: Studio III. Available from Fuld Video Project, Studio III, 370 Hawthorne Avenue, Oakland, Calif. 94609.

Correspondence

Orem, D. (1983) Vitae.

Orem, D. (1984) Personal correspondence.

Orem, D. (1988). Personal correspondence.

Interviews

Orem, D. (1984) Telephone interviews.

Orem, D. (1985) Telephone interviews.

Orem, D.E. (1987). Veterans Administration Teleconference.

Orem, D. (1988). Telephone interviews.

Secondary Sources

Book Reviews

Orem, D.E. (1971). *Nursing: Concepts of practice.*
*Canadian Nurse, 67:*47, December 1971.
*Supervisor Nurse, 3:*45-6, January 1972.
*American Journal of Nursing, 72:*1330, July 1972.

Orem, D.E. (1980). *Nursing: Concepts of practice* (2d ed.).
*Registered Nurse Association of British Columbia, 12:*25, November 1980.
*AORN Journal, 24:*776, October 1981.
*Nursing Times, 78:*1671, October 6-12, 1982.
*Journal of Advanced Nursing, 8(1):*89, January 1983.

Dissertations

Laurin, J. (1979). *Development of a nursing process-outcome model based on Orem's concepts of nursing practice for quality nursing care evaluation.* Doctoral dissertation. Catholic University of America.

Sullivan, T.J. (1979). *A self-care model of nursing practice for nursing the aged.* Doctoral dissertation. Columbia University Teachers College.

Underwood, P.R. (1978). *Nursing care as a determinant in the development of self-care behavior by hospitalized adult schizophrenics.* Doctoral dissertation. University of California, San Francisco.

Books

Chinn, P.L., & Jacobs, M.K. (1987). *Theory and nursing: A systematic approach.* St. Louis: C.V. Mosby.

Fitzpatrick, J.J., et al. (1982). *Nursing models and their psychiatric mental health applications.* Bowie, Md.: Robert J. Brady.

Hill, L., & Smith, N. (1985). *Self-care nursing.* Englewood Cliffs, N.J.: Prentice-Hall.

Fitzpatrick, J., & Whall, A. (1983). *Conceptual models of nursing: Analysis and applications.* Bowie, Md: Robert J. Brady.

Fitzpatrick, J., et al. (1982). *Nursing models and their psychiatric mental health applications.* Bowie, Md; Robert J. Brady.

Horn, B.J., & Swain, M.A. (1977). *Development of criterion measures of nursing care* (Vols. 1 and 2). University of Michigan and National Center for Health Services Research. U.S. Department of Commerce. (NTIS Publication No. 267-004 and 267-005).

Kin, H.S. (1983). *The nature of theoretical thinking in nursing.* Norwalk, Conn.: Appleton-Century-Crofts.

Leddy, S., & Pepper, J.M. (1985). *Conceptual bases of professional nursing.* Philadelphia: J.B. Lippincott.

Meleis, A.J. (1985). *Theoretical nursing's development and progress.* Philadelphia: J.B. Lippincott.

National League of Nursing (1978). *Theory development: What, why, how?* New York: N.L.N. Publication 15-1708, pp. 73-74.

Nursing Theories Conference Group, J.B. George, Chairperson, (1980). *Nursing theories: The base for professional practice.* Englewood Cliffs, N.J.: Prentice-Hall.

Parse, R.R. (1987). *Nursing Science.* Philadelphia: W.B. Saunders.

Polit, D.F., & Hungler, B.P. (1987). *Nursing Research Principles and Methods* (3d ed.). Philadelphia: J.B. Lippincott.

Torres, G. (1986). *Theoretical Foundations of Nursing.* Norwalk, Conn.: Appleton-Century-Crofts.

Winstead-Fry, P. (1986). *Case Studies in Nursing Theory.* New York: NLN.

Book Chapters

Calley, J.M., et al. (1980). The Orem self-care nursing model. In J.P. Riehl & C. Roy, *Conceptual models for nursing practice.* New York: Appleton-Century-Crofts, pp. 302-314.

Coleman, L.J. (1980). Orem's self-care nursing model. In J.P. Riehl & C. Roy, *Conceptual models for nursing practice.* New York: Appleton-Century-Crofts, pp. 315-328.

Fawcett, J. (1984). Orem's self-care model. In J. Fawcett, *Analysis and evaluation of conceptual models in nursing.* Philadelphia: F.A. Davis, pp. 175-210.

Foster, P.C., & Janssens, N.P. (1980). Dorothea E. Orem. In Nursing Theories Conference Group, J.B. George, Chairperson, *Nursing theories: The base for professional practice.* Englewood Cliffs, N.J.: Prentice-Hall, pp. 91-106.

Goldstein, N., et al. (1983). Self-care: A framework for the future. In P.L. Chinn (Ed.). *Advances in nursing theory development.* Rockville, Md.: Aspen Systems, pp. 107-121.

Horn, B.J, & Swain, M.A. (1976). An approach to development of criterion measures for quality patient care. In *Issues in evaluation research.* Kansas City: American Nurses' Association.

Horn, B.J (1978). Development of criterion measures of nursing care. (Abstract). In *Communicating nursing research* (Vol. 11: New approaches to communicating nursing research). Boulder, Col.: Western Interstate Commission for Higher Education.

Johnson, R.L. (1982). Individual psychotherapy: Relationships of theoretical approaches to nursing conceptual models. In J. Fitzpatrick, et al., *Nursing models and their psychiatric mental health applications.* Bowie, Md., Robert J. Brady, pp. 56-60.

Johnston, R.L. (1983). Orem self-care model of nursing. In J. Fitzpatrick & A. Whall, *Conceptual models of nursing, analysis and application.* Bowie, Md: Robert J. Brady, pp. 137-156.

Kinlein, M.L. (1977). *Independent nursing practice with clients.* Philadelphia, J.B. Lippincott, pp. 15-24.

Meleis, A.I. (1985). Dorothea Orem. In A.I. Meleis, *Theoretical nursing: development and progress.* Philadelphia: J.B. Lippincott, pp. 284-296.

Roy, C. (1980). A case study viewed according to different models. In J.P. Riehl & C. Roy, *Conceptual models for nursing practice.* New York: Appleton-Century Crofts, pp. 385-386.

Spangler, Z.S., & Spangler, W.O. (1983). Self-care: A testable model. In P.L. Chinn (Ed.), *Advances in nursing theory development.* Rockville, Md.: Aspen Systems, 89-105.

Stanton, M. (1980). Nursing theories and the nursing process. In Nursing Theories Conference Group, J.B. George, Chairperson, *Nursing theories: The base for professional practice.* Englewood Cliffs, N.J.: Prentice-Hall, pp. 213-217.

Sullivan, T.J. (1980). Self-care model for nursing. In *Directions for nursing in the 80's.* Kansas City: American Nurses' Association.

Underwood, P.R. (1980). Facilitating self-care. In P. Potheir (Ed.), *Psychiatric nursing: A basic text.* Boston: Little, Brown.

Thibodeau, J.A. (1983). An eclectic model: The Orem model. In J.A. Thibodeau, *Nursing models: Analysis and evaluation.* Monterey, Calif.: Wadsworth Health Sciences Division, pp. 125-140.

Articles

Allison, S. (1973). A framework for nursing action in a nurse-conducted diabetic management clinic. *Journal of Nursing Administration, 3(4)*:53-60.

Anna, D.J., et al. (1978, Nov.). Implementing Orem's conceptual framework. *Journal of Nursing Administration, 8*:8-11.

Bachscheider, J. (1974). Self-care requirement, self-care capabilities, and nursing systems in the diabetic nurse management clinic, *American Journal of Public Health, 64(12)*:1138-1146.

Bennett, J.G. (1980, March). Symposium on the self-care concept of nursing. *Nursing Clinics of North America, 15*:129-217.

Bilitski, J.S. (1981). Nursing science and the laws of health as a step in the process of theory development. *Advances in Nursing Science, 4(1)*:15-29.

Blair, C. (1985). Behavior modification in nursing practice and research: A case study. *Journal of Advanced Nursing, 10(2)*:165-168.

Bromley, B. (1980, Feb.). Applying Orem's self-care theory in enterostomal therapy. *American Journal of Nursing, 80(2)*:245-249.

Chang, B. (1980). Evaluation of health care professionals in facilitating self-care: Review of the literature as a conceptual model, *Advances in Nursing Science, 3(1)*:43-58.

Clinton, J.F., et al. (1977, Sept.). Developing criterion measures of nursing care: Case study of a process. *Journal of Nursing Administration, 7(7)*:41-45.

Crews, J. (1972). Nurse-managed cardiac clinics. *Cardiovascular Nursing, 8*:15-18.

Crockett, M.S. (1982). Self-reported coping histories of adult psychiatric and non-psychiatric subjects and controls. *Nursing Research, 31*:122. (Abstract).

Dear, M.R., & Keen, M.F. (1982). Promotion of self-care in the employee with rheumatoid arthritis. *Occupational Health Nursing, 30(1)*:32-34.

Denyes, M.J. (1982). Measurement of self-care aging in adolescents. *Nursing Research, 31*:63. (Abstract).

Dickson, G.L., et al. (1982, Oct.). Nursing theory and practice: A self-care approach. *Advances in Nursing Science, 5(1)*:29-40.

Dodd, M.J. (1984). Measuring informational intervention for chemotherapy: Knowledge and self-care behavior. *Research in Nursing and Health, 7*:43-50.

Eichelberger, K.M., et al. (1980). Self-care nursing plan: Helping children to help themselves. *Pediatric Nursing, 6(3)*:9-13.

Elstad, I. (1981, Nov. 20). A critique of the theory on self-care. *Sykepleien, 68(20)*:16-19.

Facteau, L.M. (1980, March). Self-care concepts and the care of the hospitalized child. *Nursing Clinics of North America, 15(1)*:145-155.

Fitzgerald, S. (1980, July). Utilizing Orem's self-care nursing model in designing an educational program for the diabetic. *Topics of Clinical Nursing, 2(2)*:57-65.

Fleener, K. (1979). Developing a conceptual framework. *Nursing Outlook, 27*:122-126.

Gallant, B.W., & McLane, A.M. (1979). Outcome criteria: A process for validation at the unit level. *Journal of Nursing Administration, 9(1)*:14-21.

Garvan, P., et al. (1980). Self-care applied to the aged. *New Jersey Nurse, 10(1)*:3-5.

Goodwin, J.O. (1980, Nov.-Dec.). A cross-cultural approach to integrating nursing theory and practice. *Nurse Educator 5(6)*:15-20.

Greenfield, E., & Pace, J.C. (1985). Orem's self-care theory of nursing: Practical applications to the end stage renal disease patient. *Journal of Nephrological Nursing, 2(4)*:187-193.

Harper, D.C. (1984, April). Application of Orem's theoretical construct to self-care medication behaviors in the elderly. *Advances in Nursing Science, 6(3)*:29-46.

Harris, J.K. (1980, March). Self-care is possible after cesarean delivery. *Nursing Clinics of North America, 15*:191-204.

Herrington, J.V., & Houston, S (1984, Jan). Using Orem's theory: A plan for all seasons. *Nursing and Health Care, 5(1)*:45-47.

Hoffart, N. (1982, June). Self-care decision-making by renal transplant recipients. *AANNT Journal, 9(3)*:39-47.

Hoon, E. (1986). Game playing: A way to look at nursing models. *Journal of Advanced Nursing, 11*:421-427.

Joseph, L.S. (1980, March). Self-care and the nursing process. *Nursing Clinics of North America, 15(1)*:131-143.

Kearney, B., & Fleischer, B. (1979). Development of an instrument to measure exercise of self-care agency. *Research in Nursing Health, 2*:25-34.

Kinlein, M.L. (1977). The self-care concept. *American Journal of Nursing, 4*:598-601.

Kruger, S., Shawver, M., & Jones, L. (1980). Reactions of families to the child with cystic fibrosis. *Image, 12*:67-72.

Lundh, U., Soder, M., & Warness, K. (1988, Spring). Nursing theories: A critical view. *Image, 20(1)*:36-40.

Maagard, B., & Nordström, G. (1984). Orems vårdteori [The Nursing Theory of Orem]. *Omvårdaren, 1*:16-20.

McFarland, E.A. (1980, Jan). Nursing theory: The comparison of four theoretical proposals. *Journal of Advanced Nursing, 5(10)*:3-19.

McIntyre, K. (1980). The Perry model as a framework for self-care. *Nurse Practitioner, 5(6)*:34-38.

Marten, L. (1978). Self-care nursing model for patients experiencing radical change in body image. *Journal of Obstetric, Gynecologic and Neonatal Nursing, 7(6)*:9-13.

Melnyk, K.A. (1983, May-June). The process of theory analysis: An examination of the nursing theory of Dorothea E. Orem. *Nursing Research, 32(3)*:170-174.

Michael, M.M., & Sewall, K.S. (1980, March). Use of the adolescent peer group to increase the self-care agency of adolescent alcohol abusers. *Nursing Clinics of North America, 15(1)*:157-176.

Mullin, V.I. (1980, March). Implementing the self-care concept in the acute care setting, *Nursing Clinics of North America, 15(1)*:177-190.

NLN Editorial Review Board News. (1987, December). Newark Beth Israel Medical Center adopts Orem's Self-Care Model. *Nursing and Health Care, 8(10)*: 593-594.

Nordentoft, L.S. (1981, Oct. 21). The concept of self-care defined and applied in a nursing model. *Sygeplejerskon, 81(41)*:4-6.

Perras, S.T., et al. (1982, June). The application of Orem's theory in promoting self-care in a peritoneal dialysis facility. *AANNT Journal, 9(3)*:37-39.

Piemme, J.A., & Trainor, M.A. (1977). A first-year nursing course in a baccalaureate program. *Nursing Outlook, 25(3)*:184-187.

Porter, D., & Shamian, J. (1983, Sept.). Self-care in theory and practice. *Canadian Nurse, 79(8)*:21-23.

Roberts, K.L. (1985). Theory of nursing as curriculum content. *Journal of Advanced Nursing, 10*:483-489.

Rosenbaum, J.N. (1986). Comparison of two theorists on care: Orem and Leininger. *Journal of Advanced Nursing, 11*:408-419.

Rothlis, J. (1984). The effect of a self-help group on feelings of hopelessness and helplessness. *Western Journal of Nursing Research, 6*:157-168.

Runtz, S.E., & Urtel, J.G. (1983, March). Evaluating your practice via a nursing model. *Nurse Practitioner, 8(3)*:30-32, 37-40.

Silva, M.C. (1986). Research testing nursing theory: State of the art. *Advances in Nursing Sciences, 9(1)*:1-11.

Smith, M.C. (1979, Oct.). Proposed metaparadigm for nursing research and theory development: An analysis of Orem's self-care theory. *Image, 11(3)*:5-9.

Smith, S.R. (1981, Oct.). Sound off: "Oremization," the curse of nursing. *R.N., 10*:83.

Symposium on self-care concept of nursing (1980, March). *Nursing Clinics of North America, 15(1)*: 129-217.

Toth, J.C. (1980). Effects of structured preparation for transfer on patient anxiety on leaving coronary care unit. *Nursing Research, 29*:28-34.

Valsat, S., et al. (1983, Jan. 20). Report from an Orem seminar. *Sykepleien, 70(2)*:18-19.

Walborn, K.A. (1980, March). A nursing model for the hospice: Primary and self-care nursing. *Nursing Clinics of North America, 15(1)*:205-217.

Interview

Schumacher, Lawrence (1984, April 3).

12

Evelyn Adam

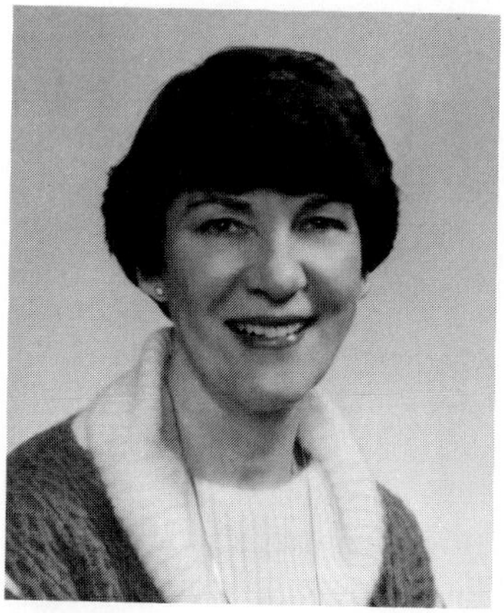

Conceptual Model for Nursing

Terri Creekmur, Janet DeFelice, Marilyn Sue Doub, Anne Hodel, Cheryl Y. Petty

CREDENTIALS AND BACKGROUND OF THE THEORIST

Evelyn Adam was born April 9, 1929, in Lanark, Ontario, Canada. She graduated from Hotel Dieu Hospital in Kingston, Ontario, in 1950 with a Diploma in Nursing. She received a B.Sc. degree in 1966 from the University of Montreal and an M.N. degree from the University of California at Los Angeles in 1971. At U.C.L.A. she met Dorothy Johnson, who she feels has "definitely been the most important influence" on her professional life.[6]

In 1979 she published her first book, *Être Infirmière* and in 1980 wrote the English version of *To Be a Nurse*. Since then, her book has been translated into Dutch (1981) and Spanish (1982). Adam has also written numerous articles on conceptual models for nursing and has coauthored several others. Professional journals publishing her articles include *Infirmière Cana-*

The authors wish to express appreciation to Evelyn Adam for editing the chapter.

dienne, Canadian Nurse, Journal of Advanced Nursing, Nursing Papers: Perspectives in Nursing, and *Journal of Nursing Education.*

Adam has been a visiting professor at several universities. She has functioned as a resource person and speaker for various professional corporations, clinical and educational settings, and national and international conventions. Since 1983, she has been a member of the review board for *Nursing Papers* and has directed the research of many graduate students since 1974. She is currently Professor of Nursing at both undergraduate and graduate levels and secretary of the nursing faculty at the University of Montreal. She is in the eighth edition of *Who's Who in the World* (1987-88). She published an article, "Nursing Theory: What It Is and What It Is Not," in *Nursing Papers: Perspectives in Nursing,* 1987.

Whereas nursing care of the elderly is a recent professional interest, promoting conceptual models for nursing has predominated since 1970. She strongly feels that "nursing practice, education, and research must be based on an explicit frame of reference specific to nursing."[6]

Adam's work makes an important distinction between a conceptual model and a theory. "A [conceptual] model is usually based on, or derives from, a theory. . . . A model, emerging from a theory, may become the basis for a new theory."[1:40] "A conceptual model, for whatever discipline, is not reality; it is a mental image of reality or a way of conceptualizing reality. A conceptual model *for* nursing is therefore a conception *of* nursing."[5:42]

Adam[4,6] accepts Roy and Roberts' definition[10:5] of a theory as "a system of interrelated propositions used to describe, predict, explain, understand, and control a part of the empirical world."

Therefore a theory is useful to more than one discipline. A conceptual model for a discipline is useful only to that particular discipline. Adam[7] believes "The day may come when nursing theory will be as useful to related disciplines as existing theories, developed in other fields, are today useful to nursing."

Adam[2:5] writes that "a conceptual model is an abstraction, a way of looking at something, an invention of the mind."

> A conceptual model for a discipline is a very broad perspective, a global way of looking at a discipline. Most of the conceptual models for nursing that we know have come from two sources: one, a theory, chosen by the author, and the other, her professional experience.[6]

A conceptual model is the precursor of a theory. The model specifies the discipline's focus of inquiry, identifies those phenomena of particular interest to nursing, and provides a broad perspective for nursing research, practice, and education. The study of phenomena that concern nursing, that is, nursing research, may lead to theories that will describe, explain, or predict those phenomena. Such theories will not be theories *of nursing* but theories *of the phenomena* that are nursing's focus of inquiry.[4:12]

Many nurses are unable to communicate clearly and explicitly their conception of the service they offer to society. Adam contends this is not because they do not have a conception of nursing but because their conceptual base is not clear. If the nurse's mental image of nursing is vague or blurred, it will therefore be difficult to put into words. The nurse will then be unable to articulate her particular role in health care and may well find that her professional activities are based on a perspective borrowed from another discipline.

Adam[1:41] states that "a model indicates the goal of our [nursing] profession—an ideal and limited goal, because it gives us direction for nursing practice, nursing education, and nursing research." Nurses who have a clear, concise conceptual base specific to nursing will be able to identify areas for theory development, prepare future practitioners of nursing, and demonstrate in their own practice nursing's contribution to health care. In this way health care will improve and the nursing profession will grow.

Although it is not necessary for every nurse to adopt the same conceptual model, it is essential that every nurse have a concise and explicit framework on which to base her work. The conceptual model is "the conceptual departure point" for her teaching, research or nursing care. Speaking figuratively, Adam places the conceptual model in the nurse's occipital lobe, known also as her visual lobe. The nurse uses a great deal of scientific knowledge as well as her experience, intuition, and creativity. In drawing on this knowledge, she is guided by her conceptual model, that is her mental image of nursing.[7]

The abstraction that is the conceptual model is linked to the reality that is nursing practice through the nursing process.[2] The data we collect depend on our conceptual base. The way we interpret the data, the plan we develop, the nursing action we choose, and the evaluation of our intervention also depend on our model. The number of steps in the nursing process is not significant because the difference is the conceptual base.[6]

In addition to the conceptual model and the nursing process, the nurse must also establish with the client what will be perceived to be a helping relationship. Adam considers this perhaps the most important component of being a nurse. It is the climate of empathy, warmth, mutual respect, caring, and acceptance that determines the effectiveness of nursing care.[2:50;7]

Adam feels that three components constitute nursing practice: the client, the nurse (with her conceptual model as a base for the nursing process), and the relationship between the client and nurse. She has created a pictorial representation of nursing practice in her books (Figure 12-1).[2:43;2:55;7]

Adam insists the helping relationship and the systematic process (which nurses have, perhaps wrongly, labeled the "nursing" process) are important to all health professionals. Nursing fits into the whole of health care as an integral component of the interdisciplinary health team. Each discipline makes a unique contribution to the promotion and preservation of health and to the prevention of health problems. Although some services overlap within this interdisciplinary health team, each discipline is present because of its distinct and specific contribution to health.

This relationship can be illustrated with a schematic flower (Figure 12-2). Each petal represents a distinct health discipline: nursing, medicine, physical therapy, speech therapy, or nutrition, for example. The center of the flower indicates the shared functions. A part of each petal is separate and distinct from the others, and the largest part of each petal represents the unique contribution of each discipline. Our conceptual model clarifies and makes explicit nursing's "petal."

Nurses currently have several conceptual models from which to choose. The decision to adopt one of the conceptual models for (not *of*) nursing is often made by considering the eventual evaluation of that particular model. Adam insists that conceptual models must be evaluated by criteria different from those used to evaluate theories. She quotes the three criteria established by Dorothy Johnson[8]:

1. Social significance: clients would be asked if the service (nursing) was significant to their health.
2. Social congruence: clients would be asked if the service (nursing) was congruent with their expectations.
3. Social utility: nurses would be asked if the conceptual model provided useful direction for education, practice, and research.

Such criteria are extrinsic to the model itself. However, in order to use these criteria the conceptual model in question must already have

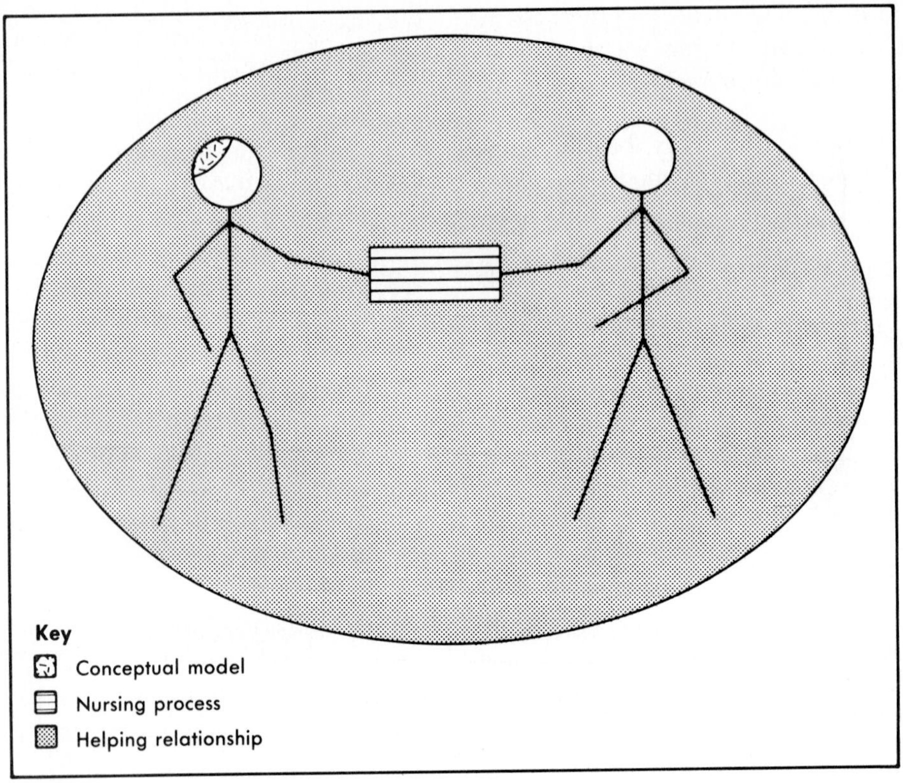

Figure 12-1. Pictorial representation of nursing practice.
From: Adam, E. (1980). *To be a nurse.* Philadelphia: W.B. Saunders Company. Reprinted by permission.

been adopted in practice, education, and research settings. A vicious cycle may develop because some nurses may hesitate to adopt a model until it has been evaluated and it cannot be evaluated until it has been adopted.* Adam recognizes a model can be evaluated intrinsically for content, logic, and other criteria that will help nurses choose one model rather than another. However, the social decisions (extrinsic criteria) constitute the definitive evaluation of the conceptual base of a service profession.[3]

Adam's conviction that every nurse should have a conceptual base specific to nursing rather than one borrowed from another discipline has led her to publish many articles and books, to speak at professional meetings, and to teach courses on this subject. She feels that the existing models are often viewed as being too abstract or too complex and therefore beyond the understanding of many nurses. Adam published *Être Infirmière* and *To Be a Nurse* to help nurses understand the writings of Virginia Henderson. She accomplished this by placing Henderson's concept of nursing within the structure of a conceptual model and by developing and refining the subconcepts identified by Henderson.

This chapter evaluates the conceptual model Adam developed in her book. The model is not a theory, but it does suggest areas for theory development.

*References 3:11; 4:16-18; 5:44; 7.

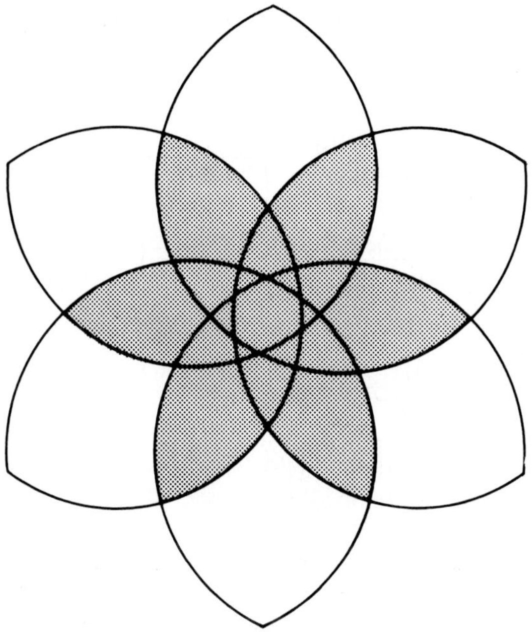

Figure 12-2. "Interdisciplinary health team."
Used with permission from Adam, E. (1983). *Être infirmière* (2d ed.). Montreal: Editions HRW Ltd.

SUMMARY OF THE CONCEPTUAL MODEL FOR NURSING

In *To Be a Nurse,* Adam explains the essential elements of a conceptual model as presented by Dorothy Johnson. She then develops Virginia Henderson's concepts within the structure of a conceptual model.*

Assumptions

The assumptions that form the theoretical foundation of Virginia Henderson's vision of nursing are drawn in part from the works of Edward Thorndike, an American psychologist, and in part from Henderson's experience in rehabilitation. There are three assumptions:

1. Every individual strives for and desires independence.
2. Every individual is a complex whole, made up of fundamental needs.
3. When a need is not satisfied, it follows that the individual is not complete, whole, or independent.

Values

The beliefs underlying Virginia Henderson's conception of nursing are also three in number.

1. The nurse has a unique function, although she shares certain functions with other professionals.
2. When the nurse takes over the physician's role, she delegates her primary function to inadequately prepared personnel.
3. Society wants and expects this service (nursing) from the nurse and no other worker is as able, or willing, to give it.

Major Units

The major units of Henderson's model[2:13-15] are:

1. The goal of nursing is to maintain or restore the client's independence in the satisfaction of his fundamental needs.
2. The client or beneficiary of the nurse's service is a whole being made up of 14 fundamental needs:
   a. Breathe normally.
   b. Eat and drink adequately.
   c. Eliminate body wastes.
   d. Move and maintain desirable postures.
   e. Sleep and rest.
   f. Select suitable clothes—dress and undress.
   g. Maintain body temperature within normal range [by adjusting clothing and modifying the environment].
   h. Keep the body clean and well groomed and protect the integument.
   i. Avoid dangers in the environment and avoid injuring others.
   j. Communicate with others in express-

*The following summary material is reprinted with permission from Adam, E. (1980). *To Be a Nurse.* Philadelphia: W.B. Saunders. pp. 13-15.

ing emotions, needs, fears, or opinions.

k. Worship according to one's faith.
l. Work in such a way that there is a sense of accomplishment.
m. Play or participate in various forms of recreation.
n. Learn, discover, or satisfy the curiosity that leads to normal development and health, and use the available health facilities.

3. The role of the nurse is a complementary-supplementary one.
4. The source of difficulty, or the probable origin of those problems known as nursing problems, is either a lack of knowledge, will, or strength.
5. The intervention: The focus, or center of attention of the nurse's action is the client's deficit or area of dependence [lack of knowledge, will, or strength].
6. The desired consequences are maintained or increased independence in the satisfaction of the 14 basic needs or, in some cases, a peaceful death.

THEORETICAL SOURCES

Adam[6] says she chose to work with Henderson's concept of nursing for two reasons. First, she felt that Henderson's work was "partly known but badly known," that is, incompletely known or understood, even though many nurses were acquainted with it. She hoped that her own publications would contribute to the recognition of Henderson's work as a useful conceptual base for nursing practice, research, and education. In addition, she felt that Henderson's work was more immediately accessible than other works, because the language was already familiar to nurses. Adam[6] "is not saying that Henderson's frame of reference is any better, or more useful, or more significant or more congruent than others. Such an evaluation has not yet been done . . . but it seems more immediately accessible."

Adam's concern for the need of an explicit conceptual model for nursing was developed when she was a student of Dorothy Johnson. It was also through Johnson that Adam became familiar with the structure of a conceptual model: assumptions, values, and major units. Adam[6;8:7-15] believes Johnson was the first nurse to avail herself of that structure, which was already being used in fields such as sociology, psychology, and mathematics.

USE OF EMPIRICAL EVIDENCE

In choosing Virginia Henderson's writings as the basis of her conceptual model, Adam accepted the scientific principles on which Henderson based her work. The chapter on Virginia Henderson discusses the contribution of Claude Bernard's principle of physiological balance and Abraham Maslow's hierarchy of needs. Because Adam did not change the basic content but merely developed it further, this empirical foundation also is unchanged.

In the previous section of this chapter the source of the structure (assumptions, values, and six major units) was identified as sociology, mathematics, and other sciences. This structure has been extensively used in several sciences so it has good reliability.

MAJOR CONCEPTS AND DEFINITIONS*

Assessment tool: instrument the professional uses in collecting information about the beneficiary; the nursing history tool; the data collection tool.

Assumption: the theoretical or scientific basis of a conceptual model; the premises which support the major units of the model.

Beneficiary: the second major unit of a conceptual model; the person or group of persons, toward whom the professional directs her activities; the client; the patient.

Change: a substitution of one thing in place of another; an alteration.

Collection of data: the first step of the nursing process; the collecting of information about the client; the client's nursing history.

---

*Reprinted with permission from Adam, E. (1980). *To Be a Nurse.* Philadelphia: W.B. Saunders. pp. 116-118.

Concept: an idea; a mental image; a generalization formed and developed in the mind.

Conception: a way of conceptualizing a reality; an invention of the mind; a mental image. Depending on its level of abstraction, a conception may be a philosophy, a theory or a conceptual model.

Conceptual Model: an abstraction or a way of conceptualizing a reality: a theoretical frame of reference sufficiently explicit as to provide direction for a particular discipline; a conception made up of assumptions, values, and major units.

Conceptual model for nursing: a mental representation, concept, or conception of nursing which is sufficiently complete and explicit as to provide direction for all fields of activity of the nursing profession.

Consequences: the sixth major unit of a conceptual model; the results of the professional's efforts to attain the ideal and limited goal.

Goal of the profession: the first major unit of a conceptual model; the end which the members of the profession strive to achieve.

Helping relationship: the interaction between the beneficiary (the helpee) and the professional (the helper) which aids the helpee to live more fully: the interpersonal exchange in which the helper illustrates such facilitating qualities as empathy, respect, and others.

Intervention: the fifth major unit of a conceptual model; the focus and modes of the professional's intervention. [In the context of the nursing process, the intervention is the fourth step (implementation of the plan of action or the nursing action itself).]

Intervention focus: part of the fifth major unit of a model; the focus or center of the professional's attention at the moment he intervenes with a client.

Intervention modes: part of the fifth major unit; the means or ways of intervening at the professional's disposal.

Major units: the six essential components of a complete and explicit conception.

Need: a requirement, a necessity.

Need, fundamental: a requirement common to all human beings, well or ill.

Need, individual: a specific, particular, or personal requirement which derives from a fundamental need.

Nursing care plan: a written plan of action; the written communication that comes from the second and third steps of the nursing process; a plan to be followed; a projection of what is to be done.

Nursing process: a methodical, systematic way of proceeding towards an action: a dynamic and logical method; a five-step process.

Practice: one of the three fields of activity of a service profession (the other two being education and research); the field of activity of the administrator and the practitioner of the service.

Problem: a difficulty to be reduced or removed.

Problem-solving method: the scientific process of solving problems; the systematic manner of proceeding used to solve problems.

Role: the third major unit of a conceptual model; the part played by the professional; the societal function of the professional.

Source of difficulty: the fourth major unit of a conceptual model; the probable origin of the client difficulty with which the professional is prepared to cope.

Values: the value system underlying a conceptual model.

MAJOR ASSUMPTIONS

In developing Henderson's work into a conceptual model, Adam[2:14] described the goal of nursing as maintaining or restoring the client's independence in the satisfaction of his 14 fundamental needs. The nurse plays a complementary-supplementary role, complementing and supplementing the client's strength, knowledge, and will.

The nurse has a unique province, although she shares certain functions with other health professionals. Society wants and expects the nurse to provide her unique service.

In this model the person is portrayed as a complex whole, made up of 14 fundamental needs. Each need has biological, physiological, and psychosociocultural dimensions. When a need is not satisfied, the person is not complete, whole, or independent. The nurse's client may also be a family or a group.[3:97-100] The concept of environment is specifically addressed in only one of the fundamental needs. However, environment is implicit in all the fundamental needs because the sociocultural dimension is integral to each need.

Health is not defined separately in *To Be a Nurse*. But Adam uses this term in discussing the goal of nursing. She says, "The goal of nursing is to maintain or to restore the client's independence in the satisfaction of his fundamental needs. This goal, congruent with the goal common to the entire health team, makes clear the nurse's specific contribution to the preservation and improvement of health."[2:14] Since an entirely satisfactory definition of health is still a subject of debate, it behooves each health discipline to make explicit its particular contribution to health.[3:95]

THEORETICAL ASSERTIONS

In the description of the conceptual model's major units, the relationships among the basic concepts can be seen in the elements Adam has labeled beliefs and values. She feels these constitute the *why* of the model and must be shared by all who use the model. Values are not subject to the criteria of *truths*, but must reflect the values of the larger society nursing wishes to serve.

1. "The nurse has a unique function, although she shares certain functions with other professionals."[2:13] The nurse must have a conceptual model in order to have a distinct professional identity and to assert herself as a colleague of the other health team members.
2. "When the nurse takes over the physician's role, she delegates her primary function to inadequately prepared personnel."[2:13] The nurse who strives to assume the physician's role will relinquish the nurse's role to some other care provider who may not have the skills and the knowledge base required for nursing.
3. "Society wants and expects this service (nursing) from the nurse and no other worker is as able, or willing to give it."[2:14] Nursing owes its existence to the fact that it fulfills a societal need, as does any service profession.

ACCEPTANCE BY THE NURSING COMMUNITY

Practice

Basing her practice on this conceptual model, the nurse is seen in a complementary-supplementary role and her goal is client independence in the satisfaction of his needs. The model serves as a guide for using the nursing process and the problem-solving method. Guided by the 14 fundamental needs, the practitioner, in whatever setting, will assess the independence of the client in need satisfaction. She will then identify his specific needs, determine the source of difficulty, and plan the intervention to complement client strength, will, or knowledge. After the care is given, it is evaluated in reference to the client objectives—have the specific needs been satisfied and has client independence been increased? A nursing problem—a client's health problem requiring a nurse's intervention—is a dependency problem in need satisfaction.[2:40] A nursing diagnosis is a specific need that is unsatisfied because of insufficient strength, will, or knowledge. Criteria for identifying specific needs have been developed.[2:73] According to Adam, the nurse "carries out the social mission of contributing to the public's improved health by working toward greater client independence."[2:66]

Education

Adam discusses the educational objectives and goals and the program content in *To Be a Nurse*. She states, "Following Henderson's concept of nursing, the nursing curriculum is planned to prepare a health worker capable of maintaining and restoring the client's independence in the satisfaction of his fundamental needs."[2:57] With this concept, a student learns the complementary-supplementary role. Adam divides the program into official and unofficial content, both of equal importance. Unofficial content "covers everything that is learned in an educational program without being taught."[2:58] Official content "is formally recognized and actually taught."[2:58] Official content is further divided into nursing and nonnursing.

According to Henderson's frame of reference, nursing content includes:

1. the goal of nursing, which is to preserve or re-establish the client's independence in the satisfaction of his basic needs.
2. the detailed description of the 14 fundamental needs, each with its biological, physiological, psychological, social, and cultural dimensions.
3. the individual variations in fundamental needs.
4. the various problems of dependence originating from a lack of strength, will, or knowledge.
5. the explanation of the complementary-supplementary role.
6. the description of the various needs of intervention.
7. the study of the desired consequences: continued or increased independence and, in certain circumstances, a peaceful death.
8. the study of the systematic process and the problem-solving method as applied to nursing.[2:58-59]

Essential subject matters, regardless of the conceptual model for nursing, are "the helping relationship, . . . the concept of health, . . . and the history of nursing."[2:59]

The theoretical courses, in the nonnursing content, include anatomy, physiology, pathology, psychology, sociology, and anthropology. In relation to Henderson's model, the first three relate to the biophysiological dimension and the last three to the psychosociocultural aspect of the fundamental needs.

Subject matter derived from the conceptual model's assumptions is "the concepts of independence and dependence; the concepts of universal and individual human needs, hierarchy of human needs, and need satisfaction; and the concept of wholeness."[2:60]

The practical aspect of nursing content consists of technical procedures and clinical experiences. Techniques are important in the complementary-supplementary role because the nurse is assisting the client in those activities that cannot be completed because of insufficient strength, will, or knowledge. Techniques help pursue the goal of client independence in the satisfaction of his needs. Adam[2:62] feels "The goal of clinical experiences is to provide the student with opportunities to help a client recover his independence in the satisfaction of his basic needs."

Although the level of education may increase, the model remains the conceptual base. The baccalaureate student's formal education will help her identify complex and subtle specific needs, find new ways of complementing and supplementing, and form and continue a helping relationship. Master's level students learn to be specialists in independence nursing or in the teaching and administration of independence nursing. Doctoral students may use the concept of independence in need satisfaction as a basis of research for theory development.

Research

Adam posed 12 questions from the conceptual model for research development. These include:

1. How can client independence be measured?
2. How can his degree of dependence be quantified?
3. What dependency problems are solved by what nursing interventions?
4. At what point must the intervention be discontinued if independence is to be promoted?
5. How can certain interventions be made more easily acceptable?
6. How can the nurse determine how much intervention is enough?
7. What dependency problems are most often encountered among selected groups—e.g., cancer patients, the aged, the mentally confused?

8. How does pain, anxiety, etc. affect independence?
9. How can linguistic barriers be overcome?
10. How can the nurse help certain ethnic or socio-economic groups to be independent?
11. How can the nurse increase client participation in health care?
12. Is the conceptual model socially useful, significant, and congruent?[2:66-67]

Adam[4] states that various clinical and educational settings in Canada are at varying stages of basing nursing care and teaching on her model and research for a small number of master's theses has been based on it. Correspondence received from Canada, the United States, and abroad indicates her books have received very favorable reviews.

LOGICAL FORM

Adam has used the structure of a conceptual model that was useful in various other sciences before being introduced into nursing. The essential elements of a model for a helping or service profession follow.

ASSUMPTIONS. The assumptions are "the suppositions that are taken for granted by those who wish to use the model; they are the 'how' of the model, its foundation."[2:6]

BELIEFS AND VALUES. The beliefs and values "constitute the 'why' of the model and are not subject to the criteria of truth." They must "reflect the value system of the larger society that the profession wishes to serve" and "be shared by the members of the profession who wish to use the model."[2:7]

MAJOR UNITS. The major units "are the 'what' of the conceptual model." They "make clear what nursing is in any setting and at any time."[2:7]

Ideal and limited goal. The ideal and limited goal of the profession is "*ideal* because it represents the ideal that all members of the profession would like to achieve and *limited* because it delineates the parameters of the profession."[2:7]

Beneficiary. The beneficiary of the professional service is "that person or group of persons toward whom the professional directs his attention." "The nurse must have a clear mental image of her client—whether he is well or ill."[2:8]

Role of the professional. The role of the professional is "the role in society played by the members of the discipline."[2:8]

Source of difficulty of the beneficiary. The source of difficulty of the beneficiary "refers to the probable origin of the client's difficulty; one with which the professional, because of his education and experience, is prepared to cope."[3:8] "The probable origin of those client problems which the nurse is prepared to solve must be made explicit."[2:9]

Intervention

Intervention focus. The focus or center of the intervention is "the focus of the professional's attention at the moment he intervenes with the client. The patient or beneficiary is perceived as an extremely complex individual; however, within that complexity only one aspect can receive all the professional's attention at any given moment. . . . No one person can do everything at the same time."[2:9]

Intervention modes. The modes of intervention "are the means the professional has at his disposal to intervene. . . . A conceptual model for nursing will indicate what means are at the nurse's disposal when she intervenes as a health professional."[2:9]

Consequences. The consequences "are the desired results of the professional activities and must be congruent with the ideal goal."[2:10]

Adam has developed Henderson's concept

of nursing into a conceptual model for nursing by placing Henderson's writings in the structure of a model. She has supplied the logical form that was less apparent in Henderson's work. Through the logical form of the resulting conceptual model, clear direction is provided to nursing practitioners, educators, and researchers.

Through the use of the structure that comprises a conceptual model and Henderson's writings, it may be said that Adam used the deductive form of logical reasoning.

FURTHER DEVELOPMENT

Although no empirical evidence has been collected for theories deriving from this model, Adam feels it could be the basis for theory development.[11:9] As with other conceptual models for nursing, this one specifies nursing's focus of inquiry. From Henderson's conceptual departure point of independence in need satisfaction, descriptive and experimental studies could be carried out to result in the identification of descriptive terms peculiar to the concept under scrutiny. The identification of descriptive terms is the first step in theory development. Possible developments might be a theory of need satisfaction or a theory of complementing knowledge or of supplementing motivation in specific client populations. Such theories would not be theories of nursing, but theories of the phenomena that concern nursing.[4]

"Nurse theorist will of course look at phenomena that interest other disciplines as well. They must, however, study them from a nursing perspective if they want to develop nursing theory."[11:9] "For example, if pain were studied from Henderson's perspective, it would be examined as a phenomenon that interferes with client independence in need satisfaction."[11:10]

In a letter of February 16, 1988, Evelyn Adam states, "Some Ontario colleges and clinical settings are showing increasing interest in basing their practice and teaching on Henderson's model as I presented it. It is still popular in Quebec and in the Atlantic provinces. Graduate students often quote it as their conceptual departure point, i.e., to justify their research project. They seldom seek to develop it."

CRITIQUE

Simplicity

The essential elements listed by Adam give the appearance of a simple conceptual model. However, on closer inspection the number of subconcepts produces a complex picture. The interrelatedness of the components necessary for the care of the whole client also adds to the complexity of the model. The concepts presented are clearly defined and easy to follow.

Generality

The assumptions, values, and major units involve nursing and clients in all aspects of society. They are not limited to age, medical diagnosis, or health care setting. Each of the 14 basic needs has biophysiological and psychosociocultural aspects.

Empirical Precision

Although testing of the model is unavailable at this time, it appears to have the potential for a high degree of empirical precision. This is related to its reality base and designated subconcepts.

Derivable Consequences

Because of the empirically based concepts and broad scope, the model is potentially applicable to nursing practice, education, and research.

Conclusion

Adam's work in developing the conceptual model is unique in that she has taken Henderson's previously existing concept of nursing and presented it within the previously existing structure of a model. The result is something more than the sum of the two. It is a complete, concise, explicit conceptual model. Adam then clarified the interrelatedness of the model, the process, and the client-nurse relationship. Making a clear distinction between model and theory, Adam explained the impact of the model on nursing research, practice, and education.

Adam[6] states that "the adoption of a conceptual model will not solve all of nursing's problems." A conceptual model makes explicit nursing's particular contribution to health care and provides nurses a professional identity and a conceptual point of departure.

It would seem that every nurse who adopts a concise and explicit conceptual model is a potential nursing theorist. A nurse who is able to articulate the scope of nursing practice would be more likely to identify areas for nursing theory development and nursing research. Imagine that the majority of nurses have an explicit conceptual model, that is, a conceptual departure point for theory development, and are able and willing to provide written documentation that would become the basis for empirical evidence. This opens the door to a marked increase in nursing theory and knowledge.

REFERENCES

1. Adam, E. (1975, Sept.). A conceptual model for nursing. *Canadian Nurse, 71*:40-41.
2. Adam, E. (1980). *To be a nurse.* Philadelphia: W.B. Saunders.
3. Adam, E. (1983). *Être infirmière* (2d ed.). Montréal: Editions HRW Ltée.
4. Adam, E. (1983). Modèles conceptuels. *Nursing Papers: Perspectives in Nursing, 15(2)*:10-21.
5. Adam, E. (1983). Frontiers of nursing in the 21st century: Development of models and theories on the concept of nursing. *Journal of Advanced Nursing, 8*:41-45.
6. Adam, E. (1984, Dec. 4). Personal interview.
7. Adam, E. (1985, April). Toward more clarity in terminology—frameworks, theories and models. *Journal of Nursing Education 24(4)*:151-155.
8. Johnson, N. (1974, Sept.-Oct.). Development of theory: A requisite for nursing as a primary health profession. *Nursing Research, 23(5)*:372-377.
9. Riehl, J.P., & Roy, C. (1974). *Conceptual models for nursing practice.* New York: Appleton-Century-Crofts, pp. 7-15.
10. Roy, C., & Roberts, S.L. (1981). *Theory construction in nursing: An adaptation model.* Englewood Cliffs, N.J.: Prentice-Hall.
11. Adam, E. (1987). Nursing theory: What it is and what it is not. *Nursing Papers: Perspectives in Nursing, 19(2)*:5-14.

BIBLIOGRAPHY

Primary Sources

Books

Adam, E. (1979). *Être infirmière.* Montréal: Editions HRW Ltée.

Adam, E. (1980). *To be a nurse.* Philadelphia: W.B. Saunders.

Adam, E. (1981). *To be a nurse.* (Dutch translation). Holland: De Tÿdstroom.

Adam, E. (1982). *To be a nurse.* (Spanish translation). Madrid: Editora Inportecnica.

Adam, E. (1983). Être infirmière (2d ed.). Montréal: Editions HRW Lteé.

Book Chapters

Adam, E. (1983). Development of models and theories on the concept of nursing, In *Health care for all: Challenge for nursing* (17th quadrennial Congress, ICN 1981). Geneva: ICN.

Adam, E. (1983). The shape of the nursing world to come: The nursing process. In *Health care for all: Challenge for nursing,* (17th quadrennial Congress, ICN 1981). Geneva: ICN.

Adam, E. (1984). Modèles conceptuels. In M. McGee (Ed.), *Theoretical pluralism in nursing science.* Ottawa: University of Ottawa Press.

Articles

Adam, E. (1975, Sept.). Un modèle conceptuel: à quoi bon? *L'infirmière Canadienne, 19(9)*:22-23.

Adam, E. (1975, Sept.). A conceptual model for nursing. *Canadian Nurse, 71(9)*:40-41.

Adam, E. (1981, Sept.), Les normes de la pratique infirmière de l'A.I.I.C.: Une interprétation. *L'Infirmière Canadienne, 23(9)*:28-29.

Adam, E. (1981, Sept.). CNA's standards for nursing practice: An interpretation. *Canadian Nurse, 77(8)*:32-33.

Adam, E. (1983). Frontiers of nursing in the 21st century: Development of models and theories on the concept of nursing. *Journal of Advanced Nursing, 8*:41-45.

Adam, E. (1983). Modèles conceptuels. *Nursing Papers: Perspectives in Nursing, 15(2)*:10-21.

Adam, E. (1984). Questions et réponses relatives au schème conceptuel de Virginia Henderson. *L'Infirmière Canadienne, 26(3)*:27-31.

Adam, E. (1985, April). Toward more clarity in terminology: Frameworks, theories, and models. *Journal of Nursing Education. 24(4)*:151-155.

Adam, E. (1987). Nursing theory: What it is and what it is not. *Nursing Papers: Perspectives in Nursing 19(2)*:5-14.

Reports

Adam, E. (1980). Programmes s'inspirant d'un modèle nursing. In *Retour aux sources.* Ottawa: A.I.I.C., pp. 27-33.

Adam, E. (1980). Implementing the curriculum based on a nursing model. In *Back to basics.* Ottawa: A.I.I.C., pp. 22-28.

Adam, E., et al. (1980). *Normes de la pratique infirmière.* Ottawa: A.I.I.C.

Adam, E., et al. (1980). *Standards for nursing practice.* Ottawa: A.I.I.C.

Adam, E. (1981). L'application d'un modele conceptuel au programme de'études collegial. Dans *Rapport du-Colloque des Techniques infirmières Partie I.* Gouvernement du Québec, pp. 49-55.

Adam, E. (1981). Leadership in nursing: The case for a conceptual model. In *Report of Annual Meeting,* CAUSN, Western Region, University of Saskatchewan. Saskatoon, Saskatchewan, pp. 1-15.

Adam, E. (1981). The case for a conceptual model. In *Proceedings from Nursing Explorations 1980,* School of Nursing, McGill University, 9 pp.

Correspondence

Adam, E. (1984, Oct. 2). Personal correspondence.

Adam, E. (1984, Nov. 1). Telephone interview.

Adam, E. (1984, Nov. 4). Telephone interview.

Adam, E. (1984, Nov. 6). Personal correspondence.

Adam, E. (1984, Nov. 12). Telephone interview.

Adam, E. (1984, Nov. 26). Telephone interview.

Adam, E. (1984, Dec. 4). Personal interview (Videotape)

Adam, E. (1988, Feb. 16) Personal correspondence.

Adam, E. (1988, April 2) Telephone interview.

Secondary Sources

Books

Chinn, P. & Jacobs, M. (1983). *Theory and nursing: A systematic approach.* St. Louis: C.V. Mosby.

Henderson, V. (1966). *The nature of nursing.* New York: Macmillan.

Articles

Henderson, V. (1964). The nature of nursing. *American Journal of Nursing, 64*:62-68.

Henderson, V. (1982). The nursing process: Is the title right? *Journal of Advanced Nursing, 7*:103-109.

Winkler, J. (1983). Conceptual models (a response to "Modèles conceptuels," by E. Adam). *Nursing Papers: Perspectives in nursing, 15(4)*:69-70.

Book Reviews

Adam, E. (1979). *Être infirmière.*
Infirmière Canadienne, 21:46, April 1979.
Infirmière Canadienne, 21:10, June 1979.
Revue de l'infirmière (Paris), 6:75, June 1979.
Revue de l'infirmière (Paris), 8:8-9, October 1979.
Infirmière enseignante (Paris), 10:11, February 1980.
Le Devoir (daily newspaper, Montreal), March 19, 1979.

Adam, E. (1980). *To be a nurse.*
Canadian Nurse, 77:50, March 1981.
Nursing Times, 77:1041, June 1981.
The Australian Nurses Journal, 11:28, October 1981.
Continuing Education in Nursing, 12:39, November-December 1981.

Other

Riehl, J.P., & Roy, C. (1974). *Conceptual models for nursing practice.* New York: Appleton-Century-Crofts.

Riehl, J.P., & Roy, C. (1980). *Conceptual models for nursing practice* (2d ed.) New York: Appleton-Century-Crofts.

Roy, C., & Roberts, S.L. (1981). *Theory construction in nursing: An adaptation model.* Englewood Cliffs, N.J.: Prentice-Hall.

13

Madeleine Leininger

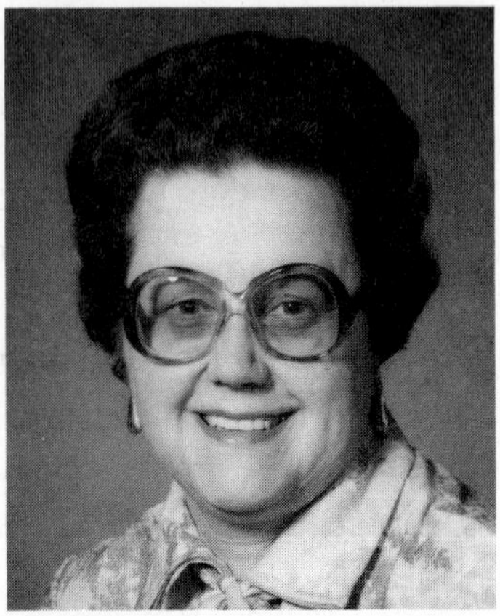

Cultural Care Theory

Sr. Judith E. Alexander, Carolyn J. Beagle, Pam Butler, Deborah A. Dougherty, Karen D. Andrews Robards, Catherine Velotta

CREDENTIALS AND BACKGROUND OF THE THEORIST

Madeleine M. Leininger is the founder of transcultural nursing and a leader in transcultural nursing and human care theory. She is the first professional nurse with graduate preparation in nursing to hold a Ph.D. in cultural and social anthropology. Born in Sutton, Nebraska, she began her nursing career by graduating from a diploma program at St. Anthony's School of Nursing in Denver, and serving as a Cadet Corps nurse while pursuing the basic nursing program. In 1950 she obtained a B.S. degree in biological science from Benedictine College, Atchison, Kansas, with a minor in philosophy and the humanistic studies. After graduation she served as an instructor, staff nurse, and head nurse on a medical-surgical unit and opened a new psychiatric unit as director of the nursing service at St. Joseph's Hospital in

The authors wish to express appreciation to Madeleine Leininger for editing the chapter.

Omaha. During this time she did advanced study in nursing, nursing administration, teaching and curriculum in nursing, and test and measurement at Creighton University in Omaha.[9]

In 1954 Leininger obtained an M.S.N. in psychiatric nursing from Catholic University of America in Washington, D.C. She then moved to the University of Cincinnati, where she began the first graduate clinical specialist program in child psychiatric nursing in the country. She also initiated and directed the first graduate nursing program in psychiatric mental health nursing at the University of Cincinnati. During this time she wrote one of the first basic psychiatric nursing texts with Hofling, entitled *Basic Psychiatric Nursing Concepts* (1960), which was published in 11 languages and used worldwide.[12]

While working in a child guidance home in the mid-1950s, Leininger identified in the staff a lack of understanding of cultural factors influencing the behavior of children. Among these children of diverse cultural backgrounds, she observed differences that deeply concerned her. Psychoanalytic theories and therapy strategies did not seem to reach children with their cultural behavior and needs. She became increasingly concerned that her interventions and those of the therapeutic staff did not appear adequate to help the children of different cultural backgrounds and lifeways. Leininger posed many questions to herself and the staff about cultural differences of the children, but she found few staff members interested in this aspect. However, about this time Margaret Mead began a visiting professorship at the Department of Psychiatry at the University of Cincinnati, and Leininger discussed with Mead the potential interrelationships between nursing and anthropology. While not getting any direct answers from Dr. Mead, she decided to pursue doctoral (Ph.D.) study at the University of Washington (Seattle) with a focus on cultural and psychological anthropology. As a doctoral student, Leininger studied the Gadsup people of the Eastern Highlands of New Guinea. She lived alone with the indigenous people for nearly two years and did an ethnographic and ethnonursing study of two villages.[4:21-44] She was able to observe not only unique features of the culture but also a number of marked differences between Western and non-Western cultures in caring and health practices. From her in-depth study and first-hand experiences with the Gadsup, she continued to develop her theory of cultural care.[4:23] From her research she was able to influence nursing students to help them understand cultural differences in human care, health, and illness with the Gadsup and other cultures in the world. She also was the major nurse leader who encouraged many students and faculty to pursue graduate studies in anthropology and to use anthropological knowledge in nursing practices.

During the 1950s and 1960s, Leininger identified several common areas of knowledge and research interests between nursing and anthropology. From this insight came the book *Nursing and Anthropology: Two Worlds to Blend,* which was the first book in transcultural nursing. The ideas presented in this book and Leininger's research studies laid the foundation for developing the field of transcultural nursing, her theory, and culturally based health care. Her second book, *Transcultural Nursing: Concepts, Theories and Practices* (1978), identified major concepts and practices in transcultural nursing and definitive ways of how the disciplines of anthropology and nursing are complementary, yet different. Her theory and conceptual framework for cultural care and health were laid in this book. During the past 30 years, Leininger[4:21-44] has further developed and explicated her transcultural care theory through the study of many cultures, both within and outside of the United States, using primarily qualitative ethnomethods to obtain *emic* (inside views) of human care.

The first course offered in transcultural nursing was in 1966 at the University of Colorado, where Leininger was a professor of Nursing and Anthropology. This marked the first joint appointment of a professor of nursing and another discipline in the United States. She also initiated and served as the director of the first nurse scientist (Ph.D.) program in the United States. In 1969 Leininger was appointed Dean and Professor of Nursing and Lecturer in Anthropology at the University of Washington. There she established the first academic nursing department on Comparative Nursing Care Systems in order to support master's and doctoral programs in transcultural nursing. Under her leadership, the Research Facilitation Office was established in 1968 and 1969. She initiated several transcultural nursing courses and guided the first individual Ph.D. program in this area. During this time, she initiated the Committee on Nursing and Anthropology (CONNA) in 1968 with the American Anthropological Association.

In 1974, she was appointed Dean and Professor of Nursing at the College of Nursing and Adjunct Professor of Anthropology at the University of Utah in Salt Lake City. At this institution she initiated master's and doctoral programs in transcultural nursing,[9] and established the first doctoral program offerings at this institution. These were the first graduate programs in the world with substantive courses and research focused specifically on transcultural nursing. She also initiated and directed a new research facilitation office at this university.

In 1981 Leininger was recruited to Wayne State University, Detroit, where she has been Professor of Nursing and Adjunct Professor of Anthropology and director of transcultural nursing offerings. She was also Director of the Center for Health Research at the university for five years. While at Wayne State, she once again developed several courses and initiated a minor in transcultural nursing at the master's level, as well as several courses and seminars for doctoral students pursuing transcultural nursing theory and research. Currently, this doctoral program has the largest number of master's and doctoral students studying transcultural nursing in the country. In addition to directing the transcultural offerings at Wayne State, Leininger teaches transcultural nursing courses in baccalaureate, master's, doctoral, and postdoctoral programs. As one of the first leaders to use qualitative research methods in the early 1960s, she has developed and continues to teach these courses at the university. She is also active in conducting research studies with several cultural groups and has completed a study of ten cultures in Michigan.

With the growing interest in transcultural nursing and health care, Leininger[12] has annually given several keynote addresses and conducted workshops and conferences nationally and internationally since 1965. Her academic vitae records nearly 600 such conferences, keynote addresses, and workshops in the United States, Canada, Europe, Pacific Islands and Asia. Many education and service settings request her consultation to understand clients, students, and faculty of diverse cultures.

As the first professional nurse to complete a doctoral degree in anthropology and to initiate several master's and doctoral nursing education programs, Leininger has many areas of expertise and interests. She has now studied at least 12 major cultures in depth and has done several ethnographic and ethnonursing studies. Besides transcultural nursing care, other related areas of interest are comparative education and administration, nursing theories, politics of nursing and health care, transcultural care, qualitative research methods, the future of nursing and health care, and nursing leadership. She initiated the National Transcultural Nursing Society Organization in 1974 and has been an active leader in this society. She also initiated the National Research Care Conferences in 1978 to help nurses focus specifically on the study of human care phenomena.[12] Leininger has gained international recognition in nursing and other related fields by her writings, research, consultation, courses, and dynamic addresses. She has energetically worked to persuade nurse educators and practitioners to incorporate transcultural nursing and culture-specific care concepts with research findings into nursing curricula and clinical practices. While very active in nursing, she has also found time to teach selected units in anthropology and to do research with anthropology colleagues since the early 1960s. She is one of the few nurses to have kept active in two disciplines and to contribute to both fields, especially in national and international conferences and association meetings.

Leininger has authored or edited 22 books. Examples of her books include *Nursing and Anthropology: Two Worlds to Blend* (1970), *Transcultural Nursing: Concepts, Theories and Practices* (1978), *Caring: An Essential Human Need* (1981), *Care: The Essence of Nursing and Health* (1984), *Qualitative Research Methods in Nursing* (1985), and *Care: Clinical and Community Uses of Care* (1988). She has published more than 265 articles and 40 chapters plus numerous films and research projects focused on transcultural nursing, human care and health phenomena, and other topics relevant to nursing and anthropology. She also served on editorial boards of 10 major publications. She is known as one of the most creative and productive authors in nursing, providing new and substantive nursing content with futuristic ideas and trends to advance nursing as a discipline and profession.

Leininger has received many awards and recognition of her accomplishments. She is listed in *Who's Who of American Women, Who's Who in Health Care, Who's Who in Community Leaders, The World's Who's Who of Women in Education, The International Who's Who in Community Services,* and *The Who's Who in International Women,* and other such listings. Her name appears on *The National Register of Prominent Americans and International Notables, International Women,* and *The National Register of Prominent Community Leaders*. She received an Honorary Doctorate of Human Letters from Benedictine College, Atchison, Kansas, in 1975, and in 1976 was presented an Award of Recognition for unique and significant contributions to the American Association of Colleges of Nursing. Leininger is a Fellow in the American Academy of Nursing and is a Fellow of the American Anthropological Society and the Society for Applied Anthropology. Her other affiliations include Sigma Theta Tau, the National Honor Society of Nursing; Delta Kappa Gamma, the National Honorary Society in Education; and the Scandinavian College of Caring Science in Stockholm. She has served as distinguished visiting scholar or lecturer in 48 universities in this country and abroad and was recently visiting professor at six universities in Sweden, in two universities in Japan, and five in Australia and New Zealand. While at Wayne State University, she has received the Board of Regents' Distinguished Faculty Award, Distinguished Researcher Award, and the President's Excellence in Teaching Award.[12]

THEORETICAL SOURCES FOR THEORY DEVELOPMENT

Leininger's theory is derived from the discipline of anthropology, but she conceptualized the theory in a unique way to be relevant to nursing. She has defined *transcultural nursing* as: a major area of nursing that focuses upon a comparative study and analysis of different cultures and subcultures in the world with respect to their caring behavior; nursing care; and health-illness vaules, beliefs, and patterns of behavior with the goal of developing a scientific and humanistic body of knowledge in order to provide culture-specific and culture-universal nursing care practices.[4:8]

The goal of transcultural nursing extends beyond an awareness state or appreciation of different cultures. It means making professional nursing knowledge and practices culturally based, conceptualized, planned, and practiced.[4:12] Leininger has stated that in time there will be "a new taxonomy of nursing practice which will reflect different kinds of nursing care which are culturally defined, classified, and tested as a guide to provide nursing care."[4:13] She predicts this to happen because culture is the broadest and the most wholistic means to conceptualize, understand, and be effective with people. In addition, she states that "transcultural nursing is becoming one of the most important, relevant, and highly promising areas of formal study research and practice because of the multicultural world in which we live."[4:14] She predicts that for nursing to be relevant to clients and the world, transcultural nursing knowledge will be imperative to guide all nursing decisions and actions.

Leininger[4:32] holds and promotes a new and different theory from the traditional theory in nursing, which usually defines *theory* as "a set of logically interrelated concepts, hypotheses or propositions which can be tested for the purpose of explaining or predicting an event, phenomenon or situation." Instead, Leininger defines *theory* as the systematic and creative way of discovering knowledge about something, or to account for some phenomenon limitedly or vaguely known. For her, nursing theory must take into account the creative discovery of individuals', families', and groups' caring behaviors, values, and beliefs based on their cultural lifeways in order to provide effective, satisfying, and culturally congruent nursing care. If nursing practices fail to recognize culturological aspects of human needs, there will be signs of less efficacious nursing care practices and dissatisfaction with nursing services.[4:33]

Leininger[4:34] developed her theory of cultural care diversity and universality upon the belief that people of different cultures can inform and best determine most of the kind of care they desire or need from professional caregivers. Because culture is the patterned lifeway of people that influences decisions and actions, the theory is directed toward nurses to grasp the world of the client and to use their viewpoints, knowledge, and practices as bases for making culturally congruent professional actions and decisions. Indeed, culture care is the broadest holistic nursing theory because it takes into account the totality of human life and existence over time, including the social structure, world view, cultural values, environmental contexts, language expressions, and folk and professional systems. These are the critical and essential bases to discover care knowledge as the essence of nursing and to practice therapeutic nursing.

USE OF EMPIRICAL EVIDENCE

For more than four decades, Leininger has held that care is the essence of nursing and the dominant, distinctive, and unifying feature of nursing.[2:13] She states that care is complex, illusive, and often embedded in social structure and other aspects of culture. She holds that there are different forms, expressions, and processes of care that are diverse, and some are universal.[2:13] Leininger favors ethnomethods as the desired and meaningful approach to study care because these methods are directed toward discovering the people's "truth" views, beliefs, and patterned lifeways. Ethnoscience is one of the rigorous ethnomethods used in anthropology to discover nursing knowledge. In the 1960s Leininger developed the ethnonursing method to specifically and systematically study nursing phenomena. Ethnonursing is focused on the systematic study and classification of nursing care beliefs, values, and practices as cognitively or subjectively known by a designated culture (or cultural representatives) through their local language, experiences, beliefs, and value system about actual or potential nursing phenomena such as care, health, and environmental factors.[4:15] Although nursing has used the words *care* and *caring* to describe its practice for more than a century, the definitions and usage are often vague and used as clichés without specific meanings to the client or even the nurse. "Indeed, the concepts about caring are some of the least understood and least studied of all human knowledge and research areas."[4:33] By means of transcultural nursing theory and ethnomethods focused on emic (insiders' views), one can get close to the discovery of care because ethnomethods are people-centered data sources and are not derived from the researcher's *etic* (or outsiders' views), beliefs, and practices. An important goal of the theory is to be able to document, know, predict, and explain systematically by field data what is diverse and universal about generic and professional care and nursing care. The general goal of transcultural nursing theory is to get to the people's emic views about care as they believe and practice care and then study this source of knowledge with the nurses' etic perspectives with the goal to provide care that fits reasonably with the client's needs and realities.

Leininger holds that "caring behavior and practices uniquely distinguish nursing from the contributions of other disciplines."[5:4] The major reasons she gives for studying care are: "First, the construct of care appears critical to human growth, development, and survival for human beings"[5:7] and has been since the beginning of human beings. The second reason is to explicate and fully understand the roles of the caregiver and care recipient in different cultures in order to provide culturally congruent care. The third reason is to preserve and use care as an essential for healing and well-being and for the survival of humans and cultures through time.[5:8] Fourth, the nursing profession has limitedly studied care in a systematic way and from the cultural perspective and has largely missed a rich epistemological and ontological base of nursing knowledge. Leininger contends care is largely an elusive phenomenon often embedded in cultural lifeways that can provide a sound basis for nurses to use care in specific therapeutic ways to maintain health, prevent illness, heal, or to help people face death. Moreover, a central thesis of her theory is that if one fully understands care, one can predict the well-being or health of individuals, families, and groups. Thus, care is viewed by Leininger as one of the most powerful concepts and distinctive phenomena of nursing. Such care concepts and forms, however, must be fully documented, understood in their meanings, and used in ways so that care becomes the major guide to nursing therapy and to explain nursing practices.

To date Leininger has studied several cultures in depth and has studied approximately 45 cultures with graduate students and faculty by using mainly qualitative ethnomethods. She has explicated 85 different care constructs in which care has different linguistic meanings, cultural experiences, and uses by the people of diverse cultures and subcultures. Many ideas related to each care construct have been identified and examined from a transcultural perspective. A taxonomy of care constructs has been identified.[12]

Leininger believes the goal of the care theory is to provide culturally congruent care. She believes nurses must work towards explicating care uses and meanings so that a culture's care, values, beliefs, and lifeways provide accurate and reliable bases for planning and effectively implementing culture-specific care, and to identify the universal features about care. She maintains that nurses cannot separate world views, social structure, and cultural beliefs (folk and professional) from health, wellness, illness, or care when working with cultures, because these factors are closely linked together. Social structure factors such as religion, politics, culture, economics, and kinship are significant forces affecting care and influencing well-being and illness patterns.

Leininger[4:56] contends that cultural blindness, shock, imposition, and ethnocentrism by nurses greatly reduce knowledge discovery and ultimately the quality of care provided to clients. Moreover, she holds that culturally congruent care is what makes clients satisfied that they received "good care," and it is the powerful healing force for health. Quality care is what clients seek most when they come for services from health care personnel and especially from the professional nurse.

MAJOR CONCEPTS AND DEFINITIONS

Leininger has developed many terms relevant to the theory, but only a few major ones are defined here. The reader can study her full theory from her books.

CARE. Care "refers to phenomena related to assistive, supportive or enabling behavior towards or for another individual (or group) with evident or anticipated needs to ameliorate or improve a human condition or lifeway."[12]

CARING. Caring "refers to *actions* directed toward assisting, supporting or enabling another individual (or group) with evident or anticipated needs to ameliorate or improve a human condition or lifeway."[12]

CULTURE. Culture "refers to the learned, shared and transmitted values, beliefs, norms and lifeway practices of a particular group that guides thinking, decisions, actions and patterned ways."[12]

CULTURAL CARE. "Cultural care refers to the cognitively known values, beliefs, and patterned expressions that assist, support or enable another individual or group to maintain well-being, improve a human condition or lifeway or face death and disabilities."[12]

CULTURAL CARE DIVERSITY. "Cultural care diversity refers to the variability of meanings, patterns, values or symbols of care that are culturally derived for health (well being) or to improve a human condition, lifeway or to face death."[12]

CULTURAL CARE UNIVERSALITY. "Cultural care universality refers to common, similar or uniform meanings, patterns, values or symbols of care that are culturally derived for health (well being) or to improve a human condition, lifeway or to face death."[12]

NURSING. Leininger[7:4-5] defines nursing as:

> a learned humanistic art and science that focuses upon personalized (individual and group) care behaviors, functions, and processes directed toward promoting and maintaining health behaviors or recovery from illness which have physical, psychocultural, and social significance or meaning for those being assisted generally by a professional nurse or one with similar role competencies.

MAJOR ASSUMPTIONS

A few major assumptions to support Leininger's transcultural care theory[7:5-6] can be stated:

1. Human caring is a universal phenomenon, but the expressions, processes, structural forms, and patterns of caring vary among cultures.
2. Caring acts and processes are essential for human birth, development, growth, survival, and peaceful death.
3. Caring is the essence of nursing and the distinct, dominant, and unifying nature of nursing.
4. Care has a biophysical, cultural, psychological, social, and environmental dimension, and the concept of culture provides the broadest means to know and understand care.
5. Nursing is a transcultural phenomenon as nurses interact with clients, staff, and other groups and requires that nurses identify and use intercultural nurse-client and system data.
6. Care behaviors, goals, and functions vary transculturally because of the social structure, world view, and cultural values of people from different cultures.
7. Self- and other care practices vary in different cultures and in different folk and professional care systems.
8. The identification of universal and nonuniversal folk and professional caring behaviors, beliefs, and practices is essential to discover the epistemological and

ontological base of nursing care knowledge.
9. Care is largely culturally derived and requires culturally based knowledge and skills for satisfying and efficacious nursing practices.
10. There can be no curing without caring, but there can be caring without curing.

In *Transcultural Nursing: Concepts, Theories and Practices,* published in 1978, Leininger[4:35-36] lists ten basic assumptions that are very similar to the ten assumptions in her 1984 publication, *Care: The Essence of Nursing and Health.*[7:5-6] The terms *culture* and *transcultural* care sources are more prevalent in her earlier works because she was in the process of discovering ethnocare data. Nine of the ten assumptions in *Care: The Essence of Nursing and Health* include the term *care*—revealing greater discovery and emphasis on care—but the assumptions are derived largely from culture data.

THEORETICAL ASSERTIONS

Leininger has developed several formulations from her transcultural nursing theory as examples to stimulate further research by nurses. These formulations are based on her ongoing inquiry, research studies, and other anthropological and nursing investigations from mainly ethnomethod studies. A major prediction of her theory is that health or well-being can be predicted by the epistemology of care. From her field studies, she has identified and made some relationship statements.

In *Transcultural Nursing: Concepts, Theories, and Practices*[4] and in other writings, she has offered several hypotheses for quantitative studies and areas of unique qualitative studies such as:[12]

1. Identifiable differences in caring values and behaviors between and among cultures lead to differences in the nursing care expectations of care-seekers.
2. Differences in caring values and norms of behavior between technologically dependent and nontechnologically dependent societies are areas of comparative inquiry.
3. As professional nurses work in strange cultures with different values about nursing care or caring behaviors, there will be overt signs of cultural conflicts and problems.
4. The greater the dependence of nursing personnel upon technological tasks and activities, the greater the signs of interpersonal distance and the fewer the client satisfactions.
5. Nursing care interventions which provide culture-specific caring practices to clients will show positive signs of client satisfaction.
6. From the study of care, beliefs, values, and practices, one can discover and predict signs of health or well-being of clients.

In *Care: The Essence of Nursing and Health,*[7:6-7] Leininger listed nine theoretical statements and some hypotheses, and she has added touches to these since the book was published in 1984.[12]

1. Intercultural differences in care beliefs, values, and practices will reflect identifiable differences in nursing care practices.
2. Cultures that highly value individualism with independence modes will show signs of self-care practices and values; whereas cultures that do not value individualism with independence modes will show limited signs of self-care practices and more signs of other-care practices.
3. There is a close relationship between caregiver and care receiver behaviors in client care outcomes.
4. Clients from different cultures can identify caring and noncaring behaviors and attitudes of nurses.
5. The greater the differences between folk care values and professional care values, the greater the signs of cultural conflict and stresses between professional caregivers and nonprofessional care receivers.
6. Technologic caring acts, techniques, and practices differ cross-culturally and have different outcomes for health and nursing care practices.
7. The greater the signs of dependency upon

technology to give care, the greater the signs of depersonalized human care to clients.

8. Symbolic forms and ritual functions of nursing care behaviors and practices have different meanings and outcomes in different cultures.
9. Political, religious, economic, kinship, and cultural values and environmental contexts greatly influence human care and predict well-being of individuals, families, and groups.

A sample of other relationship statements from Leininger's *Transcultural Nursing: Concepts, Theories, and Practices*[4:45-46;12] includes:

1. Cultures that perceive illness to be largely a personal and internal body experience (i.e., caused by physical, genetic, and intrabody stresses) tend to use more technical and physical self-care control methods (pills and physical techniques) than cultures that view illness as an extrapersonal or cultural experience.
2. Cultures that strongly emphasize caring behaviors processes tend to have more females in caring roles than males.
3. Cultures that emphasize curing behaviors and treatment processes tend to have more male curers than females.
4. Clients in need of caring services tend to seek first local (usually nonprofessional) caring persons, such as family members or friends, and only later seek professional caregivers if the client's condition is getting worse or if death is feared.
5. Ritualized ethnocaring activities that have therapeutic benefits to clients and their families tend to be largely unknown or are less valued by Western professional nurses and physicians as therapeutic.
6. Where there is marked evidence of nurturant caring behaviors in a culture, there will be less caring and more health maintenance activities. She later indicated that there will be more signs of well-being or health and less signs of illness where there is evidence of nurturant caring or the use of culture-specific care constructs.

LOGICAL FORM

Leininger's theory is derived from anthropology but reformulated to transcultural nursing with human care perspectives. She developed ethnonursing research methods and has emphasized the importance of studying people from their *emic* or local knowledge and experiences and using qualitative research methodologies. Her book *Qualitative Research Methods in Nursing* and related articles provide substantive knowledge about qualitative methods in nursing.[10]

In her own research, Leininger has been skilled in using ethnonursing, ethnographic participant-observation methods that provide a holistic approach to study human behavior in diverse environmental contexts. With this method, the researcher moves with people in their daily living activities. The nurse researcher inductively obtains data of documented descriptive and interpretive accounts from informants of observed and verified behavior to identify "the essence, nature, process, and attributes of caring behavior and therapeutic nursing care" within a culture.[4:47] This approach is important for developing basic and substantive grounded knowledge about care that can guide nursing care practices.[4:46-47]

Leininger[10] also uses the ethnoscience method as a formal and rigorous method to study nursing and human phenomena. "Ethnoscience refers to the systematic study of the way of life of a designated cultural group in order to obtain an accurate account of the people's behavior and how they perceive and know their universe."[4:76] This method involves classifying data as they reflect the people's views. Through confirming the credibility of these data with the people, a high degree of validity and reliability can be obtained about the characteristics of a culture and the theoretical formulations generated from the data. The ethnoscience method provides data that will help nurses understand the meanings of care for whatever phenomenon is studied and to explain and predict human behavior within a culture context.[4:76] In order to refine largely emic data obtained through ethnoscientific research, the researcher analyzes both emic and etic data.

"An *emic* analysis reveals the native's or a local culture's way of knowing and classifying their world."[4:78] An *etic* analysis searches for common or more universal (outside) features that may be found in more than one culture. Ultimately, universal and diverse features may be discovered through emic and etic analysis of data.[4:78]

Although other methods of research, such as hypothesis testing and experimental, can be used to study transcultural care, the method of choice depends upon the researcher's purposes, the goals of the study, and the phenomena to be studied. Creativity and the willingness of the nurse researcher to use different research methods to discover nursing knowledge are encouraged.[4:49] However, Leininger contends that qualitative ethnomethods are strongly recommended to establish an accurate and relevant body of client knowledge to advance nursing.

Leininger has developed the Sunrise Model to depict the essential components of the theory. The Sunrise Model is presented in Figure 13-1. Leininger has been refining the model since the late 1950s. It has been through various representations to convey accurately the components of the theory. This model and the full theory of cultural diversity and universality of care and health are not addressed here and only selected ideas are offered to introduce the reader to Leininger's pioneering and creative work of evolving theory through time. The Sunrise Conceptual Model is presented in *Care: The Essence of Nursing and Health, Nursing and*

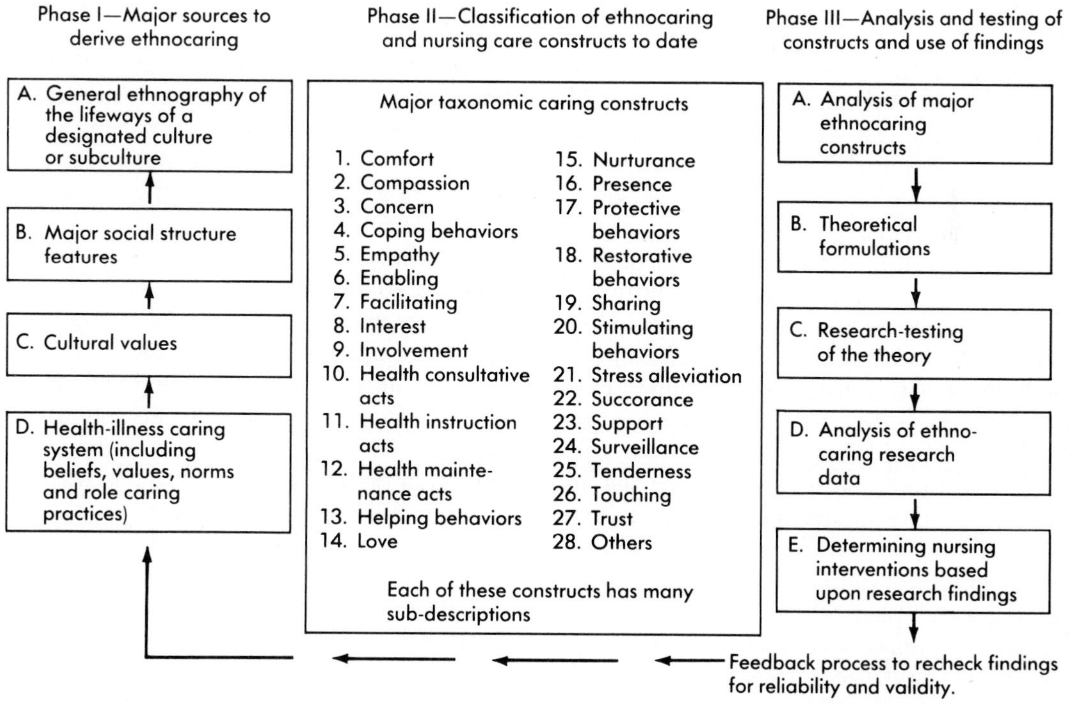

Figure 13-1. Leininger's conceptual theory and generating model to study transcultural and ethnocaring constructs. Model was developed in 1968 and reflects revisions and additions since that time. (The ethnocaring definitions are not presented here.) Data come from 30 cultures using a modified ethnoscience and ethnonursing research approach.
Used with permission from Leininger, M.M. (1981). *Caring: An essential human need.* Thorofare, N.J.: Charles B. Slack.

Health Care (1985), *Qualitative Research Methods in Nursing,* and in several other publications.

ACCEPTANCE BY THE NURSING COMMUNITY

Practice

Leininger identifies several factors for the slowness of nurses to recognize and value culture factors in nursing practices and education. First, when the theory was conceptualized, virtually no nurses were prepared in anthropology to understand transcultural concepts, models, or her theory. Most nurses had no idea about the nature of anthropology and how anthropological knowledge could contribute to human care and health behaviors. Second, although patients had long-standing and inherent cultural needs, many patients were reluctant to push health personnel to meet their cultural needs, and therefore did not demand that their cultural and social needs be recognized or met.[4:42-43] Third, until the past decade transcultural nursing articles submitted for publication were often rejected because editors did not know, value, or understand the relevance of anthropology to nursing or the idea of transcultural nursing as a new field of nursing. Fourth, the concept of care was of limited interest to nurses until the late 1970s, after Leininger had prepared a number of nurses in transcultural nursing and encouraged some nurses to pursue studies in anthropology.

More and more nurses are realizing the importance of transcultural nursing, the concept of human care, and the need to understand different cultures. Leininger[4:123] states, "We are entering a new phase of health emphasis as we examine the impact of cultural factors upon human caring, health and illness behavior." With the rise in consumer cultural identity is an accompanying increased demand for culturally sensitive and specific care and practices to assist clients of diverse cultures. Communities are becoming more multicultural, and health personnel are being expected to respond to clients' diverse cultural needs. Immigrants and people from unfamiliar cultures are generally expecting nurses to respect their cultural values, beliefs, and lifeways.

Education

The inclusion of culture and comparative care in nursing curricula began in 1966 at the University of Colorado, where Leininger was a professor of nursing and anthropology. Awareness of the relationships among culture, care, and nursing began to appear in the late 1960s, but few nurse educators were adequately prepared to teach courses on transcultural nursing. The world's first master's and doctoral programs in transcultural nursing were approved and implemented in 1977 at the University of Utah. Prior to this, Leininger had established transcultural nursing courses and a department of transcultural nursing (later cross-cultural community care) at the University of Washington while she served as dean and was active in teaching. Today, with heightened public awareness of health care costs, different cultures, and human rights, there is a greater demand for comprehensive, holistic, and multicultural client care. Leininger[4:18-21] suggests these demands have led to the need for culture-specific care and to the need to discover universal aspects of care. An urgent need remains for nurses to be educated in transcultural nursing and for well-qualified faculty prepared in transcultural nursing to teach and to do research in nursing schools in the United States and overseas.

Since 1980, an increasing number of nursing curricula emphasize transcultural nursing and care. One early program was at Cuesta College in California, which developed its nursing program with care and cultural care diversity as central themes. Course titles included Caring Concepts I & II, Caring of Families, and Professional Self-Care.[7] In the late 1980s, four master's and four doctoral programs in the United States offered transcultural nursing courses, research experiences, and guided field study experiences.[12] Leininger receives numerous requests to give workshops on human care and transcultural nursing, averaging 50 to 60 requests each year from within the United States and 12 to 20 from other countries. She can give only about 32 workshops per year because of her heavy teaching, research, consultation, and public speaking responsibilities.[12] Although this trend is encouraging, Leininger believes that more programs and courses are needed to meet the worldwide needs for transcultural nursing and to develop area specialists and generalists in transcultural nursing. The programs are also needed for certification of transcultural nursing, which is now established by the Worldwide Transcultural Nursing Society to provide safe and knowledgeable care to clients of diverse cultures. The first certified transcultural nurses were recognized in 1988.[12] More research studies related to transcultural nursing practices are being generated by faculty and graduate students. Despite the encouraging outcomes, using care as the central focus in the transcultural nursing curriculum needs further encouragement and research to validate its importance and effectiveness in client services.[11:245-248]

Research

Several research nurses are testing transcultural theories and conducting basic and advanced research studies in transcultural nursing in the United States and other countries.[4:24] Approximately 55 cultures have been studied.[12] Despite a heightened interest on the part of consumers who are supportive of research in transcultural nursing, still most of the research in transcultural nursing has not been funded by federal nursing monies. Until recently, very few transcultural grants received support unless they had a quantitative (measurement) focus. Through persistent efforts, some qualitative studies are slowly being funded. Transcultural nurses and other interested nurses have also been active contributors to international, national, regional, and local workshops in the development of conferences and instructional programs on the topic of transcultural nursing.[4:24] Through persistent ethnographic and qualitative studies in transcultural nursing in the past three decades, nurses are becoming aware of and learning to value this research. These nurses have "stimulated and maintained a stream of humanistic conscious-raising to people who know little about unfamiliar cultures in the world."[4:46]

FURTHER DEVELOPMENT

"It is reasonable to predict that all professional nurses in this country and abroad will come to recognize the need to know and use transcultural concepts in their practice, teaching, research, and consultation."[4:26] Currently, the demand for prepared transcultural nurses far exceeds the number of faculty and clinical specialists in the field. More transcultural nurse theorists, researchers, and scholars are needed to develop and synthesize the new nursing knowledge and to change unicultural norms of nursing practice to multicultural ones. "By the year 2000, it is hoped that most nurses will have a basic knowledge of a number of cultural groups in the world and an in-depth knowledge of two or three cultures."[4:28] Leininger believes transcultural nursing research will lead to some entirely new theories and different ways to conceptualize nursing education and to practice nursing. "Health disciplines will gradually become involved in transcultural studies and practices in the near future and health science courses and programs of study become established."[4:28] Because of the increased need for nurses to know and understand cultures and related nursing care needs, there is an increasing demand for transcultural nurses prepared as educators, researchers, and consultants. "It is reasonable to predict that transcultural nurse specialists . . . will (and should be) tomorrow's leaders in national and international teaching, research, and service programs."[4:28]

The present and future research in the field of transcultural nursing will enhance theoretic development and will continue to identify culture-specific and universal care constructs. According to Leininger, universal and diverse care constructs are essential to establish a substantive scientific and humanistic body of transcultural and general nursing knowledge to make nursing a worldwide profession and discipline. Leininger's theory is rapidly gaining international interest because it is holistic, relevant, and futuristic and deals with multicultural nursing care conditions and needs.[12]

CRITIQUE

Simplicity

Because the concepts of transcultural nursing theory are complex and multiple, the theory is not simple. Many questions are proposed in pursuit of a scientific body of nursing knowledge based on systematic investigation. The theoretical development and the research goals are to seek both universal and specific culturally defined care phenomena from diverse cultures and from the culture of nursing. The theory is truly transcultural, global in scope, and highly complex, requiring knowledge and appreciation of transcultural and anthropology insights. Leininger's theory is an evolving one with different but related models to guide the researcher in conceptualizing the theory and research approaches. Because of its holistic and comprehensive nature, several concepts and constructs related to social structure, environment, and language are important to understand to see how care and health are influenced by these dimensions. The theory shows multiple interrelationships of concepts and diversity of key concepts. It is a theory that requires anthropological and transcultural nursing knowledge to be used fully and accurately by nursing researchers. Once the users of the theory have conceptualized the theory, Leininger finds that undergraduate and graduate nursing students find it is highly practical, relevant, and more simple than complex.

Generality

The transcultural nursing theory does purport to demonstrate the criterion of generality, as it is a qualitatively oriented theory that is broad, comprehensive, and worldwide in scope. In fact, transcultural nursing theory addresses nursing care from a multicultural and world view perspective. It is useful and applicable to both groups and individuals with the goal of rendering culture-specific nursing care. The broad or generic concepts are organized and operationalized for study in specific cultures. The research has lead to a taxonomy of care with many subsets. Many aspects of culture, care, and health, as these factors impact upon nursing, are being studied. From this culture-specific data, a few universal care constructs are being identified. More research is needed, and a greater number of the world's cultural groups need to be studied to validate the caring constructs. The theoretical model is a guide for the study of any culture and for comparative study of several cultures. Findings from the theory use are being used in client care in a variety of health and community settings worldwide.

Empirical Precision

The transcultural nursing theory is researchable, and qualitative research has been the primary paradigm in order to discover largely unknown phenomena of care and health in diverse cultures. This qualitative approach differs from the traditional quantitative research method and renders measurement not the goal of the research. However, the ethnoscience research method is extremely rigorous and linguistically exacting in nature and outcomes. Eighty-five care constructs have been identified thus far, and more are being discovered. The important attribute is that accuracy of data derived with the use of ethnomethods or from an emic or people's viewpoint is leading to high validity and reliability of data. Ongoing and future research is hoped to lead to additional care and health findings as well as implications for ethnonursing practices and education to fit specific cultures as well as universal features. The qualitative criteria of credibility and confirmability from in-depth studies of informants and their contexts are becoming clearly evident.

Derivable Consequences

Transcultural nursing theory has outcomes that are very important for nursing. Rendering culture-specific care is a necessary and essential new goal in nursing. It places the transcultural nursing theory well within the domain of nursing knowledge acquisition and use. The theory is useful and applicable to nursing practice, education, and research. The concept of care as the primary focus of nursing, and the base of nursing knowledge and practice, is long overdue and essential to advance nursing knowledge and practices. Leininger notes that although nursing has always made claims to the concept of care, rigorous research on it has been limited. Because of its broad and multicultural focus, this theory could be the means for establishing nursing as a discipline and a profession.

REFERENCES

1. Leininger M. (1969). Conference on the nature of science and nursing. *Nursing Research, 18(5).*
2. Leininger, M. (1970) *Nursing and anthropology: Two worlds to blend.* New York: John Wiley & Sons.
3. Leininger, M. (1977). Cultural diversities of health and nursing care. *Nursing Clinics of North America, 12(1):*5-18.
4. Leininger, M. (1978). *Transcultural nursing: Concepts, theories, and practices.* New York: John Wiley & Sons.
5. Leininger, M. (1981). *Caring: An essential human need* (Proceedings of the three national caring conferences). Thorofare, N.J.: Charles B. Slack, Inc.
6. Leininger, M. (1983). Academic and professional vitae. (Current through December 1983.)
7. Leininger, M. (1984). *Care: The essence of nursing and health.* Thorofare, N.J.: Charles B. Slack, Inc.
8. Leininger, M. (1984, Oct. 19). *Transcultural care: Nursing for tomorrow.* Workshop presentation by Indiana University Alumni Association, Indiana University School of Nursing, Indianapolis.
9. Leininger, M. (1984, Oct. 19). Personal interview.
10. Leininger, M. (1985). *Qualitative research methods in nursing.* New York: Grune & Stratton.
11. MacDonald, M.R. (1984). The central construct for an associate degree nursing curriculum. In M. Leininger (Ed.), *Care: The essence of nursing and health.* Thorofare, N.J.: Charles B. Slack, Inc.
12. Leininger, M. (1988, April). Written communication with contributing author.

BIBLIOGRAPHY

Primary Sources

Books

Hofling, C.F. & Leininger, M. (1960). *Basic psychiatric concepts in nursing.* Philadelphia: J.P. Lippincott.

Leininger, M. (1970). *Nursing and anthropology: Two worlds to blend.* New York: John Wiley & Sons.

Leininger, M. (1973). *Contemporary issues in mental health nursing.* Boston: Little, Brown.

Leininger, M. (Ed.). (1974). *Health care dimensions (Vol. 1): Health care issues.* Philadelphia: F.A. Davis.

Leininger, M. (Ed.). (1975). *Health care dimensions (Vol. 2): Barriers and facilitators to quality health care.* Philadelphia: F.A. Davis.

Leininger, M. (Ed.). (1976). *Health care dimensions (Vol. 3): Transcultural health care issues and conditions.* Philadelphia: F.A. Davis.

Leininger, M. (Ed.). (1976). *Transcultural nursing care of infants and children.* Salt Lake City: University of Utah College of Nursing.

Leininger, M. (Ed.). (1978). *Transcultural nursing care of the elderly.* Salt Lake City: University of Utah College of Nursing.

Leininger, M. (Ed.). (1978). *Transcultural nursing: Concepts, theories and practices.* New York: John Wiley & Sons.

Leininger, M. (Ed.). (1979). *Transcultural nursing care of the adolescent and middle age adult.* Salt Lake City: University of Utah College of Nursing.

Leininger, M. (Ed.). (1979). *Transcultural nursing: Proceedings from four transcultural nursing conferences.* New York: Masson.

Leininger, M. (Ed.). (1980). *Cultural change, ethics and the nursing care implications.* Salt Lake City: University of Utah College of Nursing.

Leininger, M. (Ed.). (1980). *Transcultural nursing: Teaching, practice, and research.* Salt Lake City: University of Utah College of Nursing.

Leininger, M. (Ed.). (1981). *Caring: An essential human need.* Thorofare, N.J.: Charles B. Slack, Inc.

Leininger, M. (Ed.). (1984). *Care: The essence of*

nursing and health. Thorofare, N.J.: Charles B. Slack, Inc.

Leininger, M. (Ed.). (1985). *Qualitative research methods in nursing.* New York: Grune & Stratton.

Leininger, M. (Ed.). (1988). *Care: Discovery and Uses.* Detroit: Wayne State University Press.

Leininger, M. (Ed.). *Cultural Care Diversity and Universality: A Theory of Nursing.* Boston: Blackwell Publishing Co. (In progress.)

Smith, C.M., Wolf, V.C., & Leininger, M. (Eds.). (1973). *Nursing at the University of Washington, 1973-1975.* Seattle: University of Washington, Office of Publications and Department of Printing, 1973.

Book Chapters

Leininger, M. (1968). The research critique: Nature, function and art. In M. Batey (Ed.), *Communicating nursing research: The research critique.* Boulder, Col.: Western Interstate Commission on Higher Education, pp. 20-23.

Leininger, M. (1969). The young child's response to hospitalization: Separation anxiety or lack of mothering care? In M. Batey (Ed.), *Communicating nursing research.* Boulder, Col.: Western Interstate Commission on Higher Education, pp. 26-39.

Leininger, M. (1971). Anthropological approach to adaptation: Case studies from nursing. In J. Murphy (Ed.), *Theoretical issues in professional nursing.* New York: Appleton-Century-Crofts, pp. 77-102.

Leininger, M. (1973). The culture concept and its relevance to nursing. In M. Auld & L. Birum (Eds.), *The challenge of nursing: A book of readings.* St. Louis: C.V. Mosby, pp. 39-46.

Leininger, M. (1973). Primex. In M. Auld & L. Birum (Eds.), *The challenge of nursing: A book of reading.* St. Louis: C.V. Mosby, pp. 237-242.

Leininger, M. (1973). Nursing in the context of social and cultural systems. In P. Mitchell (Ed.), *Concepts basic to nursing.* New York: McGraw-Hill, pp. 37-60.

Leininger, M. (1974, Fall). Humanism, health and cultural values. In *Health care dimensions (Vol. 1): Health care issues.* Philadelphia: F.A. Davis, pp. 37-60.

Leininger, M. (1975, Spring). Health care delivery systems for tomorrow: Possibilities and guidelines. In *Health Care dimensions (Vol. 2): Barriers and facilitators to quality health care.* Philadelphia: F.A. Davis, pp. 83-95.

Leininger, M. (1976, Spring). Conflict and conflict resolutions: Theories and processes relevant to the health professions. In *Health care dimensions (Vol. 3): Transcultural health care issues and conditions.* Philadelphia: F.A. Davis, pp. 165-183.

Leininger, M. (1976, Spring). Toward conceptualization of transcultural health care systems: Concepts and a model. In *Health care dimensions (Vol. 3): Transcultural health care issues and conditions.* Philadelphia: F.A. Davis, pp. 3-22.

Leininger, M. (1976). Transcultural nursing: A promising subfield of study for nurse educators and practitioners. In A. Reinhardt (Ed.), *Current practice in family centered community nursing.* St. Louis: C.V. Mosby, pp. 36-50.

Leininger, M. (1978). Futurology of nursing: Goals and challenges for tomorrow. In N. Chaska (Ed.), *Views through the mist: The nursing profession.* New York: McGraw-Hill, pp. 379-396.

Leininger, M. (1978). Professional, political, and ethnocentric role behaviors and their influence in multidisciplinary health education. In A. Hardy & M. Conway (Ed.), *Role theory: Perspectives for health professionals.* New York: Appleton-Century-Crofts.

Leininger, M. (1981). Transcultural nursing issues for the 1980's. In J. McCloskey & H. Grace (Ed.), *Current issues in nursing.* Boston: Blackwell Scientific Publications.

Leininger, M. (1981). Women's role in society in the 80's. In *Maternal child nursing in the 80's.* Nursing perspective: A forum in honor of Katherine Kendall. College Park, Md.: University of Maryland School of Nursing.

Leininger, M. (1983). Intercultural interviews, assessments and therapy implications. In P. Pederson, (Ed.), *Interviews and assessments.* Beverly Hills, Cal.: Sage.

Leininger, M. (1988). Cultural Care and Nursing Administration, In B. Henry, C. Arndt, M. DiVincenti, & A. Marriner-Tomey (Eds.), *Dimensions of Nursing Administration.* Boston: Blackwell Scientific Publications, Inc.

Articles

Leininger, M. (1961, Oct.). Changes in psychiatric nursing. *Canadian Nurse, 57*:938-948.

Leininger, M. (1964, June). A Gadsup Village experiences its first election. *Journal of Polynesian Society 73:*29-34.

Leininger, M. (1967, April). The culture concept and its relevance to nursing. *Journal of Nursing Education, 6:*27-39.

Leininger, M. (1967, Spring). Nursing care of a patient from another culture: Japanese-American patient. *Nursing Clinics of North America, 2:*747-762.

Leininger, M. (1968, Sept.-Oct.). The research critique: Nature, function, and art. *Nursing Research, 17(5):*444-449.

Leininger, M. (1968, Nov.). Cultural differences among staff members and the impact on patient care. *Minnesota League for Nursing Bulletin, 16:*5-9.

Leininger, M. (1968, Nov.). The significance of cultural concepts in nursing. *Minnesota League for Nursing Bulletin, 16:*3-4.

Leininger, M. (1969, Jan.). Community psychiatric nursing: Trends, issues and problems. *Perspectives in Psychiatric Care, 7:*10-20.

Leininger, M. (1969, Jan.). Ethnoscience: A new and promising research approach for the health sciences. *Image, 3:*2-8.

Leininger, M. (1969, Sept.-Oct.). Conference on the nature of science in nursing. Introduction: Nature of science in nursing. *Nursing Research, 18:*388-389.

Leininger, M. (1970). Witchcraft practices and nursing therapy. *ANA Clinical Conferences.* New York: Appleton-Century-Crofts, p. 76.

Leininger, M. (1970). Some cross-cultural universal and non-universal functions beliefs and practices of food. In J. Dupont (Ed.), *Dimensions of Nutrition.* Proceedings of the Colorado Dietetic Association Conference [held in Fort Collins, Colorado, 1969]. Colorado Associated Universities Press, 1970, pp. 153-179.

Leininger, M. (1971, March). Anthropological issues related to community mental health programs in the United States. *Community Mental Health Journal, 7:*50-62.

Leininger, M. (1971, Nov.). Dean proposes educational teamwork. *Health Science Review, 1:*4.

Leininger, M. (1971, Dec.). This I believe . . . about interdisciplinary health education for the future. *Nursing Outlook, 19:*787-791.

Leininger, M. (1972). Using cultural styles of people: Conflicts and changes in the subculture of nursing. *Psychiatric Nursing Bulletin,* pp. 43-61.

Leininger, M. (1972, July). This I believe . . . about interdisciplinary health education for the future. *AORN Journal,* pp. 89-104.

Leininger, M. (1973, Winter). Health care delivery systems for tomorrow: Possibilities and guidelines. *Washington State Journal of Nursing, 45:*10-16.

Leininger, M. (1973, Spring). Witchcraft practices and psychocultural therapy with urban United States families. *Human Organization, 32:*73-83.

Leininger, M. (1973, March). An open health care system model. *Nursing Outlook, 21:*171-175.

Leininger, M. (1973, July). Primex: Its origins and significance. *American Journal of Nursing, 73:*1274-1277.

Leininger, M. (1973, Aug.). Witchcraft practices and psychocultural therapy with U.S. urban families. *Mental Health Digest, 5:*33-40.

Leininger, M. (1973, Fall). A new model: Working model for future nurse participation and utilization. *Washington State Journal of Nursing, 45:*7-15.

Leininger, M. (1973). Becoming aware of types of health practitioners and cultural imposition. *Speeches presented during the 48th Convention.* American Nurses' Association.

Leininger, M. (1974, March-April). The leadership crisis in nursing: A critical problem and challenge. *Journal of Nursing Administration, 4:*28-34.

Leininger, M. (1974, Spring). Scholars, scholarship and nursing scholarship. *Image, 6:*1-14.

Leininger, M. (1974, Dec.). Conflict and conflict resolution: Theories and processes relevant to the health professions. *American Nurse, 6:*17-21.

Leininger, M. (1974). Leadership in nursing: Challenges, concerns, and effect. *The Challenge: Rational administration in nursing and health care services,* University of Arizona, pp. 35-53.

Leininger, M. (1975, Feb.). Conflict and conflict resolution. *American Journal of Nursing, 75:*292-296.

Leininger, M. (1975, May). Transcultural nursing presents exciting challenge. *American Nurse, 5:*4.

Leininger, M. (1976, May-June). Doctoral programs for nurses: Trends, questions and projected plans. *Nursing Research, 25:*201-210.

Leininger, M. (1976, Fall). Two strange health tribes: Gnisrun and Enicidem in the United States. *Human Organization, 35:*253-261.

Leininger, M. (1976, Feb.). Caring: The essence and central focus of nursing. *American Nurses' Foundation, 12:*2-14.

Leininger, M. (1977). Cultural diversities of health and nursing care. *Nursing Clinics of North America, 12(1)*:5-18.

Leininger, M. (1977). Roles and directions in nursing and cancer nursing. *Proceedings of the Second National Conference on Cancer Nursing*. American Cancer Society.

Leininger, M. (1977). *Territoriality, power and creative leadership in administrative nursing contexts.* (Publication No. 52-1675:6-18). National League for Nursing.

Leininger, M. (1977, Nov.). Issues in nursing: A learning challenge. *Vital Signs,* 2:3. (Publication of the Student Nurses' Association, University of Utah.)

Leininger, M. (1978, March). Nursing in the future: Some brief glimpses (Part I). *Vital Signs, 2:7.*

Leininger, M. (1978, April). Nursing in the future: Some brief glimpses (Part II). *Vital Signs, 2:*8.

Leininger, M. (1978, May). Nursing in the future: Some brief glimpses (Part III). *Vital Signs, 2:9.*

Leininger, M. (1978, June). Changing foci in nursing education: Primary and transcultural care. *Journal of Advanced Nursing,* pp. 155-166.

Leininger, M. (1978, Spring). Political nursing: Essential for health and educational systems of tomorrow. *Nursing Administration Quarterly, 2(3)*:1-16.

Leininger, M. (1978, Oct.). Transcultural nursing: A new subfield to generate nursing and health care knowledge. *Scholarly Lecture Series.* University of Manitoba.

Leininger, M. (1978, Dec.). Creating and maintaining a nursing research support center. *Adelphi Report,* Adelphi University, pp. 35-60.

Leininger, M. (1978, Dec.). Transcultural nursing for tomorrow's nurse, *Imprint.*

Leininger, M. (1979, April). Health promotion and maintenance: An old transcultural challenge and a new emphasis for the health professions. Health Promotion: In *Health and Illness, Monograph #4.* Series 1978. Sigma Theta Tau.

Leininger, M. (1979). Consumer health care needs, nursing leadership and future directions. *Proceedings of the Leadership Conference.* Seattle: University of Washington, School of Nursing.

Leininger, M. (1979). Principles and guidelines to assist nurses in cross-cultural nursing and health practices. *Hope Conference Report.* Millwood, Va.: International Nursing Project Hope Health Sciences Education Center.

Leininger, M. (1979, Oct.). *Sociocultural forces impacting upon health care and the nursing profession.* NIH Annual Meeting of Nursing Departments. Washington, D.C.: National Institutes of Health.

Leininger, M. (1980, Winter) University of Utah nursing clinics. *Western Journal of Nursing Research, 2:*411.

Leininger, M. (1980, Aug.). Transcultural nursing: A new subfield. *Health Clinics International, 2:*3-4.

Leininger, M. & Shubin, S. (1980, June). Nursing patients from different cultures. *Nursing, 80:*10.

Leininger, M. (1980, Oct.). Caring: A central focus for nursing and health care services. *Nursing and Health Care, 1:*135-143, 176.

Leininger, M. (1981, July-Aug.). Woman's role in society in the 1980s. *Issues in Health Care of Women, 3(4)*:203-215.

Leininger, M. (1981, Sept.). Transcultural nursing: Its progress and its future. *Nursing and Health Care, 2(7)*:365-371.

Leininger, M. (1982, Jan.). Creativity and challenges for nurse researchers in this economic recession. *Center for Health Research News, 1:*1. (Publication of the College of Nursing, Wayne State University.)

Leininger, M. (1982, Nov.). Getting to 'Truths' or mastering numbers and research designs. *Center for Health Research News, 1:*2. (Publication of the College of Nursing, Wayne State University.)

Leininger, M. (1983, March). Creativity and challenges for nurse researchers in this economic recession. *Journal of Nursing Administration, 13:*21-22.

Leininger, M. (1983, May). Qualitative research methods: A new direction to document and discover nursing knowledge. *Center for Health Research News, 3:*2. (Publication of the College of Nursing, Wayne State University.)

Leininger, M. (1983, Aug.). Cultural care: An essential goal for nursing and health care. *Journal of Nephrology Nursing, 10:*11-17.

Leininger, M. (1983, Oct.-Dec.). Community psychiatric nursing in community mental health: Trends, issues, and problems. *Perspective Psychiatric Care, 21(4)*:139-146.

Leininger, M. (1984, March-April). Transcultural nursing: An overview. *Nursing Outlook, 32(2)*:72-73.

Leininger, M. (1984). Transcultural nursing. *Canadian Nurse, 80(11)*:41-45.

Leininger, M. (1985, April). Transcultural care diversity and universality: A theory of nursing. *Nursing and Health Care, 6(4)*:209-212.

Leininger, M. (1985, Feb.). [Translated from 'The Best of Image.' Ethnoscience: A promising research approach to improve nursing practice.] *Kango, 37(2)*:113-23.

Leininger, M. (1986). Care facilitation and resistance factors in the culture of nursing. *Topics in Clinical Nursing, 8(2)*:1-12.

Leininger, M. (1986). Care Symposium: Resources on culture (letter). *Journal of Nursing Administration, 16(6)*:35.

Leininger, M. (1986). Caring (reply letter). *Journal of Nursing Administration, 16(11)*:4.

Leininger, M. (1987). A new generation of nurses discover transcultural nursing (editorial). *Nursing & Health Care, 8(5)*:263.

Leininger, M. (1987, Summer). Response to "Infant feeding practices of Vietnamese immigrants to the Northwest United States." *Scholarly Inquiry for Nursing Practice, 1(2)*:171-174.

Leininger, M. (1988). Leininger's theory of nursing: Cultural care diversity and universality. *Nursing Science Quarterly* (Ed. Parse). Pittsburgh, Pa. (522 pp.).

Book Prefaces and Forewords

Leininger, M. (1972). Introduction. In K. Leahy, M. Cobb, & M. Jones, *Community health nursing*. New York: McGraw-Hill.

Leininger, M. (1972). Introduction. In L. Schwartz & J. Schwartz, *Psychodynamic concepts of patient care*. Englewood Cliffs, N.J.: Prentice-Hall, Inc.

Leininger, M. (1973, July). Foreword. In M. Disbrow (Ed.), *Meeting consumers' demands for maternity care*. Seattle: University of Washington Press.

Leininger, M. (1974, Fall). Preface. In M. Leininger (Ed.), *Health care issues: Health care dimensions,* Second issue, Philadelphia: F.A. Davis.

Leininger, M. (1975, Spring). Preface. In M. Leininger (Ed.), *Transcultural health care issues and conditions: Health care dimensions,* Second issue, Philadelphia: F.A. Davis.

Leininger, M. (1976, Spring). Preface. In M. Leininger (Ed.), *Transcultural health care issues and conditions: Health care dimensions,* Third issue, Philadelphia: F.A. Davis.

Leininger, M. (1978). Foreword. In J. Watson, *Nursing: The philosophy and science of caring*. Boston: Little, Brown.

Leininger, M. (1979). Foreword. In L.S. Bermosk & S.E. Porter, *Womens' health and human wholeness*. New York: Appleton-Century-Crofts.

Leininger, M. (1979). Preface. In M. Leininger, (Ed.), *Proceedings of the national transcultural nursing conferences*. New York: Masson.

Leininger, M. (1980). Foreword. *Transcultural nursing: Teaching, research, and practice*. Salt Lake City.

Leininger, M. (1981). Introduction. *Six Proceedings of the transcultural nursing conferences in 1976, 1977, 1978, 1979, 1980, 1981*. New York: Masson International Press.

Leininger, M. (1981). Preface. *Caring: An essential human need*. Thorofare, N.J.: Charles B. Slack, Inc.

Leininger, M. (1981). Preface. *Maternal child nursing in the 80's*. Nursing perspective: A forum in honor of Katherine Kendall. College Park, Md.: University of Maryland, School of Nursing.

Leininger, M. (1983). Preface. *Transcultural health and nursing references*. Thorofare, N.J.: Charles B. Slack, Inc.

Leininger, M. (1983). Preface. *Care: The essence of nursing and health*. Thorofare, N.J.: Charles B. Slack, Inc.

Leininger, M. (1983). Preface. In K. Vestal & C. McKenzie (Eds.), *High risk perinatal nursing*. Philadelphia: W.B. Saunders.

Secondary Sources

Chinn, P.L. & Jacobs, M.K. (1983). *Theory and nursing: A systematic approach*. St. Louis: C.V. Mosby.

Chinn, P.L., & Jacobs, M.K. (1987). *Theory and nursing: a systematic approach*. St. Louis: C.V. Mosby.

14

Jean Watson

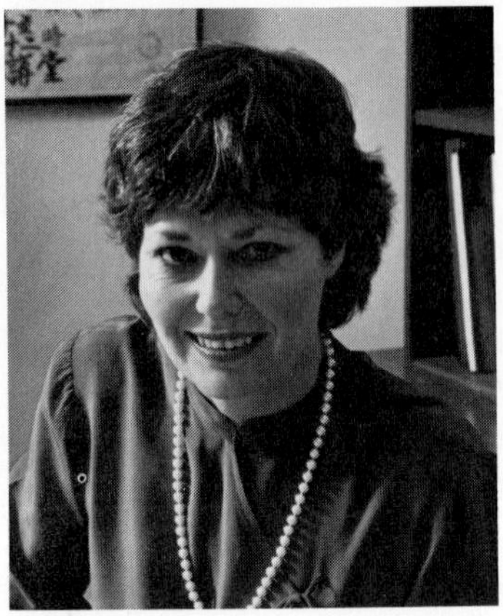

Philosophy and Science of Caring

Patricia M. Bennett, Beverly D. Porter, Rebecca S. Sloan

CREDENTIALS AND BACKGROUND OF THE THEORIST

Jean Watson was born July 21, 1940, the youngest of eight children. She is married and has two children.

Watson received a Bachelor of Science in Nursing from the University of Colorado at Boulder in 1964. She continued her education and received a Master's in psychiatric-mental health nursing from the University of Colorado at Denver in 1966. She began her nursing career as a psychiatric-mental health nurse therapist for a private group and worked with student groups at the university. In 1973 Watson received a Ph.D. in educational psychology and counseling, with a special cognate emphasis in social and clinical psychology, from the University of Colorado at Boulder.

After graduation, Watson accepted a faculty position at the University of Colorado. She also served as a founder, clinical consultant, and member of the board of the Boulder County Hospice and was active in crisis intervention and bereavement studies. She received several research grant awards to study cognitive sys-

The authors wish to express appreciation to Dr. Jean Watson for critiquing the chapter.

tems of nurses and the influence of conceptual systems on education, especially in psychosocial nursing.

A member of the University of Colorado School of Nursing faculty since 1973, Watson has been associate dean of the baccalaureate program and was director of the doctoral program and coordinator of the psychosocial mental health nursing doctoral program from 1979 to 1981. During that time she also chaired the University of Colorado Faculty Council, the academic governing body for the four-campus system. She became Dean of the School of Nursing in 1984 and was instrumental in the decision by the nursing faculty to institute a program leading to a nursing doctorate (N.D.) as the first professional degree.[6:94] Watson established the University of Colorado Center for Human Caring in the School of Nursing in 1986. The center will put Watson and other's theories of human caring into practice by "integrating the arts, humanities, and social and behavioral sciences into human care and the healing process."[8:1]

Watson has been the recipient of numerous awards and honors during her career. She received a Kennedy Foundation Award for a special short-term study in bioethics in Georgetown University's Kennedy Institute in 1977 and the Sigma Theta Tau National Honorary Nursing Society Award for Creativity in Nursing in 1980. In 1981 she was admitted as a fellow in the American Academy of Nursing. Watson was awarded a Visiting Kellogg Fellowship for study at Curtin University, Western Australia, in 1981–1982 and a faculty fellowship in the Lincoln Institute of Health Sciences, in the Royal College of Nursing in Melbourne during 1981–1982. She also received a National Science Council Award to serve as visiting lecturer-consultant at the National Taiwan University in 1982.

Watson has been a visiting nurse lecturer at Catholic University and Teachers College, Columbia University. She has been an invited Distinguished Lecturer at Hebrew University, Jerusalem, the University of Tel Aviv, and the University of Montreal, Quebec. She has received two honorary doctorates, a Doctorate of Humane Letters from Assumption College, Worcester, Massachusetts, and a Doctorate of Nursing Science from the University of Akron, Ohio. Watson has participated in National Nurse Theorist conferences and published articles and book chapters in nursing literature on research, the science of human caring, professional education, and quality health care.

While working with a group of colleagues on curriculum development, Watson was approached to publish a textbook for an integrated baccalaureate nursing curriculum. The result was what she refers to as a treatise on nursing. Published in 1979, *Nursing: The Philosophy and Science of Caring* is now treated as a theory of nursing. It was followed in 1985 by a second major work, *Nursing: Human Science and Human Care, A Theory of Nursing*. She is working on another book.

There has long been a discrepancy in nursing between theory and practice. To reduce this dichotomy, Watson proposes a philosophy and science of caring. Caring is central to nursing practice.[4:xii] It is a moral ideal rather than a task-oriented behavior and includes such elusive aspects of health as the interpersonal relationship between the nurse and client. The end is preservation of human dignity and humanity in the health care system. Watson[13:40] believes ultimate professional nursing care is the result of combined study of the sciences and the humanities culminating in a human care process between nurse and client that transcends time and space and has spiritual dimensions. The process, which is built upon an ethical human science foundation, is based on 10 carative factors of nursing.

THEORETICAL SOURCES

In addition to traditional nursing knowledge and the works of Nightingale, Henderson, Krueter, and Hall, Watson acknowledges the work of Leininger and Gadow.[13:10] She drew heavily on the sciences and the humanities in developing her framework, which has a phenomenological-existential and spiritual orientation.

Watson attributes her emphasis on the interpersonal and transpersonal qualities of congruence, empathy, and warmth to the views of Carl Rogers and recent transpersonal psychology writers. Rogers describes several incidents leading to the formulation of his thoughts on human behavior. One such episode involves his learning "that it is the *client* who knows what hurts and that the facilitator should allow the direction of the therapeutic process to come from the client."[5:11-12] Rogers[5:18-19] believed that through understanding the client would come to accept himself, an initial step toward a positive outcome. The therapist helps by clarifying and stating feelings about which the client has been unclear. To do this the therapist must be able to understand the meanings, feelings, and attitudes of the client. A warm interest has been found to facilitate understanding. Rogers presents an unpublished thesis by R.D. Quinn who studied recorded therapists' statements both in and out of context. Degree of understanding was judged to be high in both contexts and Quinn[5:44] concluded that understanding is primarily a desire to understand.

Another concept of Rogerian theory is that the therapist-client relationship is more important to the outcome than adherence to traditional methods. Rogers[5:32] states:

> In my early professional years I was asking the question, How can I treat, or cure, or change this person? Now I phrase the question in this way: How can I provide a relationship which this person may use for his own personal growth?

To support his concept Rogers notes a study by Betz and Whitehorn[1] describing the differences in degree of improvement for schizophrenic patients treated by two methods. Those patients treated by physicians who endeavored to understand the personal meaning of their patients' behavior fared better than patients of doctors who saw their clients as symptomatic of a specific diagnosis.[1:89-117;10:321-331] Additionally, J. Seeman's study[7:272-299] describes the effectiveness of psychotherapy when characterized by mutual affection and respect between the therapist and client.

Watson believes a strong liberal arts background is essential to the process of holistic care for clients. She sees the study of the humanities as an experience resulting in mind expansion, increased thinking skills, and personal growth. But Watson[10:413-416;11:244-249] describes the current status of nursing by using as an analogy the mythological Danaides, who attempted to fill a broken jar with water, only to see the water flow through the cracks. Until nursing merges theory and practice through combined study of the sciences and the humanities, similar cracks will be evident in the scientific basis of nursing knowledge.

Yalom's 11 curative factors stimulated Watson's thinking[9:xvi] about the psychodynamic and human components that could apply to nursing and caring and, consequently, to the 10 carative factors in nursing.

USE OF EMPIRICAL EVIDENCE

Watson and her colleagues have attempted to study the concept of caring by collecting data to use in classifying caring behaviors, to describe the similarities and differences between what nurses consider care and what clients consider care, and to generate testable hypotheses around the concept of nursing care. They studied responses from registered nurses, student nurses, and clients to the same open-ended questionnaire covering a variety of aspects of "(a) taking care of and (b) caring about" patients. Their findings revealed a discrepancy in the values considered most important to clients versus the student nurses versus the registered nurses. Their conclusions stressed the need for further study in order to clarify what behaviors and values are important from each viewpoint.

Their study also raised a question regarding differences in values for persons in different situations, as well as the question of meeting minimum care needs before the quality of care can be evaluated.[10:32-44]

Watson's later research into caring incorporates empirics but emphasizes methodologies that begin with nursing phenomena rather than the natural sciences.[4:344] A human science, empirical phenomenology, and transcendent phenomenology were used in her latest work. More recently she has been investigating new language, such as metaphor and poetry, to communicate, convey, and elucidate human caring and healing.[15:10-17]

MAJOR CONCEPTS AND DEFINITIONS

Watson[9:9-10] bases her theory for nursing practice on the following 10 carative factors. Each has a dynamic phenomenological component that is relative to the individuals involved in the relationship as encompassed by nursing.

FORMATION OF A HUMANISTIC-ALTRUISTIC SYSTEM OF VALUES. Humanistic and altruistic values are learned early in life but can be greatly influenced by nursing educators. This factor describes satisfaction through giving and extension of the sense of self.[9:10-12]

INSTILLATION OF FAITH-HOPE. This factor describes the nurse's role in promoting wellness by helping the client adopt health-seeking behaviors, by using the power of suggestion positively to support the client, and by developing effective nurse-client interrelationships.[9:12-16]

CULTIVATION OF SENSITIVITY TO ONE'S SELF AND TO OTHERS. Recognition of feelings leads to self-actualization through self-acceptance for the nurse and client. If a nurse is able to express her feelings, she is better able to allow others to express theirs.[9:16-19]

DEVELOPMENT OF A HELPING-TRUST RELATIONSHIP. A helping-trust relationship promotes and accepts the expression of positive and negative feelings. It involves congruence, empathy, nonpossessive warmth, and effective communication.[9:23-41]

Congruence. Congruence involves being real, honest, genuine, and authentic.[9:26-28]

Empathy. Empathy is the ability to experience, and thereby understand, the other person's perceptions and feelings and to communicate those understandings.[9:28-30]

Nonpossessive warmth. Nonpossessive warmth is demonstrated by a moderate speaking volume, a relaxed, open posture, and facial expressions that are congruent with other communications.[9:30-33]

Effective communication. Effective communication has cognitive, affective, and behavioral response components.[9:33-41]

PROMOTION AND ACCEPTANCE OF THE EXPRESSION OF POSITIVE AND NEGATIVE FEELINGS. The sharing of feelings is a risk-taking experience for both the nurse and the client. The nurse must be prepared for negative feelings. The nurse must understand that intellectual and emotional understanding of a situation are different.[9:17-48]

SYSTEMATIC USE OF THE SCIENTIFIC PROBLEM-SOLVING METHOD FOR DECISION MAKING. Use of the nursing process brings a scientific problem-solving approach to nursing care, dispelling the traditional image of nurses as the "doctor's handmaiden." The nursing process is similar to the research process.[9:51-66]

PROMOTION OF INTERPERSONAL TEACHING-LEARNING. This factor is an important concept for nursing in that it separates *caring* from *curing*. It allows the patient to be informed and thus shifts responsibility for wellness to the client. The nurse facilitates this with teaching-learning techniques that are designed to enable the client to provide self-care, determine his own needs, and provide for his own growth.[9:69-79]

PROVISION FOR A SUPPORTIVE, PROTECTIVE, OR CORRECTIVE MENTAL, PHYSICAL, SOCIOCULTURAL, AND SPIRITUAL ENVIRONMENT. Nursing must recognize that the client's environment includes external and internal variables. Change can be experienced in any aspect and requires coping. The nurse assesses and facilitates the client's coping abilities. Comfort, privacy, safety, and clean, aesthetic surroundings are important.[9:81-101]

ASSISTANCE WITH THE GRATIFICATION OF HUMAN NEEDS. The nurse recognizes the biophysical, psychophysical, psychosocial, and intrapersonal needs of herself and her client. Clients must attain the lower order needs before attaining those higher in the needs hierarchy. Food, elimination, and ventilation are lower order biophysical needs. Activity-inactivity and sexuality are lower order psychophysical needs. Achievement and affiliation are higher order psychosocial needs. Self-actualization is a higher order intrapersonal-interpersonal need.[9:105-203]

ALLOWANCE FOR EXISTENTIAL-PHENOMENOLOGICAL FORCES. Phenomenology describes data of the immediate situation that help people understand the phenomena in question.[9:208] Existential psychology is a science of human existence that employs the method of phenomenological analysis.[9:209] Watson considers this factor to be difficult to understand. It is included to provide a thought-provoking experience leading to a better understanding of ourselves and others.[9:205-215]

Watson believes nurses have the responsibility to go beyond the 10 carative factors and develop the areas of health promotion through preventive actions. This is accomplished by teaching clients behavioral changes to promote health, providing situational support, teaching problem-solving methods, and recognizing coping skills and adaptation to loss.[9:217-305]

MAJOR ASSUMPTIONS

Watson[9:8-9] states the major assumptions of her theory are:

1. Caring can be effectively demonstrated and practiced only interpersonally.
2. Caring consists of carative factors that result in the satisfaction of certain human needs.
3. Effective caring promotes health and individual or family growth.
4. Caring responses accept a person not only as he or she is now, but for what he or she may become.
5. A caring environment offers the development of potential while allowing the person to choose the best action for himself or herself at a given point in time.
6. Caring is more healthogenic than is curing. The practice of caring integrates biophysical knowledge with knowledge of human behavior to generate or promote health and to provide ministrations to those who are ill. A science of caring is therefore complementary to the science of curing.
7. The practice of caring is central to nursing.

THEORETICAL ASSERTIONS

According to Watson, nursing tries to understand how health, illness, and human behavior are interrelated. With her philosophy and science of caring, she tries to define an outcome of scientific activity in regard to the humanistic aspects of life. In other words, she attempts to make nursing an interrelationship of quality of life and death, as well as the prolongation of life.[9:xvii]

Watson believes nursing is concerned with

promoting and restoring health and preventing illness. But *health* is more than the absence of illness and is an illusive concept because it is subjective.[9:219] *Caring* is a nursing term, representing all the factors the nurse uses to deliver health care to her client. The nurse provides care to her clients through Watson's 10 carative factors.[9:6] Each carative factor describes the caring process of how a client attains, or maintains, health or dies a peaceful death. On the other hand, Watson describes *curing* as a medical term referring to elimination of disease.[9:7]

In *Nursing: The Philosophy and Science of Caring*, Watson[9:8] writes that the basic premises of a science for nursing are:

1. Caring (and nursing) has existed in every society. Every society has had some people who have cared for others. A caring attitude is *not* transmitted from generation to generation by genes. It is transmitted by the culture of the profession as a unique way of coping with its environment. Nursing has always held a caring stance in regard to other human beings. That stance has been threatened by a long history of procedure-oriented demands and the development of different levels of nursing. However, the opportunities for nurses to obtain advanced education and engage in higher-level analyses of problems and concerns in their education and practice have allowed nursing to combine its humanistic orientation with the relevant science.
2. There is often a discrepancy between theory and practice or between the scientific and artistic aspects of caring, partly because of the disjunction between scientific values and humanistic values.

Watson added the following premises for the context of human science theory development in *Nursing: Human Science and Human Care*.[13:16]

1. A philosophy of human freedom, choice, and responsibility
2. A biology and psychology of holism (nonreducible persons interconnected with others and nature)
3. An epistemology that allows not only for empirics but also for advancement of esthetics, ethical values, intuition, and process discovery
4. An ontology of time and space
5. A context of interhuman events, processes, and relationships
6. A scientific world view that is open

LOGICAL FORM

The framework is presented in a logical form. It contains broad ideas but a focused framework. It is derived from many disciplines and addresses many situations on the health-illness continuum. Watson's definition of *caring* as opposed to *curing* delineates nursing from medicine. This concept is helpful in classifying the body of nursing knowledge as a separate science.

The development of the theory since 1979 has been toward clarifying the person of the nurse and the person of the client. The other emphasis has been on existential-phenomenological and spiritual factors.

Watson's theory has foundational support from theorists in other disciplines, such as Rogers, Erikson, and Maslow. She is adamant in her support for nursing education that incorporates holistic knowledge from many disciplines and integrates humanities, art and sciences. She views the increasingly complex requirements of the health care system and nursing practice to be indicators of the need for a liberal educational background before professional education.[6:93]

ACCEPTANCE BY THE NURSING COMMUNITY

Practice

Institutions that seek to use a holistic approach to nursing care are using many aspects of Watson's theoretical commitment to caring. Nursing journals concerned with the delivery of nursing care contain increasing numbers of articles that reference Watson and incorporate the importance of caring as an essential domain of nursing.[2:25]

Education

Watson has been active in curriculum planning at the University of Colorado. Her framework is being taught in the 4-year nursing curriculum at Bellarmine College in Louisville, Kentucky. Assumption College in Worcester, Massachusetts, and other undergraduate programs also use the framework. In addition, the concepts are now widely used in nursing programs in Australia and in some programs in Sweden, Finland, and Great Britain. Watson[12] believes her theory will have more acceptance through a liberal arts college with a religious background than through the large university setting, unless the university curriculum is committed to a liberal post-baccalaureate professional nursing education.

Critics of the author's work have concentrated on the use of undefined terms, incomplete treatment of subject matter when describing the 10 carative factors, and a lack of attention to the pathophysiological aspects of nursing. Watson[9:xv] addresses these charges in the preface of her book, where she defines her intent to describe the *core* of nursing—those aspects of the nurse-client relationship resulting in a therapeutic outcome—rather than the *trim* of nursing—the procedures, tasks, and techniques employed by various practice settings. Using this focus, the framework is not limited to any nursing specialty.

Watson hopes her work will help nurses develop a meaningful philosophic base for practice.[13:50-51] A study of Watson's framework leads the reader through a thought-provoking experience by emphasizing communication skills, use of self, transpersonal growth, attention to both nurse and patient, and the human caring process that potentiates human health and healing.

Research

Watson has attempted to research her framework and to arrive at empirical data amenable to research techniques. However, this very abstract framework is difficult to study concretely. She believes that there is often a chasm between the essential qualities and subject matter of nursing and the methods we use for research.

As with her concern for uniting the liberal arts with nursing education, Watson hopes nursing research will incorporate and explore esthetics, metaphysics, empirics, and contextual methodologies.[4:343-344] The theory as presented may never be fully tested but will be clinically validated as is demonstrated by the work of Hester, Ray, and others.[3]

FURTHER DEVELOPMENTS

Nursing research has traditionally followed the *received view* format in which single-factor methodology is compared against rigorous standards of truth, operational definitions, and observational criteria.[7:413-416] Watson concludes that this methodology does not apply to the multifactorial study of nursing care. She proposes that as nursing advances in its own doctoral programs, the process of scientific development will be used on itself. Nursing research will adopt the received view, reject it, and synthesize new ideas, which will result in a new nursing model for the 1980s and 1990s.

Continued awareness of research of Watson's theory may promote widespread acceptance of her views. She has identified several critical issues for future research: conditions that foster the person as an end and not a means in a highly technological society and conditions that promote caring when humanity is threatened.[13:21] This theory should lend itself to creative research methodologies that will assist nursing in formulating a philosophical base for professional human care concepts because Watson's work is as much a philosophy as a theory.

CRITIQUE

Clarity

On the surface, Watson's theory is easily read and uses nontechnical language that provides clarity. Semantic clarity could be improved by employing precise definitions of terms. For example, nursing is defined in a variety of ways in various portions of the book. One broad definition of nursing would be helpful in understanding the thoughts of the author. Additionally, it is unclear whether Watson was speaking to the nurse's responsibilities, or to the client's responsibilities in some interactions, or to both.

Simplicity

Watson draws on a number of disciplines in formulating her theory. The reader must have an understanding of a variety of subject matters in order to understand the theory as it is presented. Therefore, this theory is not considered simple.

Generality

The scope of the framework encompasses all aspects of the health-illness continuum. In addition, the theory addresses aspects of preventing illness and experiencing a peaceful death, thereby increasing its generality.

Empirical Precision

Although the framework is difficult to study empirically, Watson draws heavily on widely accepted work from other disciplines. With this solid foundation, her views are strengthened.

Derivable Consequences

Considerable testing still needs to be undertaken, but Watson's theory can provide a useful and important metaphysical orientation for the delivery of nursing care. Watson's theoretical concepts, such as use of self, client-identified needs, the caring process, and the spiritual sense of being human, may help nurses and their clients find meaning and harmony in a period of increasing complexity.

REFERENCES

1. Betz, B.J., & Whitehorn, J.C. (1956). The relationship of the therapist to the outcome of therapy in schizophrenia. *Psychiatric Research Reports #5.* Research techniques in schizophrenia. Washington, D.C.: American Psychiatric Association.
2. Brenner, P., Boyd, C., Thompson, T., Cervantez, M., Buerhaus, P., & Leininger, M. (1986, Jan.). The care symposium: Considerations for nursing administrators. *JONA, 16(1)*:25-26.
3. Hester, N.O., & Ray, M.A. (1987). Assessment of Watson's carative factors: A qualitative research study. Paper presented at the International Nursing Research Congress. Edinburgh, Scotland.
4. Leininger, M. (1979). Preface. In J. Watson, *Nursing: The philosophy and science of caring.* Boston: Little, Brown.
5. Rogers, C.R. (1961). *On becoming a person: A therapist's view of psychology.* Boston: Houghton Mifflin.
6. Sakalys, J.A., & Watson, J. (1986). Professional education: Post-baccalaureate education for professional nursing. *Journal of Professional Nursing,* 91-96.
7. Seeman, J. (1954). Counselor judgments of therapeutic process and outcome. In C.R. Rogers & R.F. Dymond (Eds.), *Psychotherapy and personality change.* Chicago: University of Chicago Press, pp. 272-299.
8. The dean speaks out: Center for human caring established. (1986, Dec.). *The University of Colorado School of Nursing News,* pp. 1-6.
9. Watson, J. (1979). *Nursing: The philosophy and science of caring.* Boston: Little, Brown.
10. Watson, J. (1981, July). Nursing's scientific quest. *Nursing Outlook, 29:*413-416.
11. Watson, J., et al. (1979). *A model of caring: An alternative health care model for nursing practice and research.* American Nurses' Association NP-59 3W 8179190, Clinical and Scientific Sessions, Div. of Practice, Kansas City, Mo., pp.32-34.
12. Watson, J. (1984). Telephone interview.
13. Watson, J. (1985). *Nursing: Human science and health care.* Norwalk, Conn.: Appleton-Century-Crofts.

14. Watson, J. (1985). Reflections on new methodologies for study of human care. In M. Leininger (Ed.), *Qualitative methodologies on nursing.* New York: Grune and Stratton.
15. Watson, J. (1987). Nursing on the caring edge: Metaphorical vignettes. *Advances in Nursing Science, 10(1):*10-17.
16. Watson, J. (1988). Telephone interview.
17. Whitehorn, J.C., & Betz, B.M. (1954). A study of psychotherapeutic relationships between physicians and schizophrenic patients. *American Journal of Psychiatry, 111:*321-331.

BIBLIOGRAPHY

Primary Sources

Books

Taylor, R., & Watson, J. Imprint: *Human caring and human suffering: Perspectives from humanities.* Boulder, CO: Associated University Press.

Watson, J. (1979). *Nursing: The philosophy and science of caring.* Boston: Little, Brown.

Watson, J. (1985). *Nursing: Human science and health care.* Norwalk, Conn.: Appleton-Century-Crofts.

Watson, J. (1988). *Nursing: Health science and human care.* Norwalk, Conn.: Appleton-Century-Crofts. (2nd printing, New York: National League for Nursing.)

Watson, J., & Ray, M.A. (Eds.) (1988). *The ethics of care and the ethics of cure: Synthesis of chronicity.* New York: National League for Nursing.

Book Chapters

Watson, J., et al. (1979). *A model of caring: An alternative health care model for nursing practice and research.* (Publication No. NP-59 3M 8179190). Kansas City, Mo.: American Nurses' Association.

Watson, J. (1980). Self losses. In F.L. Bower & M.S. Brown, (Eds.), *Nursing and the concept of loss.* New York: John Wiley & Sons.

Watson, J. (1981). Some issues related to a science of caring for nursing practice. In M. Leininger (Ed.), *Caring: An essential human need.* Thorofare, N.J.: Charles B. Slack, Inc.

Watson, J. (1983). Delivery and assurance of quality health care: A rights based foundation. In R. Luke, J. Krueger, & R. Madrow, (Eds.), *Organization and change in health care quality assurance.* Rockville, Md.: Aspen Systems.

Watson, J. (1985). Reflections on new methodologies for study of human care. In M. Leininger (Ed.), *Qualitative Methodologies on Nursing.* New York: Grune and Stratton.

Watson, J. (1987). The dream curriculum. In NLN, *Patterns in nursing: Strategic planning for nursing education.* New York: National League for Nursing.

Watson, J. (1988). The professional doctorate as an entry level into practice. In NLN, *Perspectives in nursing, 1987-1989.* New York: National League for Nursing.

Watson, J., & Bevis, E. (1989). Coming of age for a new age. In N. Chaska (Ed.), *The nursing profession: Turning points.* New York: McGraw-Hill.

Articles

Carozza, V., Congdon, J., & Watson, J. (1978, Nov.). An experimental educationally sponsored pilot internship program. *Journal of Nursing Education, 17:*14-20.

Krysl, M., & Watson, J. (1988). Existential moments of caring: Facets of nursing and social support. *Advances in Nursing Science, 10(2):*12-17.

Sakalys, J.A., & Watson, J. (1985, Sept.-Oct.). New directions in higher education: A review of trends. *Journal of Professional Nursing,* pp. 293-299.

Sakalys, J.A., & Watson, J. (1986, Mar.-Apr.). Professional education: Post-baccalaureate education for professional nursing. *Journal of Professional Nursing,* pp. 91-96.

Watson, J. (1976, Jan.-Feb.). The quasi-rational element in conflict: A review of selected conflict literature. *Nursing Research, 25:*19-23.

Watson, J. (1976, Jan.-Feb.). Research and literature on children's responses to injections: Some general nursing implications. *Pediatric Nursing, 2:*7-8.

Watson, J. (1976, Nov.-Dec.). Research question and answer. Creative approach to researchable questions. *Nursing Research, 25:*439.

Watson, J. (1978, May-June). Conceptual systems of undergraduate nursing students as compared with university students at large and practicing nurses. *Nursing Research, 27:*151-155.

Watson, J. (1980, Spring). Response to review of Watson's book. *Western Journal of Nursing Research, 2:*514-515.

Watson, J. (1981). The lost art of nursing. *Nursing Forum, 20:*244-249.

Watson, J. (1981, Spring). Conceptual systems of

students, practitioners. *Western Journal of Nursing Research, 3:*172-192.

Watson, J. (1981, Spring). Response to "Conceptual systems of students, practitioners." *Western Journal of Nursing Research, 3:*197-198.

Watson, J. (1981, Aug.). Professional identity crisis: Is nursing finally growing up? *American Journal of Nursing, 81:*1488-1490.

Watson, J. (1981, July). Nursing's scientific quest. *Nursing Outlook, 29:*413-416.

Watson, J. (1982, Aug.). Traditional vs. tertiary ideological shifts in nursing education. *Australian Nurses' Journal, 12:*46-64.

Watson, J. (1983, Fall). The IDIR model for faculty research with students. *Western Journal of Nursing Research, 5:*301-312.

Watson, J. (1987). Nursing on the caring edge: Metaphorical vignettes. *Advances in Nursing Science, 10(1):*10-17.

Watson, J., & Carozza, V. (1978, Nov.). An experimental educationally sponsored pilot internship program. *Journal of Nursing Education, 17:*14-20.

Audiotape

Watson, J. (1987, May). *Watson's model.* Nurse theorist conference held in Pittsburgh, Pennsylvania. Audiotape available from Meetings International, 1200 Deloi Avenue, Louisville, Ky. 40217.

Videotapes

Watson, J. (1987). *Nursing theory: Circle of knowledge.* New York: National League for Nursing. Available from author, 10 Columbus Circle, New York, NY 10019.

Watson, J. (1987, May). *Watson's model.* Nurse theorist conference held in Pittsburgh, Pennsylvania. Videotape available from Meetings International, 1200 Deloi Avenue, Louisville, Ky. 40217.

Watson, J. (1989). *The nurse theorist: Portraits of excellence.* Oakland: Studio III from Fuld Video Project, 370 Hawthorne Avenue, Oakland, CA 94609.

Secondary Sources
Book Reviews

Watson, J. (1979). *Nursing: The philosophy and science of caring.*
*Nursing Outlook, 28:*45, January 1980.
*Western Journal of Nursing Research, 2:*417-418, Winter 1980.

Other Sources

Betz, B.J., & Whitehorn, J.C. (1956). The relationship of the therapist to the outcome of therapy in schizophrenia. *Psychiatric Research Reports #5.* Research techniques in schizophrenia. Washington, D.C.: American Psychiatric Association.

Brenner P., Boyd, C., Thompson, T., Cervantez, M., Buerhaus, Peter, & Leininger, M. (1986, Jan.). The care symposium: Considerations for nursing administrators. *JONA, 16(1):*25-26.

Chinn, P.L., & Jacobs, M.K. (1983). *Theory and nursing: A systematic approach.* St. Louis: C.V. Mosby.

Duldt, B.W., & Giffin, K. (1985). *Theoretical perspectives for nursing.* Boston: Little, Brown.

Hester, N.O., & Ray, M.A. (1987). Assessment of Watson's carative factors: A qualitative research study. Paper presented at the International Nursing Research Congress. Edinburgh, Scotland.

Leininger, M. (1979). Preface. In J. Watson, *Nursing: The philosophy and science of caring.* Boston: Little, Brown.

Reynolds, P.D. (1971). *A primer in theory construction.* Indianapolis: Bobbs-Merrill.

Rogers, C.R. (1961). *On becoming a person: A therapist's view of psychology.* Boston: Houghton Mifflin.

Stevens, B.J. (1979). *Nursing theory: Analysis, application, evaluation.* Boston: Little, Brown.

Whitehorn, J.C., & Betz, B.M. (1954). A study of psychotherapeutic relationships between physicians and schizophrenic patients. *American Journal of Psychiatry, 111:*321-331.

Yalom, I.G. (1975). *The theory, knowledge, and practice of group psychotherapy* (2d. ed.). New York: Basic Books.

15

Rosemarie Rizzo Parse

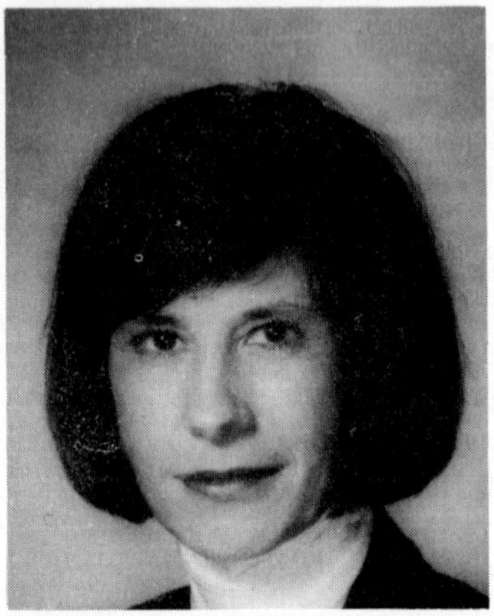

Man-Living-Health

Rickard E. Lee, Larry P. Schumacher

CREDENTIALS AND BACKGROUND OF THE THEORIST

Our lives are comprised of situations diverse in richness and magnitude. Much of what adds color to our daily existence slides by us almost unperceived. Other happenings stand out much more sharply and mark our passage through life—educational achievements, employment, close relationships, defining experiences, professional networks, academic networks.

The unfolding of Rosemarie Rizzo Parse's Man-Living-Health theory is inseparable from the lesser and greater situations that comprise her life. The idea for Man-Living-Health, Parse recalled, "began many years ago when I began to wonder and wander and ask why not? The theory itself . . . surfaced in me in Janusian fashion over the years in interrelationship with others primarily through my lived experience in nursing."[18:xiii] Numerous "predecessors, contemporaries, and successors" helped Parse see her idea more clearly.[18:xv] "Yet the theory has only just begun to be viewed and enhanced by those who take up the challenge to evolve nurs-

The author wishes to express appreciation to Rosemarie Parse for critiquing the chapter.

ing science to a higher level of complexity and specificity."[18:xiii]

Parse received her nursing education in Pittsburgh. Her master's and doctorate in nursing and higher education were earned at the University of Pittsburgh. At the time she was developing her theory, Parse was Dean of the School of Nursing at Duquesne University in Pittsburgh. At about this same time—during the 1960s and 1970s—Duquesne was regarded as the center of the existential-phenomenological movement in the United States. Dialogues she had with those in this school of thought (for example, A. van Kaam and A. P. Giorgi) stimulated and focused her thinking.

Currently, Parse is president of Discovery International, Inc., an organization she founded to promote excellence in nursing science. This firm provides consultation services, seminars, and health guidance to individuals, families, and communities. She is also Professor of Graduate Nursing and Coordinator of the Center for Nursing Research at Hunter College, City University of New York, as well as editor of the scholarly journal *Nursing Science Quarterly*.

Her research activities and interests are wide-ranging. A partial listing includes lived experiences of hope, laughter, health, aging, and quality of life.

THEORETICAL SOURCES

Parse's theoretical sources are a major reason her theory is regarded as unique for nursing.[22:181] By synthesizing the Science of Unitary Human Beings, as developed by Martha E. Rogers, and existential-phenomenological thought, as articulated by Martin Heidegger, Jean-Paul Sartre, and Maurice Merleau-Ponty, Parse pushes nursing toward an unfragmented view of Man. Man cannot be reduced to constituent systems or parts and still be understood, she declares. Man is "a living unity."[18:4]

Moreover, Parse challenges the traditional view of nursing as an emerging natural science. Rightly understood, nursing is a human science. The thrust of her approach is clear:

> A theory of nursing rooted in the human sciences is a system of interrelated concepts describing unitary man's interrelating with the environment while cocreating health. Essential to the theory is the man-environment interrelationship, coconstitution of health, the meaning unitary man gives to being and becoming, and man's freedom in each situation to choose alternative ways of becoming.[18:13]

In developing her theory, Parse used Rogers' major principles of helicy, complimentarity (now called *integrality*), and resonancy, and her corresponding concepts of energy field, openness, pattern, and organization (Rogers has recently deleted organization) and four-dimensionality. (The reader is referred to the chapter on Rogers' theory for a discussion of these principles and concepts.)

From existential-phenomenological thought, Parse drew the tenets of intentionality and human subjectivity and the corresponding concepts of coconstitution, coexistence, and situated freedom. *Intentionality* "means that in being human man is open, knows, and is present to the world. To be man, then, is to be intentional and to be involved with the world through a fundamental nature of knowing, being present and open."[18:18] Human subjectivity indicates that "Man encounters the world and is present to it in a dialectical relationship. Man grows through this relationship, giving meaning to the projects that emerge in the process of becoming. Man coparticipates in the emergence of projects through choosing to live certain values."[18:19] *Coconstitution* "refers to the idea that the meaning emerging in any situation is related to the particular constituents of that situation. . . . Man interrelates with the various views of the world and others and indeed cocreates these views by a personal presence."[18:20] *Coexistence* means that "man, an emerging being, is in the world with others. . . . Man knows self in the comprehension of dispersed concrete achievements and through the perceptions of others. Without others one would not know that one is."[18:20] *Situated freedom* indicates that "one participates in choosing the situations in which one finds oneself as well as one's attitude toward the situations."[18:20-21] Man, therefore, is always choosing. This is done on two levels: prereflectively and tacitly, and reflectively and explicitly. "In choosing ways of being with situations, one expresses value priorities."[18:21] Our choices, however, "are made without full knowledge of the outcomes yet with full responsibility for the consequences."[18:21]

USE OF EMPIRICAL EVIDENCE

"Nursing does not have practice and research traditions of its own," observed Parse. "Quantitative and qualitative methods of research used to enhance nursing science presently flow from the natural sciences and from the human sciences respectively."[20:166;21:1-5] Because Parse sees nursing as a human science, she has sought to enhance her theory by using descriptive research methodologies borrowed from the human sciences. One such methodology, phenomenology, has become increasingly important in recent years in nursing,[4:31;7:113] psychology,[18] and sociology.[5] Because of its philosophical base, this research methodology fits well with Parse's theory. It is also congruent with the importance other nurse theorists (for example, Leininger, Orlando, Patterson and Zderad, Peplau, Travelbee, Watson) have placed on understanding patients' unique perspectives in providing nursing care.[4:34] But phenomenology broadens and deepens the notion of what it means to talk about and study an individual's unique point of view.[6]

MAJOR ASSUMPTIONS

Parse creatively blended principles, tenets, and concepts from Rogers's Science of Unitary Human Beings and existential-phenomenological thought to craft the assumptions underpinning Man-Living-Health. Each assumption "connects three specific concepts in a unique way."[18:25] The three concepts Parse unites in each assumption were drawn both from Rogers and from existential phenomenology. This underscores just how firmly Parse's theoretical sources undergird her theory. "To draw upon the work of these theorists, of course, is to build upon a solid foundation and to maintain a bridge to the past necessary in the establishment of any scientific theory."[18:5]

Because Parse treats Man, environment, and health as constructs, her assumptions defy classification. (Nursing is not a concept per se; it is the scientific endeavor described by the concepts: it is the discipline itself.) Attempting to force Parse's assumptions into categories labeled Man, environment, health, and nursing would wrench them out of context and distort their meaning. Accordingly, Parse's beliefs about these pivotal topics are summarized below, following a listing of the assumptions that underpin Man-Living-Health.

Man-Living-Health: Assumptions with Related Concepts

- Man is coexisting while coconstituting rhythmical patterns with the environment. [Concepts of coconstitution, coexistence, and pattern and organization.]
- Man is an open being, freely choosing meaning in situations and bearing responsibility for decisions. [Concepts of situated freedom, openness, and energy field.]
- Man is a living unity continuously coconstituting patterns of relating. [Concepts of energy field, coconstitution, and pattern and organization.]
- Man is transcending multidimensionally with the possibles. [Concepts of openness, coconstitution, and situated freedom.]
- Health is an open process of becoming, experienced by people. [Concepts of openness, coconstitution, and situated freedom.]
- Health is a rhythmically coconstituting process of the man-environment interrelationship. [Concepts of coconstitution, pat-

tern and organization, and four-dimensionality.]

- Health is man's patterns of relating value priorities. [Concepts of pattern and organization, openness, and situated freedom.]
- Health is an intersubjective process of transcending with the possibles. [Concepts of coexistence, openness, and situated freedom.]
- Health is unitary man's negentropic unfolding. [Concepts of coexistence, energy field, and four-dimensionality.][18:34-36]

Subsequently, Parse synthesized these nine assumptions into the following three:

1. Man-Living-Health is freely choosing personal meaning in situations in the intersubjective process of relating value priorities.
2. Man-Living-Health is cocreating rhythmical patterns of relating in open interchange with the environment.
3. Man-Living-Health is cotranscending multidimensionally with the unfolding possibles.[21:10;20:161-162]

Nursing

By proposing that nursing is a human science, Parse rejects the traditional view of nursing as an emerging natural science. She contends that nursing has paralleled medicine's development, echoing its themes. "Man's participative experience with health situations has been virtually ignored," she declared. "Nursing, rooted in human sciences, focuses on Man as a living unity and Man's qualitative participation with health experiences."[18:4] For nursing to evolve as a distinct discipline, it must move away from its medical model orientation.

Parse strongly affirms nursing's responsibility to society. "The responsibility to society relative to nursing practice is guiding the choosing of possibilities in the changing health process."[18:81] Specifically, "Nursing practice is directed toward illuminating and mobilizing family interrelationships in light of the meaning assigned to health and its possibilities as languaged in the cocreated patterns of relating."[18:82] *Family,* it should be noted, is used by Parse to signify those persons with whom we have close relationships.

Man

Man is a major reason for nursing's existence. (Another major reason, of course, is health.) This has been the case since the time of Nightingale and the publication of her *Notes on Nursing.*[16] In keeping with this tradition, Parse explicitly discussed Man in her assumptions. Man is integral to her theory's concepts, principles, theoretical structures, and practice propositions—all of which flow directly from Man-Living-Health's assumptions.

For Parse, human beings evidence "a pattern of patterns of relating."[18:26] Because we exist in the world with others, we cannot not relate. "When one person encounters another person, rhythmical patterns of relating unfold as words become sentences and are shared with a certain volume at a particular tempo with unique intonation, simultaneously with a certain gaze, gesture, touch, and posture."[18:47-48] In this way, our perceptions of ourselves, others, and our situations emerge. As we live our own life stories and the historical story of our species, we grow more complex and diverse. Living simultaneously in all spheres of time—past, present, and future—we are influenced by our "ancestors, successors, and contemporaries through personal interrelationships, ideas, and future planning."[18:26] They sharpen our sensitivity to life's rhythms—its joys and sorrows, aspirations and disappointments, births and deaths. We become aware of our mortality and the possible extermination of our species. Art and music heighten our awareness of death: through them we celebrate life and the mystery it holds for us. Human beings, then, experience life as an all-at-once multidimensional experience.

Health

For Parse, health is a lived experience. It is not the absence of disease or a state of well-being, nor can it be placed on a continuum. "Man's health, then, is not a linear entity that can be interrupted or qualified by terms such as good, bad, more, or less. It is not man adapting to or coping with the environment. Such a description of health dichotomizes and denies man's unitary nature. Unitary man's health is a synthesis of values, a way of living."[18:39] Health occurs as Man "structures meaning in situations."[18:40] It is a process of being and becoming.

Environment

"Man as a pattern and organization is distinct from the pattern and organization of the environment."[18:26] But man and environment are inseparable. Interchanging energy, unfolding together toward greater complexity and diversity, influencing one another's rhythmical patterns of relating, they are a construct: Man-Environment. "Man and environment, then, interchange energy to create what is in the world, and man chooses the meaning given to the situations he creates."[18:27]

MAJOR CONCEPTS AND DEFINITIONS

From the assumptions underpinning her theory, Parse drew three thematic elements: meaning, rhythmicity, and cotranscendence. She then deduced the three principles of Man-Living-Health.

> *Principle 1:* Structuring meaning multidimensionally is cocreating reality through the languaging of valuing and imaging. The essential concepts of this principle are imaging, valuing, and languaging.[20:163-165; 18:42-50]

Meaning, the thematic element of Parse's first principle, "arises from Man's interrelationship with the world. It refers to both ultimate meaning and the meaning moments of everyday life."[18:10] Ultimate meaning is our view of life's absolute purpose. It is usually expressed in religious or philosophical language. The meaning moments of everyday life are those common happenings to which we attach varying degrees of significance. We do so through the process of imaging, "the cocreating of reality that, by its very nature, structures the meaning of an experience."[18:42]

Our worldview provides the framework for cocreating reality. Valuing "is Man's process of confirming cherished beliefs and is reflective of one's worldview. This confirming of beliefs is choosing from imaged options and owning the choices."[18:45] Languaging is expressing valued images. It encompasses all modes of self-presentation, including the rhythmical patterns of speech and movement. Our rhythmical patterns of speech and movement reflect our cultural heritage as well.[18:46-50]

> *Principle 2:* Cocreating rhythmical patterns of relating is living the paradoxical unity of revealing-concealing, enabling-limiting while connecting-separating. The essential concepts are revealing-concealing, enabling-limiting, and connecting-separating.[20:163-165; 18:50-55]

This principle's thematic element, rhythmicity, "is revealed as Man and environment move toward greater diversity. Rhythmical patterns are cocreated in the Man-environment interrelationship and are paradoxes lived all at once."[21:11] Revealing-concealing "is the simultaneous disclosing of some aspects of self and hiding of others."[18:52] When we disclose ourselves to another person, we gain knowledge about ourselves. Yet by moving in one direction, we are limited in another. This is the rhythmical pattern of enabling-limiting. "Man cannot be all possibilities at once, and, in choosing, one is both enabled and limited."[18:53] To move in one direction and not in another involves reordering relationships. "Connecting-separating . . . can be recognized as man is connecting with one phenomenon and simultaneously separating from others. . . . In separating from one phenomenon and dwelling with another, a person integrates thought, becomes more complex, and seeks new unions."[18:53-54]

> *Principle 3:* Cotranscending with the possibles is powering unique ways of originating in the pro-

cess of transforming. The essential concepts of this principle are powering, originating and transforming.[20:163-165; 18:55-67]

Cotranscendence, the thematic element of Parse's third principle, "is the process of reaching out beyond self to the not-yet."[18:12] This process "is powered through originating in transforming."[21:12] Powering "is a continuous rhythmical process incarnating one's intentions and actions in moving toward the possibilities."[18:57] Its rhythm is pushing-resisting, creating a tension, which, when changed, sometimes conflicts. When conflict surfaces, one is faced with new possibilities from which to choose in moving toward the future. Creating unique ways of living is originating. Man originates in mutual energy interchange with the environment. "Powering ways of originating is man distinguishing self from others."[18:60] Transforming is Man moving toward greater diversity through living new imaged possibilities and transcending the present. Parse calls transforming "the changing of change, coconstituting anew in a deliberate way."[18:62]

THEORETICAL ASSERTIONS

Parse's theoretical structures flow directly from Man-Living-Health's assumptions and principles. Each structure interrelates three concepts (Figure 15-1). As the purpose of the theoretical structures is to guide nursing practice and research, Parse invites their validation in these areas. Man-Living-Health's theoretical structures are:

1. Powering is a way of revealing and concealing imaging.
2. Originating is a manifestation of enabling and limiting valuing.
3. Transforming unfolds in the languaging of connecting and separating.[18:68; 20:166]

Other theoretical structures may be derived, Parse noted.

In 1987, Parse expressed her theoretical structures as practice propositions at the next lower level of abstraction. As a practice propo-

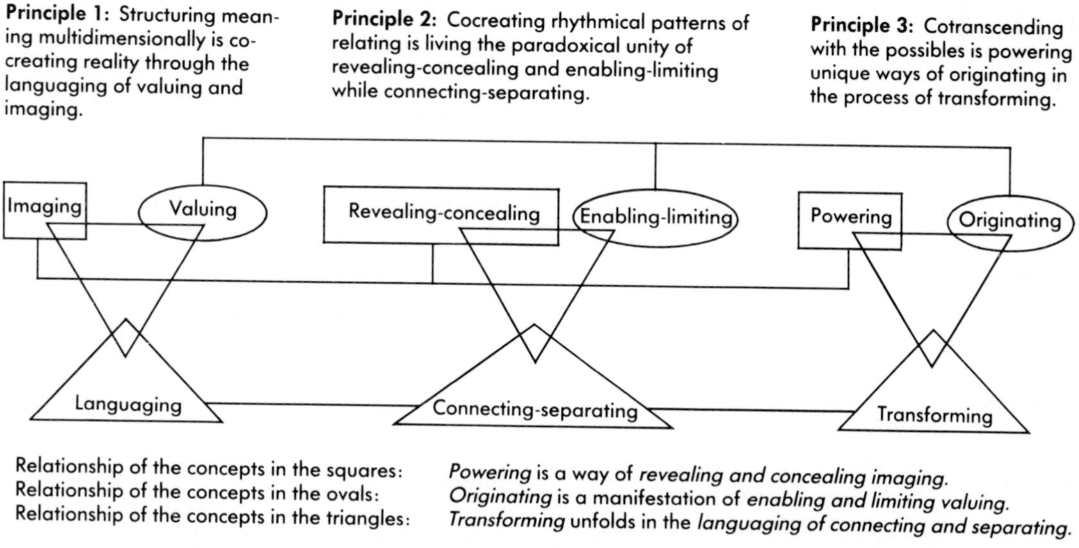
Principle 1: Structuring meaning multidimensionally is cocreating reality through the languaging of valuing and imaging.
Principle 2: Cocreating rhythmical patterns of relating is living the paradoxical unity of revealing-concealing and enabling-limiting while connecting-separating.
Principle 3: Cotranscending with the possibles is powering unique ways of originating in the process of transforming.
Imaging
Valuing
Revealing-concealing
Enabling-limiting
Powering
Originating
Languaging
Connecting-separating
Transforming
Relationship of the concepts in the squares: Powering is a way of revealing and concealing imaging.
Relationship of the concepts in the ovals: Originating is a manifestation of enabling and limiting valuing.
Relationship of the concepts in the triangles: Transforming unfolds in the languaging of connecting and separating.

Figure 15-1. Relationship of principles, concepts, and theoretical structures of Man-Living-Health.

(Used with permission from Parse, R.R. (1981). *Man-Living-Health: A theory of nursing.* New York: John Wiley & Sons, p. 69.)

sition, the first theoretical structure "can be stated as *struggling to live goals discloses the significance of the situation*"; the second as "*creating anew shows one's cherished beliefs and leads in a directional movement*"; and the third as "*changing views emerge in speaking and moving with others.*"[20:169-171] Parse cautions, however, that "the details of nursing practice can only be specified in the context of particular nurse-person and nurse-group situations."[20:170]

LOGICAL FORM

The inductive-deductive process was central to the creation of Man-Living-Health. The theory originated from Parse's lived experiences in nursing practice. She deductively crafted major components of Man-Living-Health from Rogers's Science of Unitary Human Beings and existential-phenomenological thought. By adhering rigorously to rules of logic—along with her intuitive sense—Parse methodically derived Man-Living-Health's assumptions, concepts, principles, theoretical structures, and propositions. Each assumption interrelates three foundational concepts, each principle three of Man-Living-Health's concepts, and each theoretical structure a concept from each principle.

ACCEPTANCE BY THE NURSING COMMUNITY

Practice

Man-Living-Health presents an implicit guide for practice. Parse feels that nursing based on Man-Living-Health is quite unlike nursing based on other models.[20:170-171] Winkler observed, "Basing care planning on the client's perspective of health and her/his care would encourage innovation in activities designated nursing, and acceptance of unique self-care activities."[28:292] In the original presentation of her theory, Parse discussed in detail a family situation and its implications from the perspective of her theory.[18:82-89] In the example, she viewed nursing practice as an "intersubjective participation in guiding [the family] in the choosing of possibles in the changing health process."[18:89]

Unlike some more established models, Man-Living-Health has not been used extensively in practice. Its practice methodology is evolving. Butler used the theory to change the health situation of a family facing the loss of its central figure following major neurosurgery.[3] Papers on the theory's applicability to practice have been presented in the United States and Canada.[9-12,24,26] Mitchell employed Parse's theory to guide care for an elderly woman.[15] In a replication of a study done by Parse in 1987, Santopinto is studying the difference Parse's theory makes in a practice setting.[23]

Education

Parse writes for an audience composed of graduate students in nursing, faculty in schools of nursing, and nursing administrators in university and major health care settings. Her unwavering focus, however, is on master's and doctoral students—nursing's emerging scholars. They will be the ones most likely to share or adopt her perspective and conduct much of the research needed to develop her theory further. They will also use her model for curriculum development as they gain faculty rank.

In *Man-Living-Health: A Theory of Nursing*, Parse presented a sample master's-in-nursing curriculum that incorporated the assumptions, principles, concepts, and theoretical structures of Man-Living-Health.[18:96-112] She outlined in detail this process-based curriculum, including course descriptions and course sequencing. Two courses in nursing theory are listed as focal courses in the curriculum, indicating the importance Parse attaches to theory and its development.

Research

Man-Living-Health has been validated by research. Six studies using qualitative methodologies—descriptive, phenomenological, and ethnographic—have been published.[21] In addition to validating Parse's theory, these studies complemented each other. The authors explained the complementarity thusly:

> The qualitative approach offers the researcher the opportunity to study the emergence of patterns in the whole configuration of Man's lived experiences. It is an approach in which the researcher explicitly participates in uncovering the meaning of these experiences as humanly lived.[21:3]

Man-Living-Health has embedded in it countless research questions. A research methodology specifically designed to investigate these questions is evolving.[20:172-178] To date the literature reveals little in the way of research related to Parse's theory. This is to be expected. Man-Living-Health is, after all, a young theory (it is less than 10 years old). Any theory—including this one—must be learned in detail before it can be used in research. This takes time. The qualitative research studies needed to develop the theory are another time-consuming process. Once completed, research may take up to two years before it is published. To broaden her theory's "circle of contagiousness,"[14:158] Parse has conducted several programs in which results of research studies related to her theory have been presented. A number of master's theses have been completed using Parse's theory.[19] Doctoral dissertations are beginning to be written using Man-Living-Health. For instance, Beauchamp is investigating the concept of power, specifically the decision by those who test positive for the HIV antibody to seek treatment.[2] He is being assisted in this research by Marchette.[13] Postdoctoral studies are in progress as well. Smith is investigating the lived experience of struggling through the difficulty of unemployment.[25] Liehr and Flores are studying the human experience of "living on the edge." Participants in the study are persons who have suffered at least one cardiac arrest. To understand cocreating living on the edge, the study has been expanded to include participants' spouses.[8] These studies are an important indication that more research related to Man-Living-Health will be forthcoming.

FURTHER DEVELOPMENT

We can anticipate Man-Living-Health's continuing evolution. Ongoing research is expected to refine concepts, clarify interrelationships, and lead to higher levels of theory development. As schools of nursing adopt and teach Man-Living-Health, nurses can be expected to employ it more in practice. As nurses use the theory in practice to guide patients through the changing health process, its usefulness will be more fully appreciated by society.

Unfortunately, many nurses avoid exploring this theory because of its very abstract language and philosophical base. Those who shun attempting to learn it forget that effort and discipline are required to move from "a state of understanding less to one of understanding more."[1:8] Parse, Coyne, and Smith reframed this belief specifically for nursing when they wrote:

> Learning the theory in scientific disciplines requires formal study, a reverence for quiet contemplation, and creative synthesis. Neither [Man-Living-Health] nor the methodologies presented in this work can be learned quickly. The nature of the content compels the learner to abide with the conceptualizations and study the movements in discourse required by scholars who aspire to research and theory development in nursing.[21:191]

CRITIQUE

Man-Living-Health is an abstract and complex theory. It is a theory—and not a model—because its concepts and interrelationships have received empirical validation.

Simplicity

In keeping with theoretical discourse, Man-Living-Health's major concepts are defined by Parse in highly abstract and philosophical terms. Parse's use of quotations and references in *Man-Living-Health: A Theory of Nursing* rounded out the concepts and rendered them more understandable. The examples Parse cited were clear and simple. However, a first-time reader might be tempted to dismiss them as too simple to convey the complexity inherent in her theory. To do so, though, would be a mistake; lingering with her examples and drawing them out are more beneficial. Parse's principles, theoretical structures, and practice propositions clearly set forth the interrelationships she sees operating in the world. Consistent with the expectations we have of any scientific theory, Man-Living-Health has the potential to describe, explain, and predict.

Generality

Man-Living-Health's conceptualization is broad in scope and applicable to individuals, families, or communities in change or crisis. To say, as Winkler[28:289] did, that Parse ignores biological manifestations is to miss her point: Man-Living-Health is about the unity of Man's lived experience. It is facile to talk about the biological manifestations of a physical condition and not talk about it phenomenologically. For example, when discussing chronic pain, Turk, Holzman, and Kerns stated that "a psychologically based treatment, or any treatment, must consider the patient's perspective and the phenomenology of chronic pain in developing and implementing a therapeutic regimen."[27:446] The same can be said about diabetes, asthma, or cardiovascular disease—in children and adults. Because Man-Living-Health addresses the lived experience of health, it is at the cutting edge of health care.

Empirical Precision

Parse defines Man-Living-Health's concepts denotatively and at the philosophical level of discourse. Although the concepts are highly abstract and theoretical, they can be observed in situations nurses encounter daily. But without study many nurses will not see what is going on around them. For this reason Parse's theory is exciting: it fires the imagination because it enables us to see anew. Linking it and research and practice will help us "better understand how Man chooses and bears responsibility for the rhythmical patterns of personal health."[22:201]

Derivable Consequences

Parse allies nursing and the human sciences. This is in sharp contrast to most theories of nursing, which mirror medical science. With consumers more aware of strategies for promoting their health and demanding a greater voice in its management, Parse's emphasis upon Man's participation in and responsibility for health is timely. Societal questions about the quality of life in chronic, terminal, and marginal conditions suggest the potential Parse's theory has for meeting nursing's responsibility to society by addressing these questions. "Parse's model," predicted Phillips, "will contribute to a transformation of the knowledge base of nursing and the practice of nursing from a unitary perspective. The Man-Living-Health model provides new hope that there will be greater focus in the future of [sic] the meaning and quality of life and health that transcends the disease orientation; it will deal with improved quality of life for all people as perceived by them."[22:201-202]

REFERENCES

1. Adler, M.J., & Van Doren, C. (1972). *How to read a book.* New York: Touchstone Books.
2. Beauchamp, C.J. (1988, May). Personal communication.
3. Butler, M.J. (1988). Family transformation: Parse's theory in practice. *Nursing Science Quarterly, 1(2)*:68-74.
4. Cohen, M.Z. (1987). A historical overview of the phenomenological movement. *Image, 19(1)*: 31-34.
5. Giddens, A. (1976). *New rules of sociological method.* New York: Basic Books.
6. Jennings, J.L. (1986). Husserl revisited: The forgotten distinction between psychology and phenomenology. *American Psychologist, 41*:1231-1240.
7. Knaack, P. (1984). Phenomenological research. *Western Journal of Nursing Research, 6(1)*:107-114.
8. Liehr, P. (1988, July). Personal communication.
9. Magan, S.J. (1983, Oct. 15; 1984, Jan. 28; 1985, Aug. 22-23). *Mobilizing energies in the structuring of meaning of changing health patterns.*

Paper presented at Nursing Science Symposium, Pittsburgh, Pa.; Dayton, Ohio; Nurse Theorist Conference, Edmonton, Alberta.
10. Magan, S.J. (1984, Sept. 22). *Shifting rhythms in changing health patterns.* Paper presented at Nursing Science Symposium, Pittsburgh, Pa.
11. Magan, S.J. (1986, May). *The lived experience of hopefulness: A phenomenological study.* Paper presented at Discovery International Incorporated's Nursing Science Symposium, Pittsburgh, Pa.
12. Magan, S.J. (1986, May). *The lived experience of hopefulness: A phenomenological study.* Cassette Recording No. DII-301. Louisville, Ky.: Meetings International.
13. Marchette, L. (1988, July). Personal communication.
14. Meleis, A.I. (1985). *Theoretical nursing: Development and progress.* Philadelphia: Lippincott.
15. Mitchell, G. (1986). Utilizing Parse's theory of Man-Living-Health in Mrs. M's neighborhood. *Perspectives, 10(4)*:5-7.
16. Nightingale, F. (1969). *Notes on nursing.* New York: Dover Publications. (Originally published in 1860).
17. Packer, H. (1985). Hermeneutic inquiry in the study of human conduct. *American Psychologist, 40:*1081-1093.
18. Parse, R.R. (1981). *Man-Living-Health: A theory of nursing.* New York: John Wiley & Sons.
19. Parse, R.R. (1988, July). Personal communication.
20. Parse, R.R. (Ed.). (1987). *Nursing science: Major paradigms, theories, and critiques.* Philadelphia: Saunders.
21. Parse, R.R., Coyne, A.B., & Smith, M.J. (Eds.). (1985). *Nursing research: Qualitative methods.* Bowie, Md.: Brady Communications.
22. Phillips, J.R. (1987). A critique of Parse's Man-Living-Health theory. In R.R. Parse (Ed.), *Nursing science: Major paradigms, theories, and critiques* (pp. 181-204). Philadelphia: Saunders.
23. Santopinto, M.D.A. (1988, March). Personal communication.
24. Sklar, M. (1986, May). *The experience of living in a three generational family constellation: A case study.* Cassette Recording No. DII-302. Louisville, Ky.: Meetings International.
25. Smith, M. (1988, April; 1988, July). *The lived experience of struggling through difficulty for persons who are unemployed.* Paper presented at Sigma Theta Tau–Delta Xi Research Day, Kent State University, Kent, Ohio; Wayne State University School of Nursing Summer Research Symposium, Detroit.
26. Smith, M.J. (1986, May). *The experience of being confined: A study using the emerging method.* Cassette Recording No. DII-304. Louisville, Ky.: Meetings International.
27. Turk, D.C., Holzman, A.D., & Kerns, R.D. (1986). Chronic pain. In K.A. Holroyd & T.L. Creer (Eds.), *Self-management of chronic disease: Handbook of clinical interventions and research* (pp. 441-472). Orlando: Academic Press.
28. Winkler, S.J. (1983). Parse's theory of nursing. In J. Fitzpatrick & A. Whall (Eds.), *Conceptual models of nursing: Analysis and application* (pp. 275-294). Bowie, Md.: Robert J. Brady Co.

BIBLIOGRAPHY
Primary Sources
Books

Parse, R.R. (1974). *Nursing fundamentals.* Flushing, N.Y.: Medical Examination.

Parse, R.R. (1981). *Man-Living-Health: A theory of nursing.* New York: John Wiley & Sons.

Parse, R.R., Coyne, A.B., & Smith, M.J. (1985). *Nursing research: Qualitative methods.* Bowie, Md.: Robert J. Brady.

Parse, R.R. (1987). *Nursing science: Major paradigms, theories, and critiques.* Philadelphia: Saunders.

Doctoral Dissertation

Parse, R.R. (1969). *An instructional model for the teaching of nursing, interrelating objectives and media.* (Doctoral dissertation, University of Pittsburgh.) *Dissertation Abstracts International,* 31:180A.

Book Chapters

Parse, R.R. (1978). Rights of medical patients. In C. Fisher, *Client participation in human services.* New Brunswick, N.J.: Transaction.

Parse, R.R. (1981). Caring from a human science perspective. In M.M. Leininger (Ed.), *Caring: An essential human need.* Thorofare, N.J.: Charles B. Slack, Inc.

Parse, R.R. (1988). The phenomenological research method: Its value for management science. In B. Henry, C. Arndt, M. DiVincenti, & A. Marriner-

Tomey (Eds.), *Dimensions of nursing administration: Theory, research, education, and practice.* Cambridge, Mass.: Blackwell Scientific Publications.

Parse, R.R. (1988). Parse's Man-Living-Health model and administration of nursing services. In B. Henry, C. Arndt, M. DiVincenti, & A. Marriner-Tomey (Eds.), *Dimensions of nursing administration: Theory, research, education, and practice.* Cambridge, Mass.: Blackwell Scientific Publications.

Articles

Parse, R.R. (1967, Aug.). The advantages of the ADN program. *Journal of Nursing Education, 6:*15.

Unpublished Manuscripts

Parse, R.R. (1984). *Man-Living-Health in practice.* Unpublished manuscript.

Parse, R.R. (1986). *An emerging methodology for the Man-Living-Health theory.* Unpublished manuscript.

Cassette Recordings

Parse, R.R. (Speaker). (1985). *Presentation at nurse theorist conference.* Cassette Recording No. DII-105. Louisville, Ky.: Meetings International.

Parse, R.R., & Phillips, J.R. (Speakers). (1985). *Parse's Man-Living-Health theory of nursing.* Cassette Recording No. DII-109. Louisville, Ky.: Meetings International.

Parse, R.R., Orem, D.E., Roy, C., King, I.M., Rogers, M.E., & Peplau, H.E. (Speakers). (1985). *Panel discussion with nurse theorists.* Cassette Recording No. DII-112. Louisville, Ky.: Meetings International.

Parse, R.R. (Speaker). (1986). *An emerging research methodology unique to nursing.* Cassette Recording No. DII-303. Louisville, Ky.: Meetings International.

Parse, R.R. (Speaker). (1986). *The ethnographic method.* Cassette Recording No. DII-204. Louisville, Ky.: Meetings International.

Parse, R.R. (Speaker). (1986). *The phenomenological method.* Cassette Recording No. DII-202. Louisville, Ky.: Meetings International.

Parse, R.R. (Speaker). (1986). *Quantitative and qualitative methods in nursing research.* Cassette Recording No. DII-201. Louisville, Ky.: Meetings International.

Parse, R.R. (Speaker). (1987). *Parse's theory.* Cassette Recording No. DII-403. Louisville, Ky.: Meetings International.

Parse, R.R. (Speaker). (1987). *Small group C.* Cassette Recording No. DII-411. Louisville, Ky.: Meetings International.

Parse, R.R., Peplau, H.E., King, I.M., Roy, C., Rogers, M.E., Watson, J., & Leininger, M. (Speakers). (1987). *Panel discussion with theorists.* Cassette Recording No. DII-408. Louisville, Ky.: Meetings International.

Videotape Recordings

Parse, R.R. (1985). *Presentation at nurse theorist conference.* Videotape Recording No. DII-V-105. Louisville, Ky.: Meetings International.

Parse, R.R., Orem, D.E., Roy, C., King, I.M., Rogers, M.E., & Peplau, H.E. (Speakers). (1985). *Panel discussion with nurse theorists.* Videotape Recording No. DII-V-112. Louisville, Ky.: Meetings International.

Parse, R.R. (Speaker). (1987). *Parse's theory.* Videotape Recording No. DII-V-403. Louisville, Ky.: Meetings International.

Parse, R.R., Peplau, H.E., King, I.M., Roy, C., Rogers, M.E., Watson, J., & Leininger, M. (Speakers). (1987). *Panel discussion with theorists.* Videotape Recording No. DII-V-408. Louisville, Ky.: Meetings International.

Secondary Sources

Book Reviews

Parse, R.R. (1975). *Nursing fundamentals.*
*Australian Nurses Journal, 5:*37, August 1975.

Parse, R.R. (1981). *Man-Living-Health: A theory of nursing.*
*International Journal of Rehabilitation Research, 4:*449, 1981.
*Western Journal of Nursing Research, 5:*105-106, Winter 1982.

Parse, R.R. (1986). *Nursing research: Qualitative methods.*
*Research in Nursing and Health, 9:*360-361, 1986.

Books

Chinn, P.L., & Jacobs, M.K. (1987). *Theory and nursing: A systematic approach* (2d ed.). St. Louis: C.V. Mosby.

Meleis, A.I. (1985). *Theoretical nursing: Development and progress.* Philadelphia: J.B. Lippincott.

Book Chapters

Winkler, S.J. (1983). Parse's theory of nursing. In J.J. Fitzpatrick & A.L. Whall, *Conceptual models of nursing: Analysis and application.* Bowie, Md.: Robert J. Brady.

Phillips, J. (1987). A critique of Parse's man-living-health theory. In R. Parse (Ed.), *Nursing science: Major paradigms, theories, and critiques.* Philadelphia: Saunders, pp. 181-204.

Directories and Biographical Sources

Sigma Theta Tau. (1987). *Directory of nurse researchers* (2d ed.). Indianapolis, Ind.: Author.

Articles

Butler, M.J. (1988). Family transformation: Parse's theory in practice. *Nursing Science Quarterly, 1(2)*:68-74.

Mitchell, G. (1986). Utilizing Parse's theory of Man-Living-Health in Mrs. M's neighborhood. *Perspectives, 10(4)*:5-7.

Unpublished Manuscripts

Magan, S.J. (1983, Oct. 15; 1984, Jan. 28; 1985, Aug. 22-23). *Mobilizing energies in the structuring of meaning of changing health patterns.* Paper presented at Nursing Science Symposium, Pittsburgh, Pa.; Dayton, Ohio; Nurse Theorist Conference, Edmonton, Alberta.

Magan, S.J. (1984, Sept. 22). *Shifting rhythms in changing health patterns.* Paper presented at Nursing Science Symposium, Pittsburgh, Pa.

Mitchell, G. (1987, Nov.) *Man-Living-Health in practice with the elderly.* Paper presented at Gerontological Society meeting, Washington, D.C.

Mitchell, G. (1988, July). *Man-Living-Health in practice.* Paper presented at Wayne State University Summer Research Symposium, Detroit.

Santopinto, M.D.A. (1987, May; 1988, Feb.). *A phenomenological study of the relentless drive to be ever thinner.* Paper presented at the annual convention of the Registered Nurse Association, Ontario, Canada; First Interamerican Symposium of Qualitative Nursing Research, São Paolo, Brazil.

Smith, M. (1988, April; 1988, July). *The lived experience of struggling through difficulty for persons who are unemployed.* Paper presented at Sigma Theta Tau—Delta Xi Research Day, Kent State University, Kent, Ohio; Wayne State University School of Nursing Summer Research Symposium, Detroit.

Cassette Recordings

Magan, S.J. (Speaker). (1986). *The lived experience of hopefulness: A phenomenological study.* Cassette Recording No. DII-301. Louisville, Ky.: Meetings International.

Sklar, M. (Speaker). (1986). *The experience of living in a three generational family constellation: A case study.* Cassette Recording No. DII-302. Louisville, Ky.: Meetings International.

Smith, M.J. (Speaker). (1986). *The experience of being confined: A study using the emerging method.* Cassette Recording No. DII-304. Louisville, Ky.: Meetings International.

Smith, M. (Moderator). (1986). *Panel discussion of research related to Man-Living-Health: Evaluation.* Cassette Recording No. DII-305. Louisville, Ky.: Meetings International.

Authors Citing Parse's Works

Batra, C. (1987). Nursing theory for undergraduates. *Nursing Outlook, 35(4)*:189-192.

Campbell, J. (1986). A survivor group for battered women. *Advances in Nursing Science 8(2)*:13-20.

Cohen, M.Z. (1987). A historical overview of the phenomenological movement. *Image, 19(1)*:31-34.

Counts, M.M., & Boyle, J.S. (1987). Nursing, health, and policy within a community context. *Advances in Nursing Science, 9(3)*:12-23.

Cull-Wilby, B.L., & Pepin, J.I. (1987). Toward a coexistence of paradigms in nursing knowledge development. *Journal of Advanced Nursing, 12(4)*:515-521.

Duffy, M.E. (1986). Qualitative research: An approach whose time has come. *Nursing and Health Care, 7(5)*:237-239.

Gortner, S.R., & Schultz, P.R. (1988). Approaches to nursing science methods. *Image, 20(1)*:22-24.

Haase, J.E. (1987). Components of courage in chronically ill adolescents: A phenomenological study. *Advances in Nursing Science, 9(2)*:64-80.

Moch, S.D., & Diemert, C.A. (1987). Health promotion within the nursing environment. *Nursing Administration Quarterly, 11(3)*:9-12.

Pearson, B.D. (1987). Pain control: An experiment with imagery. *Geriatric Nursing, 8(1)*:28-30.

Perry, J. (1985). Has the discipline of nursing developed to the stage where nurses do think nursing? *Journal of Advanced Nursing, 10(1)*:31-37.

Ray, M.A. (1987). Technological caring: A new model in critical care. *Dimensions of Critical Care Nursing, 6(3)*:166-173.

Reed, P.G. (1986). Religiousness among terminally ill and healthy adults. *Research in Nursing and Health, 9(1)*:35-41.

Reed, P.G. (1987). Constructing a conceptual framework for psychosocial nursing. *Journal of Psychosocial Nursing and Mental Health Services, 25(2)*:24-28.

Ruffingrahal, M.A. (1985). Qualitative methods in community analysis. *Public Health Nursing, 2(3)*:130-137.

Sarter, B. (1987). Evolutionary idealism: A philosophical foundation for holistic nursing theory. *Advances in Nursing Science, 9(2)*:1-9.

Thompson, J.L. (1985). Practical discourse in nursing: Going beyond empiricism and historicism. *Advances in Nursing Science, 7(4)*:59-71.

Uys, L.R. (1987). Foundational studies in nursing. *Journal of Advanced Nursing, 12(3)*:275-280.

Other Sources

Atran, S. (1981). Natural classification. *Social Science Information, 20(1)*:37-91.

Bargagliotti, L.A. (1983). Researchmanship: The scientific method and phenomenology. *Western Journal of Nursing Research, 5(4)*:409-411.

Benner, P. (1985). Quality of life: A phenomenological perspective on explanation, prediction, and understanding in nursing science. *Advances in Nursing Science, 8(1)*:1-14.

Bullington, J., & Karlsson, G. (1984). Introduction to phenomenological psychological research. *Scandinavian Journal of Psychology, 25(1)*:51-63.

Davis, A.J. (1973). The phenomenological approach in nursing research. In E.A. Garrison (Ed.), *Doctoral preparation for nurses with emphasis on the psychiatric field* (pp. 213-228). San Francisco: University of California Press.

Evaneshko, V., & Kay, M.A. (1982). The ethnoscience research technique. *Western Journal of Nursing Research, 4(1)*:49-64.

Giorgi, A.P. (1983). Concerning the possibility of phenomenological psychological research. *Journal of Phenomenological Psychology, 14(2)*:129-169.

Giorgi, A.P. (1984). Towards a new paradigm for psychology. *Studies in the Social Sciences, 23*:9-28.

Griffin, A.P. (1983). A philosophical analysis of caring in nursing. *Journal of Advanced Nursing Science, 8(4)*:289-295.

Heidegger, M. (1962). *Being and time.* New York: Harper & Row.

Heidegger, M. (1972). *On time and being.* New York: Harper & Row.

Jennings, J.L. (1986). Husserl revisited: The forgotten distinction between psychology and phenomenology. *American Psychologist, 41*:1231-1240.

Knaack, P. (1984). Phenomenological research. *Western Journal of Nursing Research 6(1)*:107-114.

Merleau-Ponty, M. (1956). What is phenomenology? *Cross Currents, 6*:59-70.

Merleau-Ponty, M. (1963). *The structure of behavior.* Boston: Beacon Press.

Merleau-Ponty, M. (1973). *The prose of the world.* Evanston, Ill.: Northwestern University Press.

Merleau-Ponty, M. (1974). *Phenomenology of perception.* New York: Humanities Press.

Oiler, C. (1982). The phenomenological approach in nursing research. *Nursing Research, 31(3)*:178-181.

Payne, L. (1983). Health: A basic concept in nursing theory. *Journal of Advanced Nursing Science, 8(5)*:393-395.

Polanyi, M. (1958). *Personal knowledge.* Chicago: University of Chicago Press.

Reed, P.G. (1983). Implications of the life-span developmental framework for well-being in adulthood and aging. *Advances in Nursing Science, 6(1)*:18-25.

Rogers, M.E. (1961). *Educational revolution in nursing.* New York: Macmillan.

Rogers, M.E. (1970). *An introduction to the theoretical basis of nursing.* Philadelphia: F.A. Davis.

Rogers, M.E. (1980). Nursing: A science of unitary man. In J.P. Riehl & C. Roy (Eds.), *Conceptual models for nursing practice* (2d ed., pp. 329-337). New York: Appleton-Century-Crofts.

Sartre, J.P. (1963). *Search for a method.* New York: Alfred A. Knopf.

Sartre, J.P. (1964). *Nausea.* New York: New Dimensions.

Sartre, J.P. (1966). *Being and nothing.* New York: Washington Square.

Schneider, K.J. (1986). Encountering and integrating Kierkegaard's absolute paradox. *Journal of Humanistic Psychology, 26(3)*:62-80.

Stern, P. (1980, Feb.). Grounded theory methodology. *Image, 12*:20-23.

Stevens, B.J. (1984). *Nursing theory: Analysis, application, evaluation.* Boston: Little, Brown.

Patricia Benner

16

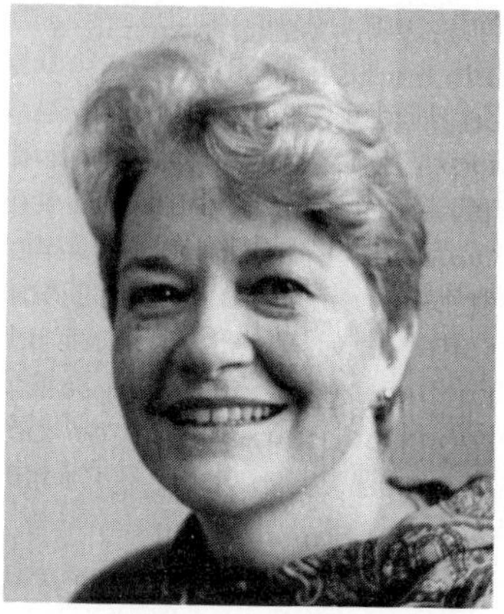

From Novice to Expert: Excellence and Power in Clinical Nursing Practice

Sr. Judith E. Alexander

CREDENTIALS AND BACKGROUND OF THE THEORIST

Patricia Benner was born in Hampton, Virginia, and spent her childhood in California, where she received her early and professional education. Majoring in nursing, she obtained a bachelor of arts degree from Pasadena College in 1964. In 1970 she earned an M.S. degree from the University of California, School of Nursing, San Francisco. In 1982 she was awarded a Ph.D. from the University of California, Berkeley, School of Education, where she majored in stress and coping.

Benner gained experience as a staff nurse for two years before assuming a head nurse position in coronary care and staff nurse positions

The author wishes to express appreciation to Patricia Benner for critiquing the chapter.

in intensive care units. Her nursing experience includes acute care nursing and visiting nurse practice. Benner has a rich background in research and began this part of her career in 1970 as a postgraduate nurse researcher in the school of nursing at the University of California, San Francisco. Since 1982 Benner has been an associate professor in the Department of Physiological Nursing at the University of California, San Francisco.

Benner acknowledges that her thinking in nursing has been greatly influenced by Virginia Henderson over the years. Henderson[19] writes that Benner's *From Novice to Expert* as clinically focused research might materially affect practice and the preparation of nurses for practice. The foreword to Benner's work *The Primacy of Caring: Stress and Coping in Health and Illness*[12] has been written by Virginia Henderson. Hubert Dreyfus, a philosophy professor at Berkeley, introduced her to phenomenology. Stuart Dreyfus, in operations research, and Herbert Dreyfus, in philosophy, developed the Dreyfus Model of Skill Acquisition, which Benner applied in her work *From Novice to Expert*.[4] She credits Jane Rubin's scholarship, teaching, and colleagueship as sources of inspiration and influence, especially in relationship to the works of Heidegger and Kierkegaard. R.S. Lazarus, with whom she worked at Berkeley, has involved her in the field of stress and coping. Judith Wrubel has been a participant and coauthor with Benner over the last 12 years, collaborating on the ontology of caring and caring practices.

Benner has published extensively and received numerous honors, including the 1984 Book of the Year award for *From Novice to Expert*. In 1985 she was inducted into the American Academy of Nurses.

Benner[8] expressed that nursing is a cultural paradox in a highly technical society and that we are slow to value and articulate caring practices. She feels that the value of extreme individualism makes it difficult to perceive the brilliance of caring in expert nursing practice.

THEORETICAL SOURCES

Benner studied clinical nursing practice in an attempt to discover and describe the knowledge embedded in nursing practice, that is, that knowledge that accrues over time in a practice discipline, and to describe the difference between practical and theoretical knowledge.[4:1] One of the first theoretical distinctions Benner made was related to theory itself. Benner stated that knowledge development in a practice discipline "consists of extending practical knowledge (know-how) through theory-based scientific investigations and through the charting of the existent 'know-how' developed through clinical experience in the practice of that discipline."[4:3] It is the description of the know-how of nursing practice that Benner has contributed.

Scientists have long distinguished interactional causal relationships as "knowing that" from "knowing how." Citing philosophers of science Kuhn and Polanyi, Benner emphasized the difference in "knowing how," a practical knowledge that may elude formulations, and "knowing that," or theoretical explanations.[4:2] "Knowing that" is the way one comes to know by establishing causal relationships between events. "Knowing how" is that skill acquisition that may defy the "knowing that," that is, one may know how prior to the development of a theoretical explanation. Benner stated that practical knowledge may extend theory or be developed ahead of scientific formulas. Nursing must develop the knowledge base of its practice (know-how) and through scientific investigation and observation begin to record and develop the know-how of clinical expertise. A dialogical relation exists between theory and practice. Theory is derived from practice and then practice is altered or extended by theory.

Dreyfus and Dreyfus' (1980; 1986) model of skill acquisition and skill development was adapted by Benner to clinical nursing practice. The Dreyfus model was developed by Stuart and Hubert Dreyfus, both professors at the University of California at Berkeley. The model is situational and describes five levels of skill acquisition and development: novice, advanced beginner, competent, proficient, and expert. The levels represent changes in aspects of skill performance, namely, a movement from reliance on abstract principles in the beginning levels to the use of past experiences as paradigms. A second change is in the learner's perception of the situation from a compilation of relevant parts to viewing it as a complete whole with certain aspects standing out as more or less important. The third transition is from that of a detached outside observer to an involved performer engaged in the situation.[4:13] "The performance level can be determined only by consensual validation of expert judges and the assessment of the outcomes of the situation."[4:293]

Benner attempted to highlight the growing edges of clinical knowledge, rather than to describe a typical nurse's day. Benner's explanation of nursing practice goes beyond the rigid application of rules and theories and instead is based on "reasonable behavior that responds to the demands of a given situation."[4:xx] The skills acquired through nursing experience and the perceptual awareness expert nurses develop as decision makers from the "gestalt of the situation" lead them to follow their hunches as they search for evidence to confirm the subtle changes they observe in patients.[4:xviii]

The concept of experience defined as the outcome when preconceived notions are challenged, refined, or refuted in the situation is based on Heidegger and Gadamer.[4:8] As the nurse gains experience, clinical knowledge becomes a blend of practical and theoretical knowledge. Expertise develops as the clinician tests and modifies principle-based expectations in the actual situation. Heidegger's influence is evident in this and in Benner's subsequent writings on the primacy of caring. Benner refutes the dualistic Cartesian descriptions of mind-body person and espouses Heidegger's phenomenological description of person as a self-interpreting being who is defined by concerns, practices, and life experiences. Persons are always situated, that is, engaged meaningfully in the context of where they are. Persons come to situations with an understanding of the self in the world. Heidegger called the kind of knowing that occurs when one is involved in the situation *practical knowledge*. Persons share background meanings, skills, and habits derived from their cultural practices. Benner and Wrubel state "skilled activity, which is made possible by our embodied intelligence, has been long regarded as 'lower' than intellectual, reflective activity" but argue that intellectual, reflective capacities are dependent on embodied knowing.[12:43] Embodied knowing and the meaning of being are premises for the capacity to care; things matter to us and "cause us to be involved in and defined by our concerns."[12:42]

While doing her doctoral studies at Berkeley, Benner was a research assistant to Richard S. Lazarus, who is known for his development of stress and coping theory. As part of Lazarus' larger study, Benner conducted a study of mid-career men's meaning of work and coping, which was published as *Stress and Satisfaction on the Job: Work Meanings and Coping of Mid-Career Men*.[3] In this study *coping* is defined as a form of practical knowledge, and it was determined that work meanings influence what is experienced as stress and what coping options are available to the individual.

Lazarus' theory of stress and coping is described as phenomenological, that is, the person is understood to constitute and be constituted by meanings. Stress is described as the disruption of meanings, and coping is what the person does about the disruption. Both doing something and refraining from doing anything about the stressful situation are ways of coping. Coping is bounded by the meanings inherent in what the person counts as stressful. The person must be understood as a "participant self" in a situation, which is shaped by reflective and nonreflective meanings and concerns. "The way the person is *in* the situation sets up different possibilities."[12:63] This key concept is used by Benner to describe clinical nursing practice in terms of nurses making a positive difference by being in the situation in a caring way.

USE OF EMPIRICAL EVIDENCE

Her early work focused on the anticipatory socialization of nurses. Benner and Kramer[10] studied the differences between nurses who worked in special care units and regular hospital units. She was a research consultant for a nursing activity study to determine the use and productivity of nursing personnel in 1974 and 1975. Concurrently she was a consultant on a study of new nurse work-entry. Benner and Benner[9] conducted a systematic evaluation of the competencies, the job-finding, and work-entry problems of new graduate nurses. Benner also studied methods of increasing teacher competencies through the use of a mobile micro-teaching laboratory.

From 1978 to 1981 she was the author and project director of a federally funded grant, "Achieving Methods of Intraprofessional Consensus, Assessment and Evaluation," known as the AMICAE Project. Out of this research, *From Novice to Expert*[4] and numerous articles have been published. Benner and Wrubel have further explained and developed the background to this study in *The Primacy of Caring: Stress and Coping in Health and Illness,* "an interpretive theory of nursing practice as it is concerned with helping patients cope with the stress of illness."[12:7] The primacy of caring is three-pronged "as the producer of both stress and coping in the lived experience of health and illness, . . . as the enabling condition of nursing practice (indeed any practice), and the ways that nursing practice based in such caring can positively affect the outcome of an illness."[12:7]

Benner has continued to conduct research in nursing practice, the nature of expert nursing care, and stress and coping in illness. Her research interests focus on the clinical practice of nursing, including study of expert skill acquisition and the nature of practical nursing knowledge. Currently she is co-investigating the nature of clinical expertise in intensive care units, coping with asthma, and ethnographic studies of patients with cancer.

Benner directed the AMICAE Project to develop evaluation methods for participating schools of nursing and hospitals in the San Francisco area. It was an interpretive descriptive study that led to the use of Dreyfus' five levels of competency to describe skill acquisition in clinical nursing practice. In describing the interpretive approach, Benner stated that a rich description of nursing practice from observation and narrative accounts of actual nursing practice provide the text for interpretation (hermeneutics). The nurses' descriptions of patient care situations in which they made a positive difference "present the uniqueness of nursing as a discipline and an art."[4:xxvi] Over 1200 nurse participants completed questionnaires and interviews and were observed by trained researchers. Twenty-one paired preceptor-preceptee interviews about patient care situations they had in common were conducted with beginning nurses and nurses who were recognized for their expertise. "The research was aimed at discovering if there were distinguishable, characteristic differences in the novice's and expert's descriptions of the same clinical incident."[4:14] Further interviews and participant observations were conducted with 51 nurse clinicians and other newly graduated nurses and senior nursing students to "describe characteristics of nurse performance at different stages of skill acquisition."[4:15] The purpose "of the inquiry has been to uncover meanings and knowledge embedded in skilled practice. By bringing these meanings, skills, and knowledge into public discourse new knowledge and understandings are constituted."[4:218]

The Dreyfus model of skill acquisition was developed as a result of studying the performance of pilots in emergency situations and chess players. In applying the model to nursing, Benner noted that skilled nursing requires a sound educational base that allows for a safer and quicker experience-based skill acquisition. Skill and skilled practice, as defined by Benner, means skilled nursing interventions and clinical judgment skills in actual clinical situations. In no case does this refer to context-free psychomotor skills or other demonstrable enabling skills outside the context of nursing practice.

Thirty-one competencies emerged from analysis of the transcripts of interviews with nurses' detailed descriptions of patient care episodes, including their intentions and interpretations of the events. From these competencies identified from actual practice situations, seven domains were inductively derived on the basis of similarity of function and intent. The seven domains of nursing practice identified were:

The helping role
The teaching-coaching function
The diagnostic and patient-monitoring function
Effective management of rapidly changing situations
Administering and monitoring therapeutic interventions and regimens
Monitoring and ensuring the quality of health care practices
Organizational and work-role competencies[4:46]

Each of these domains was described with the related competencies from the exemplars describing nursing practice.

MAJOR CONCEPTS AND DEFINITIONS

NOVICE. In the novice stage of skill acquisition from the Dreyfus model, no background understanding of the situation exists, context-free rules and attributes are required for safe performance in the situation. Benner stated that it would be unusual for a graduate nurse to be a novice. She did describe the possibility of an expert nurse in one area of practice as being a novice in another. First-year nursing students may begin at the novice stage, but this term should not be attributed to newly graduated nurses, who in most cases will perform at the level of advanced beginner.[4:296]

ADVANCED BEGINNER. The advanced beginner stage in the Dreyfus model develops when one can demonstrate marginally acceptable performance, having coped with enough real situations to note, or to have pointed out by a mentor, the recurring meaningful components of the situation. The advanced beginner has enough experience to grasp aspects of the situation.[4:291] Unlike attributes and features, aspects cannot be completely objectified because they require experience based on recognition in the context of the situation.

COMPETENT. The competent stage of the Dreyfus model is typified by considerable conscious and deliberate planning, which determines what aspects of the current and future situations are considered important and which can be ignored. At this stage, there is an increased level of efficiency.[4:292]

PROFICIENT. At the proficient stage of the Dreyfus model, the performer perceives the situation as a whole (the total picture) rather than in terms of aspects, and the performance is guided by maxims. The proficient level is a qualitative leap beyond the competent. Now the performer recognizes the most salient aspects and has an intuitive grasp of the situation based on background understanding.[4:297]

EXPERT. The fifth stage of the Dreyfus model is achieved when "the expert performer no longer relies on an analytic principle (rule, guideline, maxim) to connect her or his understanding of the situation to an appropriate action."[4:31] Benner described the expert nurse as having an intuitive grasp of the situation and as able to zero in on the accurate region of the problem without wasting consideration on a range of alternative diagnoses and solutions. The expert nurse is able to do this because of her enormous background of experience based on paradigm cases.

ASPECTS OF A SITUATION. The characteristics of the situation recognized and understood in context because of prior experience.

ATTRIBUTE OF A SITUATION. Measurable properties of a situation that can be explained without previous experience in the situation.

COMPETENCY. Competency is "an interpretively defined area of skilled performance identified and described by its intent, functions and meanings."[4:292] This term is unrelated to the competent stage of the Dreyfus model.

DOMAIN. An area of practice having a number of competencies with similar intents, functions, and meanings.

EXEMPLAR. An example of a clinical situation that conveys one or more intents, meanings, functions, or outcomes easily translated to other clinical situations.[4:293]

EXPERIENCE. Experience results when the person actively refines preconceived notions and expectations as a result of actual clinical evidence that enhances or runs counter to theoretical understanding.[4:294]

MAXIM. A cryptic description of skilled performance that requires a certain level of experience in order to recognize the implications of the instructions.[4:294]

PARADIGM CASE. A clinical experience that stands out and alters the way one perceives and understands future clinical situations.[4:296] Paradigm cases create new clinical understanding and open new clinical perspectives and alternatives.

SALIENCE. A perceptual stance of embodied knowledge whereby aspects of a situation stand out as more or less important.

MAJOR ASSUMPTIONS

Benner incorporated assumptions from the Dreyfus model, "that with experience and mastery the skill is transformed."[4:38] "This model assumes that all practical situations are far more complex than can be described by formal models, theories and text-book descriptions."[4:178]

In her subsequent writing Benner explicated the themes of nursing, person, situation and health.

Nursing

Nursing is described as a caring relationship, an "enabling condition of connection and concern."[12:4] "Caring is primary because caring sets up the possibility of giving help and receiving help."[12:4] Benner understands nursing practice as the care and study of the lived experience of health, illness, and disease and the relationships between these three.[12:8]

Person

Benner has used Heidegger's phenomenological description of person. "A person is a self-interpreting being, that is, the person does not come into the world predefined but gets defined in the course of living a life. A person also has . . . an effortless and nonreflective understanding of the self in the world."[12:41] "The person is viewed as a participant in common meanings."[12:23]

Finally the person is embodied. Benner and Wrubel[12] have conceptualized the major aspects of understanding the person must deal with as the role of the situation, the role of the body, the role of personal concerns, and the role of temporality. Together these aspects of the person make up the person in the world. This view of the person is based on the works of Heidegger,[18] Merleau-Ponty,[21] and Dreyfus.[13] Their goal is to overcome Cartesian dualism, namely, the view that the mind and body are distinct, separate entities.[25] Benner and Wrubel[12] give a central place to embodiment in their theory and defined *embodiment* as the capacity of the body to respond to meaningful situations. Based upon the work of Merleau-Ponty[21] and Dreyfus (1979), they outline five dimensions of the body: (1) the unborn complex, the unacculturated body of the fetus and newborn baby; (2) the habitual skilled body, the social learned postures, gestures, customs, and skills evident in bodily skills such as seeing, and "body language"; (3) the projective body, the way the body is set (predisposed) to act in specific situations, for example, opening a door or using a keyboard; (4) the actual projected body, one's current bodily orientation or projection in a situation; and (5) the phenomenal body, the body aware of itself, that ability to imagine and describe kinesthetic sensations. Benner and Wrubel point out that nurses attend to the body and the role of embodiment in health, illness, and recovery.

Health

Based on Heidegger and Merleau-Ponty, Benner "focuses on the lived experience of being healthy and being ill."[12:7] *Health* is defined as what can be assessed, whereas well-being is the human experience of health or wholeness. Well-being or being ill are understood as distinct ways of being in the world. Health is described as not just the absence of disease and illness. Also a person may have a disease and not experience themselves as ill, because illness is the human experience of loss or dysfunction, whereas disease is what can be assessed at the physical level.[12:8]

Situation

Benner used the term *situation* rather than *environment* because *situation* conveys a peopled environment, with social definition and meaningfulness.[12:80] She utilized the phenomenological terms of being *situated* and *situated meaning,* which are defined by the person's engaged interaction, interpretation, and understanding of the situation. Persons "enter into situations with their own sets of meanings, habits, and perspectives."[12:23] "Personal interpretation of the situation is bounded by the way the individual is *in* it."[12:84]

THEORETICAL ASSERTIONS

Benner stated that theory is crucial in order to form the right questions to ask in a clinical situation; theory directs the practitioner in looking for problems and anticipating care needs. There is always more to any situation than theory predicts.[4:178] The skilled practice of nursing exceeds the bounds of formal theory. Concrete experience provides the learning about the exceptions and shades of meaning in a situation. The knowledge embedded in practice discovers and interprets theory, precedes or extends theory, and synthesizes and adapts theory in caring nursing practice. Some of the relationship statements included in Benner's work follow:

> Discovering assumptions, expectations, and sets can uncover an unexamined area of practical knowledge that can then be systematically studied and extended or refuted.[4:8]
>
> The clinician's knowledge is embedded in perceptions rather than precepts.[4:43]
>
> Perceptual awareness is central to good nursing judgment and . . . begins with vague hunches and global assessments that initially bypass critical analysis; conceptual clarity follows more often than it precedes.[4:xviii]
>
> Formal rules are limited and discretionary judgment is used in actual clinical situations.[4:xix]
>
> Knowledge . . . accrues over time in the practice of an applied discipline.[4:1]
>
> Expertise develops when the clinician tests and refines propositions, hypotheses, and principle-based expectations in actual practice situations.[4:3]

LOGICAL FORM

The process Benner used was a qualitative descriptive study of clinical nursing practice. The Dreyfus model of skill acquisition was applied to clinical practice. An inductive approach was employed in arriving at the seven domains of nursing practice that emerged from the interpretation of the competencies in the exemplars. According to Benner, "the differences between practical and theoretical knowledge provide examples of competencies identified from the study of nursing practice; describe aspects of practical knowledge; and outline strategies for preserving and extending that knowledge."[4:2] Clinical knowledge and coping are both forms of practical knowledge that Benner seeks to understand.

ACCEPTANCE BY THE NURSING COMMUNITY

Practice

Benner has described clinical nursing practice by using an interpretive approach. Some examples of the application of her work by nurses in practice settings have been included in *From Novice to Expert*. One example described using the model as the basis for establishing a clinical ladder for promotion. Another hospital has applied the model in staff development for the new-graduate orientation program, preceptor development, and teaching experienced nurses. Symposiums focusing on excellence in nursing practice have been held for staff development, recognition, and reward and as a way of demonstrating clinical knowledge development in practice.

Fenton[16] reported the use of Benner's approach in an ethnographic study of the performance of clinical nurse specialists. She found that the nurses were functioning at an advanced level of preparation, but that "we have not yet developed accurate written and verbal descriptions of that advanced practice."[15:37] Balasco and Black[1] and Silver[22,23] used Benner's model as a basis for differentiating clinical knowledge development and career progression in nursing. The model has been adopted by a children's hospital "to identify and reward increasingly effective staff nursing practice."[1:56]

Benner has been cited numerous times by nurses writing about nursing practice concerns. She has continued to publish and apply the model in publications in professional journals.[5-7,11]

Education

Benner[2] has critiqued the concept of competency-based testing by contrasting it with the complexity of the proficiency and expert stages described in the Dreyfus model of skill acquisition and the 31 competencies. In summary, she stated, "competency-based testing seems limited to the less situational, less interactional areas of patient care where the behavior can be well defined and patient and nurse variation do not alter the performance criteria."[2:309]

Fenton[15,16] described the application of the domains of expert practice as the basis for studying the skilled performance of master's-prepared nurses. The analysis verified the performance skills of expert nurses reported in the AMICAE project and identified new areas of skilled performance and five preliminary categories relevant for curriculum evaluation in the graduate program.

Research

The above example by Fenton[15,16] presented an application of educational research. Gordon,[20] a medical anthropologist who had been a research assistant on the AMICAE project, extended the inquiry to study the formal models used in nursing practice and medicine. She concluded that formal models may serve as maps directing care and can substitute for knowledge and result in conformity. She cautions that a misuse of formal models occurs when nurses apply models without employing judgment, employ them in order to exert control, and use language from them that can cover up meanings, or not really know what they mean. Finally "formal models should be used with discretion" as tools and so as not to eclipse the relational, holistic, intuitive aspects of nursing.[4:242]

FURTHER DEVELOPMENT

Benner and Wrubel have extended the basis and interpretation of the study of clinical nursing practice in *The Primacy of Caring: Stress and Coping in Health and Illness*.[12] In this work the philosophies affecting our thinking and practice have been explored. Benner and Wrubel suggest that the adoption of a phenomenological view of person with shared meanings in the situation gives the potential for an understanding of caring and expert nursing practice and stress and coping. "Theory must be informed by real-world experience and experiments, which are in turn subject to theoretical interpretation . . . . A theory is needed that describes, interprets, and explains not an imagined ideal of nursing, but actual expert nursing as it is practiced day by day."[12:5]

Benner's application of the Dreyfus model in clinical nursing practice has provided rich descriptions of nursing as it is practiced. In the interpretation of the five levels of practice, Benner provided suggestions for matching competency to nursing practice and for the development of each stage based on experience. It is better to place a new graduate with a competent nurse preceptor who can explain nursing practice in ways that the beginner comprehends. The intuitive knowledge of the expert will elude beginners who do not have the experienced know-how to grasp the situation.

To date, the model provides concept definitions and in-depth descriptions of each from nursing practice. From these situated descriptions, 31 competencies in seven domains have been derived from actual nursing practice. By maintaining the context of these situated performances, the descriptions are holistic or synthetic, rather than procedural and elemental.[4:45] "The competencies within each domain, [are] in no way intended as an exhaustive list."[4:45] "A situation-based interpretive approach to describing nursing practice overcomes some of the problems of reductionism . . . and overcomes the problem of global and overly general descriptions based on nursing process categories."[4:46]

Dunlop explored the nursing literature related to the science of caring. She draws a distinction between a science for caring and a science of caring. "A science of caring implies that caring can be operationalized in some way as a set of behaviors which can be observed, counted or measured."[14:666] Benner has taken a hermeneutical form to uncover the knowledge embedded in clinical nursing practice. "As she does this, she is also uncovering the nursing-caring with which it is deeply intertwined."[14:668] Although useful, Dunlop noted that "it does not provide us with any universal truths about caring in general or about nursing-caring in particular—indeed it does not make any such pretension."[14:668]

CRITIQUE

Simplicity

Benner has developed an interpretive descriptive account of clinical nursing practice. The concepts are the levels of skilled practice from the Dreyfus model, including novice, advanced beginner, competent, proficient, and expert. She uses the five concepts to describe nursing practice from interviews, observations, and the analysis of transcripts of exemplars provided by the nurses. From these descriptions, 31 competencies were identified, and these were grouped into seven domains of nursing practice based on common intentions and meanings. The model is relatively simple with regard to the five stages of skill acquisition and provides a comparative guide for identifying levels of nursing practice from individual nurse descriptions and observations of actual nursing practice. The interpretations are validated by consensus. A degree of complexity is encountered in the subconcepts for differentiation between the levels of competency and the need to identify meanings and intentions. This interpretive approach is designed to overcome the constraints of the rational-technical approach to the study and description of practice. Although providing a decontextualized (i.e., object) description of the novice level of performance is possible, the limits of objectification are encountered as soon as an understanding of the situation is required for expert performance. Clinical knowledge is relational and contextual and often deals with local, specific, historical issues. To capture the contextual and relational aspects of practice, Benner uses narrative accounts of actual clinical situations and maintains that the exemplar enables the reader to recognize similar intents and meanings, even though the "objective" circumstances may be quite different.

Generality

The descriptive model of nursing practice has the potential for universal application as a framework, but the descriptions are limited by dependence upon the actual clinical nursing situations from which they must be derived. Its use is dependent upon the understanding of the five levels of competency and the ability to identify the characteristic intentions and meanings inherent at each level of practice. The model has universal characteristics in that it is not restricted by age, illness, health, or location of nursing practice. The characteristics of theoretical universality, however, imply properties of operationalization for prediction that are not a part of this perspective. Indeed, this phenomenological perspective critiques the limits of "universality" in studies of human practices.

Empirical Precision

The model was empirically tested using qualitative methodologies, and 31 competencies and seven domains of nursing practice were derived inductively. Subsequent research has been done, and there is evidence that the framework is applicable and useful in providing knowledge of the description of nursing practice. Benner stated that "if we choose only scientific, technical and organizational strategies for legitimizing expert nursing care, we will miss the primacy of caring and the central ethic of care and responsibility embedded in expert nursing practice."[8] It is precisely the use of alternative models of discovering nursing knowledge that makes it difficult to address the work of *From Novice to Expert* within a rational-empirical framework for critique. Utilizing the scientific approach, one would look for lawlike relational statements to predict practice. Nevertheless, employing the qualitative methods in an interpretive approach, Benner describes expert nursing practice in many exemplars. Positivistic science takes an alternative approach by seeking formulas and models to apply. Her work seems to be hypotheses generating rather than hypotheses testing. Benner provides no universal "how to" for nursing practice, but rather provides a methodology for uncovering and entering into the situated meaning of expert nursing care. The interpretation of the meaning and level of nursing practice will no doubt frustrate "objective" researchers who seek precision and control. The strength of the Benner model is that it is data-based research that contributes to the science of nursing.

Derivable Consequences

Benner's *From Novice to Expert*[4] model provides a general framework for identifying, defining, and describing clinical nursing practice. Benner uses a phenomenological approach to describe persons and derives meaning and abilities from interactions in life situations. Nursing is the involved interaction with persons in a caring mode. *The Primacy of Caring*[12] further develops these themes. Benner described her work as a description of the knowledge embedded in actual nursing practice. The five levels of competencies are descriptions of the practical nursing knowledge of each level in the context of the situations described. The approach to generalization is through common meanings, skills, practices, and embodied capacities rather than through general ahistorical laws. The generalizations are depicted through exemplars that demonstrate relational and contextually relevant intents and aspects of clinical knowledge. This approach takes issue with the common approaches used for universality or generalization in physics and the natural sciences and claims that the basis for generalization in clinical knowledge cannot be structural or mechanistic but rather must be based on common meanings and practices. The strategies for generalization are not based on abstraction through removing the situation or context (objectification) but rather by showing how the skilled knowledge, the intent, content, and notion of good in clinical knowledge must be depicted by exemplars that illustrate the role of the situation. Benner claims that this is not a privativistic or subjectivistic approach, but rather an attempt to overcome the limits of subject-object descriptions. Benner's work is useful in that it has framed nursing practice from the context of what nursing actually is and does, rather than from idealized theoretical descriptors that are context free.

REFERENCES

1. Balasco, E.M., & Black, A.S. (1988). Advancing nursing practice: Description, recognition, and reward. *Nursing Administration Quarterly, 12(2)*:52-62.

2. Benner, P. (1982, May). Issues in competency-based testing. *Nursing Outlook, 30(5)*:303-309.
3. Benner, P.E. (1984). *Stress on the job: Work meanings and coping of mid-career men.* New York: Praeger.
4. Benner, P. (1984). *From novice to expert: Excellence and power in clinical nursing practice.* Menlo Park, Calif.: Addison-Wesley.
5. Benner, P. (1985, Oct.). Quality of life: A phenomenological perspective on explanation, prediction, and understanding in nursing science. *Advances in Nursing Science, 8(1)*:1-14.
6. Benner, P. (1985, Feb.). The oncology clinical nurse specialist: An expert coach. *Oncology Nursing Forum, 12(2)*:40-44.
7. Benner, P. (1987, Sept.). A dialogue with excellence. *American Journal of Nursing, 87(9)*:1170-1172.
8. Benner, P. (1988). Personal correspondence.
9. Benner, P., & Benner, R.V. (1979). *The new nurses' work entry: A troubled sponsorship.* New York: The Tiresias Press.
10. Benner, P., & Kramer, M. (1972, Jan.). Role conceptions and integrative role behavior of nurses in special care and regular hospital nursing units. *Nursing Research, 21(1)*:20-29.
11. Benner, P., & Tanner, C. (1987, Jan.). Clinical judgment: How expert nurses use intuition. *American Journal of Nursing, 87(1)*:23-31.
12. Benner, P., & Wrubel, J. (1989). *The primacy of caring: Stress and coping in health and illness.* Menlo Park, Calif.: Addison-Wesley.
13. Dreyfus, H.L. (In press). *Being-in-the-world: A commentary on being and time dimension I.* Cambridge, Mass.: M.I.T. Press.
14. Dunlop, M.J. (1986). Is a science of caring possible? *Journal of Advanced Nursing, 11*:661-670.
15. Fenton, M.V. (1984). Identification of the skilled performance of master's prepared nurses as a method of curriculum planning and evaluation. In P. Benner, *From novice to expert.* Menlo Park, Calif.: Addison-Wesley, pp. 262-274.
16. Fenton, M.V. (1985). Identifying competencies of clinical nurse specialists. *Journal of Nursing Administration, 15(12)*:31-37.
17. Gordon, D.R. (1984). Research application: Identifying the use and misuse of formal nursing models in nursing practice. In P. Benner, *From novice to expert.* Menlo Park, Calif.: Addison-Wesley, pp. 225-243.
18. Heidegger, M. (1962). *Being and time.* (MacQuarrie, J. & Robinson, E., Trans.). New York: Harper and Row.
19. Henderson, V. (1989). Foreword. In P. Benner & J. Wrubel, *The primacy of caring, stress and coping in health and illness.* Menlo Park, Calif.: Addison-Wesley.
20. Lock, M., & Gordon, D.R. (Eds.). (1989). *Biomedicine examined.* Boston, Mass.: Kluwer Academic.
21. Merleau-Ponty, M. (1962). *Phenomenology of perception.* (C. Smith, Trans.). London: Routledge and Kegan Paul.
22. Silver, M. (1986). A program for career structure: A vision becomes a reality. *The Australian Nurse, 16(2)*:44-47.
23. Silver, M. (1986). A program for career structure: From neophyte to expert. *The Australian Nurse, 16(3)*:38-41.
24. Steele, S. (1986). Practice of the master's-prepared nurse in pediatrics. *Issues in Comprehensive Pediatric Nursing, 9(2)*:107-117.
25. Visintainer, M. (1988). Book review: The primacy of caring-stress and coping in health and illness. *Image: Journal of Nursing Scholarship, 20(2)*:113-114.

BIBLIOGRAPHY

Primary Sources

Books

Benner, P., & Wrubel, J. (1989). *The primacy of caring: Stress and coping in health and illness.* Menlo Park, Calif.: Addison-Wesley.

Benner, P. (1987). *Practica progresiva en enfermeria: Manual de comportamiento profesional.* (Spanish translation). Arago, 385, Barcelona: Ediciones Grijalbo, S.A.

Benner, P. (1984). *From novice to expert: Excellence and power in clinical nursing practice.* Menlo Park, Calif.: Addison-Wesley.

Benner, P.E. (1984). *Stress and job satisfaction on the job: Work meanings and coping of mid-career men.* New York: Praeger.

Benner, P., & Benner, R.V. (1979). *The new nurses' work entry: A troubled sponsorship.* New York: Tiresias Press.

Book Chapters

Allen, D., Benner, P., & Diekelmann, N. (1986). Three paradigms for nursing research-methodology implications. In P.L. Chinn (Ed.), *Nursing research methodology.* Rockville, Md.: Aspen.

Wrubel, J., Benner, P., & Lazarus, R.S. (1981). Social competence from the perspective of stress and coping. In J.D. Wine & M.D. Smye (Eds.), *Social competence.* New York: Guilford Press, pp. 61-99.

Benner, P., Roskies, E., & Lazarus, R. (1980). Stress and coping under extreme conditions. In J.E. Dimsdale (Ed.), *Survivors, victims and perpetrators: Essays on the Nazi Holocaust.* New York: Hemisphere, pp. 219-258.

Benner, P., & Kramer, M. (1977). Work shoes speak. In M. Kramer & C. Schmallenberg (Eds.), *Path to biculturalism.* Wakefield, Mass.: Contemporary Publishers, pp. 204-232.

Benner, P. (1975). Nurses in the intensive care unit. In M. Davis, M. Kramer, & A. Straus (Eds.), *Nurses in practice: A perspective on work environment.* St. Louis: C.V. Mosby, pp. 106-128.

Benner, P. (1975). Process and persistence of value transmission. In M. Davis, M. Kramer, & A. Straus (Eds.), *Nurses in practice: A perspective on work environment.* St. Louis: C.V. Mosby, pp. 166-176.

Benner, P. (1974). Reality testing a "Reality Shock" program. In M. Kramer (Ed.), *Reality shock: Why nurses leave nursing.* St. Louis: C.V. Mosby, pp. 191-215.

Articles

Benner, P. (1981, Aug.). Retaining experienced nurses is key to quality care. *The American Nurse, 13(8)*:4, 15.

Benner, P. (1982, March). From novice to expert. *American Journal of Nursing, 82(3)*:402-407.

Benner, P. (1982, May). Issues in competency-based testing. *Nursing Outlook, 30(5)*:303-309.

Benner, P. (1983, Spring). Uncovering the knowledge embedded in clinical practice. *Image: Journal of Nursing Scholarship, 15(2)*:36-41.

Benner, P. (1985, Oct.). Quality of life: A phenomenological perspective on explanation, prediction, and understanding in nursing science. *Advances in Nursing Science, 8(1)*:1-14.

Benner, P. (1985, March/April). The oncology clinical nurse specialist: An expert coach. *Oncology Nursing Forum, 12(2)*:40-44.

Benner, P. (1985). Why does nursing need a theory? *Japanese Journal of Nursing Research, 18(1)*:3-30.

Benner, P. (1985). General systems theory and nursing. *Japanese Journal of Nursing Research, 18(1)*:61-71.

Benner, P. (1985, Aug.). Preserving caring in an era of cost-containment and high technology. *Yale Nurse*, pp. 12-20.

Diekelmann, N., & Benner, P. (1985). Three paradigms for research in nursing education. *Progressions Education Research Notes, A Publication of Division I: Education in the Progressions of American Educational Research Association, 7(1)*:6-10.

Benner, P. (1986, Oct.). Advice for new graduate nurses on their first job. *The American Nurse* (invited column).

Benner, P. (1987, Sept.). A dialogue with excellence. *American Journal of Nursing, 87(9)*:1170-1172.

Benner, P., & Kramer, M. (1972, Jan./Feb.). Role conceptions and integrative role behavior of nurses in special care and regular hospital nursing units. *Nursing Research, 21(1)*:20-29.

Benner, P., & Tanner, C. (1987, Jan.). Clinical judgment: How expert nurses use intuition. *American Journal of Nursing, 87(1)*:23-31.

Benner, P., & Wrubel, J. (1982, May). Skilled clinical knowledge: The value of perceptual awareness, Part 1. *Journal of Nursing Administration, 12(5)*:11-14.

Benner, P., & Wrubel, J. (1982, June). Skilled clinical knowledge: The value of perceptual awareness, Part 2. *Journal of Nursing Administration, 12(6)*:28-33.

Benner, P., & Wrubel, J. (1982, May/June). Skilled clinical knowledge: The value of perceptual awareness. *Nurse Educator, 7(3)*:11-17.

Benner, R.V., & Benner, P. (1979, Sept./Oct.). Follow-through evaluation: A resource for curriculum planning and development. *Nurse Educator, 4(5)*:16-21.

Brandt, S., & Benner, P. (1980, March). Infection control in hospitals: What are the challenges? *American Journal of Nursing, 80(3)*:432-434.

Eaton, S., & Benner, P. (1977). Discussion stoppers in teaching. *Nursing Outlook, 25(9)*:578-583.

Marculescu, G.L., & Benner, P. [commentary]. (1987, Dec.). A dialogue with excellence: Early warning. *American Journal of Nursing, 87(12)*: 1556-1558.

Meleis, A.I., & Benner, P. (1975, May). Process vs. product evaluation? *Nursing Outlook, 23(5)*:303-307.

Videotape

Nursing theory: A circle of knowledge. (1987). New York: National League for Nursing.

Other Sources

Dreyfus, H.L., (1979). *What computers can't do.* New York: Harper and Row.

Dreyfus, H.L., & Dreyfus, S.E. (1986). *Mind over machine.* New York: The Free Press.

Dreyfus, H.L., & Rabinow, P. (1982). *Michel Foucault.* Chicago, Ill.: University of Chicago Press.

Dreyfus, S.E., & Dreyfus, H.L. (1980, Feb.). *A five-stage model of the mental activities involved in directed skill acquisition.* Unpublished report supported by the Air Force Office of Scientific Research (AFSC), USAF (Contract F49620-79-c-0063), University of California at Berkeley.

Good, B.J., & Good, M.J. Delvechio. (1982). The meaning of symptoms: A cultural hermeneutic model for clinical practice. In L. Eisenberg & A. Kleinman (Eds.). *The relevance of social sciences for medicine.* Boston, Mass.: D. Reidel.

Lazarus, R.S. (1985). The trivialization of distress. In J.C. Rosen & L.J. Solomon (Eds.), *Preventing health risk behaviors and promoting coping with illness* (Vol. 8, Vermont Conference on the Primary Prevention of Psychopathology, pp. 279-298). Hanover, N.H.: University Press of New England.

Lazarus, R.S., & Folkman, S. (1984). *Stress appraisals and coping.* New York: Springer.

Palmer, R.E. (1969). *Hermeneutics.* Evanston, Ill.: Northwestern University Press.

Polanyi, M. (1958). *Personal knowledge.* Chicago, Ill.: University of Chicago Press.

Taylor, C. (1971, Sept.). Interpretation and the sciences of man. *The Review of Metaphysics, 25(1)*:3-34, 45-51.

UNIT III

Interpersonal Relationships

17

Hildegard E. Peplau

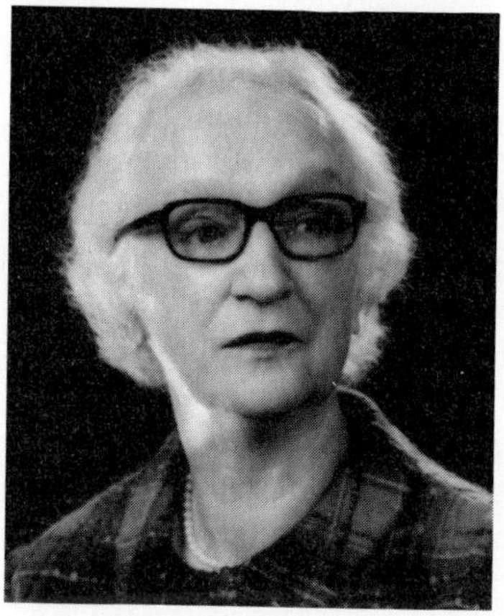

Psychodynamic Nursing

Elizabeth T. Carey, John Noll, LyNette Rasmussen, Bryn Searcy, Nancy L. Stark

CREDENTIALS AND BACKGROUND OF THE THEORIST

Hildegard E. Peplau was born September 1, 1909, in Reading, Pennsylvania. She graduated from Pottstown, Pennsylvania, Hospital School of Nursing in 1931. She received a B.A. in interpersonal psychology from Bennington College, Vermont, in 1943, an M.A. in psychiatric nursing from Teachers College, Columbia, New York, in 1947, and an Ed.D. in curriculum development from Columbia in 1953.[2]

Peplau's professional and teaching experiences have been broad and varied. She was operating room supervisor at Pottstown Hospital, and later headed the staff of the Bennington infirmary while pursuing her undergraduate degree. She did clinical work at Bellevue and Chestnut Lodge psychiatric facilities and was in contact with renowned psychiatrists Freida Fromm-Riechman and Harry Stack Sullivan. A member of the Army Nurse Corps during

The authors wish to express appreciation to Hildegard E. Peplau for critiquing the chapter.

World War II, she worked in a neuropsychiatric hospital in England.

After obtaining her master's degree at Columbia, she was invited to develop and teach in the graduate program in psychiatric nursing. She remained on the faculty 5 years. In 1954 Peplau went to Rutgers, where she developed and chaired the graduate psychiatric nursing program until her retirement in 1974.[10]

Peplau's contribution to nursing and the specialty of psychiatric nursing has been enormous, beginning in 1952 with her book *Interpersonal Relations in Nursing*. Throughout the 1950s and 1960s she conducted workshops, "abundantly sharing her knowledge and clinical skills . . . [and] encouraging nurses to use their competence . . . in a continuous, experiential and educative process."[26;31:123] She analyzed verbatim notes of sessions with medical and psychiatric patients to develop numerous lectures, articles, and workshops. She has maintained a part-time private practice since 1960 and has given many lectures throughout the United States, Canada, Africa, and South America. During the 1970s William E. Field, Jr., took copious notes on the numerous lectures Peplau delivered to psychiatric nurses. He published them for his mentor in *The Psychotherapy of Hildegard E. Peplau*. Peplau's theory and method was presented as investigative psychotherapy as it developed from 1948 to 1974.

In 1969 Peplau became executive director of the American Nurses' Association. She served as president of the ANA from 1970-1972, and as second vice-president from 1972-1974.[29] She has also served as director of the New Jersey State Nurses' Association; a member of the Expert Advisory Council of WHO; the National Nurse Consultant to the Surgeon General of the Air Force; and a nursing consultant to the United States Public Health Services, the National Institute of Mental Health, and various foreign countries.[2] She chaired the editorial board of *Perspectives in Psychiatric Care* when the journal was founded and served as chief advisor of *Nursing 74*. She is on the editorial board of the *Journal of Psychosocial Nursing*. In 1987 she was honored as the first psychosocial nurse of the year by the *Journal of Psychosocial Nursing*.

Peplau's archives are deposited in the Arthur and Elizabeth Schlesinger Library on the History of Women in America, Radcliffe College, Cambridge, Massachusetts.

THEORETICAL SOURCES

The nature of science in nursing refers to the "body of verified knowledge found within the discipline of nursing . . . [that is] mainly knowledge from the biological and behavioral sciences."[1:35] The "synthesis, reorganization, or extension of concepts drawn from the basic and applied sciences, which in their reformation tend to become new concepts," has led to the growth of nursing science.[14:292] Thus, the evolution of Peplau's theory of interpersonal relations resulted.

Peplau used knowledge borrowed from behavioral science and what can be termed the *psychological model*. Borrowing from the psychological model "enabled the nurse to begin to move away from a disease orientation to one whereby the psychologic meaning of events, feelings, and behaviors could be explored and incorporated into nursing interventions. It gave nurses an opportunity to teach patients how to experience their feelings and to explore with clients how to bear their feelings."[28:6] The conceptual framework of interpersonal relations seeks to develop the nurse's skill in using these concepts. Harry Stack Sullivan,[35] Percival Symonds,[36] Abraham Maslow,[17] and Neal Elgar Miller[18] are some of the major sources Peplau used in developing her conceptual framework. Some of the therapeutic conceptions devised by these theorists arose directly from the works of Freud[7] and Fromm.[8]

Peplau was committed to incorporating established knowledge into her conceptual framework, thus developing a theory-based nursing model. Peplau integrated theories into her model at a time when nursing theory development was relatively new.

USE OF EMPIRICAL EVIDENCE

Theories available when Peplau developed her theory described behavior within the prospectives of psychoanalytic theory, the principles of social learning, the concept of human motivation, and the concept of personality development. Peplau combined the various ideas of Maslow, Sullivan, Miller, and Symonds. These theories were initiated by the genius of Freud, Fromm, and Pavlov.[22]

Freud's hypotheses have been a rich source of research study. He emphasized the importance of motivation, conflict, and the role of the family in early childhood, and discovered the significance of the unconscious. Extensive testing of Freudian principles has been done, and his influence on later theorists' hypotheses is obvious.

Maslow's theory of human motivation is well known, and a great deal of sound research has followed its publication. Maslow[17:371] states, "The present theory must be considered to be a suggested program for future research and must stand or fall, not so much on facts available or evidence presented, as upon research yet to be done."

Miller's work focused on personality theory, adjustment mechanisms, psychotherapy, and principles of social learning. Pavlov's stimulus-response model influenced Miller's principles of social learning. Most of Miller's work consisted of developing hypotheses, the basis for research, rather than proving principles. Miller based his hypotheses on experimental studies.

Sullivan was a pioneer in the field of modern psychiatry. A comprehensive evaluation of Sullivan's work regarding personality development and interpersonal relations was written by Patrick Mullahy in 1945. Sullivan's theoretical positions in *Conceptions of Modern Psychiatry* were tested by the Washington School of Psychiatry, leading to further refinement of his theoretical positions.

MAJOR CONCEPTS AND DEFINITIONS

PSYCHODYNAMIC NURSING. Peplau defines psychodynamic nursing because her model evolves through this type of nursing. "Psychodynamic nursing is being able to understand one's own behavior to help others identify felt difficulties, and to apply principles of human relations to the problems that arise at all levels of experience."[23:xiii]

Peplau develops the model by describing the structural concepts of the interpersonal process, which are the phases of the nurse-patient relationship, and further defines the role of nurses within the relationship. She holds this to be basic to psychodynamic nursing.

NURSE-PATIENT RELATIONSHIP. Peplau describes four phases of the nurse-patient relationship. Although separate, they overlap and occur over the time of the relationship.

Orientation. During the orientation phase, the individual has a "felt need" and seeks professional assistance. The nurse helps the patient recognize and understand his problem and determine his need for help.[23:18-30]

Identification. The patient identifies with those who can help him (relatedness). The nurse permits exploration of feelings to aid the patient in undergoing illness as an experience that reorients feelings and strengthens positive forces in the personality and provides needed satisfaction.[23:30-37]

Exploitation. During the exploitation phase the patient attempts to derive full value from what is offered him through the relationship. New goals to be achieved through personal effort can be projected, and power shifts from the nurse to the patient as the patient delays gratification to achieve the newly formed goals.[23:37-39]

Resolution. Old goals are gradually put aside and new goals adopted. This is a process in which the patient frees himself from identification with the nurse.[23:39-41]

NURSE-PATIENT RELATIONSHIPS. Peplau[23] describes six different nursing roles that emerge in the various phases of the nurse-patient relationship (Figure 17-1).

Role of the stranger. The first role is the role of the stranger. Peplau states that because the nurse and patient are strangers to each other, the patient should be treated with ordinary courtesy. In other words, the nurse should not prejudge the patient, but accept him as he is. During this nonpersonal phase, the nurse should treat the patient as emotionally able, unless evidence indicates otherwise. This coincides with the identification phase.[23:44-47]

Role of resource person. In the role of the resource person, the nurse provides specific answers to questions, especially health information, and interprets to the patient the treatment or medical plan of care. These questions often arise within the context of a larger problem. The nurse determines what type of response is appropriate for constructive learning, either straightforward factual answers or providing counseling.[23:47-48]

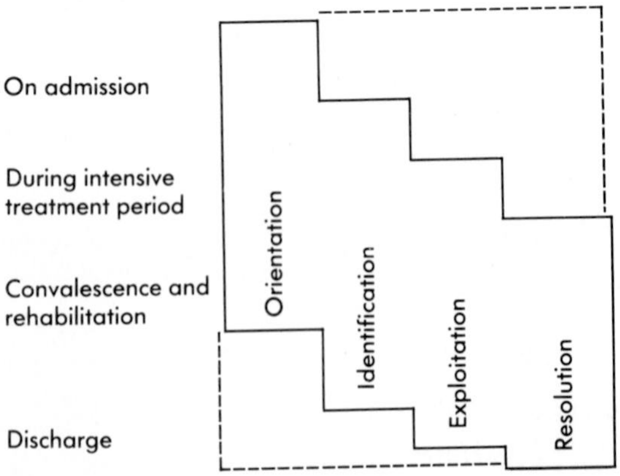

Figure 17-1. Overlapping phases in nurse-patient relationships.

Used with permission from Peplau, H.E. (1952). *Interpersonal relations in nursing*. New York: G.P. Putnam & Sons, p. 21.

Teaching role. The teaching role is a combination of all roles and "always proceeds from what the patient knows and . . . develops around his interest in wanting and ability to use . . . information."[23:48]

Peplau[24] expands on the role of teacher in later writings. She separates teaching into two categories: *instructional,* which consists largely of giving information and is the form explained in educational literature, and *experiential,* which is "using the experience of the learner as a basis from which learning products are developed."[24:98] The products of learning are generalizations and appraisals the patient makes about his experiences. This concept of learning used in the teaching role overlaps with the nurse counselor role, because the concept of learning is carried out through psychotherapeutic techniques.[25]

Leadership role. The leadership role involves the democratic process. The nurse helps the patient meet the tasks at hand through a relationship of cooperation and active participation.[23:49-51]

Surrogate role. The patient casts the nurse in the surrogate role. The nurse's attitudes and behaviors create *feeling tones* in the patient that reactivate feelings generated in a prior relationship. The nurse's function is to assist the patient in recognizing similarities between herself and the person recalled by the patient. She then helps the patient see the differences in her role and that of the recalled person. In this phase, both patient and nurse define areas of dependence, independence, and finally interdependence.[23:51-61]

Counseling role. Peplau believes the counseling role has the greatest emphasis in psychiatric nursing.[26] Counseling functions in the nurse-patient relationship by the way nurses respond to patient demands. Peplau[23:64] says the purpose of interpersonal techniques is to help "the patient remember and understand fully what is happening to him in the present situation, so that the experience can be integrated rather than dissociated from other experiences in life" (Figure 17-2).

PSYCHOBIOLOGICAL EXPERIENCES. Peplau describes four psychobiological experiences: needs, frustration, conflict, and anxiety. These experiences provide energy that is transformed into some form of action. Peplau uses nonnursing theoretical concepts to identify and explain these experiences that compel destructive or constructive responses from nurses and patients. This understanding provides a basis for goal formation and nursing interventions.[23]

MAJOR ASSUMPTIONS

Peplau[23:xii] identifies two explicit assumptions:

1. The kind of person the nurse becomes makes a substantial difference in what each patient will learn as he receives nursing care.
2. Fostering personality development toward maturity is a function of nursing and nursing education. Nursing uses principles and methods that guide the process toward resolution of interpersonal problems.

One implicit assumption was, "The nursing profession has legal responsibility for the effective use of nursing and for its consequences to patients."[23:6]

Nursing

Nursing is described as "a significant, therapeutic, interpersonal process. It functions cooperatively with other human processes that make health possible for individuals in communities." When professional health teams offer health services, nurses participate in the organization of conditions that facilitate natural ongoing tendencies in human organisms. "Nursing is an educative instrument, a maturing force that aims to promote forward movement of personality in the direction of creative, constructive, productive, personal, and community living."[23:16]

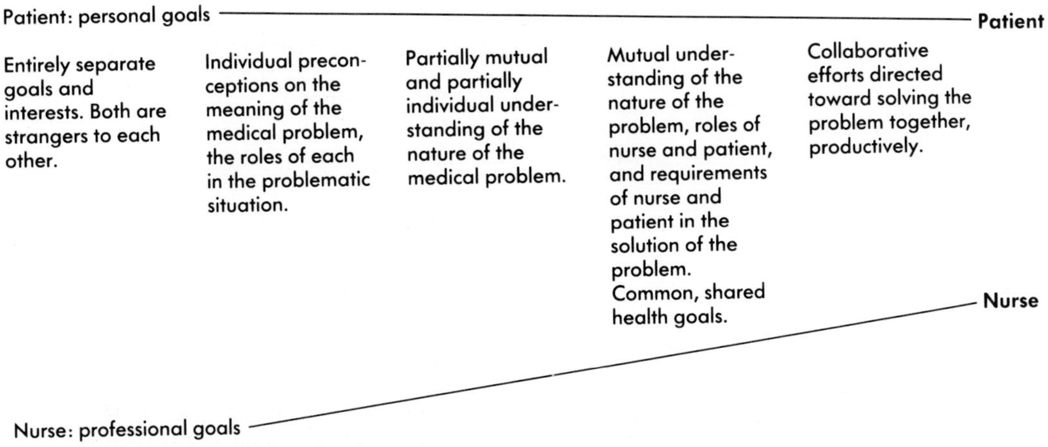

Patient: personal goals
Patient
Entirely separate goals and interests. Both are strangers to each other.
Individual preconceptions on the meaning of the medical problem, the roles of each in the problematic situation.
Partially mutual and partially individual understanding of the nature of the medical problem.
Mutual understanding of the nature of the problem, roles of nurse and patient, and requirements of nurse and patient in the solution of the problem. Common, shared health goals.
Collaborative efforts directed toward solving the problem together, productively.
Nurse
Nurse: professional goals

Figure 17-2. Continuum showing changing aspects of nurse-patient relations.
Used with permission from Peplau, H.E. (1952). *Interpersonal relations in nursing*. New York: G.P. Putnam & Sons, p. 10.

Person

Peplau defines person in terms of man. Man is an organism that lives in an unstable equilibrium.[23:82]

Health

Peplau defines health as "a word symbol that implies forward movement of personality and other ongoing human processes in the direction of creative, constructive, productive, personal, and community living."[23:12]

Environment

Peplau[23:163] implicitly defines the environment in terms of "existing forces outside the organism and in the context of culture," from which mores, customs, and beliefs are acquired. "However, general conditions that are likely to lead to health always include the interpersonal process."[23:14]

THEORETICAL ASSERTIONS

Peplau makes theoretical relationships throughout her book. In summarizing these relationships, Peplau addresses the patient-nurse relationship, the patient and his awareness of feelings, and the nurse and her awareness of feelings. She presents nursing as a maturing educative force that uses the experiential learning method for both patient and nurse (Figure 17-3).

LOGICAL FORM

The process Peplau uses is an inductive approach to theory building. Empirical generalizations are inductively established. "Induction is a type of relationship in which . . . one observes empirical events and generalizes from specific events to all similar events."[13:7] According to Peplau,[27:36] "Nursing situations provide a field of observations from which unique nursing concepts can be derived and used for the improvement of the professional's work." The selected concepts Peplau uses are organized into a larger component, forming relationships that are logical and complete. The relationships describe behaviors that occur in the nurse-patient interaction.

ACCEPTANCE BY THE NURSING COMMUNITY

Practice

Grace Sills[32:123] recalls Peplau brought "a new perspective, a new approach, a theoretically based foundation for nursing practice for therapeutic work with patients." She states, "Pep-

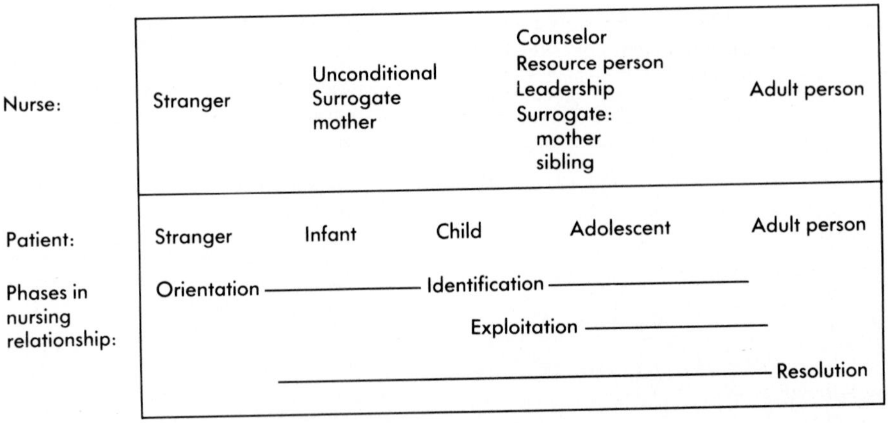

Figure 17-3. Phases and changing roles in nurse-patient relationships.
Used with permission from Peplau, H.E. (1952). *Interpersonal relations in nursing.* New York: G.P. Putnam & Sons, p. 54.

lau's work is responsible for a second order change in the nursing culture."[32:123] Peplau's ideas provided a design for the practice of psychiatric nursing with explication of the design in usable form.

Some of Peplau's ideas were not accepted in the early years, such as the concept of experiential learning for the patient and students.[32] In a panel discussion on psychotherapeutic strategies, Mertz, Mereness, and Mellow disagreed with Peplau on the methodology of psychotherapeutic functions and the role of nurse as surrogate.[30] Later criticisms of Peplau's model indicate the lack of development of social systems that would broaden the knowledge base for understanding the patient's problem.

Peplau[23] used the interpersonal and intrapersonal theories of Sullivan and Freud as the theoretical base for her model and did not take into consideration interrelationships between man and society. These concepts were later developed in general systems theory by Ludwig von Bertalanffy.[40] However, systems theory was included in the curriculum of the Rutgers graduate program in psychiatric nursing. In 1968 Peplau began the first workshop on family therapy under a grant from NIMH to the University of New Mexico.

Today, Peplau's model continues to be used by clinicians. In her article, "Peplau's Theory: An application to short term individual therapy," Linda Thompson used Peplau's model to analyze short-term individual therapy. She stated, "In working with individuals with psychological problems, the development of the interpersonal process is of the utmost importance. Without the development of a therapeutic relationship, little work could be accomplished by the nurse-counselor."[38:31]

Education

Peplau's book, *Interpersonal Relations in Nursing,* was specifically written as an aid to graduate nurses and nursing students. It was originally a hardback edition, but Macmillan printed it in paperback in 1988.

There are few early critiques of Peplau's model in the literature. Her model was designed and published in 1952, 1957, and 1962 with a particular emphasis in psychiatric nursing. The specialty journals in psychiatric nursing did not begin publication until 1963, 11 years after her model was first published. However, psychiatric nursing authors did write textbooks. Smoyak and Rouslin state that after 1952 no psychiatric nursing text could ignore Peplau's work. Peplau's impact was reflected in books in the 1950s and 1960s, such as G. Burton's *Personal, Impersonal, and Interpersonal Relations* (1959), Burd and Marshall's *Some Clinical Approaches to Psychiatric Nursing* (1963), Hofling and Leininger's *Basic Psychiatric Concepts in Nursing* (1960), and Orlando's *The Dynamic Nurse-Patient Relationship* (1961), to name but a few. Most comments on Peplau and her work were written 25 or more years after her published model. Anita O'Toole and Sheila Rouslin Welt have compiled Peplau's unpublished notes and lectures on the interpersonal theory. They have named the book *The Psychotherapy of Hildegard E. Peplau; Selected Papers.*[21]

Research

Sills[31] states that Peplau's work influenced the direction of clinical work and studies. Initial efforts to use research as a tool to develop a body of nursing knowledge were uneven in quality and quantity, and often did not explicitly recognize underlying assumptions. Early research followed the assumption that patient problems were within-the-person phenomena and were explored in nurse-patient relationship studies. This followed Peplau's conceptual model. Since the 1960s, research has shifted to "within-the-social-system" point of view, as studies have examined broader sets of relationships.

For more than 30 years Peplau's model has formed the basis for numerous applications of research methods. M.D. Thomas, J.M. Baker, and N.J. Estes[37] used Peplau's concept of anxiety as a means to constructively resolve angry feelings through experiential learning within the nurse-patient relationship. D. Hays[11] described a study teaching the concept of anxiety that is predominantly based on Peplau's concept of anxiety and used her conceptual model. Hays was a Rutgers graduate student in psychiatric nursing and was a student of Peplau's. This study is one example of Peplau's influence on new nursing leaders with graduate education in the field of psychiatric nursing. M. Topf and B. Dambacher[39] interpret the findings in their study using Peplau's role of the nurse as a stranger. A. Garrett, D. Manuel, and C. Vincent[9] cite Peplau's concept of anxiety for their operational definition of stress and its relationship to learning. In a study by F.E. Spring and H. Turk,[34] the authors develop a behavior scale using Peplau's conceptual framework and her assumption that therapeutic behavior in the nurse-patient relationship promotes experiential learning. The authors concluded that their behavior score was objective, reliable, and valid. D. Methven and R.M. Schlotfeldt,[19] who developed a tool to evaluate verbal responses, based their study on Peplau's assumption that therapeutic communication can be used to reduce or redirect anxiety.

Assumptions from Peplau's model continue to be used in current research. La Monica[15] devised an empathy instrument using Peplau's model (and work from other theorists) as a theoretical framework. She states, "The primary goal of nurses . . . is to provide services that assist in moving clients to their optimum health levels . . . and involves a helping relationship."[15:389]

The impact and significance of Peplau's conceptual model can be best described by Suzanne Lego in a thorough discussion of the history, trends, patterns, and assessment of published research that notes the direction of the one-to-one nurse-patient relationship. She states that ambiguity about the nurse-patient relationship

> abruptly ended in the literature as a result of Peplau's *Interpersonal Relations in Nursing* (1952). As she would continue to do for the next 22 years, Dr. Peplau pulled together loose, ambiguous data and put them into systematic, scientific terms that could be tested, applied, and integrated into the practice of psychiatric nursing.[16:68]

Lego states that most of the published literature describing the one-to-one nurse-patient relationship is based on theoretical concepts inspired principally by Peplau.

Peplau makes a significant contribution to the nursing community through the research done to evaluate, validate, and make more precise the Theory of Interpersonal Relations.

FURTHER DEVELOPMENT

As nursing broadens its scope, there appears to be a need for further development of Peplau's theory for use with the healthy patient, group, and community. Further development is also indicated for clients who are unable to effectively use their communication skills. Increased use of Peplau's theory in practice is needed. Continued research is needed to further refine the theory and to build on nursing's knowledge base.

CRITIQUE

Simplicity

The major focus of Peplau's theory, interpersonal relations between patient and nurse, is easily understood. The theory's basic assumptions and key concepts are defined. Of the assumptions Peplau listed, two are explicit and one is implicit. Peplau sequentially describes her four phases of the interpersonal process. The roles of the nurse and the four psychobiological experiences are clearly indicated. Her logic is based on inductive reasoning. Ideas are taken from observations of the specific and applied to the general. Peplau draws from other disciplines' theories. She is consistent with established theories and principles, such as those of Sullivan, Freud, and Maslow. Peplau deals with the relationships of the interpersonal process, nurse, patient, and psychobiological experiences. Each of these relationships is then developed, within the theory, in an understandable way. Thus, Peplau's theory can be described as meeting the evaluative quality of simplicity.

Generality

In meeting the criteria of generality, Peplau[23] states, "While clinical situations are stressed, any nurse can apply principles that are presented in any other interpersonal relationship in any other area of living." The one drawback to the theory's generality is that an interpersonal relationship must exist. The theory is adaptable only to nursing settings where there can be communication between the patient and nurse. Its use is limited in working with the comatose, senile, or newborn patient. In such situations, the nurse-patient relationship is often one-sided. The nurse and patient cannot work together to become more knowledgeable, develop goals, and mature. Even Peplau[23:41] admits, "Understanding of the meaning of the experience to the patient is required in order for nursing to function as an educative, therapeutic, maturing force." Since Peplau's theory cannot be applied to all patients, the quality of generality is not met.

Empirical Precision

Peplau provides us with a theory based on reality. The relationship between the theory and empirical data allows for validation and verification of the theory by other scientists. The definitions described by Peplau are in a middle range on a connotative-denotative continuum. Peplau operationally defines the four phases of the interpersonal process, the nurse with regard to her roles, and the patient with regard to his state of dependence. According to Duffey and Mullencamp,[5:573] "Peplau relates behavior to theory by naming and categorizing, operationalizing definitions of behavior, thematic abstractions of interaction phenomena, and diagnosis of problems and principles guiding nursing interactions." Peplau's theory can be considered empirically precise. With further research and development, the degree of precision will increase.

Derivable Consequences

In historical perspective, Peplau is one of the first theorists since Nightingale to present a theory for nursing. Therefore her work can be considered pioneering in the nursing field. "She provided nursing with a meaningful method of self-directed practice at a time when medicine dominated the health-care field."[6:44]

Peplau's work, thoughts, and ideas have touched many nurses, from students to practitioners. Although her book was published in 1952, more than three decades ago, it continues to provide direction for nursing practice, education, and research. Peplau's work has provided a significant contribution to nursing's knowledge base. The evaluative criteria of derivable consequences are unquestionably met.

REFERENCES

1. Andreoli, R.G. & Thompson, C.E. (1977, June). The nature of science in nursing. *Image, 9(2)*:32-37.
2. Belcher, J.R. & Fish, L.J. (1980). Hildegard E. Peplau. In Nursing Theories Conference Group, J.B. George, Chairperson, *Nursing theories: The base for professional nursing practice*. Englewood Cliffs, N.J.: Prentice-Hall.
3. Burd, S.F. (1963). The development of an operational definition using the process of learning as a guide. In S.F. Burd & A. Marshall (Eds.), *Some clinical approaches to psychiatric nursing*. New York: Macmillan.
4. Burton, G. (1958). Personal, impersonal, and interpersonal relations. Cited by S.A. Smoyak & S. Rouslin (Eds.) (1982), *A collection of classics in psychiatric nursing literature*. Thorofare, N.J.: Charles B. Slack.
5. Duffey, M. & Mullencamp, A.F. (1974, Sept.). A framework for theory analysis. *Nursing Outlook, 22*:570-574.
6. Fitzpatrick, J.J. & Whall, A.L. (1983). *Conceptual models of nursing, analysis and application*. Bowie, Md.: Robert J. Brady.

7. Freud, S. (1936). The problem of anxiety. In H.E. Peplau, (1952), *Interpersonal relations in nursing*. New York: G.B. Putnam's Sons.
8. Fromm, E. (1947). Man for himself. Cited by H.E. Peplau, (1952), *Interpersonal relations in nursing*. New York: G.B. Putnam's Sons.
9. Garrett, A., Manuel, D., & Vincent, C. (1976, Nov.). Stressful experiences identified by student nurses. *Journal of Nursing Education, 15(6)*:9-21.
10. Gregg, D.E. (1978). Hildegard E. Peplau: Her contributions. *Psychiatry Care, 16*:118-121.
11. Hays, D. (1961, Spring). Teaching a concept of anxiety. *Nursing Research, 10(2)*:108-113.
12. Hofling, C.K. & Leininger, M.M. (1960). Basic psychiatric concepts in nursing. Cited by S.A. Smoyak & S. Rouslin (Eds.) (1982), *A collection of classics in psychiatric nursing literature*. Thorofare, N.J.: Charles B. Slack.
13. Jacox, A. (1974, Jan.-Feb.). Theory construction in nursing: An overview. *Nursing Research, 23*:4-12.
14. Johnson, D.E. (1959). The nature of a science of nursing. *Nursing Outlook, 7*:292.
15. LaMonica, E. (1981). Construct validity of an empathy instrument. *Research in Nursing and Health, 4*:389-400.
16. Lego, S. (1980). The one-to-one nurse-patient relationship. *Perspectives in Psychiatric Care, 18(2)*:67-89. (Reprinted from Psychiatric nursing 1946-1974: A report on the state of the art. *American Journal of Nursing Co.*)
17. Maslow, A.H. & Mittleman, B. (1941). *Principles in abnormal psychology*. New York: Harper & Brothers.
18. Miller, N.E. & Dollard, J. (1941). *Social learning and initiation*. New Haven, Conn.: Yale University Press.
19. Methven, D. & Schlotfeldt, R.M. (1962, Spring). The social interaction inventory. *Nursing Research, 11(2)*:83-88.
20. Orlando, I. (1961). The dynamic nurse-patient relationship. Cited by S.A. Smoyak & S. Roustin (Eds.) (1982), *A collection of classics in psychiatric nursing literature*. Thorofare, N.J.: Charles B. Slack.
21. O'Toole, A. & Welt, S. (In press). *The psychotherapy of Hildegard E. Peplau; Selected papers*. New York: Springer
22. Pavlov, I. (1927). *Conditioned reflexes: An investigation of the physiological activity of the cerebral cortex*. London: Oxford University Press.
23. Peplau, H.E. (1952). *Interpersonal relations in nursing*. New York: G.P. Putnam's Sons.
24. Peplau, H.E. (1964). *Basic principles of patient counseling* (2d ed.). Philadelphia: Smith, Kline, & French Laboratories.
25. Peplau, H.E. (1957). Therapeutic concepts. In S.A. Smoyak & S. Rouslin (Eds.) (1982), *A collection of classics in psychiatric nursing literature*. Thorofare, N.J.: Charles B. Slack. (Reprinted from *National League of Nursing League Exchange No. 26:* Aspects of psychiatric nursing.)
26. Peplau, H.E. (1962). Interpersonal techniques: The crux of psychiatric nursing. *American Journal of Nursing, 62*:629-633.
27. Peplau, H.E. (1969). Theory: The professional dimension. In C. Norris (Ed.), *Proceedings of the first nursing theory conference*. Kansas City, Kansas, University of Kansas Medical Center, Dept. of Nursing Education.
28. Phillips, J.R. (1977, Feb.). Nursing systems and nursing models. *Image, 9(1)*:6.
29. Profile 1974, Feb. *Nursing 74, 4*:13.
30. Psychotherapeutic strategies (1968). Current concepts in psychiatric care: The implications for psychiatric nursing practice. Proceedings of the Institute on Psychiatric Nursing, cosponsored by Yale School of Nursing, Department of Psychiatric Nursing and the Community Mental Health Center Department of Nursing. In *Perspectives of Psychiatric Care, 6(6)*:271-289.
31. Sills, G.M. (1977, May-June). Research in the field of psychiatric nursing 1952-1977. *Nursing Research, 28(3)*:201-207.
32. Sills, G.M. (1978). Hildegard E. Peplau: Leader, practitioner, academician, scholar, and theorist. *Perspectives in Psychiatric Care, 16(3)*: 122-128.
33. S.A. Smoyak & S. Rouslin (Eds.) (1982). Introduction. *A collection of classics in psychiatric nursing literature*. Thorofare, N.J.: Charles B. Slack.
34. Spring, F.E. & Turk, H. (1962, Fall). A therapeutic behavior scale. *Nursing Research, 11(4)*:214-218.
35. Sullivan, H.S. (1947). Conceptions of modern psychiatry. Cited by H.E. Peplau (1952), in *Interpersonal relations in nursing*. New York: G.P. Putnam's Sons.
36. Symonds, P. (1946). *The dynamics of human ad-*

justments. New York: Appleton-Century-Crofts.

37. Thomas, M.D., Baker, J.M., & Estes, N.J. (1970, Dec.). Anger: A tool for developing self-awareness. *American Journal of Nursing, 70(12)*:2586-2590.
38. Thompson, L. (1986, Aug.). Peplau's therapy: An application to short-term individual therapy. *Journal of Psychosocial Nursing, 24(8)*:26-31.
39. Topf, M., & Dambacher, B. (1979). Predominant source of interpersonal influence in relationships between psychiatric patients and nursing staff. *Research in Nursing and Health, 2(1)*:35-43.
40. von Bertalanffy, L. (1968). *General systems theory: Foundations, development, applications.* New York: G. Braziller.

BIBLIOGRAPHY

Primary Sources

Books

Peplau, H.E. (1952). *Interpersonal relations in nursing.* New York: G.P. Putnam & Sons.

Peplau, H.E. (1964). *Basic principles of patient counseling* (2d ed.). Philadelphia: Smith, Kline, & French Laboratories.

Book Chapters

Peplau, H.E. (1969). Theory: The professional dimension. In C. Norris (Ed.), *Proceedings of the first nursing theory conference* (March 21-28). University of Kansas Medical Center, Dept. of Nursing Education, Kansas City.

Peplau, H.E. (1987). Nursing science: A historical perspective. In R. Parse, *Nursing Science: Major Paradigms, Theories, Critiques.* Philadelphia: W.B. Saunders Co.

Articles

Peplau, H.E. (1942, Oct.). Health program at Bennington College. *Public Health Nursing, 34* (10):573-575, 581.

Peplau, H.E. (1947, May). Discussion: A democratic participation technique. *American Journal of Nursing, 47(5)*:334-336.

Peplau, H.E. (1951, Dec.). Toward new concepts in nursing and nursing education. *American Journal of Nursing, 51(12):722-724.*

Peplau, H.E. (1952, Dec.). The psychiatric nurses' family group. *American Journal of Nursing, 52(12)*:1475-1477.

Peplau, H.E. (1953, Feb.). The nursing team in psychiatric facilities. *Nursing Outlook, 1(2)*:90-92.

Peplau, H.E. (1953, Oct.). Themes in nursing situations: Power. *American Journal of Nursing, 53(10)*:1221-1223.

Peplau, H.E. (1953, Nov.). Themes in nursing situations: Safety. *American Journal of Nursing, 53(11)*:1343-1346.

Peplau, H.E. (1955, Dec.). Loneliness. *American Journal of Nursing, 55(12)*:1476-1481.

Peplau, H.E. (1956). Discussion. The League Exchange No. 18: *Psychology and psychiatric nursing research,* pp. 20-22.

Peplau, H.E. (1956, Spring). Present day trends in psychiatric nursing. *Neuropsychiatry, 111(4)*:190-204.

Peplau, H.E. (1956, July 8). An undergraduate program in psychiatric nursing. *Nursing Outlook, 4*:400-410.

Peplau, H.E. (1957, July). What is experiential teaching? *American Journal of Nursing, 57(7)*:884-886.

Peplau, H.E. (1958). Educating the nurse to function in psychiatric services. *Nursing Personnel for Mental Health Programs,* Southern Regional Educational Board, Atlanta, Ga., pp. 37-42.

Peplau, H.E. (1958, Sept.). Public health nurses promote mental health. *Public Health Reports, 73(9)*:828.

Peplau, H.E. (1960). Talking with patients. *American Journal of Nursing, 60*:964-967.

Peplau, H.E. (1960, Jan.). Must laboring together be called teamwork? Problems in team treatment of adults in state mental hospitals. *American Journal of Orthopsychiatry, 30*:103-108.

Peplau, H.E. (1960, March). A personal responsibility: A discussion of anxiety in mental health. *Rutgers Alumni Monthly,* pp. 14-16.

Peplau, H.E. (1960, May). Anxiety in the mother-infant relationship. *Nursing World, 134(5)*:33-34.

Peplau, H.E. (1962). The crux of psychiatric nursing. *American Journal of Nursing, 62*:50-54.

Peplau, H.E. (1963). An approach to research in psychiatric nursing. *Training for Clinical Research in Psychiatric-Mental Health Nursing.* The Catholic University of America, pp. 5-44.

Peplau, H.E. (1963, Oct.-Nov.). Interpersonal relations and the process of adaptations. *Nursing Science, 1(4):272-279.*

Peplau, H.E. (1964). Psychiatric nursing skills and

the general hospital patient. *Nursing Forum, III, (2)*:28-37.

Peplau, H.E. (1964, Nov.). Professional and social behavior: Some differences worth the notice of professional nurses. *Quarterly, 50(4)*:23-33. (Published by the Columbia University-Presbyterian Hospital School of Nursing Alumni Association, New York.)

Peplau, H.E. (1965). The 91st day: A challenge to professional nursing. *Perspectives in Psychiatric Care, III(2)*:20-24.

Peplau, H.E. (1965, April). The heart of nursing: Interpersonal relations. *Canadian Nurse, 61(4)*: 273-275.

Peplau, H.E. (1965, Aug.). Specialization in professional nursing. *Nursing Science, 3(4)*:268-287.

Peplau, H.E. (1965, Nov.). The nurse in the community mental health program. *Nursing Outlook, 13(11)*:68-70.

Peplau, H.E. (1966). Nurse-doctor relationships. *Nursing Forum, 5(1)*:60-75.

Peplau, H.E. (1966). Nursing's two routes to doctoral degrees. *Nursing Forum, 5(2)*:57-67.

Peplau, H.E. (1966, March-April). An interpretation of the ANA position. *NJSNA-News Letter, 22(2)*:6-10.

Peplau, H.E. (1966, May-June). Trends in nursing and nursing education. *NJSNA-News Letter, 22(3)*:17-27.

Peplau, H.E. (1967, Feb.). The work of psychiatric nurses. *Psychiatric Opinion, 4(1)*:5-11.

Peplau, H.E. (1967, Nov.). Interpersonal relations and the work of the industrial nurse. *Industrial Nurse Journal, 15(10)*:7-12.

Peplau, H.E. (1968). Psychotherapeutic strategies. *Perspectives in Psychiatric Care, VI(6)*:264-289.

Peplau, H.E. (1969). Professional closeness as a special kind of involvement with a patient, client, or family group. *Nursing Forum, 8(4)*:342-360.

Peplau, H.E. (1969, Fall). The American Nurses' Association and nursing education. *Utah Nurse, 20(3)*:6.

Peplau, H. (1970, Jan.) ANA's new executive director states her views. *American Journal of Nursing, 70*:84-88.

Peplau, H.E. (1970, Summer). Professional closeness as a special kind of involvement with a patient, client or family group. *Comprehensive Nurse Quarterly, 5(3)*:66-81.

Peplau, H. (1970, Nov.-Dec.). Changed patterns of practice. *Washington State Journal of Nursing, 42*:4-6.

Peplau, H.E. (1970, Nov.-Dec.). Keynote address at the 68th annual convention of the New Jersey state nurses' association. *New Jersey Nurse, 26*:3-10.

Peplau, H.E. (1970, Dec.). ANA: Who needs it? *Nursing News, 43*:5-8.

Peplau, H.E. (1970, Dec.). What it means to be a professional nurse today. *Alabama Nurse, 24*:8-17.

Peplau, H.E. (1970, Dec.). The road ahead. *Maine Nurse, 1(3)*:3-8.

Peplau, H.E. (1971, Jan.). ANA: Who needs it? *Nursing News, 44(1)*:12-14.

Peplau, H.E. (1971). Dilemmas of organizing nurses. *Image, 4*:4-8.

Peplau, H.E. (1971, Spring). In support of nursing research. *Journal of the New York State Nurses' Association, 2*:5.

Peplau, H.E. (1971, Summer). Time of decision. *Nevada Nurses' Association Quarterly Newsletter*, pp. 1-3.

Peplau, H.E. (1971, July). Responsibility, authority, evaluation, and accountability of nursing in patient care. *Michigan Nurse, 44*:5-7.

Peplau, H.E. (1971, Sept.). The task ahead. *American Journal of Nursing, 71*:1800-1802.

Peplau, H. (1971, Nov.). The now nurse in nursing: Some problems of diversity. *Oklahoma Nurse, 46*:1.

Peplau, H.E. (1971, Nov.). What it means to be a professional nurse in today's society. *Kansas Nurse, 46*:1-3.

Peplau, H.E. (1971, Winter). Communication in crisis intervention. *Psychiatric Forum, 2*:1-7.

Peplau, H.E. (1971, Winter). Where do we go from here? *Pelican News, 27*:14-16.

Peplau, H.E. (1972, Spring). The nurse's role in health care delivery systems. *Pelican News, 28*:12-14.

Peplau, H.E. (1972, May). The independence of nursing. *Imprint, 9*:11.

Peplau, H.E. (1972, June). The president challenges nurses in address to delegates. *Kansas Nurse*, pp. 2-4.

Peplau, H.E. (1972, Nov.-Dec.) Some issues and developments that should be of concern to nurses. *New Jersey State Nurses' Association News, 2*:14-16.

Peplau, H.E. (1973, July). Meeting the challenge. *Mississippi RN, 35*:1-6.

Peplau, H.E. (1974). Creativity and commitment in nursing. *Image: Journal of Nursing Scholarship, 6*:3-5.

Peplau, H.E. (1974). Is health care a right? Affirmative response. *Image: Journal of Nursing Scholarship, 7*:4-10.

Peplau, H.E. (1974, Jan.). Nurses: Collaborate or isolate. *Pennsylvania Nurse, 29*:2-5.

Peplau, H.E. (1974, Autumn). Talking with patients. *Comprehensive Nursing Quarterly, 9(3)*:30-39.

Peplau, H.E. (1975, March-April). An open letter to a new graduate. *Nursing Digest, 3*:36-37.

Peplau, H.E. (1975, Oct.). Interview with Dr. Peplau: Future of nursing. *Japanese Journal of Nursing, 39(10)*:1046-1050.

Peplau, H.E. (1975, Oct.). Midlife crisis. *American Journal of Nursing, 75*:1761-1765.

Peplau, H.E., et al. (1976, Aug.). What future for nursing? *AORN, 24*:217-235.

Peplau, H.E. (1977, March-April). The changing view of nursing. *International Nursing Review, 24*:43-45.

Peplau, H.E. (1978, March-April). Psychiatric nursing: Role of nurses and psychiatric nurses. *International Nursing Review, 25*:41-47.

Peplau, H.E. (1980, April). New statement defines scope of practice. *American Nurse, 12(4)*:1, 8, 24.

Peplau, H. (1980, May-June). The psychiatric nurses: Accountable? to whom? for what? *Perspectives in Psychiatric Care, 18*:128-134.

Peplau, H.E. (1982, Aug.). Some reflections on earlier days in psychiatric nursing. *Journal of Psychosocial Nursing Mental Health Services, 20*:17-24.

Peplau, H.E. (1984, Jan.-Feb.). Internal versus external regulation. *New Jersey Nurse, 14*:12-14.

Peplau, H.E. (1985, Feb.). Is nursing self-regulatory power being eroded? *American Journal of Nursing, 85(2)*:140-143.

Peplau, H.E. (1987, Jan.). Tomorrow's world. *Nursing Times*: 29-32.

Peplau, H.E. (1987, May). American nurses association social policy statement: Part I. *Archives of Psychiatric Nursing, 1(5)*:301-307.

Peplau, H.E. (1988, Feb.). The art and science of nursing: Similarities, differences, and relations. *Nursing Science Quarterly, 1(1)*:8-15.

Peplau, H.E. (1988, Spring). Peplau responds. *Pacesetter* Newsletter of the American Nurses' Association Council on Psychiatric and Mental Health Nursing, *15(1)*:1-4.

Interviews

Peplau, H.E. (1985, May). Help the public maintain mental health. *Nursing Success Today, 2(5)*:30-34.

Peplau, H.E. (1985, Aug.). The power of the dissociative state. *Journal of Psychosocial Nursing, 23(8)*:31-33.

Chapters, Pamphlets, Proceedings, Reports.

Peplau, H.E. (1951). *Understanding ourselves.* Fifty-seventh annual report, National League for Nursing Education.

Peplau, H.E. (1952). *The responsibility of professional nursing in psychiatry.* Fifty-eighth annual report, National League for Nursing Education.

Peplau, H.E. (1954, Sept. 15). *Some problems of the psychiatric nursing team.* Second Annual Psychiatric Institute, New Jersey Neuropsychiatric Institute, Proceedings.

Peplau, H.E. (1956). *The yearbook of modern nursing.* New York: G.P. Putnam's Sons.

Peplau, H.E. (1958, June). Current concepts of psychiatric nursing care. *ANA Proceedings.*

Peplau, H.E. (1959). Principles of psychiatric nursing. In *American Handbook of Psychiatry* (Vol. II). New York: Basic Books.

Peplau, H.E. (1960). Ward atmosphere: Cliche or task? In *Nursing papers.* Illinois State Psychiatric Institute.

Peplau, H.E. (1962). Will automation change the nurse, nursing, or both? *Technical innovations in health care: nursing implications* (Pamphlet 5). New York: American Nurses' Association.

Peplau, H.E. (1963). Counseling in nursing practice. In E. Harms, & P. Schreiber (Eds.), *Handbook of Counseling Techniques.* New York: Pergamon.

Peplau, H.E. (1963). Leadership responsibility in toleration of stress: The leader's role in helping staff to tolerate stress. In *Conferences on preparation for leadership in psychiatric nursing service.* Department of Nursing Education, Teachers College, Columbia University, New York.

Peplau, H.E. (1963, Dec. 2-3). A personal challenge for immediate action. In AHA Conference Group in Psychiatric Nursing Practice, National Institute, Proceedings, Kansas City.

Peplau, H.E. (1967). Psychiatric nursing. In A.M. Freedman and A.I. Kaplan (Eds.), *Comprehensive textbook of psychiatry.* New York: Williams and Wilkins.

Peplau, (1968). Operational definitions and nursing practice. In L.T. Zderad & H.C. Belcher (Eds.), *Developing behavioral concepts in nursing*. SREB.

Peplau, H.E., & Smoyak, S. (1968, Nov. 14-16). Pattern perpetuation and intellectual competencies in schizophrenia. Paper presented at Conference on Schizophrenia: Current concepts and research. Waldorf Astoria, New York.

Peplau, H.E. (1969, March 20-21). *Theory: The professional dimension*. Presented at the Nursing Theory Conference, University of Kansas Medical Center, Kansas City.

Peplau, H.E. (1969). Pattern perpetuation in schizophrenia. In D. Sankar, *Schizophrenia: Current concepts and research*. Hicksville, N.Y.: PJD Publications.

Peplau, H.E. (1974). *Associate degree education for nursing: Current issues, 1974*. ANA and the professional nurse. Publication #23-1539. National League of Nursing, Dept. of Associate Degree Programs.

Videotapes

The Nurse Theorist: Portraits of Excellence: Hildegard Peplau. (1988). Oakland: Studio III. Video is available from Fuld Video Project, Studio III, 370 Hawthorne Avenue, Oakland, Cal. 94609.

Thesis

Peplau, H.E. (1953). *An exploration of some process elements which restrict or facilitate instructor-student interaction in a classroom, Type B*. Doctoral Project, Teachers' College, Columbia University.

Forewords

Peplau, H.E. (1963). In S.F. Burd & M.A. Marshall (Eds.), *Some clinical approaches to psychiatric nursing*. New York: Macmillan.

Peplau, H.E. (1963). In S. Armstrong, & S. Rouslin, *Group psychotherapy in nursing practice*. New York: Macmillan.

Peplau, H.E. (1987). In P. Martin, *Psychiatric Nursing: A Therapeutic Approach*. London: Macmillan Education Ltd.

Editorial Statements, Letters, Reactions

Peplau, H.E. (1963, Sept.). Nursing has lost its way. *Journal RN, 25(9)*:103-105.

Peplau, H.E. (1963, Jan.-Feb.) On semantics. *Perspectives in Psychiatric Care, 1*:10-11.

Letter to Editor. (1962, March). *American Journal of Nursing, 62(3)*:16, 25, 26.

Reviews

Peplau, H.E. (1955, May). Review of *The psychiatric interview* by H.S. Sullivan. *American Journal of Nursing, 55(5)*:614.

Peplau, H.E. (1957, April). Review of *The foundation of human behavior* by T. Muller. *Mental Hygiene, 41(2)*:285-286.

Peplau, H.E. (1957, Oct.) Review of *Beyond laughter* by M. Grotjohn. *American Journal of Nursing, 57(10)*:1349-1450.

Peplau, H.E. (1963). Review of *The management of the anxious patient* by Ainslic Meares. *Perspectives in Psychiatric Care, II(1), 1964*:46-47.

Peplau, H.E. (1964). Review of *More for the mind: A study of psychiatric services in Canada. Perspectives in Psychiatric Care, 11(3)*:39-42.

Peplau, H.E. (1964, Fall). Review of *Attitudes of nursing students toward direct patient care* by Sr. L.M. Vaugh, *Journal of Nursing Research, 13(4)*:348-349.

Secondary Sources

American Nurses' Association new executive director states her views. (1970, Jan.). *American Journal of Nursing, 70(1)*:84-88.

Belcher, J.R., & Fish, L.J. (1980). Hildegard E. Peplau. In Nursing Theories Conference Group, J.B. George, Chairperson, *Nursing theories: The base for professional practice*. Englewood Cliffs, N.J.: Prentice-Hall.

Burd, S.F. (1963). The development of an operational definition using the process of learning as a guide. In S.F. Burd & A. Marshall, *Some clinical approaches to psychiatric nursing*. New York: MacMillan.

Burton, G. (1958). Personal, impersonal, and interpersonal relations. Cited by S.A. Smoyak & S. Rouslin (Eds.), (1982), *A collection of classics in psychiatric nursing literature*. Thorofare, N.J.: Charles B. Slack.

Field, W.E., Jr. (Ed.). (1979). *The psychotherapy of Hildegard E. Peplau*. New Brunfels, Tex.: PSF Publications.

Fitzpatrick, J.J., & Whall, A.L. (1983). *Conceptual models of nursing: Analysis and application*. Bowie, Md.: Robert J. Brady.

Chinn, P.L., & Jacobs, M.K. (1983). *Theory and*

nursing: A systematic approach. St. Louis: C.V. Mosby.

Garrett, A., Manuel, D., & Vincent, C. (1976, Nov.). Stressful experiences identified by student nurses. *Journal of Nursing Education, 15(6)*:9-21.

Gregg, D.E. (1978, May-June). Hildegard E. Peplau: Her contributions. *Perspective Psychiatric Care, 16(3)*:118-121.

Hays, D. (1961, Spring). Teaching a concept of anxiety. *Nursing Research, 10(2)*:108-113.

Hofling, C.K. & Leininger, M.M. (1960). Basic psychiatric concepts in nursing. Cited by S.A. Smoyak, & S. Rouslin (Eds.), (1982), *A collection of classics in psychiatric nursing literature*. Thorofare, N.J.: Charles B. Slack.

Iveson, J. (1982, Nov.). A two-way process . . . theories in nursing practice . . . Peplau's nursing model. *Nursing Mirror, 155(18)*:52.

Keda, A. (1970, Winter). From Henderson to Orlando to Wiedenback: Thoughts on completion of translation of *Basic Principles of Clinical Nursing. Comprehensive Nursing Quarterly, 5(1)*:85-94.

LaMonica, E. (1981). Construct validity of an empathy instrument. *Research in Nursing and Health, 4*:389-400.

Lego, S. (1980). The one-to-one nurse-patient relationship. *Perspectives in Psychiatric Care, 18(2)*:67-89. (Reprinted from *Psychiatric Nursing 1946-1974: A report on the state of the art,* American Journal of Nursing Co.)

Marshall, J. (1963, March-April). Dr. Peplau's strong medicine for psychiatric nurses. *Smith, Kline & French Reporter, 7*:11-14.

McCarter, P. (1980, April). New statement defines scope of practice discussion with Dr. Lane and Dr. Peplau. *American Nurse, 12(4)*:1, 8, 24.

Miller, N.E. & Dollard, J. (1941). *Social learning and imitation*. New Haven, Conn.: Yale University Press.

Methven, D. & Schlotfeldt, R.M. (1962, Spring). The social interaction inventory. *Nursing Research, 11(2)*:83-88.

Nursing Theories Conference Group, J.B. George, Chairperson. (1980). *Nursing theories: The base for professional nursing practice*. Englewood Cliffs, N.J.: Prentice-Hall, pp. 73-89.

Orlando, I. (1961). The dynamic nurse-patient relationship. Cited by S.A. Smoyak & S. Rouslin, (Eds.) (1982), *A collection of classics in psychiatric nursing literature*. Thorofare, N.J.: Charles B. Slack.

Osborne, O. (1984, Nov.). Intellectual traditions in psychiatric nursing. *Journal of Psychosocial Nursing, 22(1)*:27-32.

Profile. (1974, Feb.). *Nursing 74, 4*:13.

Psychotherapeutic strategies. (1968). Current concepts in psychiatric care: The implications for psychiatric nursing practice. Proceedings of the Institute on Psychiatric Nursing, cosponsored by Yale School of Nursing, Department of Psychiatric Nursing and the Community Mental Health Center Department of Nursing. In *Perspectives of Psychiatric Care, 6(6)*:271-289.

Sills, G.M. (1977, May-June). Research in the field of psychiatric nursing 1952-1977. *Nursing Research, 28(3)*:201-207.

Sills, G.M. (1978). Hildegard E. Peplau: Leader, practitioner, academician, scholar, and theorist. *Perspectives in Psychiatric Care, 16(3)*:122-128.

S.A. Smoyak & S. Rouslin (Eds.). (1982). Introduction. In *A collection of classics in psychiatric nursing literature*. Thorofare, N.J.: Charles B. Slack.

Spring, F.E. & Turk, H. (1962, Fall). A therapeutic behavior scale. *Nursing Research, 11(4)*:214-218.

Thomas, M.D., Baker, J.M., & Estes, N.J. (1970, Dec.). Anger: A tool for developing self-awareness. *American Journal of Nursing, 70(12)*:2586-2590.

Topf, M. & Dambacher, B. (1979). Predominant source of interpersonal influence in relationships between psychiatric patients and nursing staff. *Research in Nursing and Health, 2(1)*:35-43.

Other Sources

Andreoli, R.G. & Thompson, C.E. (1977, June). The nature of science in nursing. *Image: Journal of Nursing Scholarship, 9(2)*:32-37.

Duffey, M. & Mullencamp, A.F. (1974, Sept.). A framework for theory analysis. *Nursing Outlook, 22*:570-574.

Freud, S. (1936). The problem of anxiety. Cited by H.E. Peplau, (1952), *Interpersonal relations in nursing*. New York: G.B. Putnam's Sons.

Fromm, E. (1947). Man for himself. Cited by H.E. Peplau, (1952), *Interpersonal relations in nursing*. New York: G.B. Putnam's Sons.

Jacox, A. (1974, Jan.-Feb.). Theory construction in nursing: An overview. *Nursing Research, 23*:4-12.

Johnson, D.E. (1959). The nature of a science of nursing. *Nursing Outlook, 7*:272.

Maslow, A.H. (1943, July). A theory of human motivation. *Psychological Review, 50*:370-396.

Maslow, A.H. & Mittleman, B. (1941). *Principles in abnormal psychology.* New York: Harper & Brothers.

Miller, N.E. & Dollard, J. (1941). *Social learning and imitation.* New Haven, Conn.: Yale University Press.

Mullahy, P. (1948). *Oedipus: Myth and complex.* New York: Hermitage House.

Pavlov, I. (1927). *Conditioned reflexes: An investigation of the physiological activity of the cerebral cortex.* London: Oxford University Press.

Phillips, J.R. (1977, Feb.). Nursing systems and nursing models. *Image: Journal of Nursing Scholarship, 9, (1)*:6.

Popper, K.R. (1963). *Conjectures and refutations: The growth of scientific knowledge.* New York: Basic Books.

Reynolds, P.D. (1971). *A primer in theory construction.* Indianapolis, Ind.: Bobbs-Merrill.

Solomon, A.P. (1943). Rehabilitation of patients with psychologically protracted convalescence. *Archives of Physical Therapy, 24*:270-273.

Sullivan, H.S. (1947). Concepts of modern psychiatry. Cited by H.E. Peplau (1952), *Interpersonal relations in nursing.* New York: G.B. Putnam's Sons.

Sullivan, H.S. (1948). *The meaning of anxiety in psychiatry and in life.* Washington, D.C.: William Alanson White Psychiatric Foundation.

Symonds, P. (1946). *The dynamics of human adjustment.* New York: Appleton-Century-Crofts.

von Bertalanffy, L. (1968). *General systems theory: Foundations, development, applications.* New York: Braziller.

Wertheimer, M. (1945). *Productive thinking.* New York: Harper & Brothers.

18

Joyce Travelbee
Human-to-Human Relationship Model

William H. Hobble, Theresa Lansinger, Jude A. Magers

CREDENTIALS AND BACKGROUND OF THE THEORIST

Joyce Travelbee was a psychiatric nurse practitioner, educator, and writer. Born in 1926, she completed her basic nursing preparation in 1946 at Charity Hospital School of Nursing in New Orleans. She obtained a B.S.N. Ed. from Louisiana State University in 1956 and an M.S.N. from Yale in 1959. In the summer of 1973 Travelbee began a doctoral program in Florida, but was unable to complete the program because of her untimely death later that year.[1,2,7]

Travelbee began her career as a nursing educator in 1952 by teaching psychiatric nursing at DePaul Hospital Affiliate School, New Orleans, while working on her baccalaureate degree. She also taught psychiatric nursing at Charity Hospital School of Nursing, at Louisiana State University, at New York University in New York City, and at the University of Mississippi in Jackson. In 1970 she was named Project Director at Hotel Dieu, School of Nursing in New Orleans. At the time of her death, Travelbee was the director of graduate education at Louisiana State University School of Nursing.[1,2,7]

Travelbee began publishing articles in nursing journals in 1963. Her first book, *Interpersonal Aspects of Nursing,* was published in 1966 and 1971. A second book, *Intervention in Psychiatric Nursing,* was published in 1969.

THEORETICAL SOURCES FOR THEORY DEVELOPMENT

Travelbee's experiences in her basic nursing education and initial practice in Catholic charity institutions greatly influenced the development of her theory. Travelbee believed the nursing care given patients in these institutions lacked compassion.[7] She felt nursing needed "a humanistic revolution—a return to focus on the 'caring' function of the nurse—in the caring for [and] the caring about ill persons."[9:2]

Travelbee was probably also influenced by Ida Jean Orlando, who was one of her instructors during her graduate studies at Yale. Orlan-

The authors wish to express appreciation to Leigh DeNoon, Mary Ellen Doona, Joyce Lee, and Katharine Taylor for assistance with data collection. The authors have been unable to obtain a picture of Joyce Travelbee.

do's model possesses some similarities to the model Travelbee proposes. Orlando[5:6] states, "The nurse is responsible for helping the patient avoid and alleviate the distress of unmet needs." Orlando[5:8] also states the nurse and the patient are both people who interact with each other. The similarities between the two models are shown by Travelbee's assertion that the nurse and patient interact with each other and by her definition of the purpose of nursing. Travelbee[9:7] states the purpose of nursing is to assist "an individual, family, or community to prevent or cope with the experience of illness and suffering."

Travelbee also appears to have been influenced by Viktor Frankl, a survivor of Auschwitz and other Nazi concentration camps. As a result of his experiences, Frankl[3:153] proposed the theory of Logotherapy, in which a patient "is actually confronted with and reoriented toward the meaning of his life." Travelbee[9:158] based the assumptions of her theory on the concepts of Logotherapy.

USE OF EMPIRICAL EVIDENCE

Katharine Taylor,[7] a former student and colleague of Travelbee, remembers Travelbee as a prolific reader whose office was often crammed with files of bibliography cards. Apparently, Travelbee's theory is based on the cumulation of her nursing experiences and her readings rather than the evidence of a particular research study.

MAJOR CONCEPTS AND DEFINITIONS

HUMAN BEING. "A human being is defined as a unique irreplaceable individual—a one-time-being in this world—like yet unlike any person who has ever lived or ever will live."[9:26]

PATIENT. The term *patient* is a stereotype useful for communicative economy. "Actually there are no patients. There are only individual human beings in need of the care, services, and assistance of other human beings, whom, it is believed, can render the assistance that is needed."[9:32]

NURSE. The nurse is also a human being. "The nurse possesses a body of specialized knowledge and the ability to use it for the purpose of assisting other human beings to prevent illness, regain health, find meaning in illness, or to maintain the highest maximal degree of health."[9:40]

ILLNESS. Illness is "a category and a classification."[9:49] Travelbee did not use the term *illness* as a definition of being unhealthy, but rather explored the human experience of illness. Travelbee defined illness by objective and subjective criteria. The objective criteria are determined by the outward effects of illness on the individual.[9:521] The subjective criteria refer to how a human being perceives himself as ill.[9:52]

SUFFERING. "Suffering is a feeling of displeasure which ranges from simple transitory mental, physical, or spiritual discomfort to extreme anguish, and to those phases beyond anguish, namely, the malignant phase of despairful 'not caring,' and the terminal phase of apathetic indifference."[9:62] Suffering can be placed on a continuum, such as the one in Figure 18-1.

PAIN. "Pain itself is not observable—only its effects are noted."[9:72] Pain is a lonely experience that is difficult to communicate fully to another individual.[9:72] The experience of pain is unique to each individual.

HOPE. "Hope is a mental state characterized by the desire to gain an end or accomplish a goal combined with some degree of expectation that what is desired or sought is attainable."[9:77] Hope is related to dependence on others, choice, wishing, trust and perseverance, and courage, and is future oriented.[9:78-80]

Transitory feeling of displeasure	Extreme anguish	Malignant phase of despairful not caring	Terminal phase of apathetic indifference

Figure 18-1. Continuum of suffering. (Conceptualized by Theresa Lansinger, based on Joyce Travelbee's definition.)

HOPELESSNESS. Hopelessness is being devoid of hope.[9:81]

COMMUNICATION. "Communication is a process which can enable the nurse to establish a human-to-human relationship and thereby fulfill the purpose of nursing, namely, to assist individuals and families to prevent and to cope with the experience of illness and suffering and, if necessary, to assist them to find meaning in these experiences."[9:93]

INTERACTION. "The term *interaction* refers to any contact during which two individuals have reciprocal influence on each other and communicate verbally and/or nonverbally."[9:120]

NURSE-PATIENT INTERACTION. "The term *nurse-patient interaction* refers to any contact between a nurse and an ill person and is characterized by the fact that both individuals perceive the other in a stereotyped manner."[9:120]

NURSING NEED. "A nursing need is any requirement of the ill person (or family) which can be met by the professional nurse practitioner, and which lies within the scope of the legal definition of nursing practice."[9:125]

THERAPEUTIC USE OF SELF. "The therapeutic use of self is the ability to use one's personality consciously and in full awareness in an attempt to establish relatedness and to structure nursing intervention."[9:19] It "requires self insight, self understanding, an understanding of the dynamics of human behavior, ability to interpret one's own behavior as well as the behavior of others, and the ability to intervene effectively in nursing situations."[9:19]

EMPATHY. "Empathy is a process wherein an individual is able to comprehend the psychological state of another."[9:43]

SYMPATHY. Sympathy implies a desire to help an individual undergoing stress.[8:68-69]

RAPPORT. "Rapport is a process, a happening, an experience, or series of experiences, undergone simultaneously by the nurse and the recipient of her care. It is composed of a cluster of interrelated thoughts and feelings, these thoughts, feelings and attitudes being transmitted, or communicated by one human being to another."[9:150]

HUMAN-TO-HUMAN RELATIONSHIP. "A human-to-human relationship is primarily an experience or series of experiences between a nurse and the recipient of her care. The major characteristic of these experiences is that the nursing needs of the individual (or family) are met."[9:123] "The human-to-human relationship, in nursing situations, is the means through which the purpose of nursing is accomplished."[9:119] The human-to-human relationship is established when the nurse and the recipient of her care attained a rapport after having progressed through the stages of the original encounter, emerging identities, empathy, and sympathy[9:119-120] (Figure 18-2).

MAJOR ASSUMPTIONS

Nursing

Travelbee[9:7] defines nursing as an "interpersonal process whereby the professional nurse

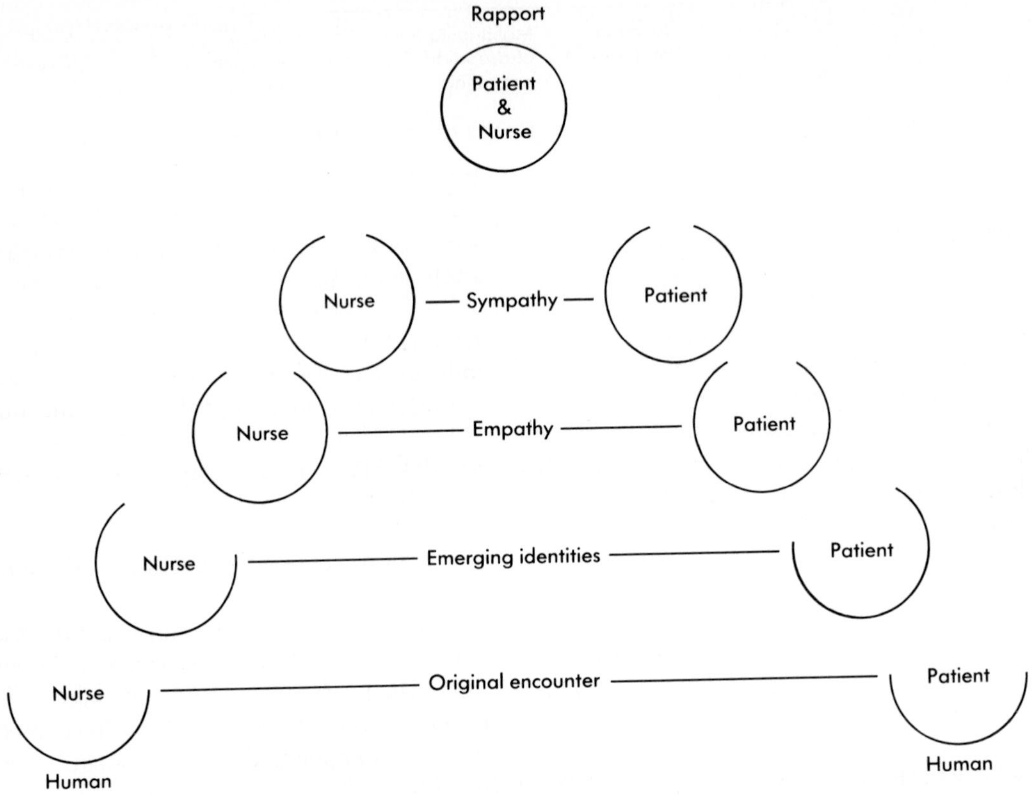

Figure 18-2. Human-to-human relationship. (Conceptualized by William Hobble and Theresa Lansinger, based on Joyce Travelbee's writings.)

practitioner assists an individual, family, or community to prevent or cope with the experience of illness and suffering and, if necessary, to find meaning in these experiences." Nursing is an interpersonal process since it is an experience that occurs between the nurse and an individual or group of individuals.[8:8]

Person

The term *person* is defined as a human being. Both the nurse and the patient are human beings. A human being is an unique, irreplaceable individual who is in the continuous process of becoming, evolving, and changing.[9:26-27]

Health

Travelbee defines health by the criteria of subjective and objective health. A person's subjective health status is how the individual perceives his health.[9:9] Objective health is "an absence of discernible disease, disability, or defect as measured by physical examination, laboratory tests, assessment by a spiritual director or psychological counselor."[9:10]

Environment

Travelbee does not explicitly define environment in the theory. She does define the human condition and life experiences encountered by all human beings as suffering, hope, pain, and illness. These human conditions can be equated to the environment.

THEORETICAL ASSERTIONS

"The purpose of nursing is achieved through the establishment of a human-to-human relationship."[9:16]

The quality and quantity of nursing care delivered to an ill human being is greatly influenced by the nurse's perception of the patient.[9:32]

The terms *patient* and *nurse* are stereotypes and only useful for communicative economy.

The roles of the nurse and patient must be transcended to establish a human-to-human relatedness.[9:33]

Illness and suffering "are spiritual encounters as well as emotional-physical experiences."[9:61]

The communication process enables "the nurse to establish a human-to-human relationship and thereby fulfill the purpose of nursing."[9:93]

"Individuals can be assisted to find meaning in the experience of illness and suffering. The meanings can enable the individual to cope with the problems engendered by these experiences."[9:158]

"The spiritual and ethical values of the nurse, or her philosophical beliefs about illness and suffering, will determine the extent to which she will be able to assist individuals and families to find meaning (or no meaning) in these difficult experiences."[9:158]

"It is the responsibility of the professional nurse practitioner to assist individuals and families to find meaning in illness and suffering (if this be necessary)."[9:158]

Human-to-human relationship

The human-to-human relationship model, shown in Figure 18-2, represents the interaction between the nurse and patient. The half circles at the point of the original encounter indicate the possibility of and need for developing the encounter into a therapeutic relationship. As the interaction process progresses toward rapport, the circles join into one full circle—representing that the potential for a therapeutic relationship has been attained.

ORIGINAL ENCOUNTER. The original encounter is characterized by first impressions by the nurse of the ill person and by the ill person of the nurse. The nurse and ill person perceive each other in stereotyped roles.[9:131]

EMERGING IDENTITIES. The emerging identities phase is characterized by the nurse and ill person perceiving each other as unique individuals. The bond of a relationship is beginning to form.[9:132]

EMPATHY. The empathy phase is characterized by the ability to share in the other person's experience. The result of the empathic process is the ability to predict the behavior of the individual with whom one has empathized.[9:137] Travelbee believed two qualities that enhanced the empathy process were similarities of experience and the desire to understand another person.[9:138]

SYMPATHY. Sympathy goes beyond empathy and occurs when the nurse desires to alleviate the cause of the patient's illness or suffering. "When one sympathizes one is involved but not incapacitated by the involvement."[9:142] The nurse is to create helpful nursing action as a result of reaching the phase of sympathy. "This helpful nursing action requires a combination of the disciplined intellectual approach combined with the therapeutic use of self."[9:149]

RAPPORT. Rapport is characterized by nursing actions that alleviate an ill person's distress. The nurse and ill person are relating as human being to human being. The ill person exhibits both trust and confidence in the nurse. "A nurse is able to establish rapport because she possesses the necessary knowledge and skills required to assist ill persons, and because she is able to perceive, respond to, and appreciate the uniqueness of the ill human being."[9:155]

LOGICAL FORM

Travelbee's theory is inductive. She has used specific nursing situations to create general ideas. Travelbee appears to follow a logical form by first defining the labels in her theory, then listing the assumptions, and finally establishing specific nursing goals.

ACCEPTANCE BY THE NURSING COMMUNITY

Practice

Travelbee believed the condition of an individual exhibiting apathetic indifference is just as critical as that of an individual who is hemorrhaging. She felt both people need emergency resuscitative measures. But an examination of patient care given by nurses today indicates the patient's physical needs still hold top priority. The acceptance and use of nursing diagnosis does appear to focus nursing care more on the total needs of the patients as compared with 20 years ago when Travelbee published her theory. However, nursing has not yet reached the humanistic revolution Travelbee proposed.

Hospice is the one area of nursing practice where the philosophy closely adheres to the tenets of Travelbee's theory. The hospice nurse attempts to develop a rapport with the patient and his significant others. Most hospice nurses agree with Elisabeth Kübler-Ross[4:2] "that death does not have to be a catastrophic, destructive thing; indeed, it can be viewed as one of the most constructive, positive, and creative elements of culture and life." One hospice nurse believes the dying person must find meaning in his death before he can ever begin to accept the actuality of his death, just as his loved ones must find meaning in his death before they can complete the grieving process.[4]

Education

Nursing education appears to have identified the need to prepare nurses to address the emotional and spiritual needs of patients. The focus of nursing education has changed from the disease entity approach, that is, signs, symptoms, and nursing intervention, to a more holistic care approach. However, basic nursing programs do not seem to adequately prepare nurses to help individuals find meaning in illness and suffering as Travelbee proposed. Travelbee's second book, *Intervention in Psychiatric Nursing: Process in the One-to-One Relationship,* has been used in various nursing programs. But this book alone does not adequately prepare nurses to help individuals find meaning in illness and suffering. Nursing programs need to offer a much broader background in communication techniques, values clarification, and thanatology to adequately prepare nurses to fulfill the purpose of nursing stated in Travelbee's theory.

Research

Some aspects of the one-to-one relationship proposed by Travelbee have been quoted by several sources in research studies. However, there does not appear to be any major research generated by Travelbee's specific theory that could stimulate further development.

FURTHER DEVELOPMENT

The recent advent of diagnostic related groups (DRGs) is creating the need to produce the highest quality nursing care by the most economical method. Tools such as patient acuity systems have been devised to determine nursing staffing patterns in accordance with the nursing needs of patients. Although this type of tool can account for the emotional needs of patients, emotional needs are not weighed as heavily as patients' physical needs. DRGs may shift the nursing focus back to solely meeting the patient's physical needs. If nurses are to prevent this, they must prove to health care administrators and health care consumers that the time taken by the nurse to meet a patient's emotional and spiritual needs is a valuable investment. Travelbee's theory could be used to provide the research data to justify this time investment. However, Travelbee's theory does not currently contain the empirical precision to support such research data. If it is to be more readily accepted, its major assumptions need to be assigned operational definitions. Once this is done, the theory could perhaps generate the data needed to facilitate further acceptance.

CRITIQUE

Simplicity

Travelbee's theory does not possess simplicity because there are many variables present. The theory is designed to help nurses appreciate not only the patient's humanness but also the nurse's humanness. To be human is to be unique; so the variables present in each phase of the human-to-human relationship will be numerous.

The definitions of terms used by Travelbee are often quite wordy. Travelbee also uses different terms for the same definition. She equates the terms *rapport, human-to-human relationship,* and *human-to-human relatedness* with the same definition. This leads to inconsistencies when labels are periodically substituted throughout the theory.

Generality

Travelbee's theory has a wide scope of application. It was primarily generated as a result of Travelbee's experience with psychiatric patients. However, the theory is not limited to use in psychiatric settings. It is applicable in all situations in which the nurse encounters ill persons in distress.

Empirical Precision

Travelbee's theory appears to have a low degree of empirical validity. Much of the lack of empirical validity can be traced to the lack of simplicity in the theory. The terms are given definitions, but these are often not operational definitions. The theory is difficult to validate with statistical data because of the lack of operational definitions.

Derivable Consequences

The usefulness of a theory is related to its ability to describe, explain, predict, and control phenomena. Travelbee's theory does explain some variables that may affect the establishment of a therapeutic relationship between nurse and patient. It also states the nurse should be able to predict the behavior of the ill person. But it lacks the ability to control phenomena of a therapeutic relationship. The lack of empirical precision also creates a lack of derivable consequences. Travelbee's theory focuses on the development of the attribute of caring. In this respect the theory can be useful, because caring is a major characteristic of the nursing profession.

REFERENCES

1. Doona, M.E. (1984, Oct.). Personal interview. (Nursing instructor, Boston College.)
2. Doona, M.E. (1984, Oct.). Telephone interview.
3. Frankl, V. (1963). *Man's search for meaning: An introduction to logotherapy.* New York: Washington Square Press.
4. Kübler-Ross, E. (1975). *Death: The final stage of growth.* Englewood Cliffs, N.J.: Prentice-Hall.
5. Orlando, I.J. (1961). *The dynamic nurse-patient relationship.* New York: G.P. Putnam.
6. Schoon, F. (1984, Oct.). Personal interview. (Hospice nurse.)
7. Taylor, K. (1984, Oct.). Telephone interview. (Former student and colleague of Joyce Travelbee.)
8. Travelbee, J. (1964, Jan.). What's wrong with sympathy? *American Journal of Nursing, 64*:68-71.
9. Travelbee, J. (1971). *Interpersonal aspects of nursing.* Philadelphia: F.A. Davis.

BIBLIOGRAPHY

Primary Sources

Books

Travelbee, J. (1966). *Interpersonal aspects of nursing.* Philadelphia: F.A. Davis.

Travelbee, J. (1969). *Intervention in psychiatric nursing: Process in the one-to-one relationship.* Philadelphia: F.A. Davis.
Travelbee, J. (1971). *Interpersonal aspects of nursing* (2d ed.). Philadelphia: F.A. Davis.
Travelbee, J. & Doona, M.E. (1979). *Travelbee's intervention in psychiatric nursing* (2d ed.). Philadelphia: F.A. Davis.

Articles

Travelbee, J. (1963, Feb.). Humor survives the test of time. *Nursing Outlook, 11*:128.
Travelbee, J. (1963, Feb.). What do we mean by rapport? *American Journal of Nursing, 63*:70-72.
Travelbee, J. (1964, Jan.). What's wrong with sympathy? *American Journal of Nursing, 64*:68-71.

Secondary Sources

Book Reviews

Travelbee, J. (1966). *Interpersonal aspects of nursing.*
Nursing Outlook, 14:77, June 1966.
American Journal of Nursing, 66:1504, July 1966.
Nursing Mirror, 122:438, August 5, 1966.
Supervisor Nurse, 2:44+, December 1971.
Nursing Outlook, 20:278, April 1972.
Journal of Nursing Administration, 3:14-15, January-February 1973.
Travelbee, J. (1969). *Intervention in psychiatric nursing: Process in the one-to-one relationship.*
American Journal of Nursing, 70:101-102, January 1970.
Nursing Outlook, 18:16, August 1970.
Nursing Mirror, 131:31, September 18, 1970.

Book Chapters

Chin, R. (1974). The utility of system models and development models for practitioners. In J. Riehl & C. Roy (Eds.), *Conceptual models for nursing practice.* New York: Appleton-Century-Crofts, pp. 46-53.
Meleis, A.I. (1985). Joyce Travelbee. In A.I. Meleis, *Theoretical nursing: Development and Progress.* Philadelphia: J.B. Lippincott, pp. 254-262.
Roy, C. (1974). Travelbee's developmental approach. In J.P. Riehl & C. Roy (Eds.), *Conceptual models for nursing practice.* New York: Appleton-Century-Crofts, pp. 267-268.
Thibodeau, J.A. (1983). An interaction model: The Travelbee model. In J.A. Thibodeau, *Nursing models: Analysis and evaluation.* Belmont, Calif.: Wadsworth, pp. 89-104.

Articles

Arnold, H.M. (1976). Working with schizophrenic patients: Guide to one-to-one relationships. *American Journal of Nursing, 76*:941-943.
Axelsson, K., Norbert, A., & Asplund, K. (1986). Relearning to eat late after a stroke by systematic nursing intervention: A case report. *Journal of Advanced Nursing, 11*:553-559.
Bullough, V.L. & Seidl, A. (1987). Attitudes on sexuality in nursing texts today and yesterday. *Holistic Nursing Practice, 1(4)*:84-92.
Cohen, Marlene Z. (1987). A historical overview of the phenomenologic movement. *Image, 19(1)*:31-34.
Fenton, M.V. (1987). Development of the scale of humanistic nursing behaviors. *Nursing Research, 36*:82-93.
Flaskerud, J.H. (1986). On "Toward a theory of nursing action: Skills and competency in nurse-patient interaction." *Nursing Research, 35*:250-252.
Freihofer, P., & Felton, G. (1976). Nursing behaviors in bereavement. *Nursing Research, 25*:332-337.
Henault, M. (1985). Un obstacle de plus pour l'enfant qui eprouve des problemes psychosociaux. *Nursing Quebec, 5(7)*:24-27.
Hinds, P.S. (1984). Introducing a definition of hope through the use of grounded theory methodology. *Journal of Advanced Nursing, 9*:357-362.
Kasch, C.R. (1986). Skills and competency in nurse-patient interaction. *Nursing Research, 35*:226-229.
Koshi, P.T. (1976). Cultural diversity in nursing curricula. *Journal of Nursing Education, 15*:14-21.
Larson, P.A. (1977). Nurse perceptions of patient characteristics. *Nursing Research, 26*:416-421.
Limandri, B.J., & Boyle, D.W. (1978). Instilling hope. *American Journal of Nursing, 78*:78-80.
McBride, A.B. (1986). Theory and research: Present issues and future perspectives of psychosocial nursing. *Journal of Psychosocial Nursing, 24(9)*:29-32.
Morse, B.W., & Vandenberg, E. (1978). Interpersonal relationships in nursing practice, interdisciplinary approach. *Communication Education, 27*:158-163.
Paul, D., Hagan, L., & Lambert, J. (1985). Au-dela du malade. *Nursing Quebec, 5(7)*:18-23.

Peterson, E.A. & Nelson, K. (1987). How to meet your clients' spiritual needs. *Journal of Psychosocial Nursing, 25(5)*:34-39.

Sarter, B. (1987). Evolutionary idealism. *Advanced Nursing Science, 9(2)*:1-9.

Schweer, S.F., & Dayani, E.C. (1973). Extended role of professional nursing: Patient education. *International Nursing Review, 20*:174+.

Sodestrom, K.E. & Martinson, I.M. (1987). Patients' spiritual coping strategies: A study of nurse and patient perspectives. *Oncology Nursing Forum, 14(2)*:41-44.

Sorgen, L.M. (1979). Student learning following an educational experience at an alcohol rehabilitation center in Saskatoon, Saskatchewan, Canada. *International Journal of Nursing Studies, 16*:41-50.

Spratlen, L.P. (1976). Introducing ethnic-cultural factors in models of nursing: Some mental health applications. *Journal of Nursing Education, 15*: 23-29.

Stetler, C.B. (1977). Relationship of perceived empathy to nurses' communication. *Nursing Research, 26*:432-438.

Stoll, R.I. (1979). Guidelines for spiritual assessment. *American Journal of Nursing, 79*:1574-1577.

Wallston, K.A., & Wallston, B.S. (1975). Role-playing simulation approach toward studying nurses decisions to listen to patients. *Nursing Research, 24*:16-22.

Wallston, K.A., Wallston, B.S., & Devellis, B.M. (1976). Effect of a negative stereotype on nurse's attitudes toward an alcoholic patient. *Journal of Studies on Alcohol, 37*:659-665.

Correspondence

Doona, M.E. (1984, Oct. 19). Personal communication.

Interviews

Doona, M.E. (1984, Oct.). Telephone interview.

Taylor, K. (1984, Oct.). Telephone interview.

Other Sources

Barrett-Lennard, G.T. (1962). Dimensions of therapist responses as causal factors in therapeutic change. *Psychological Monographs, 76*:43 (Whole No. 562).

Cartwright, R.D. & Lerner, B. (1963). Empathy, need to change, and improvement with psychotherapy. *Journal of Consulting Psychology, 27*:138-144.

Chinsky, J.M. & Rappaport, J. (1970). Brief critique of the meaning and reliability of "accurate empathy" ratings. *Psychological Bulletin, 73*:379-382.

Frankl, V. (1963). *Man's search for meaning: An introduction to logotherapy.* New York: Washington Square Press.

Kurtz, R.R. & Grummon, D.L. (1972). Different approaches to the measurement of therapist empathy and their relationship to therapy outcomes. *Journal of Consulting and Clinical Psychology, 30*:106-115.

May, R. (1953). *Man's search for himself.* New York: W.W. Norton.

McBride, M.A. (1967). Nursing approach, pain, and relief: An exploratory experiment. *Nursing Research, 16*(4):337-341.

19

Ida Jean Orlando (Pelletier)

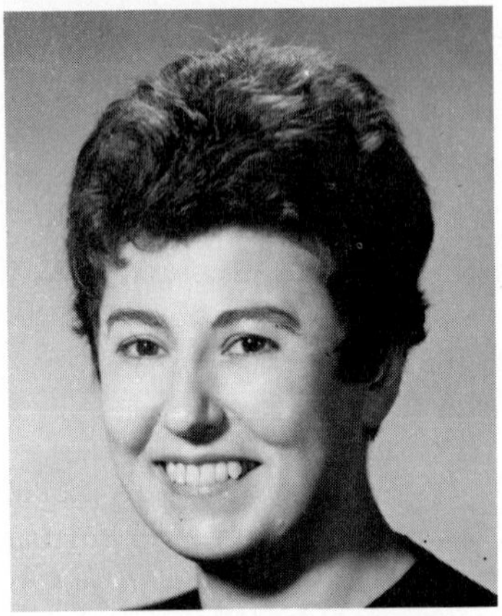

Nursing Process Theory

Ann Marriner-Tomey, Deborah I. Mills, Marcia K. Sauter

CREDENTIALS AND BACKGROUND OF THE THEORIST

Ida Jean Orlando was born August 12, 1926. In 1947 she received a diploma in nursing from New York Medical College, Flower Fifth Avenue Hospital School of Nursing in New York. She received a B.S. in Public Health Nursing from St. Johns University in Brooklyn, New York, in 1951, and an M.A. in Mental Health Consultation from Columbia University Teachers College in New York in 1954. While pursuing her education, Orlando worked intermittently, and sometimes concurrently, as a staff nurse in obstetrical, medical, surgical, and emergency nursing services. She also worked as a supervisor in a general hospital. In addition, as an assistant director of nurses, she held responsibility for a general hospital's nursing service and responsibility for teaching several courses in the hospital's nursing school.

The authors wish to acknowledge Ida Orlando Pelletier's review of the chapter and verification of this representation of her work.

After receiving her master's in 1954, Orlando went to the Yale School of Nursing in New Haven, Connecticut, for 8 years, where she was a research associate and principal project investigator on a federal project grant entitled "Integration of Mental Health Concepts in a Basic Curriculum" until 1958. The project focused on identifying factors influencing the integration of mental health principles in a basic nursing curriculum. Orlando carried out this project by observing and participating in student experiences with patients and medical, nursing, and instructional personnel throughout the basic curriculum. She recorded her observations for 3 years and then spent a fourth year analyzing the accumulated data. She reported her findings in 1958 in her first book, *The Dynamic Nurse-Patient Relationship: Function, Process and Principles of Professional Nursing Practice.* It was not published until 1961, but since then five foreign-language editions have appeared. The formulations in this book provided the foundation for Orlando's nursing theory.[22:243] During the next 4 years (1958–1961), as an associate professor and the director of the Graduate Program in Mental Health and Psychiatric Nursing, Orlando used her theory as the foundation of the program. She married Robert J. Pelletier and left Yale in 1961.

Orlando spent the years 1962–1972 as Clinical Nursing Consultant at McLean Hospital in Belmont, Massachusetts. From this position she studied the interaction of nurses with patients, other nurses, and other staff members and how these activities affected the process of the nurses' help to patients. Orlando convinced the hospital director that a training program for nurses was needed, whereupon McLean Hospital initiated one based on her theory. The nursing service of the hospital was reorganized as a result of this program.[26:45] Orlando subsequently applied for and received federal funding to evaluate training in the process discipline.

While at McLean Hospital, Orlando[27] published "The Patient's Predicament and Nursing Function" in a 1967 issue of *Psychiatric Opinion.* In 1972 she reported the 10 years of work at the hospital in her second book, *The Discipline and Teaching of Nursing Process: An Evaluative Study.*

From 1972 to 1981 Orlando lectured, served as a consultant, and conducted about 60 workshops in her theory throughout the United States and Canada. She has served on the Board of the Harvard Community Health Plan in Boston, Massachusetts, from 1972 to 1984 and on the Hospital Committee of the board from 1979 to 1985. She has since served in various capacities such as on the membership, program, and services committees.

In 1981 Orlando accepted a position as nurse educator for Metropolitan State Hospital in Waltham, Massachusetts. From 1984 until 1987 Orlando held various administrative nursing positions there. In September 1987, she became the assistant director of nursing for education and research at Metropolitan State Hospital.[28]

Orlando's nursing theory emphasizes the reciprocal relationship between patient and nurse. Both are affected by what the other says and does. Orlando[24:133] may have facilitated the development of nurses as logical thinkers rather than conformers to the medical orders of a physician. She was one of the first nursing leaders to emphasize the elements of nursing process and the critical importance of the patient's participation during the nursing process.

Orlando[28] says that her search for facts in observing nursing situations influenced her most before the development of her theory and that she derived her theory from the conceptualization of those facts. Her overall goal was to find an organizing principle for professional nursing, that is, a distinct function.[25:viii] Orlando has made a major contribution to nursing theory and practice. Her conceptualizations fulfill the criteria of theory because she presents interrelated concepts that present a systematic view of nursing phenomena; she specifies relationships among the concepts; she explains what happens during the nursing process and why; she prescribes how nursing phenomena can be controlled; and she explains how the control leads to prediction of outcome. Although nursing writers such as Fitzpatrick and Whall[16:5] do not believe any current nursing model meets the level of specificity of theory described by Ellis, Orlando's theory has considerable merit in application to practice, education, and research.

THEORETICAL SOURCES

Orlando acknowledges no theoretical sources for the development of her theory. None of her publications includes a bibliography.

USE OF EMPIRICAL EVIDENCE

Orlando synthesized facts from observations to develop her theory. She asserted that her theory was valid and applied it in her work with patients and nurses and the teaching of students. Orlando gathered a considerable amount of data before constructing her theory. She used a research process but did not follow research methodology for quantitative analysis.[13:59]

At McLean Hospital Orlando implemented the nursing process theory that she had developed at Yale. During the last three years she was there she got a research grant to do evaluative research of the training program to test what she thought had happened. She published the results in her second book.

MAJOR CONCEPTS AND DEFINITIONS

Perception. "A physical stimulation of any one of a person's five senses."[26:59]

Thought. "An idea which occurs in the mind of a person."[26:59]

Feeling. "A state of mind inclining a person toward or against a perception, thought or action."[26:59]

Action. "Observable behavior, i.e., what the individual says verbally and/or manifests nonverbally."[26:60]

MAJOR ASSUMPTIONS

Nearly all of the assumptions in Orlando's theory are implicit.

Nursing

The major assumption Orlando makes about nursing is it should be a distinct profession that functions autonomously. Although nursing has been historically aligned with medicine, and continues to have a close relationship with medicine, nursing and the practice of medicine are clearly separate professions.[25:8,12] These assumptions are reflected in Orlando's definition of the function of professional nursing.

Orlando[26:20] states that "the function of professional nursing is conceptualized as finding out and meeting the patient's immediate need for help." This may be more fully developed by Orlando's approach to nursing process, which she proposes is composed of the following basic elements: "(1) the behavior of the patient, (2) the reaction of the nurse, and (3) the nursing actions which are designed for the patient's benefit. The interaction of these elements with each other is nursing process."[25:36]

Orlando[26:7] emphasizes that inadequate patient care is "a generic manifestation of nursing's collective failure to fully articulate and exercise in its education and practice a distinct function." Another assumption Orlando[26:9] makes is that nurses should relieve physical or mental discomfort and should not add to the patient's distress. This assumption is evident in Orlando's concept of improvement in the patient's behavior as the intended outcome of nursing actions.

Person

Orlando assumes that persons behave verbally and nonverbally. Evidence of this assumption is found in Orlando's emphasis on behavior. Orlando assumes that persons are sometimes able to meet their own needs for help in some situations, but that persons become distressed when unable to do so. This is the basis for Orlando's assertion[25:22] that professional nurses should be concerned only with those persons who are unable to state the need for help clearly.

Health

Orlando[25:9] does not define health but assumes that freedom from mental or physical discomfort and feelings of adequacy and well-being contribute to health.[25:9]

Environment

Orlando does not define environment. She assumes that a nursing situation occurs when there is a nurse-patient contact and that both nurse and patient perceive, think, feel, and act in the immediate situation.

THEORETICAL ASSERTIONS

Orlando[25:8] views the professional function of nursing as finding out and meeting the immediate needs for help of the patient. This function is fulfilled when the nurse ascertains and meets the patient's immediate needs for help. Consequently Orlando's theory focuses on how to produce improvement in the patient's behavior.

A person becomes a patient requiring nursing care when he or she has unmet needs for help that cannot be met independently because of physical limitations, a negative reaction to an environment, or experiences preventing the patient from communicating needs for help.[25:11] Orlando[25:10] asserts that these limitations on the patient's ability to meet his needs are most likely to occur while the patient is receiving medical care or supervision. Thus the restrictions Orlando has frequently placed on the concept of patient can be seen as a function of the impediments persons have in meeting their needs.

Patients experience distress or feelings of helplessness as a result of unmet needs for help.[25:61] Orlando[25:46-47] believes there is a positive correlation between the length of time the patient experiences the unmet needs and the degree of distress. Therefore immediacy is emphasized throughout her theory. In Orlando's view,[25:22] when persons are able to meet their own needs, they do not feel distress and do not require care from a professional nurse. For those persons who do have a need for help, it is essential the nurse obtain correction or verification of the nurse's perceptions, thoughts, and feelings in order to determine whether the patient is in need of help.[25:29] It is the nurse's responsibility to see that "the patient's needs for help are met, either directly by her own activity or indirectly by calling in the help of others."[25:29]

Individuals in contact with each other go through an action process that involves observation of the other's behavior, the resulting thoughts and feelings about this observation and an action chosen by each individual in response to the reaction.[26:25] When the nurse acts, an action process transpires. This action process by the nurse in the nurse-patient contact is called nursing process.[26:29] The nursing process may be automatic or deliberative. Any behavior of the patient observed by the nurse must be viewed as a possible signal of distress, because it is possible for the patient to "react with distress to any aspect of an environment which was designed for therapeutic and helpful purposes."[25:17,40] Perception of patient behavior produces thoughts and feelings in the nurse. Orlando defines *reaction* as including perception, a physical stimulation of any one of a person's five senses; thought, an idea that occurs in an individual's mind; and feeling, a state of mind inclining a person toward or against a perception, thought, or feeling.[25:25] The nurse's reaction precipitates nursing actions.[25:61]

Asking the patient about the nurse's perception of the patient's behavior is more effective and less time consuming because the physical stimulus for perception has objective validity. Nursing actions that are not deliberative are automatic.[25:60] Automatic nursing actions are those having nothing to do with finding out and meeting patient's needs for help. Deliberative nursing activities are those designed to identify and meet the patient's immediate need for help and, therefore, to fulfill the professional nursing function. Deliberative nursing actions require that the nurse seek validation or correction of her thoughts and feelings with the patient before she and the patient can know what nursing action will meet the need for help.[25:41]

In her second book Orlando renamed deliberative nursing activity a *process discipline* with three specific requirements. Application of the process discipline qualifies as a *disciplined professional response*.[26:29,31] Despite this change in terminology, Orlando provides a clear procedure for nurses to ascertain and meet a patient's needs for help. First, the nurse expresses to the patient any or all of the items contained in her reaction to the patient's behavior. Second, the nurse verbally states to the patient that the expressed item belongs to the nurse by use of the personal pronoun (an "I" message). Finally, the nurse asks about the item expressed, attempting to verify or correct her perceptions, thoughts, or feelings (reaction).[26:29-30]

The value of the process discipline is in determining whether the patient feels distressed and ascertaining what help is required to relieve the distress.[25:29] Without the investigation required by the process discipline the nurse does not have a reliable data base for action.[26:32] When the nurse responds automatically, the perceptions, thoughts, and feelings of each person are not available to the other. When the nurse uses the process discipline, the perceptions, thoughts, and feeling of the nurse are available to the patient and vice versa.[26:25-27] This latter response is viewed by Orlando[25:67] as a form of "continuous reflection as the nurse tries to understand the meaning to the patient of the behavior she observed and what he needs from her in order to be helped." The nurse evaluates her actions by comparing the patient's verbal and nonverbal behavior at the end of the contact with the behavior that was present when the process started.[25:68]

LOGICAL FORM

Orlando's theory is inductive. Orlando collected records of her observations of nurse-patient situations during a 3-year period. In analyzing this material, Orlando looked for "good" versus "bad" outcomes. Good nursing outcomes were defined as those that improved the patient's behavior. Bad nursing outcomes were defined as absence of improvement. Orlando concluded that the nurse's use of the process discipline was an effective means of achieving a good outcome. On this basis, Orlando synthesized her theory.[13:34]

Using Walker and Avant's criteria[39:125-128] for theory analysis, Orlando's theory is logically adequate. Because inductive argument can produce false conclusions even when the premises are true, Orlando's conclusions seem reasonable. The structure of relationships are clear and sufficiently precise; and it is possible to represent the relationships schematically. The relationships progress from existence and conditional statements to prediction and control. The predictions Orlando makes are acceptable to the nursing profession since improvement in patient care is always valuable. There are no logical fallacies within Orlando's theory because relationships are sufficiently developed.

ACCEPTANCE BY THE NURSING COMMUNITY

Practice

Orlando's theory is clearly applicable to nursing practice, yet little evidence of acceptance by the nursing community exists in the literature. Schmidt[33:72] reported using Orlando's theory as a basis for practice in 1972. Peitchinis[29] suggested that Orlando's deliberative approach reflected the elements of the therapeutic relationship, which include expression of empathy, warmth, and genuineness. She proposed that nursing practice based on Orlando's theory would increase the therapeutic effectiveness of nursing.[29:146]

The use of Orlando's theory as a basis of

practice in the Mid Missouri Mental Health Center and in a new psychiatric unit in a general hospital in Antigonish, Nova Scotia, are other examples of use by the nursing community. Henderson[20:119] wrote in 1978 that Orlando's insistence on validation was an important contribution to the practice of nursing. More recently, Schmieding[34] reported the advantages of adopting Orlando's theory throughout a department of nursing. Implementation of Orlando's theory produced several benefits. They included increased effectiveness in meeting patient needs; improvement in decision-making skills among staff nurses, particularly in determining what constituted nursing versus nonnursing activities; more effective conflict resolution among staff nurses and between staff and physicians; and a greater sense of identity and unity among staff.[34:761]

Schmieding[36] also discusses "how specific types of actions facilitate or thwart problem identification." Using Orlando's theory, managerial responses in face-to-face contacts were analyzed. Boston's Beth Israel Hospital Division of Nursing Statement of Philosophy and Purpose represents their nursing service based on Henderson, Weidenback, and Orlando. Consequently, there is evidence that Orlando's theory is used at the patient care level, managerial level, and nursing division level.

Orlando's nursing process is confined to every immediate nurse-patient contact. Observation of the patient's verbal and nonverbal behavior provides data for determining the patient's level of distress when the process discipline is used. The nurse then takes actions to meet the patient's need for help. Finally, the nurse investigates her newer observations to learn whether the action actually relieved the distress (evaluation). If the distress is not relieved, the process begins again.

Education

Orlando's theory is a conceptual framework for the process by which professional nursing should be practiced. Orlando's process recording has made a significant contribution to nursing education. Orlando[26:32-33] found that "training" in the process discipline was necessary in order for the nurse to be able to control the nursing process and achieve improvement in the patient's behavior. She therefore developed the process recording, a tool to facilitate self-evaluation of whether or not the process discipline was used. This "systematic repetitious examination and study of the nursing process" was designed to help students learn how to express their reactions to patients and to ask for correction or verification.[26:32-33] The process recording is an educational tool still used in nursing education.

Orlando[25:vii] wrote her first book "to offer the professional nursing student a theory of effective practice." Since 1961 numerous psychiatric nursing texts have included Orlando's theory. Orlando deserves credit for providing guidelines for the nurse to use in contacts with patients. Orlando's theory was instrumental in development of the interaction theory currently used in psychiatric nursing.[3:117]

In Winder's[41] discussion of a nursing curriculum, he identifies the need to provide a "facilitating environment and implementing the caring process." He suggests that Orlando's theory provides a model for such a training process in her book *The Discipline and Teaching of Nursing Process.*

Haggerty[18] analyzed nursing students' responses to distressed patients based on Orlando's nursing process concept. Haggerty found that "emphasis on communication and psychosocial foundations in BSN curriculums may not translate into more effective exploratory skills in these students." She recommends Orlando's model for teaching BSN students to conceptualize the interactional process and its goals.

Research

Orlando's theory has enjoyed considerable acceptance by the nursing profession in the area of research and has been applied to a variety of research settings. Many of the studies have provided empirical evidence that Orlando's theoretical assertions are valid. These are discussed under Empirical Precision.

Orlando's definition of the concept *need for help* was used by K. Dracup and C. Breu[9:213] in their study of the needs of grieving spouses, and by S. Hampe[19:114] in a similar study. Orlando's *deliberative nursing* has been designated the *experimental approach* in several studies to examine its effects on a patient's distress during admission and before surgery. B. Anderson, H. Mertz, and R. Leonard[1:151] found that deliberative nursing actions promoted stress reduction during admission. J. Wolfer and M. Visintainer[42:248] demonstrated this same result with children and their parents. R. Dumas and R. Johnson[11:140] determined that preoperative exploration with patients to determine the real source of distress permitted the nurse to take appropriate action to relieve the distress, and that lower distress before surgery correlated with fewer postoperative complications. Deliberative nursing was used as the experimental nursing action by Dumas and R. Leonard[12:12] in their study of postoperative vomiting.

Haggerty,[18] as alluded to earlier, used Orlando's nursing process concept to conduct research on nursing students' responses to distressed patients. Princeton[31] tested the effects of a deliberative nursing care approach with breast-feeding mothers and their babies. These studies using the deliberative nursing approach can be considered both theory-testing and theory-generating. They have provided empirical support for Orlando's theory (theory-testing) and have produced new principles for practice, especially in the area of preoperative teaching (theory-generating).

FURTHER DEVELOPMENT

The process discipline needs to be taught and then implemented in a variety of settings. Orlando's study could be replicated to validate that the process discipline is directly related to effectiveness of a nursing system.

CRITIQUE

Clarity

Orlando's first book, *The Dynamic Nurse-Patient Relationship,* presented concepts clearly. The second book, *The Discipline and Teaching of Nursing Process,* redefined and renamed *deliberative nursing process* as *nursing process discipline.* Orlando's writing style involves defining concepts minimally at first and then developing them throughout the book. Because of the evolution of the theory the reader must be familiar with both books to evaluate her theory thoroughly.

Simplicity

As Orlando deals with relatively few concepts and their relationships with each other, her theory would be considered simple. Her theory may also be viewed as simplistic because she is able to make some predictive statements as opposed to just description and explanation. The simplicity of Orlando's theory has benefited research application.

Generality

Orlando discussed and illustrated nurse-patient contacts in which the patient is conscious, able to communicate, and in need of help. Although she did not focus on unconscious patients and groups, application of her theory to groups or unconscious patients is feasible. Actually, any other person could make use of the process discipline if educated properly. Therefore, although Orlando's theory focuses on a limited number of situations, it could be adapted to other nursing situations and other professional fields.

Empirical Precision

Two-thirds of Orlando's second book is a report of a research project designed to test the validity of her nursing formulations. A training program based on her formulations had been in progress for 3 years before the project began.[26:44] Nurses were trained to use the process discipline in nurse-patient contacts. Those nurses who became clinical nursing supervisors were trained to use the process discipline in their supervisory and other contacts as well. The following is a brief description of the research methodology.

The purpose of the project was to evaluate the effectiveness of the process discipline in the nurse's contacts at work and the effectiveness of the training program. But these evaluations could not take place before hypothetical measures for the process discipline and the effectiveness of the discipline were identified. A discipline variable was defined.[26:60] Effectiveness was determined by the presence or absence of a *helpful outcome,* as judged by two reliable outcome coders. The outcome coders compared the beginning behavior of the subject with the behavior at the end of the record.[26:76] Testing the relationship of the process discipline (in use) with the presence or absence of a helpful outcome in patient, staff, and supervisee contacts was also done. Evaluation of the training program was done by testing whether nurses increased their use of the process discipline after being trained.[26:63-66]

Two groups of nurses were included in the study. The control group consisted of "veterans"—previously trained supervisors and staff nurses. The experimental group consisted of "novices"—untrained supervisors and staff nurses. Transcripts were made of tape-recorded 10-minute periods (six for each subject) of novices' and veterans' contacts at work.

This report is extensive and detailed and may be difficult to read and interpret for those without a good understanding of statistics and research methodology. The study concludes that training in the nursing process discipline and its use achieves helpful outcomes in patient, supervisee, and staff contacts.

Although Orlando's work is difficult to understand, numerous studies by Orlando's first graduate students at Yale in the 1960s supported the validity of her theory.[1,5,6,10-15] Several that incorporated Orlando's deliberative nursing approach have already been mentioned in research application. Others, which specifically tested the usefulness of the deliberative approach, included: D. Pienschke,[30:484-489] who found that nursing intervention was more effective under conditions of open disclosure because patients' needs were perceived more accurately; M. Bochnak,[5:191-192] who found that a deliberative nursing process was more effective in relieving patients' pain; M. Dye,[14:194] who controlled for staff-patient ratios and amount of nursing time and still demonstrated that deliberative nursing actions met patient needs effectively; and J. Cameron,[6:192] who revealed that deliberative nursing actions led to the most consistent effective results in verifying patient needs.

Orlando asserts that patient distress stems from reaction to the environment that the patient cannot control alone. Dye provided empirical evidence for this assertion in her study on clarifying patient needs. She found patients experienced distress more as a reaction to the hospital setting than to their illness.[13:59]

Orlando also asserts patient distress stems from misinterpretation by the nurse of the patient's experience or from the patient's initial inability to clearly communicate the need for help. Both necessitate use of the process discipline. Two studies, one by R. Elder and the other by N. Gowan and M. Morris, provided support for this assertion. Both studies demonstrated that although patients frequently did not express their needs clearly, deliberative nursing actions alleviated the problem.[1,5,6,10-15]

Derivable Consequences

Orlando's theory is potentially beneficial in achieving valued outcomes. Identifying the patient's needs for help and the nurse's ability to meet these needs are very important to nursing practice.

Incorporating validation into the nursing process as Orlando suggests allows for maximum participation by the patient in his or her care. Several researchers have also demonstrated that the use of disciplined professional response enables the nurse to ascertain and meet the patient's needs. The study of what nurses say and do in their practice and the resulting effect displayed by the patient is valuable content for nursing education. The nursing process discipline also allows nurses to view the patient from a nursing perspective, rather than from a medical disease orientation.

REFERENCES

1. Anderson, B., Mertz, H., & Leonard, R. (1965). Two experimental tests of a patient-centered admission process. *Nursing Research, 14*:151-156.
2. Andrews, C. (1983). Ida Orlando's model of nursing. In J. Fitzpatrick & A. Whall, *Conceptual models of nursing: Analysis and application*. Bowie, Md.: Robert J. Brady, pp. 47-65.
3. Artinian, B. (1983). Implementation of the intersystem patient-care model in clinical practice. *Journal of Advanced Nursing, 8*:117-124.
4. Baron, R.A. & Byrne, D. (1977). *Social psychology: Understanding human interaction*. Boston: Allyn & Bacon.
5. Bochnak, M. (1963). The effect of an automatic and deliberative process of nursing activity on the relief of patients' pain: A clinical experiment. *Abstract in Nursing Research, 12*:191-192.
6. Cameron, J. (1963). An exploratory study of the verbal responses of the nurses in 20 nurse-patient interactions. *Abstract in Nursing Research, 12*:292.
7. Chaska, N. (1978). *The nursing profession: Views through the mist*. New York: McGraw-Hill.
8. Chinn, P. & Jacobs, M. (1983). *Theory and nursing: A systematic approach*. St. Louis: C.V. Mosby.
9. Dracup, K. & Breu, C. (1978). Using nursing research findings to meet the needs of grieving spouses. *Nursing Research, 27*:212-216.
10. Dumas, R. (1963). Psychological preparation for surgery. *American Journal of Nursing, 63*: 52-55.
11. Dumas, R. & Johnson, B. (1972). Research in nursing practice: A review of five clinical experiments. *International Journal of Nursing Studies, 9*:137-149.
12. Dumas, R. & Leonard, R. (1963). The effect of nursing on the incidence of postoperative vomiting. *Nursing Research, 12*:12-15.
13. Dye, M. (1963). Clarifying patients' communications. *American Journal of Nursing, 63*:56-59.
14. Dye, M. (1963). A descriptive study of conditions conducive to an effective process of nursing activity. *Abstract in Nursing Research, 12*:194.
15. Elder, R. (1963). What is the patient saying? *Nursing Forum, 11*:25-37.
16. Fitzpatrick, J. & Whall, A. (1983). *Conceptual models of nursing: Analysis, and application*. Bowie, Md.: Robert J. Brady.
17. Gowan, N. & Morris, M. (1964). Nurses' responses to expressed patient needs. *Nursing Research, 13*:68-71.
18. Haggerty, L. (1987). An analysis of senior nursing students' immediate responses to distressed patients. *Journal of Advanced Nursing, 12*:451-461.
19. Hampe, S. (1975). Needs of the grieving spouse in a hospital setting. *Nursing Research, 24*:113-120.
20. Henderson, V. (1978). The concept of nursing. *Journal of Advanced Nursing, 3*:113-130.
21. Larson, P., Sr. (1977). Nurse perceptions of patient characteristics. *Nursing Research, 26*:416-421.
22. McCann-Flynn, J. & Heffron, B. (1984). *Nursing: From concept to practice*. Bowie, Md.: Robert J. Brady.
23. Murray, R. & Huelskoetter, M. (1983). *Psychiatric-mental health nursing: Giving emotional care*. Englewood Cliffs, N.J.: Prentice-Hall.
24. Nursing Theories Conference Group, J.B. George, Chairperson. (1980). *Nursing theories: The base for professional practice*. Englewood Cliffs, N.J.: Prentice-Hall.
25. Orlando, I. (1961). *The dynamic nurse-patient relationship*. New York: G.P. Putnam's Sons.
26. Orlando, I. (1972). *The discipline and teaching of nursing process*. New York: G.P. Putnam's Sons.
27. Pelletier, I.O. (1967). The patient's predicament and nursing function. *Psychiatric Opinion, 4*:25-30.
28. Pelletier, I. (1984). Personal correspondence.
29. Peitchinis, L. (1972). Therapeutic effectiveness of counseling by nursing personnel. *Nursing Research, 21*:138-147.
30. Pienschke, D., Sr. (1973). Guardedness or

openness on the cancer unit. *Nursing Research, 22*:484-490.
31. Princeton, J. (1986). Incorporating a deliberative nursing care approach with breastfeeding mothers. *Health care for Women International, 7*:277-293.
32. Reynolds, P. (1971). *A primer in theory construction*. Indianapolis: Bobbs-Merrill.
33. Schmidt, J. (1972). Availability: A concept of nursing practice. *American Journal of Nursing, 72*:1086-1089.
34. Schmieding, N. (1984). Putting Orlando's theory into practice. *American Journal of Nursing, 84*:759-761.
35. Schmieding, N. (1984b). Evaluation of nurse administrators' actions. American Nurses Association Council of Nursing Administrators. *Nurse Facilitator, 10*:4.
36. Schmieding, N. (1987). Analysing managerial responses' in face-to-face contacts. *Journal of Advanced Nursing, 12*:357-365.
37. Schmieding, N. (1987). Problematic situations in nursing: Analysis of Orlando's theory based on Dewey's theory of inquiry. *Journal of Advanced Nursing, 12*:431-440.
38. Stevens, B. (1971). Analysis of structured forms used in nursing curricula. *Nursing Research, 20*:388-397.
39. Walker, L. & Avant, K. (1983). *Strategies for theory construction in nursing*. Norwalk, Conn.: Appleton-Century-Crofts.
40. Wilson, H. & Kneisel, C. (1983). *Psychiatric nursing*. Reading, Mass.: Addison Wesley.
41. Winder, A. (1984). A mental health professional looks at nursing care. *Nursing Forum, 21*:184-188.
42. Wolfer, J. & Visintainer, M. (1975). Pediatric surgical patients' and parents' stress responses and adjustment. *Nursing Research, 24*:244-255.

BIBLIOGRAPHY
Primary Sources
Books

Orlando, I. (1961). *The dynamic nurse-patient relationship*. New York: G.P. Putnam's Sons.

Orlando, I. (1972). *The discipline and teaching of nursing process*. New York: G.P. Putnam's Sons.

Book Chapters

Orlando, I. (1962). Function, process and principle of professional nursing practice. In *Integration of mental health concepts in the human relations professions*. New York: Bank Street College of Education.

Articles

Orlando, I. (1987). Nursing in the 21st century: Alternate path. *Journal of Advanced Nursing, 12*:405-412.

Pelletier, I.O. (1967). The patient's predicament and nursing function. *Psychiatric Opinion, 4*:25-30.

Correspondence

Pelletier, I.O. (1984). Personal correspondence.

Pelletier, I.O. (1985). Personal correspondence.

Pelletier, I.O. (1988). Personal correspondence.

Interviews

Pelletier, I.O. (1984). Telephone interviews.

Pelletier, I.O. (1985). Telephone interviews.

Pelletier, I.O. (1988). Telephone interviews.

Secondary Sources
Book Reviews

Orlando, I. (1961). *The dynamic nurse-patient relationship*.
AAINJ, 10:41, March, 1962.
Nursing Outlook, 10:221, April 1962.
Catholic Nurse, 10:54, June 1962.
Journal of Psychiatric Nursing, 1:65, January 1963.

Orlando, I. (1972). *The discipline and teaching of nursing process*.
Nursing Research, 22:10, January-February, 1973.
Supervisor Nurse, 4:48-49, February, 1973.
American Journal of Nursing, 73:926, May 1973.
Nursing Outlook, 21:432, July 1973.
Journal of Nursing Administration, 4:12, January-February 1974.

Dissertation

Schmieding, N. (1983). *A description and analysis of the directive process used by directors of nursing, supervisors, and head nurses in problematic situations based on Orlando's theory of nursing experience*. Doctoral dissertation. Boston: Boston University.

Book Chapters

Andrews, C. (1983). Ida Orlando's model of nursing. In J. Fitzpatrick & A. Whall, *Conceptual models of nursing: Analysis and application*. Bowie, Md.: Robert J. Brady.

Crane, M.D. (1980). Ida Jean Orlando. In Nursing Theories Conference Group, J.B. George, Chairperson, *Nursing theories: The base for professional nursing practice.* Englewood Cliffs, N.J: Prentice-Hall.

Meleis, A.I. (1985). Ida Orlando. In *Theoretical nursing: Development and progress.* Philadelphia: J.B. Lippincott.

Mertz, H. (1962). Nurse actions that reduce stress in patients. In *Emergency intervention by the nurse* (Monograph 1). New York: The American Nurses' Association.

Mills, D.I. & Sauter, M.K. (1986). Ida Jean Orlando (Pelletier). In A. Marriner, *Nursing theorists and their work.* St. Louis: C.V. Mosby.

Schmieding, N.J. (1983). An analysis of Orlando's theory based on Kuhn's theory of science. In P.L. Chinn, *Advances in nursing theory development.* Rockville, Md.: Aspen Systems.

Articles

Anderson, B., Mertz, H., & Leonard, R. (1965). Two experimental tests of a patient-centered admission process. *Nursing Research, 14*:151-156.

Artinian, B. (1983). Implementation of the intersystem patient-care model in clinical practice. *Journal of Advanced Nursing, 8*:117-124.

Beckstrand, J.A. (1980). A critique of several conceptions of practice model in nursing. *Research in Nursing and Health, 3*:69-79.

de la Cuesta, C. (1983). The nursing process: From development to implementation. *Journal of Advanced Nursing, 8*:365-371.

Diers, D. (1970). Faculty research development at Yale. *Nursing Research, 19(1)*:64-71.

Dracup, K. & Breu, C. (1978). Using nursing research findings to meet the needs of grieving spouses. *Nursing Research, 27*:212-216.

Dumas, R. (1963). Psychological preparation for surgery. *American Journal of Nursing, 63*:52-55.

Dumas, R. & Johnson, B. (1972). Research in nursing practice: A review of five clinical experiments. *International Journal of Nursing Studies, 9*:137-149.

Dumas, R. & Leonard, R. (1963). The effect of nursing on the incidence of postoperative vomiting. *Nursing Research, 12*:12-15.

Dye, M. (1963). Clarifying patients' communications. *American Journal of Nursing, 63*:56-59.

Eisler, J., Wolfer, J., & Diers, D. (1972). Relationship between need for social approval and postoperative recovery and welfare. *Nursing Research, 21*:520-525.

Elder, R. (1963). What is the patient saying? *Nursing Forum, 11*:25-37.

Elms, R. & Leonard, R. (1966). Effects of nursing approaches during admission. *Nursing Research, 15*:39-48.

Gowan, N. & Morris, M. (1964). Nurses' responses to expressed patient needs. *Nursing Research, 13*:68-71.

Haggerty, L. (1987). An analysis of senior nursing students' immediate response to distressed patients. *Journal of Advanced Nursing, 12*:451-461.

Hampe, S. (1975). Needs of the grieving spouse in a hospital setting. *Nursing Research, 24*:113-120.

Henderson, V. (1978). The concept of nursing. *Journal of Advanced Nursing, 3*:113-130.

Larson, P., Sr. (1977). Nurse perceptions of patient characteristics. *Nursing Research, 26*:416-421.

Lipson, J. & Meleis, A.I. (1983, Dec.). Issues in health care of Middle-Eastern patients. *The Western Journal of Medicine, 139*:854-861.

McGilloway, F. (1980). The nursing process: A problem solving approach to patient care. *International Journal of Nursing Studies, 17*:79-80.

Peitchinis, L. (1972). Therapeutic effectiveness of counseling by nursing personnel. *Nursing Research, 21*:138-147.

Pienschke, D., Sr. (1973). Guardedness or openness on the cancer unit. *Nursing Research, 22*:484-490.

Powers, M. & Woldridge, P. (1982). Factors influencing knowledge, research, and compliance of hypertensive patients. *Research in Nursing and Health, 5*:171-182.

Princeton, J. (1986). Incorporating a deliberative nursing approach with breastfeeding mothers. *Health Care for Women International, 7*:277-293.

Rhymes, J. (1964). A description of nurse-patient interaction in effective nursing activity. *Nursing Research, 13(4)*:365.

Schmidt, J. (1972). Availability: A concept of nursing practice. *American Journal of Nursing, 72*:1086-1089.

Schmieding, N. (1984). Putting Orlando's theory into practice. *American Journal of Nursing, 83*:759-761.

Schmieding, N. (1984b). Evaluation of nurse administrators' actions. American Nurses Association

Council of Nursing Administrators. *Nurse Facilitator, 10*:4.

Schmieding, N. (1987). Analysing managerial responses in face-to-face contacts. *Journal of Advanced Nursing, 12*:357-365.

Schmieding, N. (1987). Problematic situations in nursing: Analysis of Orlando's theory based on Dewey's theory of inquiry. *Journal of Advanced Nursing, 12*:431-440.

Silva, M. (1979). Effects of orientation information on spouses' anxieties and attitudes toward hospitalization and surgery. *Research in Nursing and Health, 2*:127-136.

Stevens, B. (1971). Analysis of structured forms used in nursing curricula. *Nursing Research, 20*:388-397.

Thibaudeau, M. & Reidy, M. (1977). Nursing makes a difference: A comparative study of the health behavior of mothers in three primary care agencies. *International Journal of Nursing Studies, 14*:97-107.

Tryon, P.A. (1963). An experiment of the effect of patients' participation in planning the administration of a nursing procedure. *Nursing Research, 12*:262-265.

Tryon, P.A. & Leonard, R.C. (1964). The effect of patients' participation on the outcome of a nursing procedure. *Nursing Forum, 3(2):79-89.*

Williamson, J. (1978). Methodologic dilemmas in tapping the concept of patient needs. *Nursing Research, 27*:172-177.

Winder, A. (1984). A mental health professional looks at nursing care. *Nursing Forum, 21:*184-188.

Wolfer, J. & Visintainer, M. (1975). Pediatric surgical patients' and parents' stress responses and adjustment. *Nursing Research, 24*:244-255.

Books

Beck, C.M., Rawlins, R., & Williams, S. (1984). *Mental health: Psychiatric nursing*. St. Louis: C.V. Mosby.

Carter, F. (1981). *Psychosocial nursing*. New York: Macmillan.

Chaska, N. (1978). *The nursing profession: Views through the mist*. New York: McGraw-Hill.

Chinn, P.L. & Jacobs, M.K. (1983). *Theory and nursing: A systematic approach*. St. Louis: C.V. Mosby.

Fitzpatrick, J. & Whall, A. (1983). *Conceptual models of nursing practice: Analysis and application*. Bowie, Md.: Robert J. Brady.

Joel, L. & Collins, D. (1978). *Psychiatric nursing: Model and application*. New York: McGraw-Hill.

McCann-Flynn, J. & Heffron, B. (1984). *Nursing: From concept to practice*. Bowie, Md.: Robert J. Brady.

Meleis, A. (1985). *Theoretical nursing: Development and progress*. Philadelphia: J.B. Lippincott.

Murray, R. & Huelskoetter, M. (1983). *Psychiatric-mental health nursing: Giving emotional care*. Englewood Cliffs, N.J.: Prentice-Hall.

Nursing Theories Conference Group, J.B. George, Chairperson. (1980). *Nursing theories: The base for professional nursing practice*. Englewood Cliffs, N.J.: Prentice-Hall.

Stuart, G. & Sundeen, S. (1983). *Principles and practice of psychiatric nursing*. St. Louis: C.V. Mosby.

Torres, G. (1986). *Theoretical foundations in nursing*. Norwalk, Conn.: Appleton-Century-Crofts.

Wilson, H., & Kneisel, C. (1983). *Psychiatric nursing*. Reading, Mass.: Addison Wesley.

Research Abstracts

Barron, M.A. (1966). The effects varied nursing approaches have on patients' complaints of pain. Abstract in *Nursing Research, 15(1)*:90-91.

Bochnak, M. (1963). The effect of an automatic and deliberative process of nursing activity on the relief of patients' pain: A clinical experiment. Abstract in *Nursing Research, 12*:191-192.

Cameron, J. (1963). An exploratory study of the verbal responses of the nurses in 20 nurse-patient interactions. Abstract in *Nursing Research, 12*:192.

Diers, D.K. (1966). The nurse orientation system: A method for analyzing the nurse-patient interactions. Abstract in *Nursing Research, 15(1)*:91.

Dye, M. (1963). A descriptive study of conditions conducive to an effective process of nursing activity. Abstract in *Nursing Research, 12*:194.

Faulkner, S. (1963). A descriptive study of needs communicated to the nurse by some mothers on a postpartum service. Abstract in *Nursing Research, 12*:26.

Fichelis, M. (1963). An exploratory study of labels nurses attach to patient behavior and their effect on nursing activities. Abstract in *Nursing Research, 12*:195.

20

Ernestine Wiedenbach

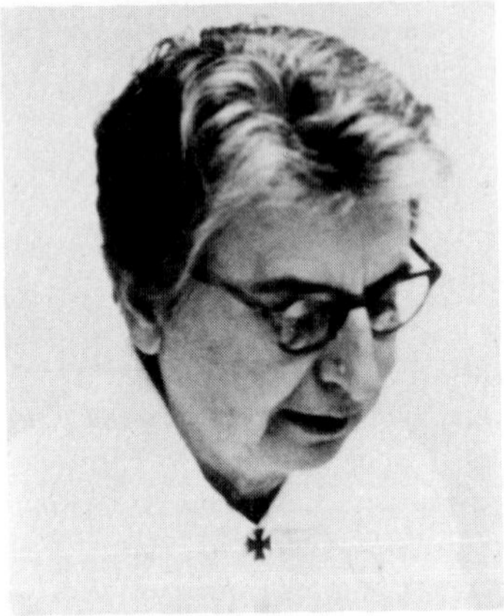

The Helping Art of Clinical Nursing

Marguerite Danko, Nancy E. Hunt, Judith E. Marich, Ann Marriner-Tomey, Cynthia A. McCreary, Margery Stuart

CREDENTIALS AND BACKGROUND OF THE THEORIST

Ernestine Wiedenbach's interest in nursing began with her childhood experiences with nurses. She greatly admired the private duty nurse who cared for her ailing grandmother and later enjoyed hearing accounts of nurses' roles in the hospital experiences of a young intern her sister was dating. Captivated by the role of the nurse, Wiedenbach enrolled in the Johns Hopkins Hospital School of Nursing after graduating from Wellesley College with a bachelor's degree in liberal arts. After completing her study at Johns Hopkins, she held a variety of positions in hospitals and public health nursing agencies in New York. She also continued her education by attending evening classes at Teachers College, Columbia University, from which she received a master's degree and a Certificate in Public Health Nursing. During this period Hazel Corbin, director of the Maternity

The authors wish to express appreciation to Catherine Martin, Janet Pezelle, and Nancy Preuss for their assistance with data collection and to Ernestine Wiedenbach for critiquing the chapter.

Center Association of New York, persuaded Wiedenbach to enroll in the Association's School for Nurse-Midwives. After completing the program, Wiedenbach practiced as a nurse-midwife in the home delivery service of the Maternity Center Association.

In addition to her practice, she also developed her academic career. She taught an evening course in advanced maternity nursing at Teachers College, wrote several articles for professional publications, and wrote a textbook on clinical nursing. She was also active in professional nursing organizations. Then in 1952 she moved from New York to Connecticut, where she was subsequently appointed to the faculty of the Yale University School of Nursing. It was out of this vast practical experience and education that she developed her model.[7:1] After a long career at Yale, she retired and moved to Florida.

THEORETICAL SOURCES

At Yale, Wiedenbach's theory development benefited from her contact with fellow faculty members. Ida Orlando Pelletier stimulated Wiedenbach's understanding of the use of self and the effect a nurse's thoughts and feelings has on the outcome of her actions. In addition, Patricia James and William Dickhoff, who taught a course in nursing theory, reviewed the manuscript for Wiedenbach's book, *Clinical Nursing—A Helping Art*. In it they identified elements of a prescriptive theory, which Wiedenbach[7] developed more fully in *Meeting the Realities in Clinical Teaching*.

USE OF EMPIRICAL EVIDENCE

At present there is no specific research supporting Wiedenbach's work. Her model was developed on the basis of her years of experience in clinical practice and teaching.

MAJOR CONCEPTS AND DEFINITIONS

PATIENT. To understand Ernestine Wiedenbach's theory, it is necessary to understand her concepts and how her definitions of common nursing terms may differ from or be similar to the current definitions of those words. She defines a patient as "any individual who is receiving help of some kind, be it care, instruction or advice, from a member of the health professions or from a worker in the field of health."[6:3] Thus, to be a patient, one does not necessarily have to be sick. Someone receiving preventive health care teaching would qualify as a patient.

NEED-FOR-HELP. Wiedenbach believed every individual experiences needs as a normal part of living. A need is anything the individual may require "to maintain or sustain himself comfortably or capably in his situation."[6:5] An attempt to meet the need is made by the intervention of help, which is "any measure or action that enables the individual to overcome whatever interferes with his ability to function capably in relation to his situation. . . . To be meaningful, help must be used by an individual and must succeed in enhancing or extending his capability."[6:5-6] Wiedenbach combines these two definitions into a more critical concept for her theory of a need-for-help.

A need-for-help is "any measure or action required and desired by the individual and which has potential for restoring or extending his ability to cope with the demands implicit in his situation."[6:6] It is crucial to the nursing profession that a need-for-help be based on the individual's perception of his own situation. If one does not perceive a need as a need-for-help, one may not take action to relieve or resolve it.

NURSE

> The nurse is a functioning human being. As such she not only acts, but she thinks and feels as well. The thoughts she thinks and the feelings she feels as she goes about her nursing are important; they are intimately involved not only in what she does, but also in how she does it. They underlie every action that she takes, be it in the form of a spoken word, a written communication, a gesture, or a deed of any kind. For the nurse whose action is directed toward

achievement of a specific purpose, thoughts and feelings have a disciplined role to play.[6:8]

PURPOSE

Purpose—that which the nurse wants to accomplish through what she does—is the overall goal toward which she is striving, and so is constant. It is her reason for being and for doing; it is the why of clinical nursing and transcends the immediate intent of her assignment or task by specifically directing her activities toward the "good" of her patient.[6:13]

PHILOSOPHY

Philosophy, an attitude toward life and reality that evolves from each nurse's beliefs and code of conduct, motivates the nurse to act, guides her thinking about what she is to do and influences her decisions. It stems from both her culture and subculture, and is an integral part of her. It is personal in character, unique to each nurse, and expressed in her way of nursing. Philosophy underlies purpose, and purpose reflects philosophy.[6:13]

PRACTICE

Overt action, directed by disciplined thoughts and feelings toward meeting the patient's need-for-help, constitutes the practice of clinical nursing. . . . It is goal-directed, deliberately carried out and patient-centered.[6:23]

Knowledge, judgment, and skills are three aspects of practice that are necessary to be effective.[6:25] Identification, ministration, and validation are three components of practice directly related to the patient's care. Coordination of resources is indirectly related to it.[6:31]

Knowledge

Knowledge encompasses all that has been perceived and grasped by the human mind; its scope and range are infinite. Knowledge may be acquired by the nurse, apart from judgment and skills, in a so-called ivory-tower setting. When acquired in this way, it has potentiality for use in directing, teaching, co-ordinating and planning care of the patient, but is not sufficient to meet his need-for-help. To be effective in meeting this need, such knowledge must be supplemented by opportunity for the nurse to function in a nurse-patient relationship with responsibility to exercise judgment and to implement skills for the benefit of the patient. Knowledge may be factual, speculative, or practical.[6:25]

Factual knowledge. "Factual knowledge is something that may be accepted as existing or as being true."[6:25-26]

Speculative knowledge. "Speculative knowledge on the other hand, encompasses theories, general principles offered to explain phenomena, beliefs or concepts, and the content of such special subject areas as the natural sciences, the social sciences, and the humanities."[6:26]

Practical knowledge. "Practical knowledge is knowing how to apply factual or speculative knowledge to the situation at hand."[6:26]

Judgment

Judgment represents the nurse's potentiality for making sound decisions. Judgment grows out of a cognitive process which involves weighing facts—both general and particular—against personal values derived from ideals, principles and convictions. It also involves differentiating facts from assumptions, and relating them to cause and effect. Judgment is personal in character; it will be exercised by the nurse according to how clearly she envisions the purpose to be served, how available relevant knowledge is to her at the time, and how she reacts to prevailing circumstances such as time, setting, and individuals. Decisions resulting from the exercise of judgment will be sound or unsound according to whether or not the nurse has disciplined the functioning of her emotions and of her mind. Uncontrollable emotions can blot out knowledge as well as purpose. Unfounded assumptions can distort facts. Although whatever decision the nurse may make represents her best judgment at the moment of making it, the broader her knowledge and the more available it is to her, and the greater her clarity of purpose, the firmer will be the foundation on which her decisions rest.[6:27]

Skills

> Skills represent the nurse's potentiality for achieving desired results. Skills comprise numerous and varied acts, characterized by harmony of movement, expression and intent, by precision, and by adroit use of self. These acts are always carried out with deliberation to achieve a specific purpose and are not goals in themselves. Deliberation and purpose, therefore, differentiate skills from nurses' actions, which, although they may be carried out with proficiency, are performed with the execution of the act as the end to be attained rather than the means by which it is reached.[6:27]

Skills may be classified as procedural or communication.

Procedural skills. "Procedural skills are potentialities for implementing procedures that the nurse may need to initiate and carry out in order to identify and meet her patients' need-for-help."[6:27-28]

Communication skills. "Communication skills are capacities for expression of thoughts and feelings that the nurse desires to convey to her patient and to others associated with his care. Both verbal and nonverbal expression may be used, singly or together, to deliver a message or to elicit a particular response."[6:28]

Identification. Identification involves individualization of the patient, his experiences, and recognition of the patient's perception of his condition.

> Activities in identification are directed toward ascertaining: (1) whether the patient has a need; (2) whether he recognizes that he has a need; (3) what is interfering with his ability to meet his need; and (4) whether the need represents a need-for-help, in other words, a need that the patient is unable to meet himself.[6:31-32]

Ministration. Ministration is providing the needed help. It requires the identification of the need-for-help and the acceptability of the help to the patient.[6:32]

Validation. "Validation is evidence that the patient's functional ability was restored as a result of the help given."[6:32]

Coordination. While striving for unity and continuity, the nurse coordinates all services provided to the patient so care will not be fragmented. Reporting, consulting, and conferring are functional elements of coordination.[6:33]

Reporting. "Reporting is the act of presenting information in written or oral form and is important in keeping others informed not only about the patient's health and social history, but also about his current condition, reaction, progress, care and plan of care."[6:33-34]

Consulting. "Consulting, the act of seeking information or of asking advice, is a means of gaining, from others, an opinion or suggestion that may help the nurse to broaden her understanding before deciding on a course of action."[6:34]

Conferring. "Conferring, the act of exchanging and comparing ideas, is most often initiated to review the patient's response to the care he has so far received, and to plan his future care."[6:35]

Art. Art is "the application of knowledge and skill to bring about desired results. . . . Art is individualized action. Nursing art, then, is carried out by the nurse in a one-to-one relationship with the patient, and constitutes the nurse's conscious responses to specifics in the patient's immediate situation."[6:36] Nursing art involves three operations: stimulus, preconception, and interpretation.[6:38-39] The nurse reacts based on those operations. "Her actions may be rational, reactionary, or deliberative."[6:40]

Stimulus. The helping process is triggered by a stimulus or the patient's presenting behavior.[6:38]

Preconception. Preconception is an expectation of what the patient may be like.

> This preconception is based on knowledge gained from a great variety of sources including the patient's chart, reports from other nurses, doctors or family members, what the nurse has read or heard of patients in similar condition, her own experiences with patients in similar condition and, finally, her recollection of previous contacts with the patient.[6:38]

Interpretation. Interpretation is comparison of perception with expectation or hope. Perception is an interpretation of the stimulus and may misinterpret the patient's behavior.[6:39]

> ***Rational action***
> Rational action is an overt act taken in response solely or mainly to the doer's immediate perception of another's action—verbal or nonverbal—or situation. In a nurse-patient relationship, the nurse's action would be called rational if she responds in a way guided by only her immediate perception of the patient's behavior—what he says, what he does, or how he appears.[6:40]
>
> ***Reactionary action***
> Reactionary action, in contrast with rational action, is an overt act taken spontaneously in response to strong feelings the doer experiences when he compares his perception of another's behavior or situation with his expectation or hope about that behavior. In a nurse-patient relationship, the nurse's action is reactionary if it is taken solely or mainly in response to her reaction, to the feelings aroused in her by comparing what she perceived as the patient's behavior with what she hoped for or expected.[6:40]
>
> ***Deliberative action***
> Deliberative action is in contrast with both rational action and reactionary action. A deliberative action is an overt act which, although not failing to take account of the doer's immediate perceptions and feeling-reactions is, nonetheless, not based solely on these perceptions or feelings. Rather, deliberative action is interaction, directed toward fulfillment of an explicit purpose and carried out with judgment and understanding of how the other means the behavior which he is manifesting either verbally or nonverbally. In a nurse-patient relationship, the nurse's action is deliberative if her overt action is based on the application—in the fulfillment of her nursing purpose—of principles of helping to gain understanding of how the patient means the behavior he is manifesting.[6:41]

FRAMEWORK OF NURSING. Limits, supports, and research provide a broad framework in which clinical nursing functions. Limits, or boundaries, in a professional service give the individual guidelines to follow in practicing that profession. Professional limits are set by the profession's code; legal limits are those found in state laws and licensing requirements; local limits are set by the hospital, agency, or individual the nurse contracts to work for; and personal limits are self-imposed by the nurse herself.[6:63-73]

Supportive facilities for the practicing nurse are nursing administration, nursing education, and nursing organizations. Although these are rarely found at the patient's bedside or in the one-to-one relationship between the nurse and patient, they are nevertheless important to the nurse by maintaining standards of quality of nursing care for the profession.[6:73-80]

Wiedenbach recognized that nursing research had not received a great deal of emphasis from the profession in the past, although more nursing research was beginning to occur. She acknowledged that such activity was essential to the growth of nursing and might even "prove to be crucial to the conservation of life and the promotion of health."[6:85]

MAJOR ASSUMPTIONS
Nursing

Nurses ascribe to an explicit philosophy. Basic to this philosophy of nursing are "(1) reverence for the gift of life; (2) respect for the dignity, worth, autonomy, and individuality of each human being; (3) resolution to act dynamically in relation to one's beliefs."[6:16] Wiedenbach identifies five essential attributes of a professional person. These characteristics are:

1. Clarity of purpose.
2. Mastery of skill and knowledge essential for fulfilling the purpose.
3. Ability to establish and sustain purposeful working relationships with others, both professional and nonprofessional individuals.
4. Interest in advancing knowledge in the area of interest and in creating new knowledge.
5. Dedication to furthering the goal of mankind rather than to self-aggrandizement.[6:2]

Person

Four explicit assumptions are stated in relation to human nature:

1. Each human being is endowed with unique potential to develop—within himself—resources which enable him to maintain and sustain himself.
2. The human being basically strives toward self-direction and relative independence and desires not only to make best use of his capabilities and potentialities but to fulfill his responsibilities.
3. Self-awareness and self-acceptance are essential to the individual's sense of integrity and self-worth.
4. Whatever the individual does represents his best judgment at the moment of his doing it.[6:17]

Health

The concept of health is neither defined nor discussed in Wiedenbach's model. The definitions of nursing, patient, and need-for-help, and the relationships among these concepts imply health-related concerns in the nurse-patient situation.

Environment

Wiedenbach does not specifically address the concept of environment. It is inferred that the environment may produce obstacles resulting in a need-for-help experienced by the person (Figure 20-1).

THEORETICAL ASSERTIONS

Identification of the patient's need-for-help involves four steps. First, the nurse uses her powers of observation to look and listen for consistencies and inconsistencies of the patient's behavior with her concept of comfort. Second, the nurse explores the meaning of the patient's behavior with him. Third, the nurse determines the cause of the patient's discomfort or incapability. Finally, the nurse determines if the patient can resolve his problem or if he has a need-for-help[6:52-57] (Figure 20-2).

Ministration of help needed involves the nurse making a plan to meet the needs and presenting it to the patient. If the patient concurs with the plan and accepts suggestions for implementing it, the nurse implements it and ministration of help needed occurs. If the patient does not concur with the plan or accept suggestions for implementation, the nurse needs to explore causes of the patient's nonacceptance. If the patient has an interfering problem, the nurse needs to explore the patient's ability to solve the problem. If the patient has a need-for-help, the nurse once again forms a plan to meet the need, presents the plan, and seeks patient concurrence with the plan and acceptance of suggestions for implementation[6:57,61] (Figure 20-3).

Validation that the need-for-help was met is important. The nurse perceives whether the patient's behavior is consistent with her concept of comfort and seeks clarification from the patient to determine if he believes his need-for-help was met. Then the nurse needs to take appropriate action based on the feedback.[6:57,62]

LOGICAL FORM

Wiedenbach developed this model through induction. The reasoning method in inductive logic begins with observation of specific instances and then combines the specifics into a

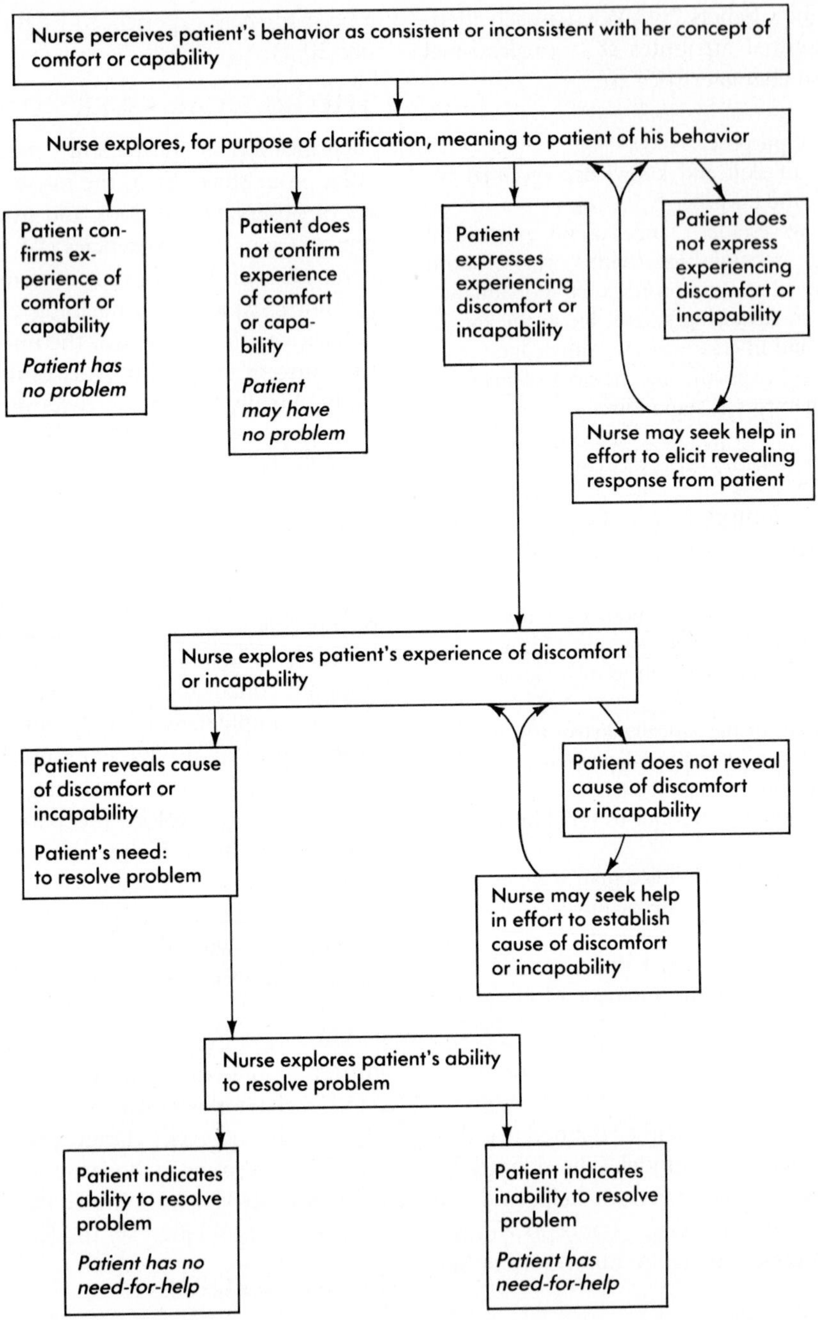

Figure 20-1. Identification of a need-for-help.
Used with permission from Wiedenbach, E. (1964). *Clinical nursing: A helping art*. New York: Springer, p. 60.

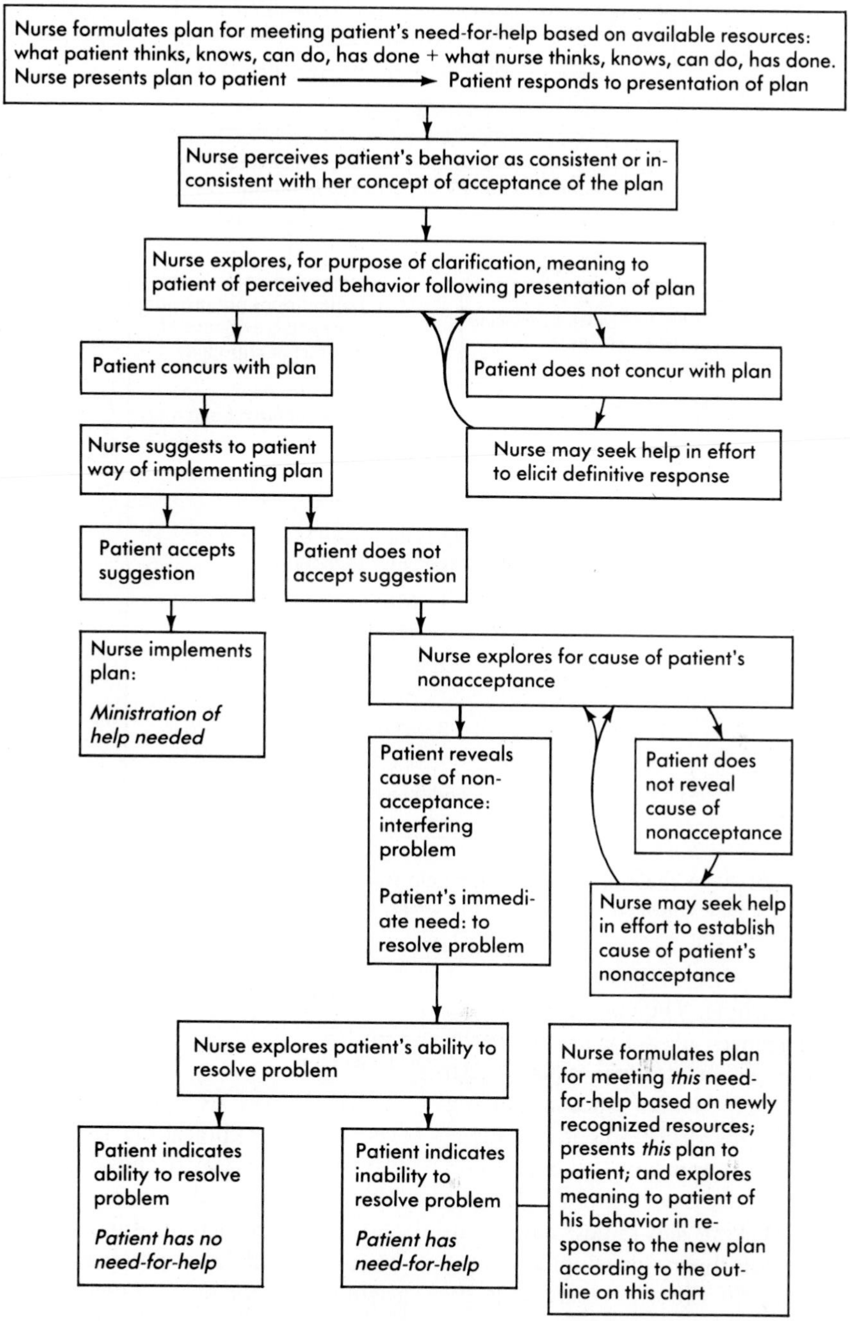

Figure 20-2. Ministration of help needed.

Used with permission from Wiedenbach, E. (1964). *Clinical nursing: A helping art*. New York: Springer, p. 61.

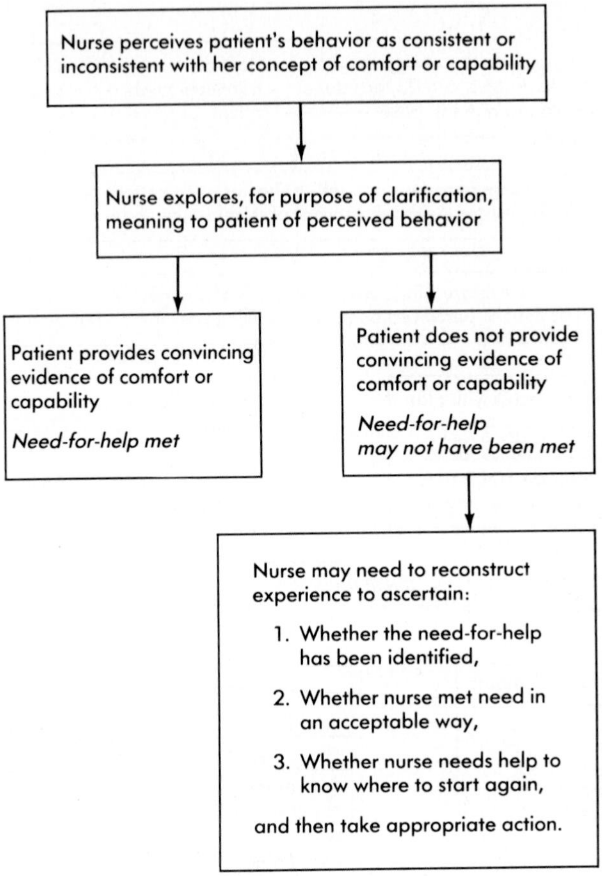

Figure 20-3. Validation that need for help was met.
Used with permission from Wiedenbach, E. (1964). *Clinical nursing: A helping art*. New York: Springer, p. 62.

more generalized whole. The common features of the specific instances allow for grouping the specifics into a larger set of phenomena.[1:61] An analysis of clinical experiences (specific nursing situations) leads to the development and interrelationships of concepts for Wiedenbach's model.[4:79]

Wiedenbach, Dickoff, and James[2] have identified four levels of theory development in a practice discipline. In order of increasing sophistication they are factor-isolating, factor-relating, situation-relating, and situation-producing. Wiedenbach[7] considers her work a situation-producing prescriptive theory.

ACCEPTANCE BY THE NURSING COMMUNITY

Practice

Today, nurses are applying Wiedenbach's concepts to their clinical practice more so than did nurses in the 1950s and 1960s. According to Wiedenbach,[7:23] the practice of clinical nursing "is an overt action, directed by disciplined thoughts and feelings toward meeting the patient's need for help." Drawing from her many years of experience as a nurse midwife, she published "Childbirth as Mothers Say They Like It." In this article Wiedenbach noted that mothers wanted childbirth to be as natural as possible. In addition, mothers wanted instructions on childbirth, father participation, full participation in the labor and delivery process, and rooming-in with their infant in the postpartum periods.[5:417-421] But not until the 1970s were some or most of these needs for help met. In the 1980s the health care industry provided the supposedly unique concept of Family Centered Care, which Wiedenbach addressed some 20 years ago.

Education

Wiedenbach[6:75] proposed that nursing education serves the practice of nursing in four major ways:

1. It is responsible for the preparation of future practitioners of nursing;
2. It arranges for nursing students to gain experience in clinical areas of the hospital or in the homes of patients;
3. Its representatives may function in the clinical area and work closely with the staff; and
4. It offers educational opportunities to the nurse for special or advanced study.

Application of Wiedenbach's model to clinical practice requires the nurse to have a sound knowledge of the normal and pathological states, a thorough understanding of human psychology, competence in clinical skills, and the ability to initiate and maintain therapeutic communication with patient and family. Also, the nurse must develop sound clinical judgment in decision making about patient care and be able to interpret the patient's behavior. These skills require a general education for nurses.

Today, many nursing schools are meeting this need for general education. Students are prepared with two years of courses in the humanities, biological science, and the social sciences, followed by two years in nursing science. This curriculum prepares a generalist in professional nursing and serves as the basis for graduate study.

Wiedenbach[6:78] saw graduate study as a means "for nurses to extend the personal limits of their practice and to realize, to a greater degree than before, their potentialities for creative and imaginative practice within the area of their responsibility in the total field of health." Today's focus on graduate education is much the same as Wiedenbach's. It is directed toward preparing advanced practitioners who are competent, self-directed, and concerned with the exploration of practice, issues, and problems of health care in a selected area of nursing.

Research

Before the development of Wiedenbach's model, nursing research focused more on the medical model than on a nursing model. But in Wiedenbach's model the focus of nursing research is to be related to the patient's response to the health care experience. Her model would support research designed to promote family relationships, to control factors responsible for disabling conditions, and to foster sound health care practices. Although not specifically based on Wiedenbach's model, numerous nursing research studies have been carried out in those areas. The results of those studies have been reported in nursing periodicals such as *Nursing Research.* Because of these nursing studies, nurses are better able to meet the patient's need for help.

FURTHER DEVELOPMENT

Wiedenbach is a pioneer in the writing of nursing theory. Her model of clinical nursing is one of the early attempts to systematically describe what it is that nurses do and what nursing is all about. It needs to be further developed by more clearly defining the concepts of health and environment. In addition, the component of nursing art needs to be identified in an operational way.

CRITIQUE

Wiedenbach's model evolved out of a desire to describe the practice of professional nursing. Her theory was influenced by Ida Orlando Pelletier and the philosophy of Dickoff and James, who were her colleagues at Yale University. Hers was one of the earlier nursing theories developed.

Clarity

Wiedenbach's model meets the criterion of clarity in that the concepts and definitions are clear, consistent, and intelligible.

Simplicity

There are too many relational statements for the theory to be classified as a simple theory. The concepts include the need-for-help, nursing practice, and nursing art. All of these concepts are interrelated, equal in importance, and have no meaning aside from their interaction.[5:76] Relationships between the major components can be linked, but it is difficult to diagram some of the concepts in the model. In addition, the concepts describe or explain phenomenon but do not predict.

Generality

The scope of the concepts of patient (person), nursing, and need-for-help are very broad and thus possess generality. However, the concept of need-for-help is based on the patient's recognition of his or her need for help. This concept is not applicable to the infant, comatose patient, or many other physiologically or psychologically incompetent persons. Also, the assumption that all nurses do not share a similar philosophy of nursing lessens the generality of the model.

Empirical Precision

Substantiation of a theory is accomplished through research, and thus the usefulness of the theory is determined. In Wiedenbach's model, the criterion is only partially met. The concepts of nursing practice and need-for-help are operationally defined and measurable. However, the concept of need-for-help is not always applicable. Also, within this theory is an attempt to operationally define nursing art. Therefore, it would be difficult to test this theory.

However, the potential exists for research to be done with this model. J. Fawcett believes three steps must be taken before the model can be tested. "First, the model must be formulated; second, a theory must be derived from the model; and third, operational definitions must be given to the concepts, and hypothesis derived."[3:26]

Derivable Consequences

Derivable consequences refer to the overall effect of the theory and its importance to nursing research, practice, and education. Wiedenbach's model fulfills the purpose for which it was developed: to describe professional practice. The theory focuses on nurse-patient interactions and regards the patient from a holistic point of view. Wiedenbach's work influenced the work of other early scholars, including Orlando and Peplau.

As one of the early nursing theorists, Wiedenbach made an important contribution to the nursing profession.

REFERENCES

1. Chinn, P.L. & Jacobs, M.K. (1983). *Theory and nursing: A systematic approach*. St. Louis: C.V. Mosby.
2. Dickoff, J.J., James, P.A., & Wiedenbach, E. (1968, Nov.-Dec.). Theory in a practice discipline: Practice-oriented theory. *Nursing Research, 17*:545-554.
3. Fawcett, J. (1984). *Analysis and evaluation of conceptual models of nursing*. Philadelphia: F.A. Davis.
4. Raleigh, E. (1983). Wiedenbach's model. In J. Fitzpatrick & A. Whall, *Conceptual models of nursing analysis and application*. Bowie, Md.: Robert J. Brady.
5. Wiedenbach, E. (1949, Aug.). Childbirth as mothers say they like it. *Public Health Nursing,* 5:417-421.
6. Wiedenbach, E. (1964). *Clinical nursing: A helping art*. New York: Springer.
7. Wiedenbach, E. (1984, Spring). Written interview.

BIBLIOGRAPHY
Primary Sources
Books

Wiedenbach, E. (1958). *Family-centered nursing.* New York: G.P. Putnam's Sons.

Wiedenbach, E. (1964). *Clinical nursing: A helping art.* New York: Springer.

Wiedenbach, E. (1969). *Meeting the realities in clinical teaching.* New York: Springer.

Wiedenbach, E. & Falls, C.E. (1978). *Communication: Key to effective nursing.* New York: Tiresias.

Book Chapters

Wiedenbach, E. (1973). The nursing process in maternity nursing. In J.P. Clausen, et al., *Maternity nursing today.* New York: McGraw-Hill.

Articles

Dickoff, J.J., James, P.A., & Wiedenbach, E. (1968, Sept.-Oct.). Theory in a practice discipline I: Practice-oriented discipline. *Nursing Research, 17:* 415-435.

Dickoff, J.J., James, P.A., & Wiedenbach, E. (1968, Nov.-Dec.). Theory in a practice discipline II: Practice-oriented research. *Nursing Research, 17:*545-554.

Wiedenbach, E. (1940, Jan.). Toward educating 130 million people: A history of the nursing information bureau. *American Journal of Nursing, 40:*13-18.

Wiedenbach, E. (1949, Aug.). Childbirth as mothers say they like it. *Public Health Nursing, 5:*417-421.

Wiedenbach, E. (1960, May). Nurse-midwifery, purpose, practice, and opportunity. *Nursing Outlook, 8:*256.

Wiedenbach, E. (1963, Nov.). The helping art of nursing. *American Journal of Nursing, 63:*54-57.

Wiedenbach, E. (1965, Dec.). Family nurse practitioner for maternal and child care. *Nursing Outlook, 13:*50.

Wiedenbach, E. (1968, May). Genetics and the nurse. *Bulletin of the American College of Nurse Midwifery, 13:*8-13.

Wiedenbach, E. (1968, June). The nurse's role in family planning: A conceptual base for practice. *Nursing Clinics of North America, 3:*355-365.

Wiedenbach, E. (1970, May). Nurses' wisdom in nursing theory. *American Journal of Nursing, 70:*1057-1062.

Wiedenbach, E. (1970, Sept.-Oct.) Comment on beliefs and values: Basis for curriculum design. *Nursing Research, 19:*427.

Correspondence

Wiedenbach, E. (1984, Spring). Personal correspondence.

Wiedenbach, E. (1988, Spring). Personal correspondence.

Interviews

Wiedenbach, E. (1984, May 31). Telephone interview.

Secondary Sources
Book Reviews

Wiedenbach, E. (1958). *Family-centered maternity nursing.*
*Childbirth, 5:*229-230, November 1958.
*Nursing Outlook, 7:*193, April 1959.
*American Journal of Nursing, 59:*663, May 1959.
*Medical World News, 9:*82, January 19, 1968.
*Briefs, 32:*27, February 1968.
*Hospital Progress, 49:*98, July 1968.
*Nursing Outlook, 16:*71, August 1968.
*American Journal of Nursing, 68:*1758, August 1968.
*Obstetrics and Gynecology, 32:*446, September 1968.
*Nursing Journal of India, 60:*38, January 1969.

Wiedenbach, E. (1964). *Clinical nursing: A helping art.*
*Nursing Outlook, 12:*16, September 1964.
*Nursing Mirror, 119:*70, October 16, 1964.
*Journal of American Association of Nurse Anesthetists, 32:*401+, December 1964.
*Canadian Nurse, 61:*83, February 1965.
*Catholic Nurse, 13:*34, June 1965.
*American Journal of Nursing, 65:*62, July 1965.

Wiedenbach, E. (1969). *Meeting the realities in clinical teaching.*
*Association of Operating Room Nurses, 10:*155. November 1969.

Wiedenbach, E. & Falls, C.E. (1978). *Communication: Key to effective nursing.*
*Occupational Health Nursing, 26:*54, July 1978.
*Supervisor Nurse, 9:*244, September 1978
*American Journal of Nursing, 78:*1976, November 1978

*California Nurse, 74:*28, March-April 1979.
*Nursing Times, 75:*588-589, April 5, 1979.

News Releases

Presentation of Hattie Hemschemeyer Award: 24th annual meeting of the American College of Nurse Midwives. *Journal of Nurse-Midwifery, 24:*35-36.

Books

Chinn, P.L. & Jacobs, M.K. (1983). *Theory and nursing: A systematic approach.* St. Louis: C.V. Mosby.

Fawcett, J. (1984). *Analysis and evaluation of conceptual models of nursing.* Philadelphia: F.A. Davis.

Yale University School of Nursing Index Staff. (1969) *Nursing studies index* (Vol. 4). Philadelphia: J.B. Lippincott.

Book Chapters

Bennett, A.M. & Foster, P.C. (1980). Ernestine Wiedenbach. In Nursing Theories Conference Group, J.B. George, Chairperson, *Nursing theories: The base for professional nursing practice.* Englewood Cliffs, N.J.: Prentice-Hall, pp. 138-149.

Meleis, A.I. (1985). Ernestine Wiedenbach. In A.I. Meleis, *Theoretical nursing: Development and progress.* Philadelphia: J.B. Lippincott, pp. 263-274.

Menke, E.M. (1983). Critical analysis of theory development in nursing. In N.L. Chaska (Ed.), *The nursing profession: A time to speak.* New York: McGraw-Hill, pp. 416-426.

Raleigh, E. (1983). Wiedenbach's model. In J. Fitzpatrick & A. Whall, *Conceptual models of nursing analysis and application.* Bowie, Md.: Robert J. Brady, pp. 67-85.

Walker, L.O. (1983). Theory and research in the development of nursing as a discipline: Retrospect and prospect. In N.L. Chaska (Ed.), *The nursing profession: A time to speak.* New York: McGraw-Hill, pp. 406-415.

Articles

Barnard, K. (1981). Perinatal parental behavior: Nursing research and implications for newborn health—closing. *Birth Defects, 17:*285.

Roberts, J. (1981). Maternal positions in labor: Analysis in relation to comfort and efficiency. *Birth Defects, 17:*97.

Schmidt, W. & Valadian, I. (1964). A bookshelf on maternal-child health. *American Journal of Public Health, 54:*551.

Sheldon, R.S. (1974). Consolidation of hospital obstetric services. *Medical Clinics of North America, 58:*885.

Thompson, J.B. (1981). Nurse midwives and health promotion during pregnancy. *Birth Defects, 17:*29.

Wooden, H.E. (1965). Infection control in family-centered maternity care. *Obstetrics and Gynecology, 25:*232.

Other Sources

Eisler, J., Wolfer, J.A., & Diers, D. (1972). Relationship between the need for social approval and postoperative recovery welfare. *Nursing Research, 21(5):*520-525.

Larson, P.A. (1977). Nurse perception of client illness. *Nursing Research, 26*(6):416-421.

Leonard, R.C., Skipper, J.K., & Woolridge, P.J. (1967). Small sample field experiments for evaluating patient care. *Health Services Research, 2(1):*47-50.

Rickleman, B.L. (1971). Bio-psycho-social linguistics: A conceptual approach to nurse-patient interaction. *Nursing Research, 20(5):*398-403.

Shields, D. (1978). Nursing care in labor and patient satisfaction. A descriptive study. *Journal of Advances in Nursing, 3:*535-550.

Wolfer, J. & Visintainer, M. (1975). Pediatric surgical patients' and parents' stress responses and adjustment. *Nursing Research, 24(4):*244-255.

Joan Riehl Sisca

21

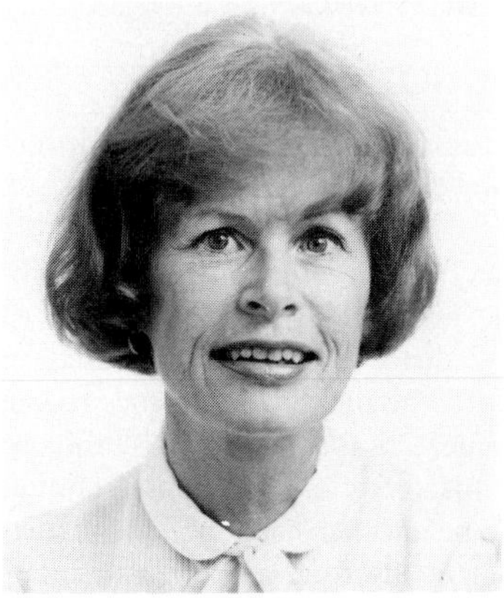

Symbolic Interactionism

Donna J. Crawford, Alta J.H. Gochnauer, Deborah Hissa, Kathleen Millican Miller

CREDENTIALS AND BACKGROUND OF THE THEORIST

Although Joan Riehl was born in Davenport, Iowa, she spent most of her childhood and young adult life in a Chicago suburb. She attended the University of Illinois in Urbana and Chicago where she obtained her B.S.N. After graduation she worked as a clinical instructor, a supervisor, and an in-service director in Texas and in California before returning to college for her master's degree in nursing. After receiving her M.S.N. from UCLA, Riehl taught pediatric nursing at California State University for three years before joining the faculty at the University of California in Los Angeles. There she began teaching theoretical concepts and their application. Two major professional events resulted from this instruction. First, she began writing nursing textbooks on conceptual models to use for teaching graduate students, and she began to identify her own theoretical

The authors wish to express appreciation to Dr. Joan Riehl Sisca for critiquing the chapter.

framework. Her interest resulted in doctoral study at UCLA in sociology, which afforded the opportunity to pursue the knowledge base needed to develop the particulars of her model. Symbolic interactionism is the foundation upon which this model is built. Role theory and self-concept are components of the theory. They constituted her dissertational investigation for her Ph.D., which she received in 1980.

Like many nurses who attend graduate school, Riehl worked part-time to maintain her clinical and research skills. The positions she held during this period included being a staff nurse in medical-surgical and psychiatric nursing and in the ICU-CCU, and being a supervisor in a gerontological hospital in Southern California. She also worked as a research assistant and coordinator in several research projects at the University of California at Los Angeles.

After graduation, Riehl moved to San Antonio, Texas. While there she taught sociology, psychiatric nursing, and mental health concepts as a lecturer in the Department of Social Science at the University of Texas and as an associate professor in the Division of Nursing at Incarnate Word College. She also served as a research evaluator on a government grant that examined numerous variables regarding the R.N. to B.S.N. student. When the three-year grant in Texas was completed, Riehl was named Chairperson of the Department of Nursing at the Harrisburg Area Community College in Harrisburg, Pennsylvania.

In 1985, Riehl became an associate professor at the graduate level in the Department of Nursing at Indiana University of Pennsylvania. She serves as the graduate coordinator for the M.S.N. program and is responsible for teaching master's-prepared students theoretical foundations, research, curriculum theory and practice, ethical, legal and political dimensions of health care, family theory and practice, and administration theory and practicum. Riehl continues to receive national and international recognition as a pioneer and leader for publishing in the field of nursing theory.

Riehl is a member of numerous professional organizations. They include the National League of Nursing, American Nurses' Association, the ANA Council of Nurse Researchers, Sigma Theta Tau, the American Sociological Association, and the American Association for the Advancement of Science.

THEORETICAL SOURCES

Riehl's theory is derived from symbolic interactionism (SI). In SI theory,

> interaction occurs between human beings who interpret or define each others' actions instead of merely reacting to them. The response is based on the meaning which the individual attaches to the action. Human interaction is mediated by the use of symbols, by interpretation, or by ascertaining the meaning of one another's action. This mediation is equivalent to inserting a process of interpretation between the stimulus and the response in the case of human behavior.[3:8]

Consequently, Riehl claims several theoretical sources from sociology and social psychology, including George Mead, Herbert Blumer, Arnold Rose, L. Edward Wells, Gerald Marwell, and Robert E.L. Faris.

EMPIRICAL EVIDENCE

During the past 50 years, the SI theory has been supported by numerous empirical studies. Many theoretical sources, including those mentioned above, have illustrated the utility of this theory and have contributed to further refinement and clarification of its components. Blumer[1:viii] eloquently states, "It is my conviction that an empirical science necessarily has to respect the nature of the empirical world that is its object of study. In my judgment symbolic interactionism shows that respect for the nature of human group life and conduct."

MAJOR CONCEPTS AND DEFINITIONS

Riehl's theory and model adapt four key concepts from the SI theory described by Blumer.[1:50] In addition, Riehl employs the "me" and "I" concepts developed by Mead. Last, she identifies role reversal and sick role as examples of the concept.

PEOPLE. "People, individually and collectively, are prepared to act on the basis of the meaning of the objects that comprise their world."[1:50] In the Riehl model, the term *people* includes the patient, the nurse, other health care professionals, and the patient's family and friends. Riehl[5:17] describes the nurse as one who knows her capabilities, is self-directed, and assumes more than one role in a given period.

ASSOCIATION. "The association of people is necessarily in the form of a process in which they are making indications to one another and interpreting each other's indications."[1:50] Riehl summarizes this as the defining process of role taking, a social-psychological concept instituted by Mead. Role taking occurs when an individual cognitively internalizes another person's perceptions of reality in varied situations.[5:352] Hence, the formative meanings of actions arise from this reciprocal interaction. The nurse-patient interface is an example of this interaction.

SOCIAL ACTS. "Social acts, whether individual or collective, are constructed through a process in which the actors note, interpret, and assess the situations confronting them."[1:50] Riehl[3:46] states, "Their interpretation of these situations influence their social acts toward each other." She expounds on the interpretive phase as described by Faris, in which a delayed response promotes clear thought, reduced frustration, and prospective learning.[5:354] This concept correlates to Riehl's method of process recordings, which allows the nurse to assess and respond more appropriately to a patient's behavior.

INTERLINKAGES. "The complex interlinkages of acts that comprise organizations, institutions, division of labor, and networks of interdependency are moving and not static affairs."[1:50] From this concept Riehl derives that patient assessment is a dynamic process that often necessitates the use of several resources in meeting patient's needs, particularly in long-term care.

ME. Riehl defines *me* synonymously with a role taker in a given situation. In other words, the me learns and assumes the attitudes of others. This is a concept used in the development of one's behavior as well as a method of understanding another's actions.

I (SELF-CONCEPT). Riehl defines *I,* or *self-concept,* as the individual's total behavioral perceptions, reflecting the summation of roles. She states, "The self-concept refers to a global, relatively constant self-perception that an individual holds and it changes only gradually."[3:64]

ROLE REVERSAL. Role reversal is an example of a potential consequence resulting during the interaction between nurse and patient. Riehl[5:355] defines role reversal as an inadvertent situation in which "the patient assumes the therapeutic role while the nurse becomes the recipient of the care." Rectification of this situation may require assistance from a third person.

SICK ROLE. Riehl defines the *sick role* "as the position one assumes when one perceives himself as ill."[10] There may be a problem "when a patient is reluctant to part with the sick role."[5:355] As with role reversal, this situation suggests the need of additional resources for the patient's rehabilitation.

MAJOR ASSUMPTIONS

Riehl relates Arnold Rose's genetic and analytic assumptions to nursing and uses them in her derived theory. Rose divides his assumptions into two categories. The first, genetic assumptions, deals with only the child. The second is the analytic assumptions, which focus on all ages of man other than the child.

Genetic Assumptions

Rose cites the following four genetic assumptions applicable to the SI theory.

1. "Society—a network of interacting individuals—with its culture—the related meanings and values by means of which individuals interact—precedes any existing individual."[5:353]
2. "The process by which socialization takes place can be thought of as occurring in three stages."[5:353] These stages are:
   a. "The infant is habituated to a certain sequence of behaviors and events through a psychogenic process such as trial and error."[5:353]
   b. "When the habit is blocked, the image of the incomplete act arises in the infant's mind and he thus learns to differentiate the object . . . in that act by a symbol."[5:353]
   c. "As the infant acquires a number of meanings he uses them to designate to others, and to himself, what he is thinking."[5:353]
3. "The individual is socialized into the general culture and also into various subcultures."[5:353]
4. "While some groups and personal meanings and values may be dropped and become lower on the reference-relationship scale, they are not lost or forgotten."[5:353]

Analytic Assumptions

The five analytic assumptions pertaining to the SI theory according to Rose follow.

1. "Man lives in a symbolic as well as in a physical environment and can be stimulated to act by symbols as well as by physical stimuli."[5:351]
2. "Through symbols, man has the capacity to stimulate others in ways other than those in which he himself is stimulated."[5:351] Riehl[5:351] states that role taking, a concept included under this assumption, is important in nursing.
3. "Through communication of symbols, man can learn huge numbers of meanings and values—and hence ways of acting—from other men."[5:351] Riehl summarizes that as a result of this assumption man's behavior is not learned through trial and error or through conditioning, but rather through symbolic communication.[5:351] "According to the SI theory, an individual's perception of how others evaluate him is more important in forming his self-concept than the actual evaluation that others hold."[3:12] Riehl[5:351] explains that it can be deduced from this assumption that "through the learning of a culture, or subculture, men are able to predict each other's behavior and gauge their own behavior accordingly."
4. "The symbols—and the meanings and values to which they refer—do not occur in isolated bits, but in large and complex clusters."[5:351] This assumption refers to man's role. As defined in the discussion of concepts, the "me" is the role-taker and the "I," or self-concept, is the perception of the person as a whole. "Since the 'me' is made up of the attitudes of others, these others can take this role and predict an individual's behavior in a given capacity."[3:351] Consequently, a person is able to gain insight into another's problem by taking the other's role, anticipating how he will act, and implementing a plan of action to help him accomplish his goal.[5:352]
5. "Thinking is the process by which possible symbolic solutions and other future courses of action are examined, assessed for their relative advantages and disadvantages in terms of the values of the individual, and chosen for action or rejected."[5:352] Riehl discusses two major points involving this assumption. First, the assumption encompasses the four steps of the nursing process: "nursing assessment, diagnosis, planned intervention, and evaluation of action."[5:352] Second, she points out, "Since meaning arises in the process of interaction between two persons, and individuals differ,

even the most carefully thought out plan may go awry."[5:352]

THEORETICAL ASSERTIONS

Riehl has identified several theoretical assertions in her model. These include:

1. "The premise that social action is built up by the acting unit through the process of noting, interpreting, etc., implies how social action should be studied."[5:354] Riehl identifies the acting unit as the individual.
2. "According to Blumer (1969), in order to treat and analyze social action, one must observe the process by which it is constructed." Riehl[5:354] identifies "one" as the nurse, who must view the social action as the individual sees it.
3. "Since the self-concept is an integral part of this model, the nurse must continue to develop self-insight through self evaluation regarding his/her own actions to understand end results of interactions with others."[8,9]
4. "The goal of action is to guide the patient in maintaining/regaining a higher level of wellness to improve the quality of life and to gain insight during life's journey regardless of the health problem."[10] "The goal of action is based upon a key factor of SI, which is taking the role of the others."[5:354] Riehl[5:354] identifies three methodological approaches the nurse uses to achieve this goal. The first approach, role taking, allows the nurse to understand why the patient does what he does. The second method entails interpretation of these actions. The third involves the use of process recordings. Riehl does not advocate recording all interactions, but she does recommend recordings be used until the nurse is able to respond effectively during on-the-spot interactions.
5. "It must be realized that it is not completely possible to take the role of the other, but genuine attempts to do so convey understanding of the other's position."[7,9]
6. "Three additional elements must be included to meet the requirements of an effective conceptual model for nursing, namely, the source of difficulty, the intervention, and the consequences."[5:354] Riehl[6,8] equates the source of difficulty with the nursing diagnosis, and the intervention with the plan of care arrived at after role taking, interpretation, and process recordings.
7. The eclipse shown in her model (Figure 21-1), "should never be complete, however, because maintaining a certain distance is essential for the preservation of the individuality of each person."[5:356] As the nurse and patient gain knowledge and insight from their interactions, the circles in the model move toward each other and form an ecliptical image. However, Riehl[5,8] emphasizes that if the circles form a complete eclipse, objectivity and independence will be lost.

LOGICAL FORM

Riehl's theory uses deductive and inductive logic. It is deductive because Riehl draws relationships between nursing and the SI theory. Her statements are consistent with Mead's concepts of role taking and self-concept. Her theoretical assertions deduced from Rose's assumptions demonstrate further consistency. This allows for easy identification of the interrelationships between the theoretical components, and thus enhances the generation of hypotheses for empirical testing. It is inductive because Riehl utilizes SI as a foundation upon which to build and develop her concepts into a nursing theory.[10]

ACCEPTANCE BY THE NURSING COMMUNITY

Practice

Riehl's theory is becoming more widely accepted in the United States and is used fairly

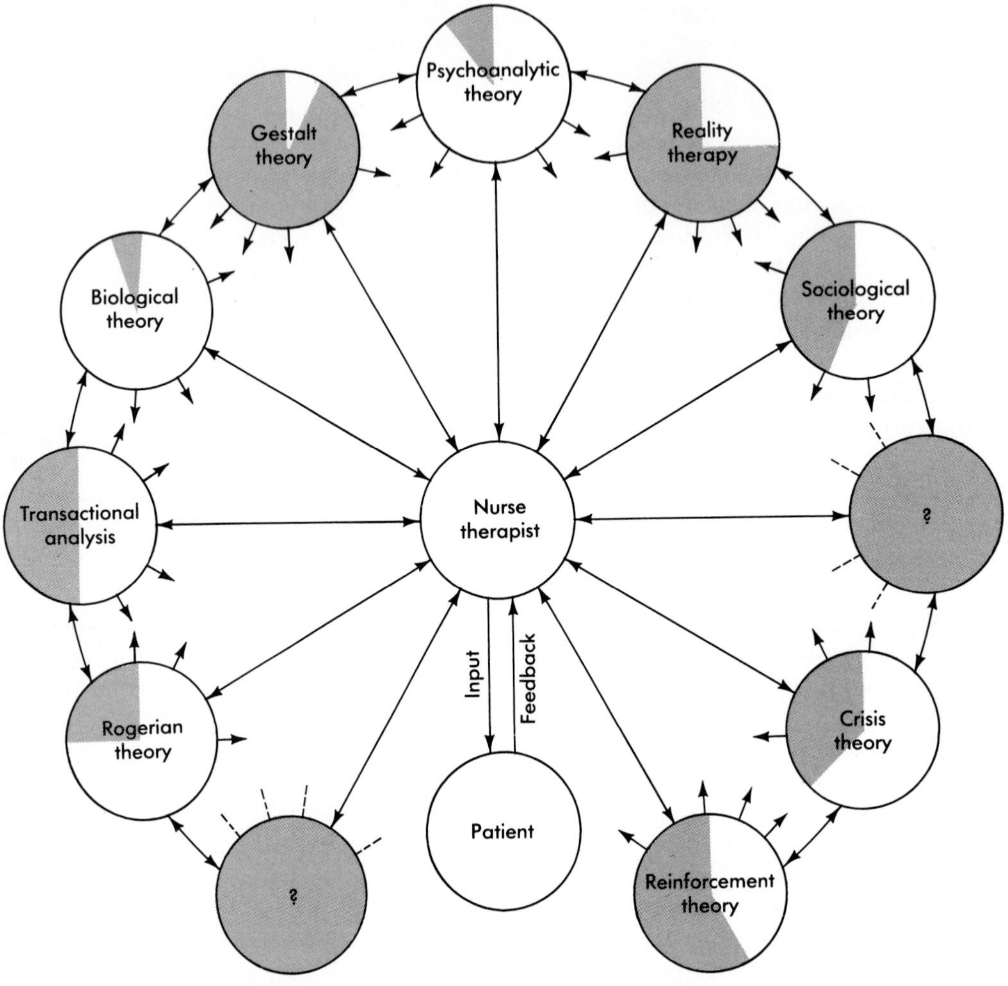

Figure 21-1. Schematic representation of model.
Used with permission from Preisner, J.M. (1980). A proposed model for the nurse therapist, In J.P. Riehl and C. Roy, *Conceptual models for nursing practice.* New York: Appleton-Century-Crofts. p. 363.

extensively in Canada, England, Japan, and the Middle East.[10] It has been considered a middle range theory in nursing.[2:13] Middle range constitutes a relatively broad scope of phenomena. However, Riehl's theory and model have been found applicable to all age groups and in a variety of clinical settings.[4]

As Figure 21-1 illustrates, Riehl views the nurse therapist and the patient as actively exchanging information and gleaning knowledge. This is accomplished through mutual role taking in conjunction with the nurse selecting and using known theoretical approaches. The unshaded areas of the model indicate active processes in the relationship, while the arrows represent the complex interdependencies of these elements, allowing for continual reassessment and evaluation.

Riehl's model provides a realistic approach for nursing practice in any situation where the focus is on role interaction in the nurse-patient relationship. Preisner demonstrates the applicability of Riehl's model in the psychiatric setting.[5:362-371] The nurse selects from multiple theories, therapies, and allied health disciplines in planning and implementing effective nursing interventions.

Wood demonstrates the use of role taking in a patient's hospital admission.[5:357-361] The nurse interprets the patient's response to the new environment and thereby helps the patient acquire the necessary perceptual changes or new roles in the health care system.

The nursing implications are evident yet not restrictive to the interaction between the nurse and patient. The role interaction framework may also be effective in nurse-nurse relationships (nursing management, for example), nurse-physician dyads, nurse-patient-family triads, and other interactive situations. However, the model's emphasis is on the nurse-patient-family relationships.

Education

The SI theory has long been prevalent among schools of sociology and psychology. The Riehl interaction model was introduced to the nursing discipline in 1980. The number of educational institutions that have incorporated it into their nursing curriculum is uncertain. The Riehl Interaction Model was considered as part of the organizing framework of the curriculum at both Harrisburg Area Community College and Indiana University of Pennsylvania.

In addition, interaction models as a group are moderately employed in B.S.N. programs.[5:396-398] Nursing is presently concerned with developing a distinct body of knowledge and delineating its professional role. Riehl's model, which focuses on the therapeutic processes in the nurse-patient and nurse-patient-family relationships, continues to contribute to these goals.

Research

The earliest research relevant to Riehl's theory can be found in her own doctoral dissertation. This study examines autistic children's ability to role take as compared with their "normal" siblings. It implicates a positive correlation between the level of development of self-concept and the ability to role take.

The generation of implications for further research is inherent in empirical studies. Riehl makes several suggestions for further testing dealing specifically with autistic children, such as investigating their perceptions of their parent's treatment of them and simply increasing the sample size to study more variables in this population. Examples of other recommendations include applying this study to other handicapped children and developing more tools for measuring self-conception.

The most recent research on Riehl's theory and model supports their applicability to a wide variety of patients and clinical settings. These studies include use of the model with pregnant women, with adults in a medical clinic and the concept of personal space, with diabetic children and their self-esteem, with patients being transported by helicopter to acute care settings, and with a woman in postpartum psychosis.[4] Continued research is needed for Riehl's theory to gain credibility, acceptance, and future application.

FURTHER DEVELOPMENT

In operationalizing her model, Riehl has developed an assessment tool in the form of a matrix with the mnemonic FANCAP down the left side and the parameters physiological, psychological, sociological, cultural, and environmental across the top. With this approach, each factor intersects with each parameter and is therefore addressed (Figure 21-2). After analyzing the collected data and making a diagnosis, a plan of care is made with the patient and/or family. The diagnosis and plan of care are prioritized (nurse with patient and/or family) and evaluated after

	Physiological	Psychological	Sociological	Cultural	Environmental
Fluids					
Aeration					
Nutrition					
Communication					
Activity					
Pain					

Figure 21-2. Riehl Interaction Model Assessment Tool. (Drawn by Deborah Hissa from description given by Riehl.)

implementation. This tool has been tested and Riehl indicates that it is valid and reliable.[4]

Riehl has introduced an interesting and valuable model of SI to nursing. She has included further development of her theory in her third edition of *Conceptual Models for Nursing Practice*.

More explicit definitions of many concepts in the current model, including *I, me, process recordings,* and *SI* itself are needed for in-depth descriptions in regard to the relationship statements between Blumer's concepts and nursing, and between Rose's assumptions and nursing. Furthermore, the theoretical assertions require refinement for lucidity and depth.

As a therapeutic nursing approach, Riehl's theory merits the involvement of the profession for progress in its development, understanding, and validation. Abundant potential for both nursing research and subsequent contributions to the theory seems to lie particularly in the psychiatric nurse setting. This testing may also generate new information. "Theory development is important to the growth of any discipline" and should be pursued.[5:3]

CRITIQUE

Complexity

The Riehl interaction model contains several key concepts and theoretical relationships; thus, it is complex. With the future development of concepts and relationships, this level of complexity will increase.

Generality

Riehl's interaction model is generalizable to the broad scope of nursing. However, in a situation with a nonresponsive comatose patient, this application may be limited to information and interpretations obtained from the patient's family and friends.

Empirical Precision

The derived concepts from Blumer and Mead have been defined explicitly and grounded in observable reality within their parent discipline. Riehl does not clarify all her concepts with denotative definitions and therefore obscures the means for accurate testability. For this reason, a high degree of empirical precision is not present.

Derivable Consequences

Riehl's interaction model employs the nursing process in implementing nursing care. Emphasis is on the nurse assessing and interpreting the patient's actions and then making predictions about the patient's behavior in order to plan interventions with the patient and his family. Furthermore, the evaluation phase in the theory, regarding potential patient problems, presents important nursing implications. The theory's usefulness is evident not only in the delivery of nursing care, but also in delineating the nurse's professional role.

Summary

Riehl is continuing the development of her nursing theory, which is derived from SI. SI, as defined by Blumer, involves the interaction that transpires between people who "interpret or define each other's actions instead of just relating to them."[5:350] Riehl uses Rose's genetic and analytic assumptions as her own. She identifies Blumer's concepts, the I and Me concepts of Mead, and the role reversal and sick role concepts in describing her model.

Using these assumptions and concepts, Riehl relates nursing to the SI theory. She believes that the nurse must view the actions of the individual as he perceives them. By role playing, explicitly or implicitly the nurse is able to understand why the patient does what he does and is thus better able to identify the source of difficulty, or nursing diagnosis. Then, having interpreted the patient's action and studied the process recordings, the nurse is able to intervene with a plan of care. The plan of care involves helping the patient and/or family assume roles they have used in the past, or are currently using, to cope with the present illness. The evaluation process is then used to determine the success of this role taking. Riehl views this dynamic process as one that changes daily, requiring continuous assessment by both the nurse and the patient.

Although testing of Riehl's theory within the science of nursing has occurred only since 1985, its contribution to nursing is apparent.

REFERENCES

1. Blumer, H. (1969). *Symbolic interactionalism: Perspective and method*. Englewood Cliffs, N.J.: Prentice-Hall.
2. Kim, H.S. (1983). *The nature of theoretical thinking in nursing*. Norwalk, Conn.: Appleton-Century-Crofts.
3. Riehl, J.P. (1980). *The self-conception and role relationships of autistic children: A symbolic interactionist perspective*. Doctoral dissertation. Los Angeles: University of California, Department of Sociology.
4. J. Riehl (Ed.). (In press). *Conceptual models for nursing practice* (3d ed.). Norwalk, Conn.: Appleton and Lange.
5. J.P. Riehl & C. Roy (Eds.). (1980). *Conceptual models for nursing practice* (2d ed.). New York: Appleton-Century-Crofts.
6. Riehl Sisca, J. (1984). Telephone interviews.
7. Riehl Sisca, J. (1985). Telephone interviews.
8. Riehl Sisca, J. (1984). Personal correspondence.
9. Riehl Sisca, J. (1985). Personal correspondence.
10. Riehl Sisca, J. (1988). Personal correspondence.

BIBLIOGRAPHY

Primary Sources

Books

J.P. Riehl & J.W. McVay (Eds.). (1973). *The clinical nurse specialist: Interpretations*. New York: Appleton-Century-Crofts.

J.P. Riehl & C. Roy (Eds.). (1974). *Conceptual models for nursing practice*. New York: Appleton-Century-Crofts.

J.P. Riehl & C. Roy (Eds.). (1980). *Conceptual models for nursing practice* (2d ed.). New York: Appleton-Century Crofts.

J. Riehl Sisca (Ed.). (1985). *The science and art of self-care*. East Norwalk, Conn.: Appleton-Century-Crofts.

J. Riehl (Ed.). (In press). *Conceptual models for nursing practice* (3d ed.). Norwalk, Conn.: Appleton and Lange.

Book Chapters

Chrisman, M. & Riehl, J.P. (1974). The systems-developmental stress model. In J.P. Riehl & C. Roy (Eds.), *Conceptual models for nursing practice*. New York: Appleton-Century-Crofts.

McVay, J.W., Riehl, J.P., & Chen, S. (1973). The clinical nurse specialist as perceived by the deans of baccalaureate and higher degree programs. In J.P. Riehl & J.W. McVay (Eds.), *The clinical nurse specialist: Interpretations*. New York: Appleton-Century-Crofts.

Riehl, J.P. (1973). Role change and resistance: The baccalaureate student as practitioner. In J.P. Riehl & J.W. McVay (Eds.), *The clinical nurse specialist:*

Interpretations. New York: Appleton-Century-Crofts.

Riehl, J.P. (1974). Application of interaction theory. In J.P. Riehl & C. Roy (Eds.), *Conceptual models for nursing practice.* New York: Appleton-Century-Crofts.

Riehl, J.P. & Roy, C. (1974). Conceptual models in nursing: Use of nursing models in education, research, and service. In J.P. Riehl & C. Roy (Eds.), *Conceptual models for nursing practice.* New York: Appleton-Century-Crofts.

Riehl, J.P. & Roy, C. (1974). Discussion of a unified nursing model. In J.P. Riehl & C. Roy (Eds.), *Conceptual models for nursing practice.* New York: Appleton-Century-Crofts.

Riehl, J.P. & Roy, C. (1974). The nature and history of models: Models related to theory: Use of models in other fields; and history of nursing models. In J.P. Riehl & C. Roy (Eds.). *Conceptual models for nursing practice.* New York: Appleton-Century-Crofts.

Riehl, J.P. & Roy, C. (1974). Toward a unified nursing model. In J.P. Riehl & C. Roy (Eds.), *Conceptual models for nursing practice.* New York: Appleton-Century-Crofts.

Riehl, J.P. & Roy, C. (1980). The nature of nursing models. In J.P. Riehl & C. Roy (Eds.), *Conceptual models for nursing practice* (2d ed.). New York: Appleton-Century-Crofts.

Riehl, J.P. (1980). Nursing models in current use. In J.P. Riehl & C. Roy (Eds.), *Conceptual models for nursing practice* (2d ed.). New York: Appleton-Century-Crofts.

Riehl, J.P. (1980). The Riehl interaction model. In J.P. Riehl & C. Roy (Eds.), *Conceptual models for nursing practice* (2d ed.). New York: Appleton-Century-Crofts.

Riehl, J.P. & Roy, C. (1980). A unified model of nursing. In J.P. Riehl & C. Roy (Eds.), *Conceptual models for nursing practice* (2d ed.). New York: Appleton-Century-Crofts.

Skolny, M.A. & Riehl, J.P. (1974). Hope: Solving patient and family problems by using a theoretical framework. In J.P. Riehl & C. Roy (Eds.), *Conceptual models for nursing practice.* New York: Appleton-Century-Crofts.

Riehl Sisca, J. (1985). Orem's general theory of nursing: An interpretation. In J. Riehl Sisca (Ed.), *The science and art of self-care.* East Norwalk, Conn.: Appleton-Century-Crofts.

Riehl Sisca, J. (1985). Determining criteria for graduate and undergraduate self-care curriculums. In J. Riehl Sisca (Ed.), *The science and art of self-care.* East Norwalk, Conn: Appleton-Century-Crofts.

Riehl Sisca, J. (1985). Epilogue: Future implications for the science and art of self-care. In J. Riehl Sisca (Ed.), *The science and art of self-care.* East Norwalk, Conn.: Appleton-Century-Crofts.

Riehl, J. (In press). The Riehl interaction model. In J. Riehl (Ed.), *Conceptual models for nursing practice* (3d ed.). East Norwalk, Conn.: Appleton and Lange.

Riehl, J. (In press). Prologue and epilogue chapters. In J. Riehl (Ed.), *Conceptual models for nursing practice* (3d ed.). East Norwalk, Conn.: Appleton and Lange.

Riehl, J. (In press). Preface and introductions to each unit. J. Riehl (Ed.), *Conceptual Models for Nursing Practice* (3d ed.). East Norwalk, Conn.: Appleton and Lange.

Articles

Riehl, J.P. (1965). The effect of naturally occurring pain on the galvanic skin response and heart rate: A clinical study. *American Nurses' Association Regional Clinical Conference, 3:*16-23.

Riehl, J.P. & Chambers, J. (1976, July). Better salvage for the stroke victim. *Nursing, 6:*24-31.

Riehl Sisca, J. (1981, Aug.). Preparing to take the state board exams. *California Nurse, 77:*5.

Riehl Sisca, J. (1982). Nontraditional RN-BSN programs for ethnic minority students: A research paradigm. *Journal of Nursing Education, 21*(8):75.

Riehl Sisca, J. & Kerr, J. (1984). Passing the state board examination. *Journal of Nursing Education, 23*(8):358-360.

Professional Papers

Riehl, J.P. (1965). *The effect of naturally occurring pain on the galvanic skin response and heart rate: A clinical study.* Master's thesis. Los Angeles: University of California, Department of Nursing.

Riehl, J.P. (1980). *The self-conception and role relationships of autistic children: A symbolic interactionist perspective.* Doctoral dissertation. Los Angeles: University of California, Department of Sociology.

Secondary Sources

Book Reviews

J.P. Riehl & J.W. McVay (Eds.). (1973). *The clinical nurse specialist: Interpretations.*
*The Canadian Nurse, 69:*38, November 1973.
*Nursing Outlook, 21:*689-690, November 1973.
*Nursing Research, 23:*76-77, January-February 1974.
*American Journal of Nursing, 74:*960, May 1974.
*Hospitals, 48:*36, May 16, 1974.
*Nursing Mirror, 141:*72, October 2, 1975.

J.P. Riehl & C. Roy (Eds.). (1974). *Conceptual models for nursing practice.*
*The Canadian Nurse, 76:*48, December 1980.
*Nursing Times, 77:*825, May 7, 1981.
*Nursing Research, 30:*379, November-December 1981.
*American Journal of Nursing, 82:*696, April 1982.
*The Nursing Clinics of North America, 21:*461-471, September 1986.

J.P. Riehl & C. Roy (Eds.). (1980). *Conceptual models for nursing practice.*
*The Journal of Advanced Nursing, 11:*197-202, November 1986.

Books

Chinn, P.L. & Jacobs, M.K. (1983). *Theory and nursing: A systematic approach.* St. Louis: C.V. Mosby.

Kim, H.S. (1983). *The nature of theoretical thinking in nursing.* Norwalk, Conn.: Appleton-Century-Crofts.

A. Marriner (Ed.). (1986). *Nursing theorists and their work.* St. Louis: C.V. Mosby.

Meleis, A.J. (1985). *Theoretical development and progress.* Philadelphia: Lippincott.

L.H. Nicoll (Ed.). (1986). *Perspectives on nursing theory.* Boston: Little, Brown, & Co.

Walker, L.O. & Avant, K. (1983). *Strategies for theory construction in nursing.* Norwalk, Conn.: Appleton-Century-Crofts.

Book Chapters

Preisner, J.M. (1980). A proposed model for the nurse therapist. In J.P. Riehl & C. Roy (Eds.), *Conceptual models for nursing practice* (2d ed.). New York: Appleton-Century-Crofts. pp. 362-371.

Wood, M.J. (1980). Implementing the Riehl interaction model in nursing administration. In J.P. Riehl & C. Roy (Eds.), *Conceptual models for nursing practice* (2d ed.). New York: Appleton-Century-Crofts, pp. 357-361.

Correspondence

Curriculum vitae of Joan Riehl Sisca, revised November 1984.

Curriculum vitae of Joan Riehl Sisca, revised 1987.

Riehl Sisca, J. (1984, Nov. 2). Personal correspondence.

Riehl Sisca, J. (1985). Personal correspondence.

Riehl Sisca, J. (1988, April). Personal correspondence.

Interviews

Riehl Sisca, J. (1984, Oct. 10). Telephone interview.

Riehl Sisca, J. (1984, Oct. 17). Telephone interview.

Riehl Sisca, J. (1984, Nov. 30). Telephone interview.

Riehl Sisca, J. (1985). Telephone interview.

Other Sources

Blumer, H. (1969). *Symbolic interactionism: Perspective and method.* Englewood Cliffs, N.J.: Prentice-Hall.

Faris, R.E.L. (1964). *Handbook of modern sociology.* Chicago: Rand McNally.

Mead, G.H. (1934). *Mind, self, and society* (C.V. Morris, Ed.). Chicago: University of Chicago.

Rose, A.M. (1962). *Human behavior and social processes.* Boston: Houghton Mifflin.

Wells, L.E. & Marwell, G. (1976). *Self-esteem: Its conceptualization and measurement.* Beverly Hills: Sage Publications.

22

Helen C. Erickson, Evelyn M. Tomlin, Mary Ann P. Swain

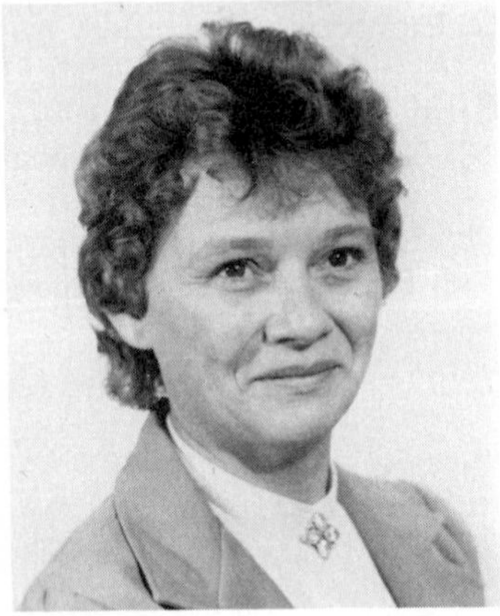

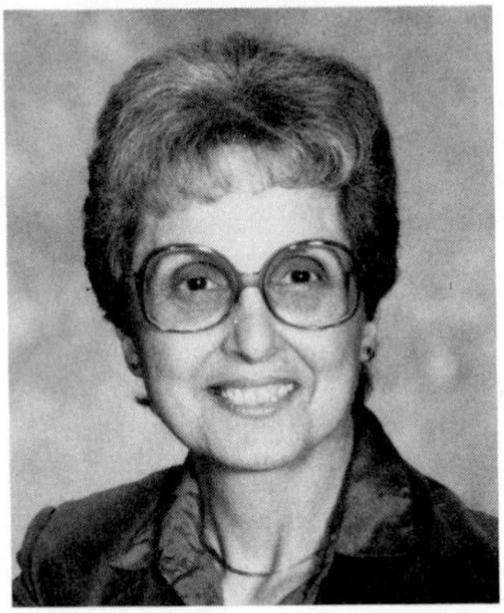

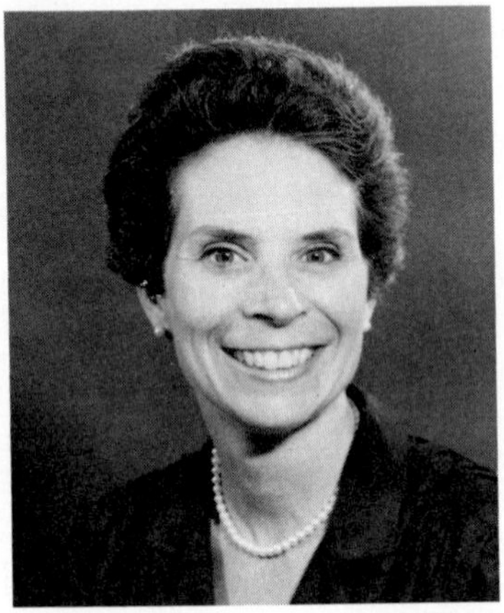

Modeling and Role-Modeling

Jane A. Caldwell-Gwin, Lisa A. Carr, Brenda Kay Harmon, Connie Rae Jarlsberg, Judy McCormick, Kathryn W. Noone

CREDENTIALS AND BACKGROUND OF THE THEORISTS

Helen Erickson

Helen Erickson received a diploma from Saginaw General Hospital, Saginaw, Michigan, in 1957. Her degrees include a Bachelor of Science in Nursing in 1974, a Master of Science in Psychiatric Nursing in 1976, and a Doctor of Educational Psychology in 1984, all from the University of Michigan.

Erickson's professional experience began in the emergency room of the Midland Community Hospital in Midland, Texas, where she was the head nurse for two years. She then worked in Mt. Pleasant, Michigan, as night supervisor

The authors wish to express appreciation to Helen C. Erickson, Evelyn M. Tomlin, and Mary Ann P. Swain for critiquing the chapter.

of nursing in the State Home for the Handicapped. She was then Director of Health Services at the Inter American University in San German, Puerto Rico, from 1960 to 1964. On her return to the United States, she worked as a staff nurse at both St. Joseph's and University Hospitals in Ann Arbor, Michigan. Erickson later served as a psychiatric nurse consultant to the Pediatric Nurse Practitioner Program at the University of Michigan. Her academic career began as a teaching assistant in the RN Studies program at the University of Michigan School of Nursing, where she later served as Chairperson of the Undergraduate Program and Interim Dean for Undergraduate Studies.

Erickson was an assistant professor of Nursing at the University of Michigan from 1978 to 1986, and is currently an adjunct assistant professor of Nursing there. In 1986, Erickson left Michigan to go to the University of South Carolina College of Nursing. Initially she served as Assistant Dean for Academic Programs, and later held the position of Associate Dean for Academic Affairs. Since 1988, Dr. Erickson has been a Professor of Nursing at the University of Texas in Austin. Erickson has also maintained an independent nursing practice since 1976.

Erickson is a member of the American Nurses Association, American Nurses' Foundation (The Charter Club), American Public Health Association, Texas Nurses Association, National League for Nursing, Sigma Theta Tau, and the Institute for the Advancement of Health. In addition, she has served as president of the Society for the Advancement of Modeling and Role-Modeling from 1986 to 1990. She was the chairperson of the First National Symposium on Modeling and Role-Modeling (1986) and served on the planning committee for the Second National Conference in 1988.

She has been listed in *Who's Who Among University Students*. She received the Sigma Theta Tau Rho Chapter Award of Excellence in Nursing in 1980, the Amoco Foundation Good Teaching Award in 1982, and was accepted into ADARA, a university honor society, in 1982.

Erickson is actively researching the Modeling and Role-Modeling theory and has presented numerous seminars and papers on various aspects of the theory both nationally and internationally.

She has served as a consultant in the implementation of the theory into clinical practice at the University of Michigan Medical Center in the surgical area and has consulted with faculty in various schools of nursing and service agencies that have considered adopting the theory into their curriculum and practice.[5,6,9,10]

Evelyn Tomlin

Evelyn Tomlin's nursing education began in Southern California. She attended Pasadena City College, Los Angeles County General Hospital School of Nursing, and the University of Southern California, where she received her Bachelor of Science in Nursing. She received a Master of Science in Psychiatric Nursing from the University of Michigan in 1976.

Tomlin's professional experiences are varied, beginning when she was a clinical instructor at Los Angeles County General Hospital School of Nursing in Surgical Nursing, Maternal and Premature Infant Nursing. She later lived in Kabul, Afghanistan, where she taught English at the Afghan Institute of Technology. In addition, she also served as school nurse and family nurse practitioner to the overseas American and European communities with which she was associated, a role that included attending more than 40 home deliveries with a Certified Nurse Midwife. After the establishment of medical services and a hospital at the United States Embassy Hospital, Tomlin functioned as relief staff nurse at the hospital. When she returned to the United States, she was employed by the Visiting Nurse Association as a staff nurse in Ann Arbor, Michigan. She then functioned as the coordinator and clinical instructor for student practical nurses. She has been a staff nurse in a coronary care unit and was briefly the head nurse of the emergency room at St. Joseph's Mercy Hospital in Ann Arbor. She has also been an assistant professor in the RN Studies Program at the University of Michigan School of Nursing. She has served as the mental health consultant to the Pediatric Nurse Practitioner Program at the University of Michigan. For 8 years she was Assistant Professor of Nursing in the fundamentals area at the University of Michigan.

Tomlin was among the first 14 nurses in the United States to be certified by the American Association of Critical Care Nurses. With several colleagues, she opened one of the first offices for independent nursing practice in Michigan. She continues to maintain her independent practice begun in 1976.

Tomlin is a member of the American Nurses Association, the Illinois Nurses Association, Sigma Theta Tau Rho Chapter, the California Scholarship Federation, and the Philathian Society. She has presented programs incorporating a variety of nursing topics into the Modeling and Role-Modeling theory and paradigm, with an emphasis on clinical applications.

In late 1985, Tomlin moved with her husband to Big Rock, Illinois, where she enjoys teaching small community and nursing groups. Tomlin is currently editing the newsletter of the Society for the Advancement of Modeling and Role-Modeling.[19,20]

Mary Ann Swain

Mary Ann Swain's educational background is in psychology. She received her Bachelor of Arts in psychology from DePauw University in Greencastle, Indiana, and her Master of Science and doctoral degrees from the University of Michigan, both in the field of psychology.

Swain has taught psychology research methods and statistics as a teaching assistant at DePauw University and later as a lecturer and an associate professor of Psychology in Nursing at the University of Michigan. She became Director of the Doctoral Program in Nursing in 1975 and served in that capacity for one year. She was Chairperson of Nursing Research from 1977 to 1982 and is currently Professor of Nursing Research at the University of Michigan. In 1983, Swain became Associate Vice President for Academic Affairs at the University of Michigan.

Swain is a member of the American Psychological Association and an associate member of the Michigan Nurses' Association. She has developed and taught classes of psychology, research, and nursing research methods. She has collaborated with nurse researchers on various projects, including health promotion among diabetics, and influencing compliance among hypertensive patients, and has worked with Erickson to develop a model for assessing potential adaptation to stress, which is significant to the Modeling and Role-Modeling theory.

Swain received the Alpha Lambda Delta, Psi Chi, Mortar Board, and Phi Beta Kappa awards while at DePauw University. In 1981, she was recognized by the Rho Chapter of Sigma Theta Tau for Contributions to Nursing and in 1983, became an honorary member of Sigma Theta Tau.[16,17]

THEORETICAL SOURCES

The theory, Modeling and Role-Modeling, uses psychological, cognitive, and biological theories as the theoretical base for the observations the theorists make regarding similarities and differences among individuals. The works of Abraham Maslow, Erik Erikson, Milton H. Erickson, Jean Piaget, George Engel, and Hans Selye are salient in the development of this theory.

Erickson, Tomlin, and Swain note a correspondence between their clinical observations and Abraham Maslow's growth principle and theory of human needs. "Maslow states that all people want to be the best they can possibly be; unmet basic needs interfere with holistic growth whereas satisfied needs promote growth."[12:45] The theorists believe that unmet basic needs can lead to initiation or aggravation of physical or mental illnesses.

The work of Erik Erikson describing the

eight stages of psychosocial development provides another source of the development of this theory. Erikson's stages represent developmental tasks. As an individual resolves each task, strengths are gained that contribute to character and health. "The utility of Erikson's theory is the freedom we may take to view aspects of people's problems as uncompleted tasks. This perspective provides a hopeful expectation for the individual's future since it connotes something still in progress."[12:62-63]

The cognitive developmental theory of Jean Piaget provides the basis for considering one of the ways individuals are alike: the development of thinking. The theorists believe that chronologically older individuals who do not develop the last stage of cognitive development, the formal operations stage, have encountered impediments in their learning process.[12:68]

The theorists identify object attachment-loss and grief theory as important in the development of their concept of Affiliated-Individuation. The works of Winnicott, Klein, Mahler, and Bowlby have provided the vast majority of the literature related to this concept.[12:68] Object relations theory is a theory of attachment that progresses from an infant's attachment to its mother, to attachment to objects such as teddy bears and blankets in childhood, and finally to more abstract attachments in adulthood, such as an educational degree. According to the theorists, "research supports the notion that object attachment is vital for adaptive coping."[12:69]

The work of Selye and Engel provides the background theory for the beliefs the theorists hold regarding the stress response. Selye's theory is a biophysical one, whereas Engel's is psychosocial. The synthesis of these theories has led to the development of the Adaptive Potential Assessment Model (APAM). The focus of the APAM is the ability of the individual to mobilize resources when confronted with stressors rather than the adaptation process. This was first developed by Erickson (1976) and published by Erickson and Swain in 1982.[10]

The final theoretical source for the development of Modeling and Role-Modeling are the psychiatric and hypnotic techniques of Milton H. Erickson. He urged Helen Erickson to "Model the client's world, understand it as they do, then role-model the picture the client has drawn—building a healthy world for them."[7]

USE OF EMPIRICAL EVIDENCE

The Adaptive Potential Assessment Model identifies three different coping potential states: arousal, equilibrium (adaptive and maladaptive), and impoverishment. Each of these states represents a different potential to mobilize self-care resources.[12:80] "Movement among the states is influenced by one's ability to cope [with ongoing stressors] and the presence of new stressors."[12:80-81] Nurses can use this model to predict an individual's potential to mobilize self-care resources in response to stress.

The Adaptive Potential Assessment Model (Figures 22-1 and 22-2) has been tested by two of the theorists. Data from the study support the classification model. "This classification model distinguishes individuals in states of stress from those in nonstress states."[11:99] "While this study statistically supports the proposed classification model, the sample size prohibits generalizations. Replication with a larger sample . . . would provide the data necessary to further develop the adaptive potential model."[11:100-101]

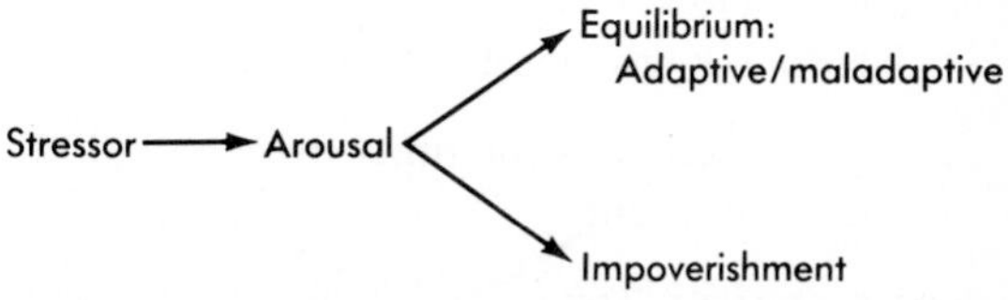

Figure 22-1. Adaptive potential assessment model.

From Erickson, H.C., Tomlin, E.M., & Swain, M.A.P. *Modeling and role-modeling: A theory and paradigm for nursing.* (1983). p. 81. Reprinted with permission of Prentice-Hall, Englewood Cliffs, N.J.

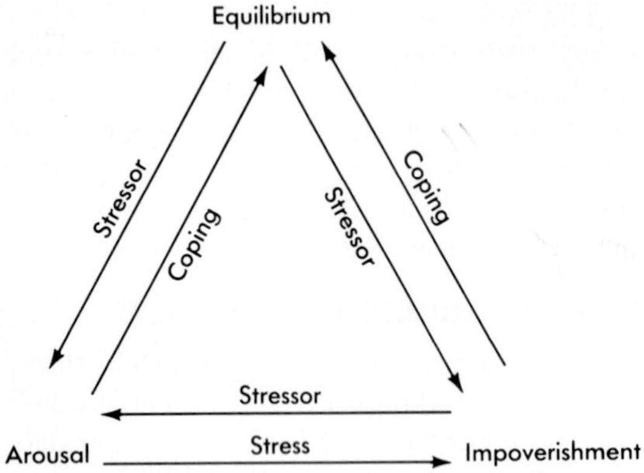

Figure 22-2. An illustration of the dynamic relationship among the states of the adaptive potential assessment model.
From Erickson, H.C., Tomlin, E.M., & Swain, M.A.P. *Modeling and role-modeling: A theory and paradigm for nursing*. (1983.) p. 82. Reprinted with permission of Prentice-Hall, Englewood Cliffs, N.J.

MAJOR CONCEPTS AND DEFINITIONS

The theory and paradigm modeling and role-modeling contains multiple concepts. These are defined as follows:

MODELING

> The act of Modeling, then, is the process the nurse uses as she develops an image and understanding of the client's world—an image and understanding developed within the client's framework and from the client's perspective. . . . The art of Modeling is the development of a mirror image of the situation from the client's perspective. . . . The science of Modeling is the scientific aggregation and analysis of data collected about the client's model.[12:95]

"Modeling occurs as the nurse accepts and understands her client."[12:96]

ROLE-MODELING

> The art of Role-Modeling occurs when the nurse plans and implements interventions that are unique for the client. The science of Role-Modeling occurs as the nurse plans interventions with respect to her theoretical base for the practice of nursing. . . . Role-Modeling is . . . the essence of nurturance. . . . Role-Modeling requires an unconditional acceptance of the person as the person is while gently encouraging and facilitating growth and development at the person's own pace and within the person's own model.[12:95]

"Role-Modeling starts the second the nurse moves from the analysis phase of the nursing process to the planning of nursing interventions."[12:95]

NURSING

> Nursing is the holistic helping of persons with their self-care activities in relation to their health. This is an interactive, interpersonal process that nurtures strengths to enable development, release, and channeling of resources for coping with one's circumstances and environment. The goal is to achieve a state of perceived optimum health and contentment[12:49]

Nurturance

> Nurturance fuses and integrates cognitive, physiological, and affective processes, with the aim of assisting a client to move toward holistic health. Nurturance implies that the nurse seeks to know and understand the client's personal model of his or her world and to appreciate its value and significance for that client from the client's perspective.[12:48]

Unconditional acceptance

> Being accepted as a unique, worthwhile, important individual—with no strings attached—is imperative if the individual is to be facilitated in developing his or her own potential. The nurse's use of empathy helps the individual learn that the nurse accepts and respects him or her as is. The acceptance will facilitate the mobilization of resources needed as this individual strives for adaptive equilibrium.[12:49]

PERSON. People are alike because of their holism, lifetime growth and development, and their Affiliated Individuation. They are different because of their inherent endowment, adaptation, and self-care knowledge.

How people are alike

Holism. "Human beings are holistic persons who have multiple interacting subsystems. Permeating all subsystems are the inherent bases. These include genetic makeup and spiritual drive. Body, mind, emotion, and spirit are a total unit and they act together. They affect and control one another interactively. The interaction of the multiple subsystems and the inherent bases creates holism: Holism implies that the whole is greater than the sum of the parts."[12:44-45]

Basic needs. "All human beings have basic needs that can be satisfied, but only from within the framework of the individual."[12:58] "Basic needs are only met when the individual perceives that they are met."[12:57]

Lifetime development. Lifetime development evolves through psychological and cognitive stages.

Psychological stages. "Each stage represents a developmental task or decisive encounter resulting in a turning point, a moment of decision between alternative basic attitudes (for example, trust versus mistrust or autonomy versus shame and doubt). As a maturing individual negotiates or resolves each age-specific crisis or task, the individual gains enduring strengths and attitudes that contribute to the character and health of the individual's personality in his or her culture."[12:61]

Cognitive stages. "Consider how thinking develops rather than what happens in psychosocial or affective development. . . . Piaget believed that cognitive learning develops in a sequential manner and he has identified several periods in this process. Essentially, there are four periods: sensorimotor, preoperational, concrete operations, and formal operations."[12:63-64]

Affiliated-Individuation. "Individuals have an instinctual need for affiliated-individuation. They need to be able to be dependent on support systems while simultaneously maintaining independence from these support systems. They need to feel a deep sense of both the 'I' and the 'we' states of being and to perceive freedom and acceptance in both states."[12:47]

How people are different

Inherent endowment. "Each individual is born with a set of genes that will to some extent predetermine appearance, growth, development, and responses to life events. . . . Clearly, both genetic makeup and inherited characteristics influence growth and development. They might influence how one perceives oneself and one's world. They make individuals different from one another, each unique in his or her own way."[12:74-75]

Adaptation. "Adaptation occurs as the individual responds to external and internal stressors in a health and growth-directed manner. Adaptation involves mobilizing internal and external coping resources. No subsystem is left in jeopardy when adaptation occurs."[12:47]

Mind body relationships. "We are all biophysical, psychosocial beings who want to develop our potential, that is, to be the best we can be."[12:70]

Self-care. Self-care involves the use of knowledge, resources, and action.

> *Self-care knowledge.* "At some level a person knows what has made him or her sick, lessened his or her effectiveness, or interfered with his or her growth. The person also knows what will make him or her well, optimize his or her effectiveness or fulfillment (given circumstances), or promote his or her growth."[12:48]
>
> *Self-care resources.* Self-care resources are "the internal resources, as well as additional resources, mobilized through self-care action that help gain, maintain, and promote an optimum level of holistic health."[12:254-255]
>
> *Self-care action.* Self-care action is "the develop-

ment and utilization of self-care knowledge and self-care resources."[12:254]

MAJOR ASSUMPTIONS

Nursing

"The nurse is a facilitator, not an effector. Our nurse-client relationship is an interactive, interpersonal process that aids the individual to identify, mobilize, and develop his or her own strengths."[12:48]

Person

A differentiation is made between patients and clients in this theory. A patient is given treatment and instruction; a client participates in his own care. "Our goal is for nurses to work with clients."[12:21] "A client is one who is considered to be a legitimate member of the decision-making team, who always has some control over the planned regimen, and who is incorporated into the planning and implementation of his or her own care as much as possible."[12:20]

Health

"Health is a state of physical, mental, and social well-being, not merely the absence of disease or infirmity. It connotes a state of dynamic equilibrium among the various subsystems [of a holistic person]."[12:46]

Environment

"Environment is not identified in the theory as an entity of its own. The theorists see environment in the social subsystems as the interaction between self and others both cultural and individual. Biophysical stressors are seen as part of the environment."[7]

THEORETICAL ASSERTIONS

The theoretical assertions of Modeling and Role-Modeling are based on the linkages between completion of developmental tasks and basic need satisfaction; between basic need satisfaction, object attachment and loss, and developmental tasks; and the relationship between the ability to mobilize coping resources and need satisfaction. Three generic theoretical assertions that constitute a number of theoretical linkages implied in the theory but less specifically delineated are:

1. "The degree to which developmental tasks are resolved is dependent on the degree to which human needs are satisfied."[12:87]
2. "The degree to which needs are satisfied by object attachment depends on the availability of those objects and the degree to which they provide comfort and security as opposed to threat and anxiety."[12:90]
3. "An individual's potential for mobilizing resources—the person's state of coping according to the APAM [Adaptive Potential Assessment Model]—is directly associated with the person's need satisfaction level."[12:91]

LOGICAL FORM

The theory, Modeling and Role-Modeling, is formulated by the use of retroductive thinking. The theorists go through all four levels of theory development and then recycle from inductive to deductive to inductive to deductive.[7] The theoretical sources were used to validate clinical observations. Clinical observations were tested in light of the theoretical bases. These sources were synthesized with their observations, which enabled Erickson, Tomlin, and Swain to develop a "multi-dimensional new theory and paradigm—Modeling and Role-Modeling."[7]

The theorists label Modeling and Role-Modeling a theory and paradigm. This is a valid label because Modeling and Role-Modeling meets the five functions of a paradigm as identified by Merton,[15:70] who said paradigms "provide a compact arrangement of central concepts and their interrelations that are utilized for description and analysis." The theorists provide a clear presentation of their central concepts and build on the relationships as they described them. "Paradigms lessen the likelihood of inadvertently introducing hidden assumptions and concepts, for each new assumption and concept must be either logically derived from previous components or explicitly introduced into it."[15:71] Erickson, Tomlin, and Swain build on previous components as their paradigm is developed, each component being logically derived from clinical observations or based in theory. "Third, paradigms advance the cumulation of theoretical interpretation."[15:71] It appears the assumptions and concepts made by the theorists allow for interpretation in multiple clinical and research situations in which the concepts may be applied, thereby expanding the theory base of nursing. "Paradigms promote analysis rather than description of concrete details."[15:71] Modeling and Role-Modeling promotes analysis of significant concepts. The interrelationships among the concepts can also be empirically examined because they have broad applicability, and lend themselves to multiple research questions. "Fifth, paradigms make for codification of qualitative analysis in a way that approximates the logic if not the empirical rigor of quantitative analysis."[15:71] Erickson states that a qualitative approach has been used to form concepts. Based on that approach, scales were built using deductive logic to test those concepts.[7] The methods used will become available for replication of studies as they are published.

ACCEPTANCE BY THE NURSING COMMUNITY

Practice

Publication of the books *Modeling and Role-Modeling: A Theory and Paradigm for Nursing* and a chapter on Self-care in *Introduction to Person-Centered Nursing,* as well as publication of research studies based on the theory, have exposed practicing nurses to this theory. Currently, nurses on surgical units at the University of Michigan Medical Center are using an assessment tool based on the theory Modeling and Role-Modeling. The tool is used to gather information to identify the clients' need assets, deficits, developmental residual, attachment-loss, and grief status, and potential therapeutic interventions. (See Appendix A.)[3,10,14]

The theorists have spoken prolifically on their theory and have held one-to-one consultations that exposed nurses from various practice and educational backgrounds to the theory. Nurses in critical care, mental health, and hospices are using the theory. Erickson[7] has noted that what seemed to be a revolutionary idea as recently as 7 to 8 years ago—"calling for the client to be the head of the Health Care Team"—is rapidly gaining acceptance, as is the notion that nurses can practice nursing independently. According to Erickson,[7] negative responses to the theory came from individuals who cannot accept the idea of "listening to the client first" or who do not take the concept of holism seriously.

Education

The theory is introduced into the curriculum in the sophomore year at the University of Michigan School of Nursing and is required for returning R.N. students as well. Faculty members at several nursing schools have contacted Erickson regarding the use of the theory in their curricula.

Introduction to Person-Centered Nursing, with a chapter on "Self-care" by Tomlin, is being used as a text in various schools of nursing and is expanding exposure to the theory concepts.

Research

Erickson and Swain continue to research the Modeling and Role-Modeling Theory. A study recently completed was entitled "Modeling and Role-Modeling: Testing Nursing Theory." A current research activity involves validating the self-care knowledge construct.[6] The initial study provided evidence that psychosocial factors are significantly related to physical health problems. A follow-up study (1988) supported these findings. Key concepts include perceived support, perceived control, hope for the future, and satisfaction with daily life. The 1988 study was authored by Erickson, S. Lock, and Swain.[10]

The theorists identify several other research projects that are tests of the theory. Several doctoral students at the University of Michigan School of Nursing are pursuing various research questions based in the theory. A research study is under way at the University of Michigan Medical Center by three nurses who have hypothesized that length of hospital stay correlates with stages of development. A nursing assessment tool developed by D. Finch, J. Campbell, and M. Hunt was used to measure a patient's psychosocial development and to relate developmental status to the length of hospitalization and the number of health problems identified during hospitalization. The results show that the balance of trust-mistrust accounts for a large percent of the variance in the length of hospitalization. There was no significant relationship between psychosocial coping skills and number of health problems identified.[13,14]

The Adaptive Potential Assessment Model has recently been validated in a research study conducted by Dr. Janet Barnfather at the University of Michigan.[1,2] In addition, several other doctoral students are currently using Modeling Role-Modeling as a basis for their dissertations.[9] Although there is currently a lack of published work that substantiates the theory, this does not adequately reflect the research being done. More empirical evidence supporting the theory will be forthcoming.

FURTHER DEVELOPMENT

This theory is in its infancy; therefore, there is much potential for further development. Currently the theory is gaining national and international attention. One reason for this increased attention is the founding of the Society for the Advancement of Modeling and Role-Modeling. The Society was formed in order to develop a network of colleagues who could advance the development and application of the Modeling and Role-Modeling theory. One of the goals is to promote continued research related to the theory. The Society's first National Symposium was held in 1986 and has met biennially thereafter. At the 1988 conference held at Hilton Head, South Carolina, the membership chair announced that society members came from 12 different states.[10] The conference is a forum for researchers, educators, and practitioners to disseminate knowledge pertaining to the Modeling Role-Modeling theory and paradigm.[10] Currently, little published data related to the theory exists. Erickson[7] states, "Every part of it [the theory] needs further development. . . . There are a thousand research questions in that book. . . . You can take any one statement we make and ask a research question about it. . . . Modeling and Role-Modeling has only begun."

EVALUATION OF THE THEORY

Clarity

Erickson, Tomlin, and Swain present their theory clearly. Definitions in the theory are denotative, with the concepts explicitly defined. They use everyday language and offer many examples to illustrate their meaning. Their definitions and assumptions are consistent, and there is a logical progression from assumptions to assertions.

Simplicity

The theory appears simple at first. However, on closer inspection, it becomes complex. It is based on biological and psychological theories and several of the theorists' own assumptions. The interactions among the major concepts, assumptions, and assertions add depth to the theory and increase its complexity.

Generality

Because its major assumptions that deal with developmental tasks, basic needs satisfaction, object attachment and loss, and adaptive potential are broad enough to be applicable in multiple diverse nursing situations, the theory is generalizable to all nursing and client situations. The theorists cite many examples of the applicability of their concepts, both in clinical practice and research. It may be argued that the theory lacks applicability in the pediatric or comatose population. But we believe the theory is applicable in these situations, although it may take some creativity on the part of the clinician to make those applications. Modeling and Role-Modeling is generalizable to all aspects of professional nursing practice.

Empirical Precision

Empirical precision is increased if the theory has operationally defined concepts, identifiable subconcepts, and denotative definitions. The major concepts, Modeling and Role-Modeling, are reality-based, which makes them more empirical than general. Definitions in the theory are denotative, making it possible to test empirically the concepts identified. The theorists provide an outline for collecting, analyzing, and synthesizing data, and guidelines for implementing their theory based on the client's model. These explicit guidelines increase the empirical precision of the theory by allowing any practitioner to test the theory using these tools.

Chinn and Jacobs[4:42] state, "Empirical precision is necessarily increased with research testing." Data reflecting research testing of the theory is not currently readily available; however, as has been stated, studies are ongoing. We believe Modeling and Role-Modeling will gain empirical precision when data become available for critical analysis. The theorists recognize the need for further research of their theory and encourage practicing nurses to do it.[7]

Derivable Consequences

One of the many challenges facing the profession of nursing is the development of a unique, scientific knowledge base. One aid in this process is the use of nursing theory as a basis for professional practice. Erickson, Tomlin, and Swain's theory of Modeling and Role-Modeling can provide the stimulus to accomplish this goal.

Although this is a relatively recent theory, it is gaining recognition in the nursing community. As interest grows, additional research supporting its theoretical statements will be generated. Many nurses are engaged in research based on this theory. Publication of the findings will lend credence to the theoretical propositions.

Chinn and Jacobs state a theory should be evaluated in terms of its derivable consequences. The derivable consequences can be determined by examining whether or not the theory guides research, directs practice, generates new ideas, and differentiates the focus of nursing from other professions.[4:142] In terms of these criteria, this theory does appear to possess inherent value, although the scope is undeterminable at this time. As the theory matures, the extent of its merit and worth will become evident. However, one thing can undoubtedly be said. Erickson, Tomlin, and Swain's theory of Modeling and Role-Modeling encourages, as well as challenges, nurses to practice theory-based nursing.

REFERENCES

1. Barnfather, J.S. (1988, March). Personal correspondence.
2. Barnfather, J.S. (1988). *Mobilizing coping resources related to basic need status in healthy, young adults.* Doctoral dissertation, the University of Michigan.
3. Campbell, J., Finch, D., Allport, C., Erickson, H.C., & Swain, M.A.P. (1985). A theoretical approach to nursing assessment. *Journal of Advanced Nursing, 10:*111-115.
4. Chinn, P.L. & Jacobs, M.K. (1983). *Theory and nursing: A systematic approach.* St. Louis: C.V. Mosby.
5. Erickson, H.C. (1984, Oct.) Curriculum vitae.
6. Erickson, H.C. (1988, Feb.). Curriculum vitae.
7. Erickson, H.C. (1984, Nov. 5). Telephone interview.
8. Erickson, H.C. (1984, Nov. 7). Telephone interview.
9. Erickson, H.C. (1988, March 30). Telephone interview.
10. Erickson, H.C. (1988). Personal correspondence.

11. Erickson, H.C. & Swain, M.A. (1982). A model for assessing potential adaptation to stress. *Research in Nursing and Health, 5:*93-101.
12. Erickson, H.C. Tomlin, E.M., & Swain, M.A. (1983). *Modeling and role-modeling: A theory and paradigm for nursing.* Englewood Cliffs, N.J.: Prentice-Hall.
13. Finch, D. (1987). *Testing a theoretically based nursing assessment.* Doctoral dissertation. The Unversity of Michigan.
14. Finch, D. (1988, March). Personal correspondence.
15. Merton, R.K. (1968). *Social theory and social structure.* New York: The Free Press.
16. Swain, M.A. (1984, Oct.). Curriculum vitae.
17. Swain, M.A.P. (1988, Feb.). Curriculum vitae.
18. Tomlin, E.M. (1982). Self-care. In J. Lindberg, M. Hunter, & A. Pruszewski, *Introduction to person-centered nursing.* Philadelphia: J.B. Lippincott.
19. Tomlin, E.M. (1984, Oct.). Curriculum vitae.
20. Tomlin, E.M. (1988, Feb.) Curriculum vitae.

BIBLIOGRAPHY

Primary Sources

Books

Erickson, H.C., Tomlin, E.M., & Swain, M.A. (1983). *Modeling and role-modeling: A theory and paradigm for nursing.* Englewood Cliffs, N.J.: Prentice-Hall.

Raush, H., et al. (1974). *Communication, conflicts, and marriage.* San Francisco: Jossey-Bass.

Book Chapters

Erickson, H.C. (1977). Communication in nursing. In *Professional nursing matrix: A workbook.* Ann Arbor, Mich.: Media Library, University of Michigan, pp. 1-150.

Tomlin, E.M. (1983). Self-care. In J. Lindberg, M. Hunter, & A. Kruszewski, *Introduction to person-centered nursing.* Philadelphia: J.P. Lippincott, pp. 51-60.

Articles

Campbell, J., Finch, D., Allport. C., Erickson, H.C., & Swain, M.A.P. (1985). A theoretical approach to nursing assessment. *Journal of Advanced Nursing, 10:*111-115.

Erickson, H. & Swain, M.A. (1977). The utilization of a nursing care model for treatment of essential hypertension. 56 Supp. III (1977, Oct.): 145. Circulation. (Abstract).

Erickson, H. & Swain, M.A. (1982, June). A model for assessing potential adaptation to stress. *Research in Nursing and Health, 5:*93-101.

Schulman, B.A. & Swain, M.A. (1980, Jan.). Active patient orientation. *Patient Counseling and Health Education, 2:*32-37.

Steckel, S. & Swain, M.A. (1977, Dec.). The use of written contracts to increase adherence. *Hospitals, 51:*81-84.

Swain, M.A. & Steckel, S. (1981, March). Influencing adherence among hypertensive. *Research in Nursing and Health, 4:*213-222.

Tomlin, E.M. (1953, Oct.). Los Angeles Program for Premature Infant Care (Section III). *Nursing Outlook, 1:*568-569.

Thesis

Erickson, H. (1976). *Identification of states of coping utilizing physiological and psychological data.* Master's thesis. The University of Michigan.

Dissertations

Erickson, H. (1984). *Self-care knowledge: Relationships among the concepts of support, hope, control, and satisfaction with daily life.* Doctoral dissertation, the University of Michigan.

Correspondence

Erickson, H.C. (1984, Oct.). Curriculum vitae.
Erickson, H.C. (1988, Feb.). Curriculum vitae.
Erickson, H.C. (1988). Personal correspondence.
Swain, M.A. (1984. Oct.). Curriculum vitae.
Swain, M.A.P. (1988, Feb.). Curriculum vitae.
Tomlin, E.M. (1984, Oct.). Curriculum vitae.
Tomlin, E.M. (1988, Feb.). Curriculum vitae.

Interviews

Erickson, H. (1984, Nov. 5). Telephone interview.
Erickson, H. (1984, Nov. 7). Telephone interview.
Erickson, H.C. (1988, March 30). Telephone interview.

Secondary Sources

Book Reviews

Erickson, H.C., Tomlin, E.M., & Swain, M.A.P. (1983). *Modeling and role-modeling: A theory and paradigm for nursing.*

*American Journal of Nursing, 83:*1355, September 1983.
*Nursing and Health Care, 4:*413, September 1983.
*Nursing Outlook, 32:*116, February 1984.

Dissertations

Barnfather, J.S. (1988). *Mobilizing coping resources related to basic need status in healthy, young adults.* Doctoral dissertation, the University of Michigan.

Finch, D. (1987). *Testing a theoretically based nursing assessment.* Doctoral dissertation, the University of Michigan.

Correspondence

Barnfather, J.S. (1988, March). Personal correspondence.

Finch, D. (1988, March). Personal correspondence.

Other Sources

Bowlby, J. (1958). The nature of the child's tie to his mother. *International Journal of Psychoanalysis, 39:*89-97.

Bowlby, J. (1960). Child care and the growth of love. In M. Haimowitz & N. Haimowitz, *Human development* (2d ed.). New York: Thomas Y. Crowell. pp. 155-166.

Bowlby, J. (1961). Childhood mourning and its explications for psychiatry. *American Journal of Psychiatry, 118:*481-498.

Bowlby, J. (1961). Process of mourning. *International Journal of Psychoanalysis, 42:*317-340.

Bowlby, J. (1969). *Attachment.* New York: Basic Books.

Bowlby, J. (1973). *Separation.* New York: Basic Books.

Bowlby, J. (1980). *Loss.* New York: Basic Books.

Bowlby, J., Robertson, J., & Rosenbluth, D. (1952). A two-year-old goes to the hospital. *The Psychoanalytic Study of the Child, 7:*89-94.

Chinn, P.L. & Jacobs, M.K. (1983). *Theory and nursing: A systematic approach.* St. Louis: C.V. Mosby.

Engel, G.S. (1962). *Psychological development in health and disease.* Philadelphia: Saunders.

Erikson, E. (1960). The case of Peter. In M. Haimowitz & N. Haimowitz, *Human development.* (2d ed.). New York: Thomas Y. Crowell, pp. 355-359.

Erikson, E. (1960). Identity versus self-diffusion. In M. Haimowitz & N. Haimowitz, *Human development* (2d ed.). New York: Thomas Y. Crowell, pp. 766-770.

Erikson, E. (1963). *Childhood and society.* New York: W.W. Norton.

Erickson, H. (1986). Synthesizing clinical experiences: A step in theory development. Ann Arbor, Mich.: Biomedical Communications.

Haley, J. (1973). *Uncommon therapy: The psychiatric techniques of Milton H. Erickson, M.D.* New York: W.W. Norton.

Klein, M. (1952). Some theoretical conclusions regarding the emotional life of the infant. In J. Riviere, *Developments in psycho-analysis.* London: Hogarth Press, pp. 198-236.

Mahler, M.S. (1967). On human symbiosis and the vicissitudes of individuation. *Journal of the American Psychoanalytic Association, 15:*740-763.

Mahler, M.S. & Furer, M. (1968). *On human symbiosis and the vicissitudes of individuation* (Vol. I). *Infantile psychosis.* New York: International Universities Press.

Maslow, A.H. (1936). The need to know and the fear of knowing. *The Journal of General Psychology, 68:*111-25.

Maslow, A.H. (1968). *Toward a psychology of being* (2d ed.). New York: D. Von Nostrand.

Maslow, A.H. (1970). *Motivation and personality* (2d ed.). New York: Harper & Row.

Merton, R.K. (1968). *Social theory and social structure.* New York: The Free Press.

Piaget, J. (1952). *The origins of intelligence in children.* New York: International Universities Press.

Piaget, J. (1974). The pathway between subjects' recent life changes and their near-future illness reports: Representative results and methodological issues. In B.S. Dohrenwend & B.P. Dohrenwend, *Stressful life events: Their nature and effects.* New York: John Wiley & Sons, pp. 73-86.

Piaget, J. & Inhelder, B. (1969). *The psychology of the child.* New York: Basic Books.

Selye, H. (1974). *Stress without distress.* Philadelphia: Lippincott.

Selye, H. (1976). *The stress of life* (2d ed.). New York: McGraw-Hill.

Selye, H. (1979). Further thoughts on stress without distress. *Resident and Staff Physician, 25:*125-134.

Winnicott, D.W. (1953). Transitional objects and transitional phenomena: A study of the first not-me possession. *International Journal of Psychoanalysis, 34:*89-97.

Winnicott, D.W. (1965). The theory of the parent-infant relationship. In D.W. Winnicott, *The maturational processes and the facilitating environment.* London, Hogarth Press.

APPENDIX A. ASSESSMENT TOOL BASED ON MODELING AND ROLE-MODELING

I. Description of Situation
   A. Primary source (patient)
   B. Secondary sources (nursing and family)

II. Expectations
   A. Primary source
   B. Secondary sources

III. Support Resources
   A. Primary source
   B. Secondary sources

IV. Strengths
   A. Primary source
   B. Secondary sources

V. Geographical Data

VI. Health Status
   A. Primary source
   B. Secondary sources

23

Kathryn E. Barnard

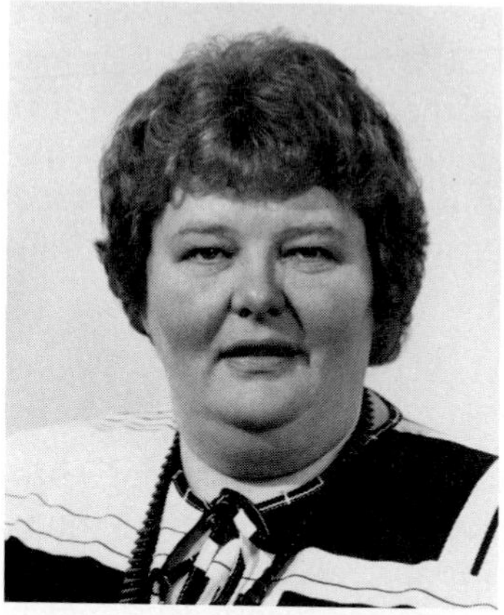

Parent-Child Interaction Model

Jill K. Baker, Debra A. Borchers, Debra Trnka Cochran, Karla G. Kaltofen, Nancy Orcutt, Elizabeth Godfrey Terry, Cynthia A. Wesolowski, Lorraine A. Yeager

CREDENTIALS AND BACKGROUND OF THE THEORIST

Kathryn E. Barnard was born April 16, 1938, in Omaha, Nebraska. In 1956 she enrolled in a prenursing program at the University of Nebraska and graduated with a Bachelor of Science in Nursing in June 1960. Upon graduation, she continued at the University of Nebraska in part-time graduate studies. That summer she accepted an acting head nurse position and in the fall became an assistant instructor in pediatric nursing.[8] In 1961 Barnard moved to Boston, Massachusetts, where she enrolled in a Master's program at Boston University. She also worked as a private duty nurse. After earning her Master's of Science in Nursing in June 1962 and a certificate of Advanced Graduate Specialization in Nursing Education, she accepted a position as an instructor in maternal and child nursing at the University of

The authors wish to express appreciation to Dr. Elizabeth Choi for her assistance with data collection and to Dr. Kathryn E. Barnard for critiquing the chapter.

Washington in Seattle. In 1965 she was named Assistant Professor. She began consulting in the area of mental retardation, and coordinated training projects for nurses in child development and the care of children with mental retardation and handicaps. Barnard became the project director for a research study to develop a method for nursing child assessment in 1971. The following year she earned a Ph.D. in the Ecology of Early Childhood Development from the University of Washington.[7:1-2]

In 1972 Barnard accepted a position at the University of Washington as a professor in parent-child nursing. From May 1985 to May 1986, Barnard was an adjunct professor of Psychology at the University of Washington. She was appointed Associate Dean for Academic Affairs at the University of Washington School of Nursing in 1987.[17:3]

Since 1972 she has been the principal investigator of 18 research grants and coinvestigator of one research grant. In addition to these research efforts, Barnard has provided consultation, presented lectures internationally, and served on multiple advisory boards. She has published articles in both nursing and nonnursing journals since 1966. Her books include a four-part series on child health assessment, two editions related to teaching the mentally retarded/developmentally delayed child, and her most recent work focusing on families of vulnerable infants.[7:2-14]

Barnard[4:4] is a member of the American Nurses' Association, where she has served on the Executive Committee for the Division on Maternal and Child Health Nursing. She is also an active member of ten other national organizations, including The Society for Research in Child Development, Sigma Theta Tau, the National League for Nursing, and the American Academy of Nursing.* She has served on numerous advisory boards and committees of these professional organizations.[17:7-8]

In 1969 Barnard was presented with the Lucille Petry Leone Award by the National League for Nursing for her outstanding contribution to nursing education.[15:9] Since then she has been honored by several other associations, including the American Nurses' Association's Maternal and Child Health Nurse of the Year Award, which was presented at the 1984 convention.[16:242] In 1987 Barnard was named Nurse Scientist of the Year by the Council of Nurse Researchers of the American Nurses' Association. She was the recipient of two research awards from Sigma Theta Tau in that same year.[17:9]

THEORETICAL SOURCES FOR THEORY DEVELOPMENT

Although Barnard cites various nursing theorists, such as Florence Nightingale, Virginia Henderson, and Martha Rogers, their direct influence on her research and theory development is uncertain.[10:193-194;4:208]

Barnard refers to the Neal Nursing Construct, which has four expressions of health and illness: cognition, sensation, motion, and affiliation. Neal worked on a construct for practice and Barnard and her associate developed measures related to the period of infancy. Barnard later stated, "In reviewing both the Maryland construct and the Washington research, we were impressed with how the design and results of the Nursing Child Assessment Project (NCAP) fit into the [Neal] construct."[10:195-196]

Barnard credits Florence Blake for the beliefs and values making up the foundation of current nursing practice. She describes Blake as:

> a great pediatric nursing clinician and educator [who] turned our minds toward an orientation on the patient rather than the procedure. Blake saw the principal function of parenthood and nursing to be the capacity to establish and maintain constructive and satisfying relationships with others. She amplified for nursing important acts such as mother-infant attachment, maternal care, and separation of child from parents. She helped nursing understand the importance of the family.[10:194]

*7:8; 18:268; 17:7-8.

Many of Dr. Barnard's publications were coauthored by writers such as D. King and A.W. Pattullo, indicating a variety of influences. Barnard also published a book, entitled *Teaching the Mentally Retarded Child: A Family Care Approach,* with Marcene L. Powell. Four years later they developed a second edition, *Teaching Children with Developmental Problems: A Family Care Approach.* Of greater influence were the coinvestigators and consultants of the Nursing Child Assessment Project, which includes Sandra Eyres, Charlene Snyder, and Helen Bee Douglas.[9:IV] Barnard[8] states she was influenced by child development theorists such as J. Piaget, J.S. Brunner, L. Sander, and T.B. Brazelton, in addition to nursing theorists.

USE OF EMPIRICAL EVIDENCE

Many researchers' findings were used as Barnard's work centering around the parent-child interaction evolved. Barnard used T. Berry Brazelton's work as well as Bettye Caldwell's. Once it was determined that the interaction/adaptation between parent and child was the area to focus on, Barnard[9:6] used the research findings of many, such as H. Als, M.F. Waldrup and J.D. Goering, and L.M.S. Dubowitz. Their findings added to the growing body of usable knowledge that could be brought to bear on the task of developing tools to adequately assess that important interactional aspect of early child development.

In addition to tapping others' research, Barnard conducted her own. She began her research in 1968 by studying mentally and physically handicapped children and adults. In the early 1970s she studied the activities of the well child and later expanded her study to include methods of evaluating growth and development of children. She also initiated a 10-year series of research projects to examine the effects of stimulation on sleep states in premature infants. The majority of these research studies were funded by grants from the U.S. Department of Health, Education, and Welfare.[7:5]

In 1976 Barnard was awarded a grant by HEW to determine "the most effective ways of disseminating research with the use of media including communication satellite."[127:5] This led to the evolution of the Nursing Child Assessment Satellite Training Project. In 1977 Barnard began researching methods for disseminating information about newborns and young children to parents. Projects have been funded by the National Foundation of the March of Dimes and Johnson & Johnson baby products. Barnard recently participated in a publication for parents entitled, "The Many Facets of Touch," which was also funded by Johnson & Johnson.

Today, Barnard continues to study the mother-infant relationship. Her most recent research projects examine the nurse's role in relation to high-risk mothers and high-risk infants.[7:6]

The Nursing Child Assessment Project (NCAP) formed the basis for Barnard's Child Health Assessment Interaction Theory. This was a longitudinal study "to identify poor [child development] outcomes before they occur and to examine the variability of the screening and assessment measures over time."[12:16] The study population included 193 infants and their parents. Using various assessment scales and interviewing tools, the child and his or her parental relationships were assessed at six stages: prenatally, postnatally, at 1 month, 4 months, 8 months, and 1 year of age. Additional funds were obtained to continue the project by reassessing the child and parent at 2 years of age, and again when the children were in the second grade.[12:16]

MAJOR CONCEPTS AND DEFINITIONS

A major focus of Barnard's work was the development of assessment tools to evaluate child health, growth, and development while viewing the parent and child as an interactive system. Barnard stated the parent-infant system was influenced by individual characteristics of each member and that the individual characteristics were also modified to meet the needs of the system. She defines modification as adaptive behavior. The interaction between parent and child is diagrammed in the Barnard Model in Figure 23-1.

Barnard[2:9-12] has defined the terms in the diagram as follows:

> *Infant's clarity to cues.* To participate in a synchronous relationship, the infant must send cues to his/her caregiver. The skill and clarity with which these cues are sent will make it either easy or difficult for the parent to "read" the cues and make the appropriate modification of his/her own behavior. Infants send cues of many kinds: sleepiness, fussiness, alertness, hunger and satiation, and changes in body activity, to name a few. Ambiguous or confusing cues sent by an infant can interrupt a caregiver's adaptive abilities.
>
> *Infant's responsiveness to the caregiver.* Just as the infant must "send" cues so that the parent can modify his/her behavior, the infant must also "read" cues so that he/she can modify his/her behavior in return. Obviously, if the infant is unresponsive to the behavioral cues of his/her caregivers, adaptation is not possible.
>
> *Parent's sensitivity to the child's cues.* Parents, like infants, must be able to accurately read the cues given by the infant if they are to appropriately modify their behavior. . . . There are also other influences on the parents' sensitivity. Parents who are greatly concerned about other aspects of their lives, such as occupational or financial problems, emotional problems, or marital stress may be unable to be as sensitive as they would be otherwise. Only when these stresses are reduced are some parents able to "read" the cues of their young children.
>
> *Parents' ability to alleviate the infant's distress.* Some cues sent by the infant signal that assistance from the parent is needed. . . . The effectiveness of parents in alleviating the distress of their infants depends upon several factors. First, they must recognize that distress is occurring. . . . Second, they must know (or figure out) the appropriate action which will alleviate distress. . . . Finally, they must be available to put this knowledge to work.
>
> *Parent's social and emotional growth-fostering activities.* . . . The ability to initiate social and emotional growth-fostering activities depends upon more global parent adaption. The parent needs to be able to play affectionately with the child, engage in social interactions such as those associated with eating, and to provide appropriate social reinforcement of desirable behaviors. To do these things the parent must be aware of the child's level of development and be able to adjust his/her behavior accordingly. . . . This depends as much upon the parent's available energy as on his/her knowledge and skill.
>
> *Parent's cognitive growth fostering activities.* . . . It has been shown in a number of studies that cognitive growth is facilitated by providing stimulation which is just above the child's level of understanding. To do this, the parent must have a good grasp of the child's present level of understanding . . . and the parent also have the energy available to use these skills.

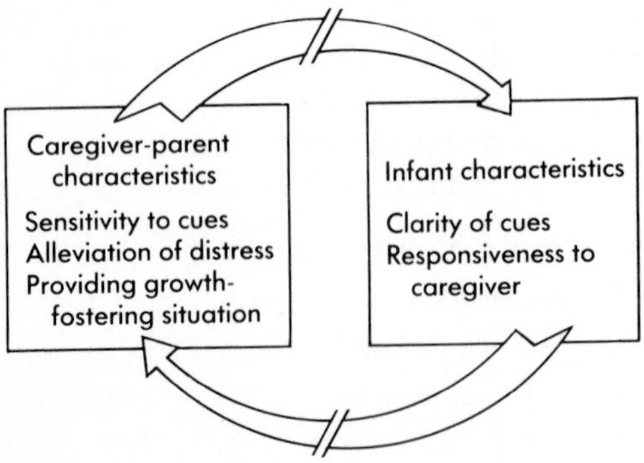

Figure 23-1. The Barnard model.
Used with permission from Barnard, K.E., et al. (1977). *The nursing child assessment training study guide: Program learning manual.* p. 8.

As the NCAP continued, Barnard's model became the foundation for her Child Health Assessment Interaction Theory. Three major concepts form the basis of this theory.

CHILD. In describing the child, Barnard[12:16] used the characteristics of "newborn behavior, feeding and sleeping patterns, physical appearance, temperament and the child's ability to adapt to his/her caregiver and environment."

MOTHER. *Mother* refers to the child's mother or caregiver and his or her important characteristics. The mother's characteristics include her "psychosocial assets, her concerns about her child, her own health, the amount of life change she experienced, her expectations for her child, and most important, her parenting style and her adaptional skills."[12:17]

ENVIRONMENT. The environment represents the environment of both child and mother. Characteristics of the environment include "aspects of the physical environment of the family, the father's involvement and the degree of parent mutuality in regard to child rearing."[12:17]

MAJOR ASSUMPTIONS

Nursing

Except for nursing, Barnard does not define her major assumptions. In 1966 she defined *nursing* as "a process by which the patient is assisted in maintenance and promotion of his independence. This process may be educational, therapeutic, or restorative: it involves facilitation of change, most probably a change in the environment."[1:629] Five years later, in a 1981 keynote address to the first International Nursing Research Conference, she defined nursing as "the diagnosis and treatment of human responses to health problems."[6:2]

Person

When Barnard describes a person or human being, she speaks of the ability "to take in auditory, visual, and tactile stimuli but also to make meaningful associations from what he takes in."[11:15] This term includes infants, children, and adults.

Health

Although Barnard does not define health, she describes the family "as the basic unit of health care."[5:210] In the *Nursing Child Assessment Satellite Training Study Guide,* she states, "In health care, the ultimate goal is primary prevention."[2] Barnard emphasizes the importance of striving to reach one's maximum potential. She believes "We must promote new values in American society, which up to now has valued not health, but the absence of disease."[17:9] She wrote the definition for the scope of practice on maternal child health.

Environment

Environment is an essential aspect of Dr. Barnard's theory. In *Child Health Assessment, Part 2: The First Year of Life,* she states, "In essence, the environment includes all experiences encountered by the child: people, objects, places, sounds, visual and tactile sensations."[9:53] She makes a distinction between the animate and inanimate environments. "The inanimate environment refers to the objects available to the child for exploration and manipulation. The animate environment includes the activities of the caretaker used in arousing and directing the young child to the external world."[9:53]

THEORETICAL ASSERTIONS

Barnard's Child Health Assessment Interaction Theory is based on 10 theoretical assertions. They are:[12:6-7]

1. In child health assessment the *ultimate* goal is to identify problems at a point before they develop and when intervention would be most effective.
2. Environmental factors, as typified by the process of parent-child interaction, are important for determining child health outcomes.
3. The caregiver-infant interaction provides information that reflects the nature of the child's ongoing environment.
4. The caregiver brings a basic style and level of skills that are enduring characteristics; the caregiver's adaptive capacity is more readily influenced by responses of the infant and her environmental support.
5. In the adaptive parent-child interaction, there is a process of mutual modification in that the parent's behavior influences the infant or child and in turn the child influences the parent so that both are changed.
6. The adaptive process is more modifiable than

the mother's or infant's basic characteristics; therefore, in intervention the nurse should lend support to the mother's sensitivity and response to her infant's cues rather than trying to change her characteristics or styles.
7. An important quality of promoting the child's learning is in permitting child-initiated behaviors and in reinforcing the child's attempt at a task.
8. A major issue for the nursing profession is support of the child's caregiver during the first year of life.
9. Interactive assessment is important in any comprehensive child health care model.
10. Assessment of the child's environment is important in any child health assessment model.

The Child Health Assessment Interaction Model was developed to illustrate Barnard's theory (Figure 23-2). "The smallest circle represents the child and his/her important characteristics. . . . The next largest circle represents the mother or caregiver and his/her important characteristics. . . . The largest circle represents the environment of both the child and mother."[12:16-17]

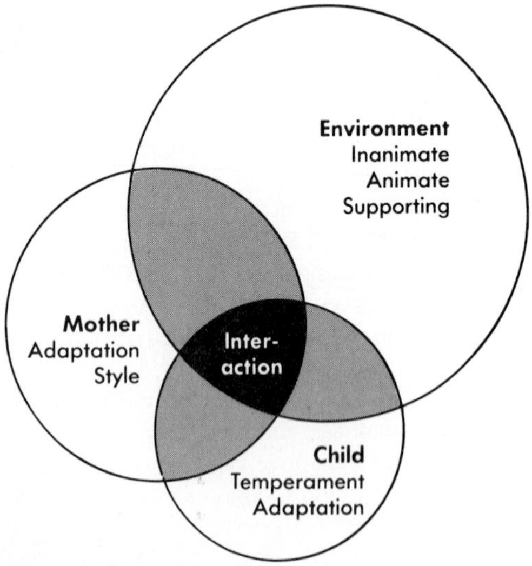

Figure 23-2. Child health assessment interaction model.

Used with permission from Barnard, K.E., et al. (1977). *The nursing child assessment training study guide: Program learning manual.* p. 19.

Those portions of the model where two circles overlap represent interaction between the two concepts. The dark center area represents interaction among all three concepts. Barnard's theory focuses on this crucial mother-child-environment interactive process. The Nursing Child Assessment Project used this as the theoretical basis for the study of potential screening and assessment methods to be used with young children.[12:17]

LOGICAL FORM

According to Chinn and Jacobs,[13:61] "In inductive logic the reasoning method relies on observing particular instances and then combining those particulars into a larger whole." Inductive logic is the form Barnard used in developing her Child Health Assessment Interaction Theory. This theory was an outcome of the investigation and findings of the Nursing Child Assessment Project. Barnard concluded the most important aspect of child health assessment was the interaction and adaptation that occurs between parent and child.

ACCEPTANCE BY THE NURSING COMMUNITY

Practice

The nursing satellite training project prepared about 4,000 nurses to use a series of standard assessment instruments. The exactness of the preparation in interrater reliability has increased observation skills applicable to other aspects of nursing. Now nurses use the assessment tools and their skills throughout the nation and in foreign countries.

Education

The nursing satellite training project initially used satellite communications and later videotaped classes to teach nurses how to use a series of standard assessment instruments. The concept of interrater reliability has encouraged nurses to share their knowledge and observations with co-workers. The explicitness of the observations has made the task of educating others easier.

Research

One of the outcomes of the contract to develop accurate assessment tools was the creation of a research project. The purpose of the satellite training program was to quickly disseminate current research findings. Barnard is continuing to refine the assessment scales and continues to receive funds for research. She is well recognized for her work, having been cited in the Citation Indices at least 35 times between 1976 and 1984. She has received awards recognizing her work from several organizations, including the American Nurses' Association, the American Public Health Association, and the Nurses' Association of the American College of Obstetricians and Gynecologists.

FURTHER DEVELOPMENT

The greatest deficit of Barnard's theory is lack of clarity. Barnard does not explicitly define her major assumptions about nursing, person, health, and environment. Although the identification of major concepts is implied through the Nursing Child Health Assessment Interaction Model, Barnard fails to clearly define these concepts. This is an area requiring further development.

In the Child Health Assessment Interaction theory, the mother is identified as a major concept, while the father is included in the description of the environment. Although this may accurately describe the father's role in most families, a problem exists when the father assumes the role of primary caregiver. In these instances, Barnard's theory needs modification.

Barnard says her future endeavors will focus on further investigation of the child, his or her parents, and the environment. She plans to continue work in the area of teaching parents how to improve interaction skills with their children. From 1982 to 1988 she conducted research involving the high-risk infant. In 1987 she began a study to develop a nursing model for preterm infant follow-up.[17:6] Although Barnard's theory is a micro theory, she does not intend to broaden her scope. Rather, she will be looking more closely at individual variables and how these affect a child's development.[8]

CRITIQUE

Clarity

Clarity in general refers to the lucidness and consistency of the theory. . . . An extremely important aspect of semantic clarity is that of definition of concepts.[13:133] Barnard does not identify or define her theoretical concepts. Rather, she describes and implies the definitions of these concepts. "In a theory with structural clarity, concepts are interconnected and organized into a coherent whole."[13:136] By using Barnard's Child Health Assessment Interaction Model, it is relatively easy for the reader to understand the interrelationships of her theoretical concepts. Barnard is consistent in the use of an inductive form of logic.

Simplicity

The Child Health Assessment Interaction Model is a simple way of communicating the main focus of Barnard's work as it relates to the parent-child interaction and the development of accurate assessment tools. However, there are several identified characteristics for both concepts and assertions, and consequently the complexity is great. It must also be noted that the research necessary to define and support the assertions is complex.

Generality

Barnard's work with the interactive focus between parent and child is not generalizable to nursing. The original work was done on interactions between parent and child during the child's first 12 months of life. Subsequent work lengthened the time period of the child assessment to 36 months. However, one can currently only generalize to parent-child interactions in the first 3 years of life. The parent-child interaction model approaches midrange theory as defined by Chinn and Jacobs.[13] Despite the narrow scope, Barnard's theory is applicable, not only to nursing but also to other disciplines that deal with the parent-child relationship.

Empirical Precision

There is much research included in Barnard's original work. She also used alternate research concurrently to validate test results obtained by one set of raters who made home visits with test results obtained by a set of testers from another discipline. Further development of the feeding and teaching assessment tools demonstrated test-retest reliability and validity of the original scales. Original video tapes were rescored using the revised scales.

Derivable Consequences

More than 2000 nurses have been trained to use the standardized assessment scales with 85% interrater reliability. Nurses across the nation and in other countries utilize the observational skills in daily practice.[14]

Throughout her writings, Barnard emphasizes the need for strong links between nursing research, theory, and practice. She indicates, "There has been no more exciting time in nursing than now. We have the clinical, research, scholarship, administrative, and educational expertise so carefully developed over the past years."[18:252] In discussing research, she states "We simply must attempt to be in closer alignment with practice from the beginning."[18:169] In the Nursing Child Assessment Satellite Training Project, she identifies her goal as the dissemination of research findings and the application of these findings to practice. This is a prime example of Barnard's efforts to link research, theory, and practice.

REFERENCES

1. Barnard, K.E. (1966, Dec.). Symposium on mental retardation. *Nursing Clinics of North America, 1*:629-630.
2. Barnard, K.E. (1979, Sept. 20). Child advocates must help parents, too. *The American Nurse, 11*:4.
3. Barnard, K.E. (1980, July). Knowledge for practice: Directions for the future. *Nursing Research, 29*:208-212.
4. Barnard, K.E. (1982, Summer). The research cycle: Nursing, the profession, the discipline. *Western Journal of Nursing Research, 4*:1-12.
5. Barnard, K.E. (1984). Curriculum vitae.
6. Barnard, K.E. (1984, Nov.). Cassette tape interview.
7. Barnard, K.E., & Eyres, S.J. (Eds.). (1979). *Child health assessment, part II: The first year of life.* Hyattsville, Md.: U.S. Department of Health, Education, and Welfare.
8. Barnard, K.E., & Neal, M.V. (1977, May-June). Maternal-child nursing research: Review of the past and strategies for the future. *Nursing Research, 26*:193-200.
9. Barnard, K.E., & Powell, M.L. (1972). *Teaching the mentally retarded child: A family care approach.* St. Louis: C.V. Mosby.
10. Barnard, K.E., et al. (1977). *The nursing child assessment satellite training study guide,* Unpublished program learning manual, 1977.
11. Chinn, P., & Jacobs, M. (1983). *Theory and nursing: A systematic approach.* St. Louis: C.V. Mosby.
12. Goldman, B. (Ed.). (1984, March-April). Ross Public Health Currents 24(2).
13. Kathryn E. Barnard presented with the Lucille Petry Leone Award at NLN annual convention. *Washington State Journal of Nursing, 41*:9
14. Kathryn E. Barnard presented with the Maternal and Child Health Nurse of the Year Award, 1983, at ANA annual convention. (1984). *Nursing Outlook, 32*:242.
15. Kathryn E. Barnard presented with the 1983 Martha May Eliot Award of the American Public Health Association, Maternal and Child Health Section. (1984, March-April). *Public Health Currents, 24*:7-10.
16. King, D., Barnard, K.E., & Hoehn, R. (1981, March). Disseminating the results of nursing research. *Nursing Outlook, 29*:164-169.
17. Barnard, K.E. (1987, Oct.). Curriculum vitae.
18. Barnard, K.E. (1985). Rituals that integrate nursing practice, education, and research. In K.E. Barnard & G.R. Smith (Eds.), *The second*

annual symposium in nursing faculty practice. American Academy of Nursing.

BIBLIOGRAPHY

Primary Sources

Books

Barnard, K.E. (Ed.). (1983). *Structure to outcome: Making it work.* Kansas City, Mo.: American Academy of Nursing.

Barnard, K.E. (1984). *Social support and families of vulnerable infants.* White Plains, N.Y., March of Dimes Birth Defects Foundation.

Barnard, K.E. & Brazelton, T.B. (Chairpersons). (1984). *The many facets of touch.* Somerville, N.J., Johnson & Johnson.

Barnard, K.E., & Douglas, H.B. (Eds.). (1974). *Child health assessment, part I: A literature review.* Bethesda, Md.: U.S. Department of Health, Education and Welfare.

Barnard, K.E., & Erickson, M.L. (1976). *Teaching children with developmental problems: A family care approach* (2d ed). St. Louis: C.V. Mosby.

Barnard, K.E., & Eyres, S.J. (Eds.). (1979). *Child health assessment, part II: The first year of life.* Hyattsville, Md.: U.S. Department of Health, Education, and Welfare.

Barnard, K.E., & Powell, M.L. (1972). *Teaching the mentally retarded child: A family care approach.* St. Louis: C.V. Mosby.

Book Chapters

Barnard, K.E. (1973). Nursing. In J. Wortis (Ed.), *Mental retardation and developmental disabilities: An annual review.* New York: Brunner-Mazel.

Barnard, K.E. (1975). Infant programming. In R. Koch (Ed.), *Proceedings of confidence on Down's syndrome.* New York: Brunner-Mazel.

Barnard, K.E. (1976). The state of the art: Nursing and early intervention with handicapped infants. In T. Tjossem (Ed.), *Proceedings of 1974 president's committee on mental retardation meeting on infant intervention.* Baltimore, Md.: University Park Press.

Barnard, K.E. (1978). Introduction to parent-infant interaction studies. In G.P. Sackett (Ed.), *Observing behavior* (Vol. I): *Theory and application in mental retardation.* Baltimore, Md., University Park Press.

Barnard, K.E. (1979). How focusing on the family changes the health care system. In T.B. Brazelton & V.C. Vaughan (Eds.), *The family: Setting priorities.* New York: Science & Medicine.

Barnard, K.E. (1980). How nursing care may influence prevention of development delay. In E.J. Sell (Ed.), *Follow-up of the high risk newborn: A practical approach.* Springfield, Ill.: Charles C Thomas.

Barnard, K.E. (1980). Sleep organization and motor development in prematures. In E.J. Sell (Ed.), *Follow-up of the high risk newborn: A practical approach.* Springfield, Ill.: Charles C Thomas.

Barnard, K.E. (1980). How nursing care may influence prevention of development delay. In E.J. Sell (Ed.), *Follow-up of the high risk newborn: A practical approach.* Springfield, Ill.: Charles C Thomas.

Barnard, K.E. (1981). An ecological approach to parent-child relations. In C.C. Brown (Ed.), *Infants at risk: Assessment and intervention.* Johnson & Johnson Pediatric Round Table.

Barnard, K.E. (1981). General issues in parent-infant interaction during the first years of life. In D.L. Yeung (Ed.), *Essays of pediatric nutrition.* Ontario, Canada: The Canadian Science Committee on Food and Nutrition, Canadian Public Health Association.

Barnard, K.E. (1981). The nursing role in the promotion of child development. In M. Tudor (Ed.), *Child development.* New York: McGraw-Hill.

Barnard, K.E. (1981). A program of temporarily patterned movement and sound stimulation for premature infants. In V.L. Smeriglio (Ed.), *Newborns and parents: Parent-infant contact and newborn sensory stimulation.* Hillsdale, N.J.: Lawrence Erlbaum Associates, pp. 31-48.

Barnard, K.E. (1984). Nursing research in relation to infants and young children. In H. Werley & J. Fitzpatrick (Eds.), *Annual review of nursing research* (Vol. 1). New York: Springer, pp. 3-25.

Barnard, K.E. (1985). Rituals that integrate nursing practice, education and research. In K.E. Barnard & G.R. Smith (Eds.), *The second annual symposium in nursing faculty practice.* American Academy of Nursing.

Barnard, K. (1986). Major issues in program evaluation. In *Program evaluation: Issues, strategies and models.* Washington, D.C.: National Center for Clinical Infant Programs.

Barnard, K.E. (1987). Paradigms for intervention: Infant state modulation. In N. Gunzenhauser (Ed.), *Infant stimulation: For whom, what kind, when, and how much?* Skillman, N.J.: Johnson & Johnson Baby Products Company, pp. 129-136.

Barnard, K.E., Bee, H.L., & Hammond, M.A. (1984). Home environment and cognitive development in a health, low-risk sample: The Seattle study. In A. Gottfried (Ed.), *Home environment and early cognitive development*. New York: Academic.

Barnard, K.E., Booth, C.L., Mitchell, S.K., & Telzow, R.W. (1988). Newborn nursing models: A test of early intervention to high-risk infants and families. In E. Hibbs (Ed.)., *Children and families: Studies in prevention and intervention*. New York: International Universities Press.

Barnard, K.E. & Brazelton, T.B. (Eds.). (1987). Touch: The foundation of experience. National Center for Clinical Infant Programs, Monograph No. 4.

Barnard, K.E., et al. (1977). Premature infant refocus. In Mittler, P. (Ed.), Research to practice in mental retardation: Biomedical aspects, Vol. 3, I.A.S.S.M.D.

Barnard, K.E., Eyres, S.J., Lobo, M., & Snyder, C. (1983). An ecological paradigm for assessment and intervention. In T.B. Brazelton & B. Lester (Eds.), *New Approaches to developmental screening of infants*. New York: Elsevier.

Barnard, K.E., Hammond, M.A., Mitchell, S.K., Booth, C.L., Spietz, A., Snyder, C., & Elsas, T. (1985). Caring for high-risk infants and their families. In M. Green (Ed.), *The psychological aspects of the family*. Lexington, Mass.: Lexington Books.

Barnard, K.E., Magyary, D.L., Booth, C.L., & Eyres, S.J. (1987). Longitudinal design: Considerations and application to nursing research. In M. Cahoon (Ed.), *Recent advances in nursing: Research methodology*. Edinburgh: Churchill Livingstone.

Barnard, K.E., Hammond, M.A., Booth, C.L., Bee, H.L., Mitchell, S.K., & Spieker, S.J. (In press). Measurement and meaning of parent-child interaction. In F.J. Morrison, C.E. Lord, & D.P. Keating (Eds.), *Applied developmental psychology*, Vol. III. New York: Academic Press.

Mitchell, S.K., et al. (1985). Prediction of school problems and behavior problems in children followed from birth to age eight. In W.K. Frankenburg, R.N. Emde & J. Sullivan (Eds.). *Early identification of children at risk: An international perspective*. New York: Plenum Press.

Mitchell, S.K., Magyary, D., Barnard, K.E., Sumner, G.A., & Booth, C.L. (1988). A comparison of home-based prevention programs for families of newborns. In L.A. Bond & B. Wagner (Eds.), *Families in Transition: Primary prevention programs that work*. Beverly Hills, Cal.: Sage.

Articles

Barnard, K.E. (1966, April-May). New four-part training project is developed. *Children Limited, 15:*2.

Barnard, K.E. (1966, Dec.). Symposium on mental retardation. *Nursing Clinics of North America, 1:*629-630.

Barnard, K.E. (1968, Feb.). Teaching the mentally retarded child is a family affair. *American Journal of Nursing, 68:*305-311.

Barnard, K.E. (1969, Oct.). Are professionals educable? *Alabama Journal of Medical Sciences, 6:*388-391.

Barnard, K.E. (1973, Dec.). The effect of stimulation on the sleep behavior of the premature infant. *Communicating Nursing Research, 6:*12-33.

Barnard, K.E. (1975, Oct.). Trends in the care and prevention of developmental disabilities. *American Journal of Nursing, 75:*1700-1704.

Barnard, K.E. (1976, Oct.). Predictive nursing: The baby and parents. *Health Care Dimensions, 3:*185-202.

Barnard, K.E. (1977, Aug. 15). A challenge for nursing care. *The American Nurse, 9:*4.

Barnard, K.E. (1978, March-April). The family and you. *American Journal of Maternal Child Nursing, 3:*82-83.

Barnard, K.E. (1979, Sept. 20). Child advocates must help parents, too. *The American Nurse, 11:*4.

Barnard, K.E. (1980, July). Knowledge for practice: Directions for the future. *Nursing Research, 29:*208-212.

Barnard, K.E. (1981, May-June). The research question. *American Journal of Maternal Child Nursing, 6:*211.

Barnard, K.E. (1981, July-August). Breast-feeding is best for U.S. babies, too. *The American Nurse, 13:*44.

Barnard, K.E. (1981, July-August). Research designs: Descriptive method. *American Journal of Maternal Child Nursing, 6:*243.

Barnard, K.E. (1981, Sept.-Oct.). Research designs: Experimental method. *American Journal of Maternal Child Nursing, 6:*321.

Barnard, K.E. (1981, Nov.-Dec.). Research designs: The historical method. *American Journal of Maternal Child Nursing, 6:*391.

Barnard, K.E. (1982, Jan.-Feb.). Research designs: Sampling. *American Journal of Maternal Child Nursing, 7:*15.

Barnard, K.E. (1982, March-April). Measurements: Reliability. *American Journal of Maternal Child Nursing, 7:*101.

Barnard, K.E. (1982, May-June). Measurement: Validity. *American Journal of Maternal Child Nursing, 7:*165.

Barnard, K.E. (1982, Summer). The research cycle: Nursing, the profession, the discipline. *Communicating Nursing Research, 15:*1-12.

Barnard, K.E. (1982, Summer). The research cycle: Nursing, the profession, the discipline. *Western Journal of Nursing Research, 4:*1-12.

Barnard, K.E. (1982, July-Aug.). Measurement descriptive statistics. *American Journal of Maternal Child Nursing, 7:*235.

Barnard, K.E. (1982, Sept.-Oct.). Determining the focus of nursing research. *American Journal of Maternal Child Nursing, 7:*299.

Barnard, K.E. (1982, Nov.-Dec.). Determining the role of nursing. *American Journal of Maternal Child Nursing, 7:*36.

Barnard, K.E. (1983, Jan.). Social policy statement can move nursing ahead. *The American Nurse, 15:*4, 14.

Barnard, K.E. (1983, Jan.-Feb.). The case study method: A research tool. *American Journal of Maternal Child Nursing, 8:*36.

Barnard, K.E. (1983, March-April). Identifying potential nursing research areas. *American Journal of Maternal Child Nursing, 8:*117.

Barnard, K.E. (1983, May-June). Nursing diagnosis: A descriptive method. *American Journal of Maternal Child Nursing, 8:*223.

Barnard, K.E. (1983, July-Aug.). Formulation of hypotheses. *American Journal of Maternal Child Nursing, 8:*263.

Barnard, K.E. (1983, Sept.-Oct.). Informed consent. *American Journal of Maternal Child Nursing, 8:*327.

Barnard, K.E. (1983, Nov.-Dec.). Control groups. *Maternal Child Nursing, 8:*431.

Barnard, K.E. (1984). Nursing research related to infants and young children. *Annual Review of Nursing Research, 1:*3-25.

Barnard, K.E. (1984, Jan.-Feb.). The family as a unit of measurement. *American Journal of Maternal Child Nursing, 9:*21.

Barnard, K.E. (1984, March-April). Commonly understood outcomes. *American Journal of Maternal Child Nursing, 9:*99.

Barnard, K.E. (1984, March-April). Children: Our greatest national resource. *Public Health Currents, 24:*8-10.

Barnard, K.E. (1984, May-June). Knowledge development. *American Journal of Maternal Child Nursing, 9:*175.

Barnard, K.E. (1984, July-Aug.). Planning experiments. *American Journal of Maternal Child Nursing, 9:*247.

Barnard, K.E. (1984, Sept.-Oct.). Determining relationships. *American Journal of Maternal Child Nursing, 9:*345.

Barnard, K. (1985). Blending the art and science of nursing. *Maternal-Child Nursing, 10(1):*63.

Barnard, K. (1985). Planning the analysis. *Maternal-Child Nursing, 10(2):*139.

Barnard, K. (1985). Retention of research sample. *Maternal-Child Nursing, 10(3):*214.

Barnard, K. (1985). Seeking approval of conducting research. *Maternal Child Nursing, 10(4):*292.

Barnard, K. (1985). Seeking funds for research. *Maternal-Child Nursing, 10(6):*424.

Barnard, K. (1985). Studying patterns of behavior. *Maternal-Child Nursing, 10(5):*358.

Barnard, K. (1985). Supportive measures for high-risk infants and families. *Birth Defects, 20(5):*291-329.

Barnard, K.E. (1986). Research utilization: The clinician's role. *Maternal-Child Nursing, 11(3):*224.

Barnard, K.E. (1986). Research utilization: The researcher's responsibilities. *Maternal-Child Nursing, 11(2):*150.

Barnard, K.E. (1986). Writing a research proposal. *Maternal-Child Nursing, 11(1):*76.

Barnard, K.E., & Bee, H.L. (1983). The impact of temporarily patterned stimulation on the development of preterm infants. *Child Development, 54:*1156-1167.

Barnard, K.E., & Bee, H.L. (1984). Developmental changes in maternal interactions with term and preterm infants. *Infant Behavior and Development, 7:*101-113.

Barnard, K.E., Bee, J.L., & Hammond, M.A. (1984). Developmental changes in maternal interactions with term and preterm infants. *Infant Behavior and Development, 1:*101-113.

Barnard, K.E., & Blackburn, S. (1985). Making a case for studying the ecologic niche of the newborn. *Birth Defects, 21(3):*71-88.

Barnard, K., Boothe, C., Johnson, C., & Crowley, N. (1985). Infant massage and exercise: Worth the effort? *Maternal-Child Nursing, 10(3):*184-189.

Barnard, K.E., & Collar, B.S. (1973, Feb.). Early diagnosis, interpretation and intervention: A commentary on the nurse's role. *Annals of the New York Academy of Science, 205:*373-382.

Barnard, K.E., et al. (1976). Predictive nursing: The baby and parents. *Health Care Dimensions, 31(1):*185-202.

Barnard, K.E., Hammond, M.A., Sumner, G.A., Kang, R., Johnson-Crowley, N., Snyder, C., Spietz, A., Blackburn, S., Brandt, P., Magyary, D. (1987). Helping parents with preterm infants: Field test of a protocol. *Early Child Development and Care, 27(2):*56-290.

Barnard, K.E., & Neal, M.V. (1977, May-June). Maternal-child nursing research: Review of the past and strategies for the future. *Nursing Research, 26:*193-200.

Barnard, K.E., Snyder, C., & Spietz, A. (1984). Supportive measures for high-risk infants and families. In K.E. Barnard, et al. (Eds.), *Social support and families of vulnerable infants. Birth Defects: Original Article Series* (Vol. 20, No. 5). White Plains, N.Y.: March of Dimes Birth Defects Foundation.

Bee, H.L., et al. (1982). Prediction of IQ and language skill from perinatal status, child performance, family characteristics, and mother-infant interaction. *Child Development, 53:*1134-1156.

Bee, H.L., et al. (1984). Predicting intellectual outcomes: Sex differences in response to early environmental stimulation. *Sex Roles, 10.*

Bee, H.L., Hammond, M.A., Eyres, J.J., Barnard, K.E., & Snyder, C. (1986). The impact of parental life change in the early development of children. *Research in Nursing and Health, 9(1):*64-74.

Booth, C.L., Lyons, N.B., & Barnard, K.E. (1984). Synchrony in mother-infant interaction: A comparison of measurement methods. *Child Study Journal, 14:*95-114.

Hammer, S.L., & Barnard, K.E. (1966, Nov.). The mentally retarded adolescent: A review of the characteristics and problems of 44 non-institutionalized adolescent retardates. *Pediatrics, 38:*845-857.

Jacox, A., Lang, N., & Barnard, K.E. (1982, Oct.). Four nurses describe "dramatic" changes in education. *The American Nurse, 9:*8.

Kang, R., & Barnard, K. (1979). Using the neonatal behavioral assessment scale to evaluate premature infants. *Birth Defects: Original Article Series, XV* (7):119-144. The National Foundation. New York: Alan R. Liss.

King, D., Barnard, K.E., & Hoehn, R. (1981, March), Disseminating the results of nursing research. *Nursing Outlook, 29:*164-169.

Mitchell, S.K., Barnard, K.E., Booth, C.L., et al. (1986). The natural alliance of psychology and nursing: Substance as well as practice (commentary). *American Psychologist, 41(10):*1170.

Murray, B.L., & Barnard, K.E. (1966, Dec.). The nursing specialist in mental retardation. *Nursing Clinics of North America, 1:*631-640.

Pattullo, A.W., & Barnard, K.E. (1968, Dec.). Teaching menstrual hygiene to the mentally retarded. *American Journal of Nursing, 12:*2572-2575.

Snyder, C., Eyres, S.J., & Barnard, K.E. (1979, Nov.-Dec.). New findings about mothers' antenatal expectations and their relationship to infant development. *American Journal of Maternal Child Nursing, 4:*354-357.

Whitney, L., & Barnard, K.E. (1966, June). Implications of operant learning theory for nursing care of the mentally retarded. *Mental Retardation, 4:*3.

Unpublished Papers

Barnard, K.E. (1967, April). Nursing and mental retardation: A problem solving paper. U.S. Public Health Service, Mental Retardation Division, pp. 1-70.

Barnard, K.E. (1967, April). Planning for learning experiences in university affiliated centers. Proceedings of the 4th National Workshop for Nurses in Mental Retardation, U.S. Children's Bureau.

Barnard, K.E. (1975). Predictive nursing care. In *Proceedings of perinatal nursing conference,* sponsored by University of Washington School of Nursing and Maternal and Child Health Services, HSMHA, Seattle, Washington.

Barnard, K.E. (1976, Feb.). A perspective on where we are in early intervention programs. Adapted from a Keynote Address at a conference on "The Nursing Role in Early Intervention Programs for Developing Disabled Children," sponsored by the

University of Utah College of Nursing Division of Continuing Education and Utah State Division of Health, Denver, Colorado.

Barnard, K.E. (1977). Nursing child assessment satellite training fact sheet.

Barnard, K.E., Principal Investigator. Models of newborn nursing services. Grant #NU-00719. Division of Nursing, Bureau of Health Professions, Health Resources Administration, Public Health Service, Department of Health and Human Services. July 7, 1979-June 30, 1982.

Barnard, K.E., Principal Investigator. Clinical nursing model for infants and their families. National Institute of Mental Health, Alcohol, Drug Abuse, and Mental Health Administration, Public Health Service, Department of Health and Human Services. Grant submitted May 1981.

Barnard, K.E., Principal Investigator. Premature infant refocus. Grant #MC-R-530348. Maternal and Child Health and Crippled Children's Services, Bureau of Community Health Services, Health Services Administration, Public Health Service, Department of Health and Human Resources. Sept. 1, 1974-April 30, 1981.

Barnard, K.E. (1981). Critical issues: Support of the caregiver Maternal Child Nursing in the 80s: Nursing Perspective. A Forum in Honor of Katherine Kendall. School of Nursing, University of Maryland.

Barnard, K.E., & Bee, H.L. The assessment of parent-infant interaction by observation of feeding and teaching.

Barnard, K.E., & Bee, H.L. (1981, Sept.). Premature infant refocus. Final report on Grant #MC-R-530348. Prepared for the Maternal and Child Health and Crippled Children's Services Research Grants Program, Bureau of Community Health Services, HSA, PhS, DHHS.

Barnard, K.E., & Hoehn, R.E. (1978, Dec.). Nursing child assessment satellite training. In R.A. Duncan, (Ed.), Biomedical communications experiments, Lister Hill National Center for Biomedical Communications, Dept. of HEW, Public Health Service.

Barnard, K.E., & Kelly, J.F. (1980, May). Infant intervention: Parental consideration. State of art paper. Guidelines for Early Intervention Programs. Based on a conference Health Issues in Early Intervention Programs, Washington, D.C. Sponsored by College of Nursing, University of Utah, and School of Public Health, University of Hawaii. Office for Maternal & Child Health, Department of Health and Human Services.

Barnard, K.E., Lendzion, A., & Moser, J. (1974). Final report on the measuring interactions project, technical report #3, The first three years: Programming for atypical infants and their families. New York: United Cerebral Palsy Association.

Barnard, K.E., & Powell, M. (1967, April). Planning for learning experiences in university affiliated centers. Proceedings of the 4th National Workshop for Nurses in Mental Retardation, U.S. Children's Bureau.

Barnard, K.E., & Summer, G.A. (1981, June). The health of women with fertility-related needs. In L.V. Klerman (Ed.), Research priorities in maternal and child health: Report of a conference, Brandeis University, Waltham, Mass.

Barnard, K.E., et al. (1977). The nursing child assessment satellite training study guide. Program learning manual.

Barnard, K.E., et al. (1983, Dec.). Newborn nursing models. Final report on Grant #R01-NU-00719. Prepared for the Division of Nursing, Bureau of Manpower, Health Resources Administration, Department of Health and Human Services.

Bee, H.L., et al. (1981, April). Parent-child interaction during teaching in abusing and nonabusing families. Paper presented at the biennial meetings of the Society for Research in Child Development, Boston, Mass.

Eyres, S.J., Barnard, K.E., & Gray, C.A. Child health assessment, part III: 2-4 years.

Hammond, M.A., et al. (1983, July). Child health assessment, part IV: Follow-up at second grade. Final report of Grant #R01-NU-00816 prepared for Division of Nursing, Bureau of Health Professions, Health Resources and Services Administration, U.S. Public Health Service.

Interview

Barnard, K.E. (1984, Nov.). Cassette tape interview.

Correspondence

Barnard, K.E. Curriculum vitae. (1984, Sept.).

Barnard, K.E. Curriculum vitae. (1987, Oct.).

Videotapes

Videotape. (1984, July 27). NAACOG Invitational Research Conference, Indianapolis, Indiana.

Videotape Services, Nursing Child Assessment Satellite Training.

Secondary Sources

Book Chapters

Disbrow, M.A. (1983). Conducting interdisciplinary research: Gratifications and frustrations. In N.L. Chaska, *The nursing profession: A time to speak.* New York: McGraw-Hill.

Menke, E.M. (1983). Critical analysis of theory development in nursing. In N.L. Chaska, *The nursing profession: A time to speak.* New York: McGraw-Hill.

Book Reviews

Barnard, K.E., & Douglas, H.B. (Eds.). (1974). *Child health assessment, part I: A literature review.*
*Journal of Continuing Education in Nursing, 6:*52, November-December 1975.
*Nursing Mirror, 141:*71, October 2, 1975.
*RN, 38:*122, September 1975.

Barnard, K.E., & Erickson, M.L. (1976). *Teaching children with developmental problems: A family care approach* (2d ed.).
*American Journal of Nursing, 77:*499, March 1977.
*Canadian Nurse, 73:*46, July 1977.

Barnard, K.E., & Powell, M.L. (1972). *Teaching the mentally retarded child: A family care approach.*
*American Journal of Nursing, 73:*729, April 1973.
*Canadian Nurse, 69:*54, March 1973.

Research Abstracts

Barnard, K.E. (1972, Oct.). The effect of stimulation on the duration and amount of sleep and wakefulness in the premature infant. *Dissertation Abstracts International, 33:*2167-2168.

News Releases

Kathryn E. Barnard named in *National Nursing Directory* (1982). Rockville, Md.: Aspen Systems.

Kathryn E. Barnard named in *Sigma Theta Tau Directory of Nurse Researchers* (1983). Indianapolis, Indiana: Sigma Theta Tau.

Kathryn E. Barnard named in *Directory of Nurses with Doctoral Degrees* (1984). St. Louis: Missouri: American Nurses Association.

Kathryn E. Barnard presented with the Lucille Petry Leone Award at NLN annual convention. (1969, May-June). *Washington State Journal of Nursing, 41:*9.

Kathryn E. Barnard presented with the Maternal and Child Health Nurse of the Year Award for 1983 at ANA annual convention. (1984). *Nursing Outlook, 32:*242.

Kathryn Elaine Barnard presented with the 1983 Martha May Eliot Award of the American Public Health Association, Maternal and Child Health Section. (1984, March-April). *Public Health Currents, 24:*7-8.

Other Sources

Als, H. (1976, May). Personal communication.

Brazelton, T.B. (1973). *The neonatal behavioral assessment scale.* London: William Heinemann; Philadelphia: J.B. Lippincott.

Brunner, J.S. (1956). *A study of thinking.* New York: John Wiley & Sons.

Brunner, J.S. (1966). *Studies in cognitive growth.* New York: John Wiley & Sons.

Caldwell, B.M. (1965). *Daily program II: A manual for teachers.* Washington, D.C.: Office of Economic Opportunity.

Caldwell, B.M. (1967). What is the optimal learning environment for the young child? *American Journal of Orthopsychiatry, 37:*8-21.

Caldwell, B.M. (1968). On designing supplementary environments for early child development. *BAEYC Reporter 10:*1-11.

Caldwell, B.M. (1970). *Instruction manual inventory for infants* (Home Observation for Measurement of the Environment). Little Rock, Ark.

Caldwell, B.M. (1970). The rationale for early intervention. *Exceptional Children, 36:*717-726.

Caldwell, B.M. (1971, Feb. 20). A timid giant grows bolder. *Saturday Review,* pp. 47-66.

Caldwell, B.M. (1971). Impact of interest in early cognitive simulation. In H. Rie (Ed.), *Perspectives in psychopathology.* Chicago: Aldine-Atherton.

Caldwell, B.M. (1973). Do young children have a quality life in day care? *Young Children, 28:*197-208.

Caldwell, B.M. (1972). Infant day care: Fads, facts, and fancies. In R. Elardo and B. Pagan (Eds.), *Perspective on infant day care.* Orangeburg, S.C.: Southern Association on Children under Six.

Caldwell, B.M. (1972). Kramer school: Something for everybody. In S.J. Braun and E.P. Wards (Eds.), *History and theory of early childhood education.* Worthington, Ohio, Charles A. Jones.

Caldwell, B.M., & Elardo, R. (1972). Innovative op-

portunities for school psychologists in early childhood education. *School Psychology Digest, 1:*8-16.
Caldwell, B.M., et al. (1963). Mother-infant interaction in monomatric and polymatric families. *American Journal of Orthopsychiatry, 33:*653-664.
Caldwell, B.M., & Richmond, J.B. (1968). The children's center in Syracuse, New York. In L.L. Dittman (Ed.) *Early child care: The new perspectives.* New York: Atherton.
Caldwell, B.M., & Smith, L.E. (1970). Day care for the very young: Prime opportunity for primary prevention. *American Journal of Public Health, 60:*690-697.
Caldwell, B.M., et al. (1970). Infant day care and attachment. *American Journal of Orthopsychiatry, 40:*397-412.
Dubowitz, L.M.S., et al. Clinical assessment of gestational age in the newborn infant. *Pediatrics, 77:*1-10.
Piaget, J. (1962). *Judgment and reasoning in the child.* New York: Humanities. (Reproduction of 1928 ed.).
Piaget, J. (1976). *The grasp of consciousness: Action and concept in young children.* Cambridge, Mass.: Harvard University Press.
Piaget, J (1983). *The child's perception of physical causality.* New York: Adren Lib. (Reproduction of 1930 ed.).
Waldrop, M.F., & Goering, J.D. (1971). Hyperactivity and minor physical anomalies in elementary school children. *American Journal of Orthopsychiatry, 41(4):*602-607.

24

Ramona T. Mercer

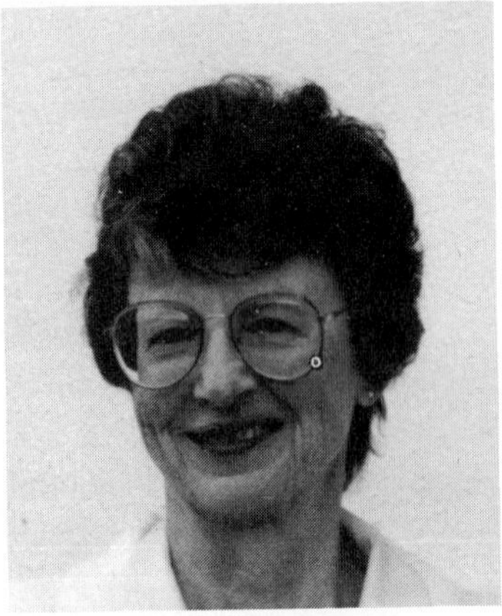

Maternal Role Attainment

Alberta M. Bee, Stephanie Oetting

CREDENTIALS AND BACKGROUND OF THE THEORIST

Ramona T. Mercer began her nursing career in 1950, when she was graduated from St. Margaret's School of Nursing, Montgomery, Alabama. She was graduated with the L.L. Hill Award for Highest Scholastic Standing. In the ten years that followed, she worked as a nurse, head nurse, and instructor in the areas of pediatrics, obstetrics, and contagious diseases before returning to school in 1960. She completed a Bachelor of Science degree in Nursing in 1962, graduating with distinction, from the University of New Mexico, Albuquerque. She went on to earn an M.S.N. in Maternal Child Health from Emory University in 1964 and then a Ph.D. in Maternity Nursing from the University of Pittsburgh in 1973.

From 1961 through 1963, while pursuing studies in nursing, Mercer worked as a clinical instructor. In 1964 she was awarded the HEW Public Health Service Nurse Trainee Award and was inducted into Sigma Theta Tau. From 1964 to 1971 she was an assistant professor of Maternal Child Health Nursing at Emory Uni-

The authors with to express appreciation to Ramona T. Mercer for critiquing the chapter.

versity. During this time she was again awarded an HEW Public Health Service Nurse Trainee Award and also the Bixler Scholarship for Nursing Education and Research, Southern Regional Board.

Mercer moved to California in 1973 and accepted the position of Assistant Professor, Department of Family Health Care Nursing at the University of California, San Francisco. She held that position until 1977, at which time she was promoted to associate professor. In 1983 she accepted a position as a professor in the same department and remained in that role until her retirement in 1987.

In early research efforts, Mercer focused on the behaviors and needs of breastfeeding mothers, mothers with postpartum illness, and mothers bearing infants with defects. The results were published in several articles and led to the writing of *Nursing Care for Parents at Risk,* which was published in 1977 and received an *American Journal of Nursing* Book of the Year Award in 1978. This prior research led Mercer to study mothers of various ages, family relationships, and antepartal stress as related to familial relationships and the maternal role. A portion of that work, concerning teenage mothers over the first year of motherhood, resulted in the book *Perspectives on Adolescent Health Care,* which in 1980 also received an *American Journal of Nursing* Book of the Year Award. In 1986, Mercer's work on mothers at various ages was drawn together in *First-time Motherhood: Experiences From Teens to Forties*. In the twenty years that have followed her first publication in 1968, she has published three books, articles in both nursing and nonnursing journals, six book chapters, and many abstracts, forewords, editorials, and book reviews.

As of 1988, Mercer maintained membership in seven professional organizations, including the American Nurses' Association and the American Academy of Nursing, and has been an active member on many national committees. Since 1983 she has been the associate editor of *Health Care for Women International,* and she serves on the review panel for *Nursing Research, Research in Nursing and Health,* and the *Western Journal for Nursing Research.* She has also served as a reviewer for numerous grant proposals. Additionally, she has been very actively involved in various capacities with regional, national, and international scientific and professional meetings and workshops.

Other honors and awards she has received include: Maternal Child Health Nurse of the Year Award by the National Foundation March of Dimes and American Nurses' Association, Division of Maternal Child Health Practice in 1982; Fourth Annual Helen Nahm Lecturer, University of California, San Francisco, School of Nursing in 1984; ASPO/Lamaze National Research Award in 1987; and in 1988 the Distinguished Research Lectureship Award, Western Institute of Nursing, Western Society for Research in Nursing.

THEORETICAL SOURCES

Mercer received her Ph.D. from the University of Pittsburgh where her mentor Reva Rubin was a professor and director of graduate programs in Maternity Nursing.

Early in Mercer's research, she drew from Mead's interactionist theory of self and Von Bertalanffy's general systems theory. As her research developed into attainment of the maternal role, she also combined the work of Werner and Erikson with Burr and associates' theory to develop a theoretical framework of role theory from an interactionist approach. Reva Rubin's research on maternal role attainment and Mercer's own research conducted on the different variables affecting the maternal role were also major theoretical sources.

Mercer used a large number of measurement tools to test the variables under investigation in her maternal role research: To measure early postpartum and the first-month attachment, she used E.R. Broussard and Hartner's prediction of neonatal outcomes and perceptions work, and later she used the Degree of Bothersome Inventory to measure stress related to infant behavior. Samko and Schoenfeld's measurement tool was adapted by Mercer and Marut to a 29-item questionnaire to assess the effect of the perception of the birth experience. Leifer's How I Feel About My Baby questionnaire was used to measure attachment at 1, 4, 8, and 12 months. She also used Leifer's Child-Trait Checklist at 1 month because of its representation of the claiming behaviors described by Gottlieb (1978), Robson and Moss (1970), and Rubin (1961, 1972).[9:342] Gratification of the maternal role was measured by an adaptation of Russell's (1974) Gratification Checklist. Maternal behavior was measured by Disbrow and associates' (1977, 1982). Ways Parents Handle Irritating Behavior Scale was originally used for discriminating between abusive and nonabusive parents. Maternal behavior in Mercer's studies, as observed by the raters, was measured by an adaptation from Blank's (1974) scale.

To measure social stress, Mercer used the Life Experience Survey constructed by Sarason, Johnson, and Siegel (1978). She also used the Checklist of Bothersome Factors to reflect infant stress in the transition to parenthood developed by Hobbs (1965), who revised it for a replicated study (Hobbs and Cole, 1976). A seven-item subscale, derived from Hobbs Checklist, relating to change in the mate relationship, was utilized during the eight-month test period. An adaptation of Burr and associates' (1979) Scale of Role Strain was used as a reflection of stress in the role of parenting at 4, 8, and 12 months. Mercer also used a 12-item empathy scale from Stotland's 96-item scale by Disbrow's Child Abuse prediction project (Hansen et al, 1978).

To measure maternal rigidity, she used a 15-item scale constructed by Larsen (1966). Maternal temperament was measured by using Thomas, Mittelman, and Chess's (1982) 140-item Early Adult Life Temperament Questionnaire. This questionnaire was chosen because of "its high isomorphism with the Carey Infant Temperament Questionnaire that was used to measure infant temperament" (Carey 1970, Carey and McDevitt, 1978).[9:350] The Tennessee Self Concept Scale (TSCS) was selected by Mercer to measure maternal self-concept, personality integration, and personality disorders in her research subjects. Two measures, the Parent Child-Rearing Attitude Scales developed by Disbrow and associates (1977) and the Maternal Attitude Scale (MAS) developed by Cohler and associates (1970), were used for those variables.

In her research in antepartum stress on the family, she used Rowe's family development approach, as well as the work of R.B. Hyman and P. Woog, C.D. Speilberger and associates, J.E. Ware, L. Radloff, G. Smilkstein and associates, and M.S. Cranley, R.A. Hunt's Locke-Wallace Marital Adjustment Scale was used in the assessment of antepartal stress on parental relationships.

EMPIRICAL EVIDENCE

Mercer's theory is based on the evidence of her research spanning 15 years. Many other researchers' findings were also used in the formulation of the Maternal Role Attainment theory. The work of Reva Rubin on maternal role attainment stimulated Mercer's initial interest. The focus of Mercer's work, however, went beyond the "traditional" mother to encompass adolescents, older mothers, ill mothers, mothers with defective children, families experiencing antepartal stress, parents at high risk, and mothers who had c-section deliveries. Rubin also dealt with role attainment from the point of the acceptance of the pregnancy to 1-month postpartum; Mercer looked beyond that period to how the maternal role was attained from delivery to 12 months postpartum.

In Mercer's "Theoretical Models for Studying the Effect of Antepartum Stress on the Family," an extensive theoretical framework (not included in this chapter) was used to develop three models that would predict the effect of that particular stress on family functioning. These models identified relationships between important variables as seen in the review of the literature.[16:339] The intent of these models was to stimulate and guide future research on the topic.

The terms in Figure 24-1 were defined by Mercer as follows:

Antepartum stress. "A complication of pregnancy or at-risk condition (pregnancy risk) and negatively perceived life events."[16:339]

Family. "A dynamic system which includes subsystems—individuals (mother, father, fetus/infant) and dyads (mother-father, mother-fetus/infant, and father-fetus/infant) within the overall family system."[16:339]

Self-esteem. "An individual's perception of how others view one and self acceptance of the perception."[16:341]

Social support. "The amount of help actually received, satisfaction with that help, and the persons (network) providing that help."[16:341]

Health status. "The mother's and father's perception of their prior health, current health, health outlook, resistance-susceptibility to illness, health worry concern, sickness orientation and rejection of the sick role."[16:342]

SOM (sense of mastery). "The extent to which one's life chances are regarded to be under one's own control as opposed to being fatalistically ruled."[16:340]

Anxiety. "A trait in which there is specific proneness to perceive stressful situations as dangerous or threatening."[16:342]

Depression. "Having a group of depressive symptoms, and in particular the affective component of the depressed mood."[16:342]

Dyad relationships between parents. "Perception of the mate relationship that includes intended and actual values, goals and agreements between the two."[16:343]

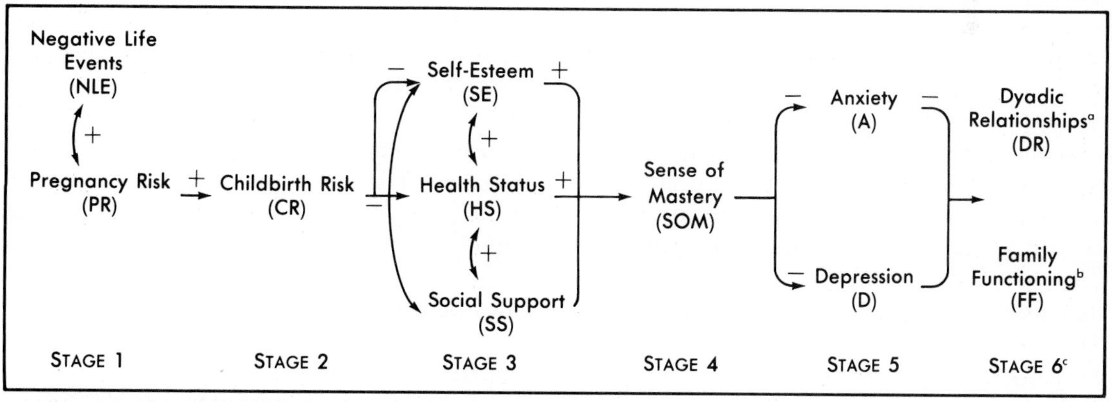

[a] Three models may be tested for dyadic relationships (DR), mother–father, mother–infant, and father–infant, from each parent's perspective.
[b] A model may be tested for family functioning (FF) from each parent's perspective.
[c] Stage 1 is hypothesized to predict Stage 2, which predicts Stage 3, and so on; in a longitudinal model such as the one proposed from pregnancy through 8 months postpartum, DR and FF will be added to the model at Stages 7, 8, 9, and 10, i.e., birth, 1, 4, and 8 months.

Figure 24-1. Theoretical Models: Effect of Antepartum Stress on Dyadic Relationships and Family Functioning.

Dyadic relationships between parent-fetus. "Includes attachment behaviors of giving of self, differentiation of self from fetus, role-taking, and attribution of characteristics of fetus."[16:343]

Dyadic relationships between parent-infant. "Parental-rated feelings about their infant and interactions with their infants."[16:343]

Family functioning. "The parent's satisfaction with family parameters of adaptation, partnership, growth, affection and resolve."[16:344]

Indirect effects. "Effects that impact on the outcome variable through another variable."[16:340]

The "straight arrows in the models are the researchers' hypotheses of a causal effect; the arrowheads point toward the influenced variable and indicate a direct effect. . . . The curved arrows with points at both ends represent correlations between two variables that are not considered predictive. Positive and negative signs indicate positive and inverse relationships."[16:340]

Model one represents the specific variables affecting health status. Model two ends with the predicted effect on the dyad relationships and is identical to the model presented here, except this model also includes the predicted effects on family functioning. This research was finalized as a grant report for the National Center for Nursing Research, National Institute of Health, and has been reported in three publications. The report was coauthored by S.L. Ferketich, K.A. May, J. DeJoseph, and D. Sollied in 1987.

MAJOR CONCEPTS AND DEFINITIONS

Mercer bases her theory for maternal role attainment on the following factors:

MATERNAL ROLE ATTAINMENT. An interactional and developmental process occurring over a period of time, during which the mother becomes attached to her infant, acquires competence in the care-taking tasks involved in the role, and expresses pleasure and gratification in the role.[9:2-6]

MATERNAL AGE. Chronological and developmental.[10:25]

PERCEPTION OF BIRTH EXPERIENCE. A woman's perception of her performance during labor and birth.[14:202]

EARLY MATERNAL-INFANT SEPARATION. Separation from the mother after birth due to illness and/or prematurity.[14:202]

SOCIAL STRESS. Positively and negatively perceived life events; personal and marital stress, high life-change scores, and illness.[15:251]

SOCIAL SUPPORT. A term that has been used widely and indiscriminately without adequate definition. Mercer uses four types of support as cited in the literature by House (1981).[15:251]

Emotional Support. "Feeling loved, cared for, trusted, and understood."[9:14]

Informational Support. "Helps the individual help herself by providing information that is useful in dealing with the problem and/or situation."[9:14]

Physical Support. A direct kind of help.[15:251]

Appraisal Support. "A support that tells the role taker how she is performing in the role; it enables the individual to evaluate herself in relationship to others' performance in the role."[9:14]

PERSONALITY TRAITS. Maternal traits of temperament, empathy, and rigidity.[10]

SELF-CONCEPT (SELF-REGARD). "The overall perception of self that includes self-satisfaction, self-acceptance, self-esteem, and congruence or discrepancy between self and ideal self."[9:18]

CHILD-REARING ATTITUDES. How parents reported they handled irritating child behaviors, parent-child interaction, empathy, and parent-child communication.[9:19]

HEALTH STATUS. Maternal illness associated with pregnancy.[9:304]

GRATIFICATION. As voiced by subject mothers and the measurement obtained on the gratification scale.[9]

INFANT TEMPERAMENT. An easy versus a difficult temperament, it is related to whether the infant sends hard-to-read cues, leading to feelings of incompetence and frustration in the mother.[9:76]

INFANT HEALTH STATUS. Illness causing maternal-infant separation, interfering with the attachment process.[9:76]

MAJOR ASSUMPTIONS

For maternal role attainment, Mercer stated the following assumptions:[9:24-25]

1. A relatively stable "core self," acquired through life-long socialization, determines how a mother defines and perceives events; her perceptions of her infant's and others' responses to her mothering, along with her life situation, are the real world she responds to.
2. In addition to the mother's socialization, her developmental level and innate personality characteristics also influence her behavioral responses.
3. The mother's role partner, her infant, will reflect the mother's competence in the mothering role via growth and development.

Nursing

Mercer does not define *nursing* but refers to nursing as a science emerging from a "turbulent adolescence to adulthood."[5] Nurses are the health professionals having the most "sustained and intense interaction with women in the maternity cycle."[5] Nurses are responsible for "promoting the health" of families and children; nurses are "pioneers" in developing and sharing assessment strategies for these clients.[4]

Obstetrical nursing, according to Mercer, is the diagnosis and treatment of women's and men's responses to actual or potential health problems during pregnancy, childbirth, and the postpartum period.[8:29]

Person

Mercer does not specifically define *person* but refers to the "self" or "core-self."[7:198] Self, when used by Mercer, is in reference to the mother. She views the self as separate from the roles that are played. Through maternal individuation a woman may regain her own "personhood" as she extrapolates her "self" from the mother-infant dyad.[9:295] The core self evolves from a culture context and determines how situations are defined and shaped.[7:198]

Health

In her theory Mercer defines *health status* as the mother's and father's perception of their prior health, current health, health outlook, resistance-susceptibility to illness, health worry concern, sickness orientation, and rejection of the sick role. Health status of the newborn is the extent of pathology present and infant health status by parental rating of overall health.[9:342] The health status of a family is negatively affected by antepartum stress. Health status is an important indirect influence on satisfaction with relationships in childbearing families.

Environment

In Mercer's work she does not define *environment*. She does, however, address the individual's culture, mate, family and/or support network, and size of that network as it relates to maternal role attainment.[9:50] A mate's love, support, and nurturance were important factors in enabling a woman to mother her child. The responses of mates, parents, other relatives, and friends are closely evaluated by the role taker. Supportive responses provided sanction for their mothering role and seemed to communicate confidence in their ability to mother. The mate, parents, family, and friends were also identified as sources of coping and help for the new mother.[9:14-17]

THEORETICAL ASSERTIONS

1. Increased age appears to be an asset in child-care behavior.[3:73-77]
2. Age differences also reflect developmental differences. The older the woman, the more experience she has had in acquiring new roles.[3:73-77]
3. Competency in moving to new roles is enhanced by greater knowledge and earlier experiences.[3:73-77]
4. The maternal role is socially accepted as an adult role that is inappropriate for the psychologically immature teenager.[3:73-77]
5. The impact of events during labor and delivery has the potential to affect a mother's self-esteem and early interaction behaviors with her infant positively or negatively.[3:73-77]
6. Social stress has been related to complications of pregnancy and parenting.[3:73-77]
7. A relationship exists between the woman's support system and her mothering.[3:73-77]
8. The woman's ego strength, self-confidence, and nurturant qualities have been observed to be basic determinants of her capacity as a mother.[3:73-77]
9. Maternal illness during pregnancy or birth affects the woman's self-esteem and drains energy that would otherwise be available for mothering.[3:73-77]
10. Child-rearing attitudes, how parents handle irritating child behaviors, parent-child interaction, and parent-child communication all sharply differentiated between abusive and nonabusive parents.[3:73-77]
11. Mothers rating high in adaptive maternal behavior have been observed to have infants with easy temperaments.[30:73-77]
12. Culture and socioeconomic level affect the maternal role.[30:73-77]
13. The maternal role may be attained in twelve months.[9:266]

LOGICAL FORM

Mercer used both deductive and inductive logic in developing the theoretical framework for studying factors that influence maternal role attainment in the first year of motherhood.

Deductive logic is demonstrated in her use of works from other researchers and disciplines. Both role and developmental theories and the work of R. Rubin on Maternal Role Attainment provided a base for the framework.

Mercer also used inductive logic in the development of her maternal role attainment theory. Through practice and research, she observed adaptation to motherhood from a variety of circumstances. She noted that differences existed in adaptation to motherhood when maternal illness complicated the postpartum, when a child with a defect was born, and when a teenager became a mother. These observations directed the research about those situations and subsequently the development of her theoretical framework.

ACCEPTANCE BY THE NURSING COMMUNITY

Practice

When considering practice using Mercer's framework, a clinical practice was set up using part of the concepts in the research conducted by Neeson, Patterson, Mercer, and May, "Pregnancy Outcomes for Adolescents Receiving Prenatal Care by Nurse Practitioners in Extended Roles."

The concepts theorized by Mercer have been used by nursing in multiple obstetrical textbooks. She is often cited as taking the work by Rubin and expanding its utilization. Her theory is extremely practice oriented.

Education

As previously stated, Mercer's work has appeared extensively in nursing texts, not just as it relates to maternal role attainment, but each individual piece of research is used and valued.

Research

Mercer has tested factors that she theorized and/or hypothesized have an impact on maternal attainment. She has done extensive literature reviews and formulated questions and models that guide future research.

Mercer has written articles on nursing research and stated her belief that nursing research is the bridge to excellence in practice. She also advocates the involvement of students in faculty research, with faculty serving as mentors.

During her tenure at the University of California, she chaired committees and was a committee member for numerous graduate theses and/or dissertations. Her work was used as the basis for at least eight graduate students' topics of research.[11]

The theoretical framework for the correlational study exploring differences between three age groups for first-time mothers (ages 15-19, 20-29, and 30-42) has been tested in part by others, including Lorraine Walker and associates, University of Texas, Austin, and reported in *Nursing Research.* Angela B. McBride wrote, "Maternal role attainment has been a fundamental concern of nursing since the pioneering work of Mercer's mentor, Rubin, almost two decades ago. It is now becoming the research-based, theoretically sound construct that nurse researchers have been searching for in their analysis of the experience of new mothers."[2:72]

Collaborative research with a graduate student and a junior faculty member in 1977 and 1978 led to the development of a highly reliable, valid instrument that measured attitudes about the labor experience. Over 60 researchers have requested permission to use the instrument.[11]

FURTHER DEVELOPMENT

Mercer believes that areas in need of further development and research are: the mate relationship, that is, finding a tool that accurately reflects the dyadic relationship; investigating maternal role attainment among younger adolescents; developing more reliable and valid measurements of social support; and extending measurements into pregnancy, especially with the adolescent population.[9:335-336] She also believes that further investigation into family dynamics and situational events that occur simultaneously with maternal role attainment is necessary.[7]

In her book *First-Time Motherhood: Experiences from Teens to Forties,* she presents a model of four phases occurring in the process of maternal role attainment during the first year of motherhood. The four phases are labeled as follows: the physical recovery phase, occurring from birth to 1 month; the achievement phase from 2 to 4 or 5 months; the disruption phase occurring from 6 to 8 months; and finally the reorganization phase from after the eighth month and still in process at 1 year.[9:299-314] Additionally, adaptation to the maternal role is proposed to occur at three levels—biologic, psychologic, and social—which are interacting and interdependent throughout the phases. These phases and levels of adaptation are briefly described and applied to her research on maternal role attainment. This model appears very logical and useful but is in need of further explanation, exposure, and development.

Additionally, research could investigate the

application of this framework to multigravidas and extend the time frame beyond the first year. An interesting study would be whether differences exist in maternal role attainment among mothers conceiving and rearing children from multiple gestations (i.e., twins, triplets) when compared with mothers rearing only one child. More explicit definitions of concepts and a greater consistency in labeling some concepts would benefit the reader. However, in 1988, having retired, Mercer did not plan to continue with further development and research on the theoretical framework for studying maternal role attainment.[13] She is writing reports from her later research that focuses on the perinatal family, women's development, and intergenerational influences on both.

CRITIQUE

Clarity

The concepts, variables, and relationships are not explicitly defined but rather described and implied. They are, however, theoretically defined and operationalized. The operational and theoretical definitions are consistent. Some interchanging of terms and labels used to identify concepts (e.g., adaptation and attainment, social support and support network) can create some confusion for the reader. Additionally, *maternal role attainment* is not consistently defined and thus obstructs clarity. Overall, the concepts, assumptions, and goals are organized into a logical and coherent whole, and understanding the interrelationships among the concepts is relatively easy.

Simplicity

In spite of numerous concepts and relationships, the theoretical framework for Maternal Role Attainment organizes a rather complex phenomenon into an easily understood and useful form. The theory is predictive in nature and thus readily lends itself to guide practice.[1:142] Concepts are not specific to time and place, and so are abstract, but are described and operationalized to the extent that meanings are not easily misinterpreted. However, note that the research completed to define and support the theoretical relationships was very complex, largely due to the great number of concepts.

Generality

Mercer's work on Maternal Role Attainment has very limited application. Concepts, assumptions, and relationships are more concrete than abstract, thus limiting the generalizability of the framework. The framework is confined to use with first-time mothers, the mother-child dyad, and a time span covering only the first year of motherhood. However, Mercer's work has done much to broaden the range of application of previously existing theories on maternal role attainment, as her studies have spanned various developmental levels and situational contexts, whereas others have not.

Empirical Precision

Mercer's work was derived from extensive research efforts. The concepts, assumptions, and relationships are grounded predominantly in empirical observations and are congruent. The degree of concreteness and the completeness of operational definitions further increases the empirical precision.[1:144] The theoretical framework for exploring differences between age groups of first-time mothers lends itself well to further testing and is being used by others, as previously discussed in the acceptance section of this chapter.

Derivable Consequences

The theoretical framework for Maternal Role Attainment in the first year has proven to be useful, practical, and valuable to nursing. Mercer's work is repeatedly utilized in research, practice, and education. The framework is also readily utilizable to any discipline that works with mothers and children in the first year of motherhood. McBride wrote, "Dr. Mercer is the one who developed the most complete theoretical framework for studying one aspect of parental experience, namely, the factors that influence the attainment of the maternal role in the first year of motherhood."[2:72]

According to Chinn and Jacobs, nursing theory should "differentiate the focus of nursing from other service professions."[1:145] By combining the social, psychologic, and biologic sciences, Mercer achieves this criteria.

Throughout her career, Mercer has consistently linked research to practice. Implications for nursing and/or nursing interventions are addressed and provide the bond between research and practice in most of her works. She believes that nursing research is the "bridge to excellence" in nursing practice.[6]

REFERENCES

1. Chinn, P.L., & Jacobs, M.K. (1987). *Theory and nursing: A systematic approach*. St. Louis: C.V. Mosby.
2. McBride, Angela B. (1984). The experience of being a parent. *Annual Review of Nursing Research, 2:*63-81.
3. Mercer, R.T. (1981). A theoretical framework for studying factors that impact on the maternal role. *Nursing Research, 30:73-77.*
4. Mercer, R.T. (1981). Foreword. In C. Kehoe (Ed.), *The Cesarean Experience*. New York: Appleton-Century-Crofts.
5. Mercer, R.T. (1982). Foreword. In S. Hummenick (Ed.), *Assessment evaluation: A clinical and technical review of selected assessment strategies for use in the health care of families in pregnancy and early parenting years*. New York: Appleton-Century-Crofts.
6. Mercer, R.T. (1984). Nursing research: The bridge to excellence in practice. *Image: The Journal of Nursing Scholarship, 16(2):*47-51.
7. Mercer, R.T. (1985). The process of maternal role attainment over the first year. *Nursing Research, 34:*198-204.
8. Mercer, R.T. (1985). Obstetric nursing research: Past, present, and future. *Birth Defects: Original Article Series, 21(3):*29-70.
9. Mercer, R.T. (1986). *First-time motherhood: Experiences from teens to forties*. New York: Springer.
10. Mercer, R.T. (1986). The relationship of developmental variables to maternal behavior. *Research in Nursing & Health, 9:*25-33.
11. Mercer, R.T. (1987, Feb.). Curriculum vitae.
12. Mercer, R.T. (1988). Curriculum vitae.
13. Mercer, R.T. (1988). Telephone interview.
14. Mercer, R.T., Hackley, K.C., & Bostrom, A. (1983). Relationship of psychosocial and perinatal variables to perception of childhood. *Nursing Research, 32(4):*202-207.
15. Mercer, R.T., Hackley, K.C., & Bostrom, A. (1984). Social support of teenage mothers. *Birth Defects: Original Article Series, 20(5):*245-290.
16. Mercer, R.T., May, K.A., Ferketich, S., & DeJoseph, J. (1986). Theoretical models for studying the effect of antepartum stress on the family. *Nursing Research, 35:*339-346.
17. Slager-Ernest, S.E., Hoffman, S.J., & Beckman, C.J.A. (1987). Effects of a specialized prenatal adolescent program on maternal and infant outcome. *Journal of Obstetric, Gynecologic and Neonatal Nursing, 19(6):*422-429.

BIBLIOGRAPHY

Primary Sources

Books

Mercer, R.T. (1977). *Nursing care for parents at risk*. Thorofare, N.J.: Charles B. Slack, Inc.

Mercer, R.T. (1979). *Perspectives on adolescent health care*. Philadelphia: J.B. Lippincott.

Mercer, R.T. (1986). *First-time motherhood: experiences from teens to forties*. New York: Springer.

Mercer, R.T., Nichols, E.G., & Doyle, G. (In press). *Transitions in the life cycle of women: A comparison of mothers and nonmothers*. New York: Springer.

Articles

Highley, B.L., & Mercer, R.T. (1978). Safeguarding the laboring woman's sense of control. *MCN, The American Journal of Maternal Child Nursing, 4:*39-41.

Marut, J.S., & Mercer, R.T. (1979, Sept-Oct.). A comparison of primiparas' perception of vaginal and cesarean birth. *Nursing Research, 28:*260-266.

Marut, J.S., & Mercer, R.T. (1981). The cesarean birth experience: Implications for nursing. *Birth Defects: Original Article Series, 17:*129-152.

(Mercer) Evans, R.T. (1968). Needs identified among breastfeeding mothers. *ANA Clinical Sessions* (pp. 162-171). New York: Appleton-Century-Crofts.

Mercer, R.T. (1973, Spring). One mother's use of negative feedback in coping with her infant with a defect. *Maternal-Child Nursing Journal, 2:29-37.*

Mercer, R.T. (1974, March-April). Mothers' responses to their infants with defects. *Nursing Research, 23*:133-137.
Mercer, R.T. (1974). Two fathers' early responses to the birth of a daughter with a defect. *Maternal-Child Nursing Journal, 3*:77-86.
Mercer, R.T. (1974). A focus on field methodology as a method of research in nursing practice. *Occasional Papers in Nursing Research, University of California, San Francisco, 2*:14-17.
Mercer, R.T. (1975). Responses of mothers to the birth of an infant with a defect. *ANA Clinical Sessions* (pp. 340-349). New York: Appleton-Century-Crofts.
Mercer, R.T. (1976). Mothering at sixteen. *MCN, The American Journal of Maternal Child Nursing, 1*:44-52.
Mercer, R.T. (1977, July). Postpartum illness and the acquaintance-attachment process. *American Journal of Nursing, 77*:1174-1178.
Mercer, R.T. (1977, Nov.). Crisis: A baby is born with a defect. *Nursing 77, 7*:45-47.
Mercer, R.T. (1978). Internal and external constraints on teenage mothering. *Research in Education, 13(8)*.
Mercer, R.T. (1979, Sept.-Oct.). She's a multip: She knows the ropes. *MCN, The American Journal of Maternal Child Nursing, 4*:301-304.
Mercer, R.T. (1980, Jan.-Feb.). Teenage motherhood: The first year. Part I, The teenage mothers' views and responses. Part II, How their infants fared. *Journal of Obstetric, Gynecologic, and Neonatal Nursing, 9*:16-27.
Mercer, R.T. (1980). Commentary on maternal identification and infant care: A theoretical perspective. *Western Journal of Nursing Research, 2*:700-702.
Mercer, R.T. (1981, March-April). A theoretical framework for studying factors that impact on the maternal role. *Nursing Research, 30*:73-77.
Mercer, R.T. (1981, Sept.-Oct.). The nurse and maternal tasks of early postpartum. *MCN, The American Journal of Maternal Child Nursing, 6*:341-345.
Mercer, R.T. (1981). Factors impacting on the maternal role the first year. *Birth Defects: Original Article Series, 17*:233-252.
Mercer, R.T. (1983, June). Assessing and counseling teenage mothers during the perinatal period. *Nursing Clinics of North America, 8*:293-301.
Mercer, R.T. (1984, Spring). Nursing Research: The bridge to excellence in practice. *Image: The Journal of Nursing Scholarship, 16(2)*:47-51.
Mercer, R.T. (1984). Commentary on subject mortality: Is it inevitable? *Western Journal of Nursing Research, 6*:336-337.
Mercer, R.T. (1984, June). Challenges during the first year of motherhood. *The Fourth Helen Nahm Lecture.* San Francisco: University of California, School of Nursing.
Mercer, R.T. (1984). Student involvement in faculty research: A mentor's view. *Western Journal of Nursing Research, 6(4)*:433-437.
Mercer, R.T. (1984). Health of the children of adolescents. *Adolescent Family, Report of Fifteenth Ross Roundtable on Critical Approaches to Common Pediatric Problems.* Columbus, Ohio: Ross Laboratories (pp. 60-66).
Mercer, R.T. (1985, July-Aug.). The relationship of the birth experience to later mothering behavior. *Journal of Nurse Midwifery, 30(4)*:204-211.
Mercer, R.T. (1985, July-Aug.). The process of maternal role attainment over the first year. *Nursing Research, 34(4)*:198-204.
Mercer, R.T. (1985). Obstetrical nursing: Past, present, and future. *Birth Defects: Original Article Series, 21(3)*:29-70.
Mercer, R.T. (1985). Teenage pregnancy as a community problem. *Annual Review of Nursing Research, 3*:49-76.
Mercer, R.T. (1985). The relationship of age and other variables to gratification in mothering. *Health Care for Women International, 6*:295-308.
Mercer, R.T. (1986). Predictors of maternal role attainment at one year post-birth. *Western Journal of Nursing Research, 8(1)*:9-32.
Mercer, R.T. (1986). The relationship of developmental variables to maternal behavior. *Research in Nursing & Health, 9*:25-33.
Mercer, R.T. (1987). The mentor and research outcomes. *Search: Improved Nursing Care Through Research, 11(2)*:1-2.
Mercer, R.T. (Spring, 1988). P's and Q's of monitoring and maintaining a research career. *Community Nursing Research,* Volume 21. *Nursing: A socially responsible profession.* Boulder, Col.: Western Institute of Nursing, pp. 21-31.
Mercer, R.T., & Ferketich, S.L. (1988). Stress and social support as predictors of anxiety and depression during pregnancy. *Advances in Nursing Science, 10(2)*:26-39.

Mercer, R.T., Ferketich, S.L., May, K., DeJoseph, J., & Sollid, D. (1988). Further exploration of maternal and paternal fetal attachment. *Research in Nursing & Health, 11*:83-95.

Mercer, R.T., Ferketich, S.L., DeJoseph, J., May, K., & Sollid, D. (1988, September, October). Effect of stress on family functioning during pregnancy. *Nursing Research, 37(5)*:268-275.

Mercer, R.T., Hackley, K.C., & Bostrom, A.G. (1983, July-Aug.). Relationship of psychosocial and perinatal variables to perception of childbirth. *Nursing Research, 32*:202-207. Reprinted (1984) in *Taiwan Nursing Digest, 106(21)*:100-104.

Mercer, R.T., Hackley, K.C., & Bostrom, A. (1984). Adolescent motherhood: Comparisons of outcome with older mothers. *Journal of Adolescent Health Care, 4*:7-13.

Mercer, R.T., Hackley, K.C., & Bostrom, A. (1984). Social support of teenage mothers. *Birth Defects: Original Article Series, 20(5)*:245-290.

Mercer, R.T., & Highley, B.L. (1978). Maternity specialization: Where are the challenges? In M.R. Spaulding (Ed.), *Report of Conference on Crisis in Maternal-Child Nursing Leadership* (pp. 63-75). Richmond, Va.: Medical College of Virginia, School of Nursing.

Mercer, R.T., May, K.A., Ferketich, S., & DeJoseph, J. (1986, Nov.-Dec.). Theoretical models for studying the effect of antepartum stress on the family. *Nursing Research, 35(6)*:339-346.

Mercer, R.T., Nichols, E., & Doyle, G. (1988). Transitions over the life cycle: A comparison of mothers and nonmothers. *Nursing Research, 37*:144-151.

Mercer, R.T., & Stainton, M.C. (1984). Perceptions of the birth experience: A cross-cultural comparison. *Health Care for Women International, 5*:28-47.

(Mercer) Evans, R.T., Thigpen, L., & Hamrick, M. (1969, Jan.-Feb.). Exploration of factors involved in maternal physiological adaptation to breastfeeding. *Nursing Research, 18(1)*:28-33.

Neeson, J.D., Patterson, K.A., Mercer, R.T., & May, K.A. (1983, June). Pregnancy outcome for adolescents receiving prenatal care by nurse practitioners in extended roles. *Journal of Adolescent Health Care, 4*:94-99.

Slavazza, K.L., Mercer, R.T., Marut, J.S., & Shnider, S.M. (1985, July-Aug.). Differences in maternal perceptions of anesthesia, analgesia for vaginal childbirth. *Journal of Obstetric, Gynecologic, and Neonatal Nursing, 14(4)*:321-329.

Correspondence

Mercer, R.T. (1988, Jan.). Curriculum vitae.

Mercer, R.T. (1988, Feb.). Revised curriculum vitae.

Grant Reports

Mercer, R.T., Hackley, K.C., & Bostrom, A. Factors having an impact on maternal role attainment the first year of motherhood. Grant #MC-R-05-060435. Maternal and Child Health (Social Security Act, Title V), San Francisco: Department of Family Health Care Nursing, University of California, San Francisco. (1982).

Mercer, R.T., Ferketich, S.L., May, K.A., DeJoseph, J., & Sollid, D. Antepartum stress: Effects on family health and functioning. Grant #R01 NR 01064. National Center for Nursing Research, National Institutes of Health, San Francisco: Department of Family Health Care Nursing, University of California, San Francisco. (1987).

Book Chapters

Mercer, R.T. (1981). Potential effects of anesthesia and analgesia on mother-infant attachment process of cesarean mothers. In C. Kehoe (Ed.), *The Cesarean Experience.* New York: Appleton-Century-Crofts.

Mercer, R.T., & Marut, J.S. (1981). Comparative viewpoints: Cesarean versus vaginal birth. In D.D. Affonso (Ed.), *Impact of cesarean childbirth.* Philadelphia: F.A. Davis.

Mercer, R.T. (1981). Reaction of parents following cesarean delivery. In S. Rosno (Ed.), *A humanistic approach to cesarean childbirth.* San Jose, Cal.: Cesarean Birth Control International, Inc.

Mercer, R.T. (1983). Parent-infant attachment. In L.J. Sontegard, K.M. Kowalski, & B. Jennings (Eds.), *Women's Health,* Vol. II *Childbearing.* New York: Grune & Stratton.

Mercer, R.T. (1987). Adolescent pregnancy. In L.J. Sontegard, K.M. Kowalski & B. Jennings (Eds.), *Women's Health:* Vol. III *Crisis and Illness in Childbearing.* Orlando: Grune & Stratton.

Mercer, R.T. (1988). Theoretical perspectives on the family. In Gilliss, B. Highley, B. Roberts, & I. Martinson (Eds.), *Toward a Science of Family Nursing.* Menlo Park, Cal.: Addison-Wesley.

Abstracts

Hackley, K., & Mercer, R.T. (1981). Variables correlating with the mother's perception of her neonate early postpartum and at one month. *Proceedings Nurses' Association of American College of Obstetrics and Gynecologists, Third National Meeting, San Francisco, March 29-April 4, 1981.* Libertyville, Ill: Hollister, Inc.

Hackley, K.C., Mercer, R.T., & Bostrom, A. (1982). Motherhood in the 30s: A preview of their experiences. *Western Journal of Nursing Research, 4(3)*:61. Also in: *Communicating Nursing Research, 15*:61.

Mercer, R.T. (1986). Needs identified among breastfeeding mothers. *American Journal of Nursing, 68*:1274-1275.

Mercer, R.T. (1974). Responses of five multigravidae to the event of the birth of an infant with a defect. *Dissertation Abstracts International, 34:(10).*

Mercer, R.T. (1979). Internal and external constraints on teenage mothering. Resources in Women's Educational Equity, *ERIC Documents.*

Mercer, R.T., Hackley, K., & Bostrom, A. (1980). Maternal age and role attainment at one month postpartum. *Nursing Research Advancing Clinical Practice for the 80's.* San Francisco: Department of Nursing Service, Stanford University Hospital, and Symposia Medicus.

Mercer, R.T. (1980). Teenage mothering. *Perinatal Press, 4(5)*:71.

Mercer, R.T., & Hackley, K. (1981). Factors correlated with the primipara's perception of her labor and delivery experience. *Proceedings Nurses' Association of American College of Obstetrics and Gynecologists, Third National Meeting, San Francisco, March 29-April 4, 1981.* Libertyville, Ill: Hollister, Inc.

Mercer, R.T. (1982). The changing family. *Proceedings Seventh Annual March of Dimes Perinatal Nursing Conference, March 22 & 23, 1982.* Mead Johnson Nutritional Division.

Mercer, R.T., & Hackley, K. (1982). Factors correlating with maternal age early postpartum. *Nursing Research, 31*:188.

Mercer, R.T. (1982). The early postpartum days: Expectations versus realities. *Pediatric Nursing Currents, 29(1)*:1-2.

Mercer, R.T., Hackley, K.C., & Bostrom, A. (1982). Adolescent mothers: Their assets and deficits. *Western Journal of Nursing Research, 4*:59. Also in: *Communicating Nursing Research, 15*:59.

Mercer, R.T., Hackley, K.C., & Bostrom, A. (1983). Impact of motherhood after thirty. *Communicating Nursing Research, 16*:51-52.

Mercer, R.T., Hackley, K.C., & Bostrom, A. (1983, April). Comparison of mothering behaviors. *Maternal and Child Health Technical Information Series,* 8-9.

Mercer, R.T. (1983) Predictors of gratification for mothers 30 and older. *Proceedings Council on Nurse Researchers Conference, Minneapolis, September 21-23.* American Nurses' Association.

Mercer, R.T. (1983). The relationship of attitudes toward the birth experience and mothering behaviors. *Journal of Adolescent Health Care, 4*:212.

Mercer, R.T. (1984). Predictors of maternal role attainment at one year post birth. *Western Journal of Nursing Research, 6(3)*:62.

Mercer, R.T., & Hackley, K.C. (1984). A comparison of employed and unemployed mothers' responses and attitudes. *Western Journal of Nursing Research, 6(3)*:61.

Mercer, R.T., Ferketich, S., May, K., & DeJoseph, J. (1987). A comparison of maternal and paternal responses during pregnancy. *Proceedings Council of Nurse Researchers Conference, Arlington, Va., October 13-16,* American Nurses' Association.

Mercer, R.T., Nichols, E.G., & Doyle, G. (1987). Transitions in the life cycle of women: Mothers and nonmothers. *Proceedings Sigma Theta Tau International Biennial Conference, San Francisco, November 10,* Sigma Theta Tau International.

Mercer, R.T., Ferketich, S., May, K., DeJoseph, J., & Sollid, D. (1987). Maternal and paternal responses in high- and low-risk pregnancies. Symposium. *Proceedings Sigma Theta Tau International Biennial Conference, San Francisco, November 10,* Sigma Theta Tau International.

Audiovisuals

Beland, J.W., & Mercer, R.T. (1975). The crisis of loss, TIO, Psychiatric-Mental-Health Nursing. *American Journal of Nursing* Company, Educational Services Division.

Forewords

Foreword. (1981). In C. Kehoe (Ed.), *Nursing management in cesarean births.* New York: Appleton-Century-Crofts.

Foreword. (1982). In S. Hummenick (Ed.), *Assessment evaluation: A clinical and technical review of selected assessment strategies for use in the health care of families in pregnancy and early parenting years.* New York: Appleton-Century-Crofts.

Foreword. (1986). In J.D. Neeson & K.A. May (Eds), *Comprehensive maternity nursing.* Philadelphia: J.B. Lippincott.

Letters to Editor

Mercer, R.T. (1984). Eight stages of a doctoral dissertation. *Nursing Research, 23:*435-436.

Mercer, R.T. (1976). Preparation of the breast for breastfeeding. *Nursing Research, 25:*222.

Mercer, R.T. (1977). Moving out of the nursing ghetto. *MCN, The American Journal of Nursing, 2:*65.

Book Reviews

Mercer, R.T. (1983). *Parenting reassessed: A nursing perspective. American Journal of Nursing, 83:*963.

Mercer, R.T. (1985). *Maternal Identity and the Maternal Experience. American Journal of Nursing, 85:*103-104.

Secondary Sources

Articles

Barnard, K.E., & Neal, M.V., Maternal child nursing research: Review of the past and strategies for the future. *Nursing Research, 26:*193-200.

Cranley, M.S., Hedahl, K.J., & Pegg, S.H. (1983). Women's perceptions of vaginal and cesarean deliveries. *Nursing Research, 32(1):*10-15.

Crawford, G. (1982). A theoretical model of support network conflict experienced by new mothers. *Nursing Research, 34:*100-102.

Curry, M.A. (1982). Maternal attachment behavior and the mother's self-concept: The effect of early skin-to-skin contact. *Nursing Research, 32(2):*73-78.

Gift, A.G., & Palmer, M.H. (1987). Planning clinical nursing research with a geriatric population. *Clinical Nurse Specialist, 1(2):*56, 87.

Hawkins, J.W. (1986). Did we do all we could? *American Journal of Nursing, 86:*158.

Lederman, R.P., Weingarten, C.T., & Lederman, E. (1981). Postpartum self-evaluation questionnaire: Measures of maternal adaptation. *Birth Defects: Original Article Series, 17(6):*201-231.

Lin, R.C. (1986). A project for facilitating maternal adaptation with Chinese adolescent mothers in Taiwan. *Health Care For Women International, 7(4):*311-327.

Lipson, J.G., & Tilden, V.P. (1980). Psychological integration of the cesarean birth experience. *American Journal of Orthopsychiatry, 50(4):*598-609.

Majewski, J.L. (1986). Conflicts, satisfactions, and attitudes during transition to the maternal role. *Nursing Research, 35(1):*10-14.

Proctor, S.E. (1986). A developmental approach to pregnancy prevention with early adolescent females. *Journal of School Health, 56(8):*313-321.

Sadler, L.S., & Catrone, C. (1983). The adolescent parent: A dual developmental crisis. *Journal of Adolescent Health Care, 4(2):*100-105.

Sims-Jones, N. (1986). Back to the theories: Another way to view mothers of prematures. *MCN, The Journal of Maternal Child Nursing, 11(6):*394-397.

Slager-Ernest, S.E., Hoffman, S.J., & Beckman, C.J.A. (1987). Effects of a specialized prenatal adolescent program on maternal and infant outcomes. *Journal of Obstetric, Gynecologic and Neonatal Nursing, 16(6):*422-429.

Spivak, H., & Weitzman, M. (1987). Social barriers faced by adolescent parents and their children. *Journal of Adolescent Health Care, 258:*1500-1504.

Walker, L.O., Crain, H., & Thompson, E. (1986). Maternal role attainment and identity in the postpartum period: Stability and change. *Nursing Research, 35(2):*68-71.

Walker, L.O., Crain, H., & Thompson, E. (1986). Mothering behavior and maternal role attainment during the postpartum period. *Nursing Research, 35(6):*322-355.

Wasserman, G.A., & Rhiasom, A. (1985). Maternal withdrawal from handicapped toddlers. *Journal of Child Psychology and Psychiatry and Allied Disciplines, 26:*381-387.

White, M., & Dawson, C. (1981). Impact of the at-risk infant on family solidarity. *Birth Defects, 17:*253-284.

Yoos, L. (1987). Perspectives on adolescent parenting: Effect of adolescent egocentrism on the maternal-child interaction. *Journal of Pediatric Nursing, 2(3):*193-200.

Zuskar, D.M. (1987). The psychological impact of prenatal diagnosis of fetal abnormality: Strategies for investigation and intervention. *Women Health, 12:*91-103.

Other Sources

Burr, W.R., Leigh, G.K., Day, R.D., & Constantine, J. (1979). Symbolic interaction and the family. In W.R. Burr, R. Hill, F.I. Nye, & I.L. Reiss (Eds.), *Contemporary theories about the family* Vol. 2 (pp. 42-111). New York: Free Press.

Erikson, E.H. (1959). Identity and the life cycle. *Psychological Issues* (Monograph). 1(1):1-171.

Mead, G.H. (1934). *Mind, self and society.* Chicago: University of Chicago Press.

Rowe, G.P. (1966). The developmental conceptual framework to the study of the family. In F.I. Nye & F.M. Berardo (Eds.), *Emerging conceptual frameworks in family analysis* (pp 198-222). New York: Macmillan Co.

Rubin, R. (1967). Attainment of the maternal role: Part I. Processes. *Nursing Research, 16:*237-245.

Rubin, R. (1967). Attainment of the maternal role: Part II. Models and referrants. *Nursing Research, 16:*342-346.

Rubin, R. (1977). Binding in the postpartum period. *Maternal-Child Nursing Journal, 6:*67-75.

Rubin, R. (1984). *Maternal identity and the maternal experience.* New York: Springer.

Von Bertalanffy, L. (1968). *General Systems Theory.* New York: George Braziller.

Werner, H. (1957). The concept of development from a comparative and organismic point of view. In D.H. Harris (Ed.), *The concept of development* (pp. 125-148). Minneapolis: University of Minnesota.

APPENDIX A: SUPERVISED DOCTORAL DISSERTATIONS: UNIVERSITY OF CALIFORNIA, SAN FRANCISCO, CALIFORNIA, SCHOOL OF NURSING

1980-1984

Virden, Susan B., *The effect of information about infant behavior on primiparas' maternal adequacy* (Chair).

Howe, Carole L., *Psychosocial maturity and adolescent sexual behavior and attitude* (Chair).

Tilden, Virginia P., *The relationship of single status during pregnancy to life stress, social support and emotional disequilibrium.*

Corbin, Juliet C., *Protective governing: Strategies for managing a pregnancy-illness* (Chair).

Hoevet, Gail L., *The relationship of a facial defect and separation history with security, attachment behavior, exploration, and object permanence in the one-year-old infant.*

1984-1986

Millor, Georgia K., *Children's temperaments and parent-child interactions in child abuse families* (Chair).

Majewski, Janice, *Transitions to parenthood: Impact of perceived role conflict on transition to the maternal role* (Chair).

Stevens, Marcia, *Adolescents' coping with hospitalization.*

Zachariah, Rachel, *Intergenerational attachment and well being during pregnancy* (Chair).

Stainton, Colleen, *The development of cue sensitivity between mother and infant* (Chair).

Elsayed, Yousria, *The 40-day postpartum period among Arab American women.*

Olshansky, Ellen, *The meaning of infertility and strategies used in coming to terms with it.*

Sammons, Lucy, *Maternal anxiety, somatic symptoms, marital adjustment, and family relationships in second pregnancy* (Chair). Received the Distinguished Dissertation Award, School of Nursing, 1986.

Randell, Brooke, *Maternal self perception: The impact of the adult mother-daughter relationship* (Chair in progress).

Johnson, Rebecca, *Impact of physical and social environment on maternal adaptation* (Chair in progress).

Donaldson, Nancy, *Early postpartum maternal adaptation: The effect of weekly telephone-based nursing intervention* (in progress).

UNIT IV

Systems

Dorothy E. Johnson

25

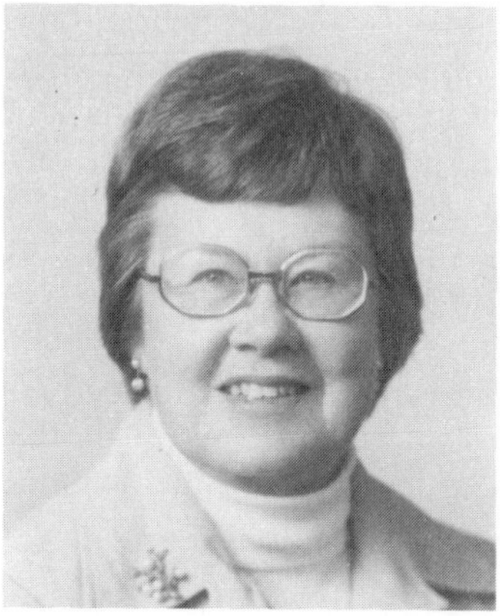

Behavioral System Model

Sharon S. Conner, Jude A. Magers, Judith K. Watt

CREDENTIALS AND BACKGROUND OF THE THEORIST

Dorothy E. Johnson was born Aug. 21, 1919, in Savannah, Georgia. She received her A.A. from Armstrong Junior College in Savannah, Georgia, in 1938; her B.S.N. from Vanderbilt University in Nashville, Tennessee, in 1942; and her M.P.H. from Harvard University in Boston in 1948.

Most of Johnson's professional experiences involved teaching, although she was a staff nurse at the Chatham-Savannah Health Council from 1943 to 1944. She has been an instructor and an assistant professor in pediatric nursing at Vanderbilt University School of Nursing. From 1949 until her retirement in 1978 and subsequent move to Florida, Johnson was an assistant professor of pediatric nursing, an associate professor of nursing, and a professor of nursing at the University of California in Los Angeles.

In 1955 and 1956 Johnson was a pediatric nursing advisor assigned to the Christian Medical College School of Nursing in Vellore, South India. In addition, from 1965 to 1967

The authors wish to express appreciation to Cynthia J. Allen, Sharon Evick, and Glenda Mitchell for their assistance with data collection, and to Dorothy E. Johnson for critiquing the chapter.

she chaired the committee of the California Nurses' Association that developed a position statement on specifications for the clinical specialist. Johnson's publications[21] include 4 books, more than 30 articles in periodicals, and many reports, proceedings, and monographs.

Of the many honors she has received, the ones Johnson[20] is proudest of are the 1975 Faculty Award from graduate students, the 1977 Lulu Hassenplug Distinguished Achievement Award from the California Nurses' Association, and the 1981 Vanderbilt University School of Nursing Award for Excellence in Nursing. She is pleased that her behavioral system model has been found useful in furthering the development of a theoretical basis for nursing, but says her greatest source of satisfaction has come from following the productive careers of her students.

THEORETICAL SOURCES

Johnson's behavioral system theory springs from Nightingale's belief that nursing's goal is to help individuals prevent or recover from disease or injury.[24:117] The science and art of nursing should focus on the patient as an individual and not on the specific disease entity.

Johnson used the work of behavioral scientists in psychology, sociology, and ethnology to develop her theory. Talcott Parsons is acknowledged specifically in early developmental writings presenting concepts of the behavioral system model.[10:3] She relies heavily on the systems theory and uses concepts and definitions from A. Rapoport, R. Chin, and W. Buckley.[19:208] The structure of the behavioral system theory is patterned after a systems model; a system is defined as consisting of interrelated parts functioning together to form a whole. In her writings, Johnson conceptualizes man as a behavioral system in which the functioning outcome is observed behavior. An analogy to the behavioral system theory is the biological system theory, which states that man is a biological system consisting of biological parts and that disease is an outcome of biological system disorder.

Developing the theory from a philosophical perspective, Johnson[19:207] writes that nursing contributes by facilitating effective behavioral functioning in the patient before, during, and following illness. She uses concepts from other disciplines, such as social learning, motivation, sensory stimulation, adaptation, behavioral modification, change process, tension, and stress to expand her theory.

Johnson notes that although the literature indicates others support the idea that man is a behavioral system, as far as she knows, the idea is original with her. Knowledge of the parts of the behavioral system is supported in the behavioral sciences, but the empirical literature supporting the notion that the behavioral system is a whole has yet to be developed. In the biological system, knowledge of the parts precedes knowledge of the whole.[19:208]

EMPIRICAL EVIDENCE

Some of the concepts Johnson has identified and defined in her theory are supported in the literature. Leitch and Escolona point out that tension produces behavioral changes and that the manifestation of tension by an individual depends on both internal and external factors.[12:66] Johnson[9:292] uses the work of Selye, Grinker, Simmons, and Wolff to support the idea that specific patterns of behavior are reactions to stressors from biological, psychological, and sociological sources, respectively. Johnson[10:8] suggests a difference in her model from Selye's conception of stress. Johnson's concept of stress "follows rather closely Caudill's conceptualization; i.e., that stress is a process in which there is interplay between various stimuli and the defenses erected against them. Stimuli may be positive in that they are present, or negative in that something desired or required is absent."[10:7-8] Selye "conceives stress as 'a state manifested by the specific syndrome which consists of all the nonspecifically induced changes within a biologic system.'"[10:8]

In *Conceptual Models for Nursing Practice,* Johnson describes seven subsystems that comprise her behavioral system. To support the attachment-affiliative subsystem, she uses the work of Ainsworth and Robson.[19:210] Heathers, Gerwitz, and Rosenthal have described and explained dependency behavior, another subsystem defined by Johnson.[19:212-213] The response systems of ingestion and elimination, as described by Walike, Mead, and Sears, are also parts of Johnson's behavioral system.[19:213] The work of Kagan and Resnik is used to support the sexual subsystem.[19:213] The aggressive subsystem which functions to protect and preserve, is supported by Lorenz and Feshbach.[19:213] According to Atkinson, Feather, and Crandell, physical, creative, mechanical, and social skills are manifested by achievement behavior, another subsystem identified by Johnson.[19:214]

MAJOR CONCEPTS AND DEFINITIONS

BEHAVIOR. Johnson accepts the definition of *behavior* as expressed by the behavioral and biological scientists: the output of intraorganismic structures and processes as they are coordinated and articulated by and responsive to changes in sensory stimulation. She focuses on behavior affected by the actual or implied presence of other social beings that has been shown to have major adaptive significance.[19:207-208]

SYSTEM. Using Rapoport's 1968 definition of system, Johnson[19:208] states, "A system is a whole that functions as a whole by virtue of the interdependence of its parts." She accepts Chin's statement that there is "organization, interaction, interdependency, and integration of the parts and elements."[19:208] In addition, man strives to maintain a balance in these parts through adjustments and adaptations to the forces impinging on them.

BEHAVIORAL SYSTEM. A behavioral system encompasses the patterned, repetitive, and purposeful ways of behaving. These ways of behaving form an organized and integrated functional unit that determines and limits the interaction between the person and his environment and establishes the relationship of the person to the objects, events, and situations within his environment. Usually the behavior can be described and explained. Man as a behavioral system tries to achieve stability and balance by adjustments and adaptations that are successful to some degree for efficient and effective functioning. The system is usually flexible enough to accommodate the influences affecting it.[19:208-209]

Subsystems. Because the behavioral system has many tasks to perform, parts of the system evolve into subsystems with specialized tasks. A subsystem is "a minisystem with its own particular goal and function that can be maintained as long as its relationship to the other subsystems or the environment is not disturbed."[19:221] The seven subsystems identified by Johnson are open, linked, and interrelated. Motivational drives direct the activities of these subsystems, which are continually changing because of maturation, experience, and learning. The systems described appear to exist cross-culturally and are controlled by biological, psychological, and sociological factors. The seven identified are attachment-affiliative, dependency, ingestive, eliminative, sexual, achievement, and aggressive.[19:209-212]

Attachment-affiliative subsystem. The attachment-affiliative subsystem is probably the most critical, because it forms the basis for all social organization. On a general level, it provides survival and security. Its consequences are social inclusion, intimacy, and formation and maintenance of a strong social bond.[19:212]

Dependency subsystem. In the broadest sense, the dependency subsystem promotes helping behavior that calls for a nurturing response. Its consequences are approval, attention or recognition, and physical assistance. Developmentally, dependency behavior evolves from almost total dependence on other to a greater degree of dependence on self. A certain amount of interdependence is essential for survival of social groups.[19:213]

Biological subsystems. The biological subsystems of ingestion and elimination "have to do with when, how, what, how much, and under what conditions we eat, and when, how, and under what conditions we eliminate."[19:213] These responses are associated with social and psychological as well as biological considerations.[19:213]

Sexual subsystem. The sexual subsystem has the dual functions of procreation and gratification. Including, but not limited to, courting and mating, this response system begins with the development of gender role identity and includes the broad range of sex role behaviors.[19:214]

Aggressive subsystem. The aggressive subsystem's function is protection and preservation. This follows the line of thinking of ethologists such as Lorenz[4] and Feshbach[23] rather than the behavioral reinforcement school of thought. It holds that aggressive behavior is not only learned, but has a primary intent to harm others. However, society demands that limits be placed on modes of self-protection and that people and their property be respected and protected.[19:213]

Achievement subsystem. The achievement subsystem attempts to manipulate the environment. Its function is control or mastery of an aspect of self or environment to some standard of excellence. Areas of achievement behavior include intellectual, physical, creative, mechanical, and social skills.[19:214]

Equilibrium. Johnson states that equilibrium is a key concept in nursing's specific goal.[10] It is defined "as a stabilized but more or less transitory, resting state in which the individual is in harmony with himself and with his environment."[12:65] "It implies that biological and psychological forces are in balance with each other and with impinging social forces."[11:11] It is "not synonymous with a state of health, since it may be found either in health or illness."[11:11]

Tension. "The concept of tension is defined as a state of being stretched or strained and can be viewed as an end-product of a disturbance in equilibrium."[10:10] Tension can be constructive in adaptative change or destructive in inefficient use of energy, hindering adaptation and potential structural damage.[10:10] Tension is the cue to disturbance in equilibrium.[11:15]

Stressor. Internal or external stimuli that produce tension and result in a degree of instability are called *stressors*. "Stimuli may be positive in that they are present; or negative in that something desired or required is absent. [Stimuli] . . . may be either endogenous or exogenous in origin [and] may play upon one or more of our linked open systems."[11:13] The open linked systems are in constant interchange. The open linked systems include the physiological, personality, and meaningful small group (e.g., the family) systems as well as the larger social system.[11:13]

ASSUMPTIONS
Nursing

Nursing, as perceived by Johnson, is an external force acting to preserve the organization of the patient's behavior while the patient is under stress by means of imposing regulatory mechanisms or by providing resources.[24:118] An art and a science, it supplies external assistance both before and during system balance disturbance and therefore requires knowledge of order, disorder, and control.[19:209;17:207] Nursing activities do not depend on medical authority but are complementary to medicine.

Person

Johnson[19:209] views man as a behavioral system with patterned, repetitive, and purposeful ways of behaving that link him to the environment. Man's specific response patterns form an organized and integrated whole.[16:207] *Person* is a system of interdependent parts that requires some regularity and adjustment to maintain a balance.[19:208]

Johnson[19:208] further assumes that a behavioral system is essential to man and when strong forces or lower resistance disturb behavioral system balance, man's integrity is threatened.[24:126] Man's attempt to reestablish balance may require an extraordinary expenditure of energy, which leaves a shortage of energy to assist biological processes and recovery.[24:126]

Health

Johnson perceives health as an elusive, dynamic state influenced by biological, psychological, and social factors. Health is a desired value by health professionals and focuses on the person rather than the illness.[24:119]

Health is reflected by the organization, interaction, interdependence, and integration of the subsystems of the behavioral system.[19:208] Man attempts to achieve a balance in this system, which will lead to functional behavior. A lack of balance in the structural or functional requirements of the subsystems leads to poor health. When the system requires a minimal amount of energy for maintenance, a larger supply of energy is available to affect biological processes and recovery.[24:126]

Environment

In Johnson's theory the environment consists of all the factors that are not part of the individual's behavioral system but that influence the system and some of which can be manipulated by the nurse to achieve the health goal for the patient.[24:126] The individual links himself to and interacts with the environment.[10] The behavioral system attempts to maintain equilibrium in response to environmental factors by adjusting and adapting to the forces that impinge upon it. Excessively strong environmental forces disturb the behavioral system balance and threaten the person's stability. An unusual amount of energy is required in order for the system to reestablish equilibrium in the face of continuing forces.[24:126] When the environment is stable, the individual is able to continue with his successful behaviors.

THEORETICAL ASSERTIONS

Johnson's behavioral system theory addresses two major components: the patient and nursing (Figure 25-1). The patient is a behavioral system with seven interrelated subsystems.

Each subsystem can be described and analyzed in terms of structure and functional requirements. The four structural elements that have been identified include: (1) drive, or goal; (2) set, predisposition to act; (3) choice, alternatives for action; and (4) behavior.[19:210-211]

Each of the subsystems has the same functional requirements: protection, nurturance, and stimulation.[24:123] The system and subsystems tend to be self-maintaining and self-perpetuating as long as internal and external conditions remain orderly and predictable. If the conditions and resources necessary to their functional requirements are not met, or the interrelationships among the subsystems are not harmonious, dysfunctional behavior will result.[19:212]

The responses by the subsystems are developed through motivation, experience, and learning and are influenced by biological, psychological, and social factors.[19:209] The behavioral system attempts to achieve balance by adapting to internal and environmental stimuli. The behavioral system is made up of "all the patterned, repetitive, and purposeful ways of behaving that characterize each man's life."[19:209] This functional unit of behavior "determines and limits the interaction of the person and his environment and establishes the relationship of the person with the objects, events, and situations in his environment."[19:209] The behavioral

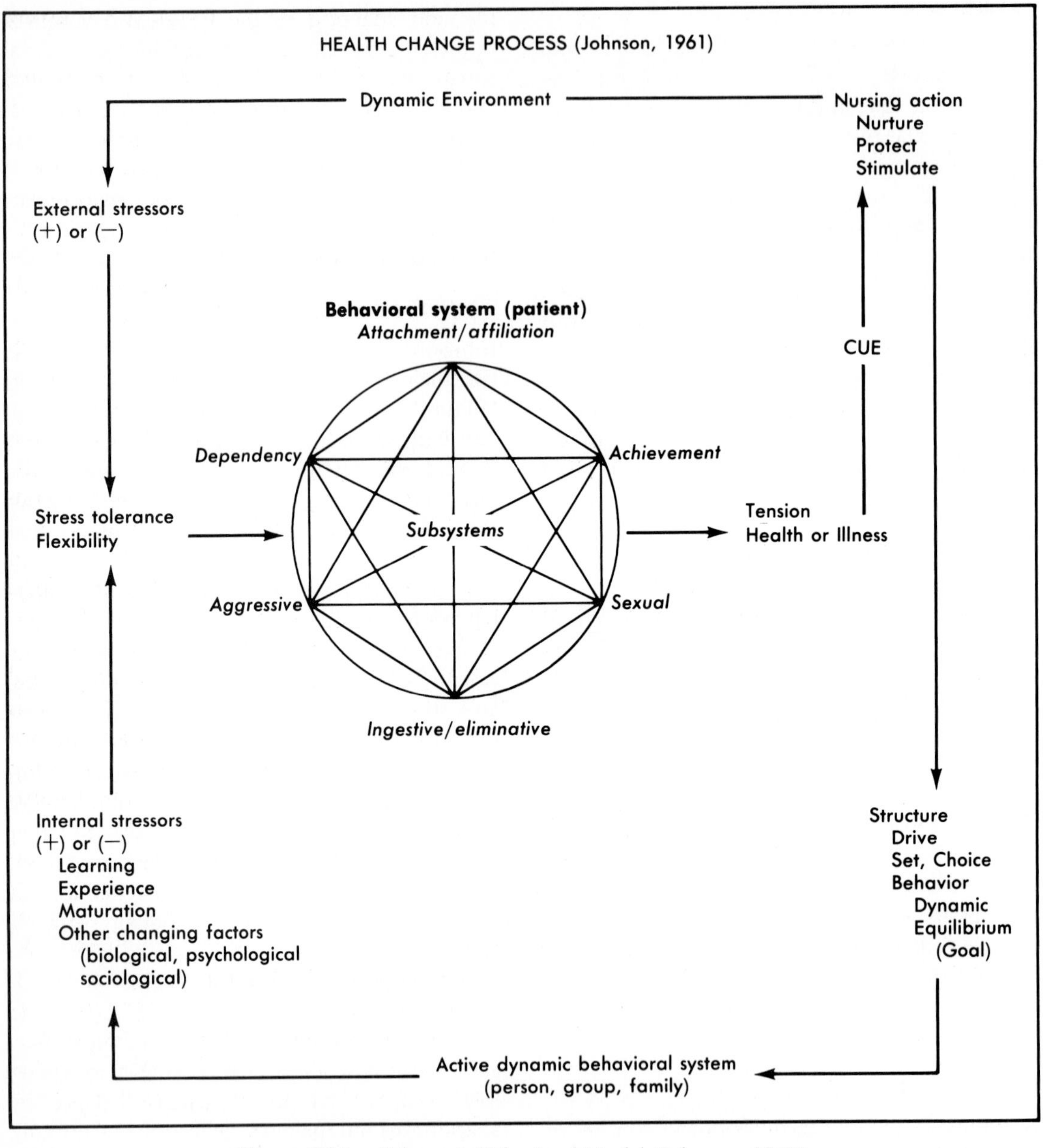

Figure 25-1. Johnson's Behavioral Model (Johnson, 1961).
Conceptualized by Jude A. Magers.

system manages its relationship with its environment.[19:209] The behavioral system appears to be active and not passive. The nurse is external to and interactive with the behavioral system.

A state of instability in the behavioral system results in a need for nursing intervention. Identification of the source of the problem in the system leads to appropriate nursing action that results in the maintenance or restoration of behavioral system balance.[24:129] Nursing is seen as an external regulatory force that acts to restore the balance in the behavioral system.[19:214]

LOGICAL FORM

By observing specifics in her practice, nursing literature, and research, Johnson has used the logical form of inductive reasoning to develop her theory. She states that a common core exists in nursing, which practitioners use in many settings and with varying populations.[8:200] Johnson used her observations of behavior over many years to formulate a general theory of man as a behavioral system.

ACCEPTANCE BY THE NURSING COMMUNITY

Practice

According to Johnson,[19] the behavioral system theory provides direction for practice, education, and research. Because the goal of the theory is to maintain and restore balance in the patient by helping him achieve a more optimal level of functioning, a goal also valued by nursing, the theory is acceptable to nursing. Knowledge of the behavioral system theory allows the nurse to be aware of the importance of providing a constant supply of protection, nurturing, and stimulation.

In 1974 Judy Grubbs[5:245,250] adapted the theory to the nursing process by developing an assessment tool and a nursing process sheet based on the seven subsystems. Questions and observations related to each subsystem provided powerful tools with which to collect important data. By using these tools, the nurse can discover other choices of behavior that will enable the patient to accomplish his goal of health.

That same year Bonnie Holaday[6:256] used the theory as a model to develop an assessment tool when caring for children. This tool allowed the nurse to objectively describe the child's behavior and to guide nursing action. Holaday concluded that the user of Johnson's theory was provided with a guide for planning and giving care based on scientific knowledge.

In 1980 Antionette Rawls[26:14-15] presented her attempt to use and evaluate the Johnson behavioral system theory in clinical practice. She used the theory to systematically assess a patient who was facing the loss of function in one arm and hand. Rawls concluded that Johnson's theory provided a tool that predicted the results of nursing intervention, formulated standards for care, and administered holistic care.

Johnson does not use the term *nursing process*. The concepts of assessment, disorders, treatment, and evaluation are referred to in a variety of works by Johnson. "For the practitioner, conceptual models provide a diagnostic and treatment orientation, and thus are of considerable practical import."[15:2]

The nursing process becomes applicable in the behavioral system model when behavioral malfunction occurs "that is in part disorganized, erratic, and dysfunctional. Illness or other sudden internal or external environmental change is most frequently responsible for such malfunctions."[19:212] "Assistance is appropriate at those times the individual is experiencing stress of a health-illness nature which disturbs equilibrium, producing tension."[10:6]

Johnson implies that the initial nursing assessment begins when the cue tension is observed and signals disequilibrium.[10:10] Sources for assessment data can be through history taking, testing, and structural observations.[19:211]

"The behavioral system is thought to determine and limit the interaction between the person and his environment."[15:3] This suggests that nursing assessment is not reactive. Nor is its accuracy or quantity of data controlled by the nurse. It is controlled by the patient (system). The only observed part of the subsystems structure is behavior. The nurse must be able to access information related to goals, sets, and choices that make up the structural subsystems. "One or more of [these] subsystems is likely to be involved in any episode of illness, whether in an antecedent or a consequence way or simply in association, directly or indirectly with the disorder or its treatment."[15:3] Accessing the data is critical to accurate statement of the disorder.

Johnson stated that nursing research would need to "identify and explain the behavioral system disorders which arise in connection with illness, and develop the rationale for the means of management."[15:7] Johnson does not define specific disorders but does state two general categories of disorders based on relationship to the biological system.[15:7]

Disorders are "those which are related tangentially or peripherally to disorder in the biological system; that is, they are precipitated simply by the fact of illness or the situational context of treatment; and . . . those [disorders] which are an integral part of a biological system disorder in that they are either directly associated with or a direct consequence of a particular kind of biological system disorder or its treatment."[15:7]

The "means of management"[15:7] or interventions do consist in part to the provision of nurturance, protection, and stimulation.[19:212] The nurse may provide "temporary imposition of external regulatory and control mechanisms, such as inhibiting ineffective behavioral responses, and assisting the patient to acquire new responses."[15:6] Johnson suggests techniques may include "teaching, role modeling, and counseling."[19:211] If a problem or disorder is anticipated, preventive nursing action is appropriate with adequate methodologies.[19:214]

The outcome of nursing intervention is behavioral system equilibrium. "More specifically, equilibrium can be said to have been achieved at that point at which the individual demonstrates a degree of constancy in his pattern of functioning, both internally and interpersonally."[10:9] The evaluation of the nursing process is based upon whether or not it made "a significant difference in the lives of the persons involved."[19:215]

Education

Carol Loveland-Cherry and Sharon Wilkerson[24:133] analyzed Johnson's theory and concluded that it has utility in nursing education. A curriculum based on man as a behavioral system would have definite goals and straightforward course planning. Study would center on the patient as a behavioral system and its dysfunction, which would require use of the nursing process. In addition to an understanding of systems theory, the student would need knowledge in the biological fields and emphasis on psychology and sociology.

Research

The behavioral system theory leads the researcher in one of two directions. One researcher might investigate the functioning of the system and subsystems by focusing on the basic sciences, while another researcher might concentrate on investigating problem-solving activities as they influence the behavioral system.[24:132]

Nurse researchers have demonstrated the usefulness of Johnson's theory in clinical practice. Beverly Small[28:264] used Johnson's theory as a conceptual framework to use when caring for visually impaired children. By evaluating and comparing the perceived body image and spacial awareness of normally sighted children with those of visually impaired children, Small found that the sensory deprivation of visual impairment affected the normal development of the child's body image and the awareness of his body in space. She concluded that when the human system is subjected to excessive stress, the goals of the system cannot be maintained.

Karla Damus[3:276] tested the validity of Johnson's theory by comparing SGPT values in patients exposed to hepatitis B with the number of nursing diagnoses. Damus correlated the physiological disorder of elevated SGPT values with behavioral disequilibrium and found that disorder in one area reflected disorder in another area.

Believing the model has potential in preventive care, Majesky[25] used it to construct a tool to measure patient indicators of nursing care. Holaday, Rawls, and Stamler[29] have done research using one subsystem.

FURTHER DEVELOPMENT

Although Johnson's behavioral system theory seems to focus on man as a passive being, Johnson believes people are active beings seeking constantly not only to adjust to their environments but also to adjust environments to the end of better functioning for themselves. She also views the behavioral system as active rather than merely reactive.[20] Because the model allows for this belief, work can be done regarding it.

The theory has been associated primarily with individuals. Johnson believes groups of individuals can be considered as groups of interactive behavioral systems. Use of her theory with families and other groups needs more visibility.[14]

As a result of the current emphasis on health promotion and maintenance and on illness and injury prevention, the theory could be developed further by recognizing behavior disorders in these areas.

> It should be noted that preventive nursing, i.e., to prevent behavioral system disorder, is not the same as preventive medicine, i.e., to prevent biological system disorders; and that disorders in both cases must be identified and explicated before approaches to prevention can be developed. At this point not even medicine has developed very many specific preventive measures (immunizations for some infectious diseases, and protection against some vitamin deficiency diseases are notable exceptions). There are a number of general approaches to better health, of course—adequate nutrition, safe water, exercise, etc.—which are applicable contributing to prevention of some disorders. Small wonder then that preventive nursing remains to be developed, and this is true no matter what model or theory for nursing is used.[20]

Further development could identify nursing actions that would facilitate appropriate functioning of the system toward disease prevention and health maintenance. Instead of spending energy developing nursing interventions for the consequences of disequilibrium, nurses need to determine how to intervene with the precursors of disequilibrium in order to prevent a crisis in health.

How can Johnson's theory be used in community health nursing? Assuming that a community is a geographical area, a subpopulation, or any aggregate of people, and assuming that a community can benefit from nursing interventions, the behavioral system framework can be applied to community health. A community can be described as a behavioral system with interacting subsystems that have structural elements and functional requirements. Communities have goals, norms, choices, and actions in addition to needing protection, nurturance, and stimulation. The community reacts to internal and external stimuli, which result in functional or dysfunctional behavior. An example of an external stimulus is health policy and an example of dysfunctional behavior is a high infant mortality. Somewhere between is the behavioral system, consisting of yet undefined subsystems that are organized, interacting, interdependent, and integrated. Biological, psychological, and sociological factors also impact on community behavior.

CRITIQUE

Simplicity

Johnson's theory is relatively simple in relation to the number of concepts. Man is described as a behavioral system composed of seven subsystems. Nursing is an external regulatory force. However, the theory is potentially complex because of the number of possible interrelationships between and among the behavioral system and its subsystems and the forces impinging on them. However, at this point only a few of the potential relationships have been explored.

Generality

Johnson's theory is relatively unlimited when applied to sick individuals. But it has not been used as much with well individuals or groups. Johnson perceives man as a behavioral system comprised of seven subsystems, aggregates of interactive behavioral systems. The role of nursing in nonillness situations is not clearly defined in the theory, but Johnson does address it.[24:132]

Empirical Precision

Empirical precision is difficult to achieve when a theory contains highly abstract concepts and has only potential generality. Empirical precision can improve when subconcepts that are well defined and have reality indicators are introduced. The units and the relationships between the units in Johnson's theory are consistently defined and used. However, Johnson's theory has only a moderate degree of empirical precision because the highly abstract concepts need to be better defined. Throughout Johnson's writings terms such as *balance, stability and equilibrium, adjustments and adaptations, disturbances, disequilibrium,* and *behavioral disorders* are used interchangeably, which confounds their meanings. The introduction of subsystems improves the theory's empirical precision.

Derivable Consequences

The theory should guide practice, education, and research, generate new ideas, and differentiate nursing from other professions. Johnson's theory guides nursing practice, education, and research. Because of the many interacting concepts it generates new ideas for practice and research. By focusing on behavior rather than biology, the theory clearly differentiates nursing from medicine although the concepts overlap with the psychosocial professions.

Johnson's behavioral systems theory provides a conceptual framework for nursing education, practice, and research. It has generated many questions for research and continues to be used as a basis for the development of curricula. Practitioners and patients have judged the resulting nursing actions to be satisfactory.[19:215] The theory has potential for continued utility in nursing in order to achieve valued nursing goals.

REFERENCES

1. Chin, R. (1961). The utility of system models and developmental models for practitioners. In K. Benne, et al. (Eds.), *The planning for change.* New York: Holt, Rinehart & Winston.
2. Chinn, P.L., & Jacobs, M.K. (1983). *Theory and nursing: A systematic approach.* St. Louis: C.V. Mosby.
3. Damus, K. (1980). An application of the Johnson behavioral system model for nursing practice. In J.P. Riehl & C. Roy (Eds.), *Conceptual models for nursing practice* (2d ed.). New York: Appleton-Century-Crofts.
4. Feshback, S. (1970). Aggression. In P. Mussen (Ed.), *Carmichael's manual of child psychology* (3d ed.). New York: John Wiley & Sons.
5. Grubbs, J. (1980). An interpretation of the Johnson behavioral system model for nursing practice. In J.P. Riehl & C. Roy (Eds.), *Conceptual models for nursing practice* (2d ed.). New York: Appleton-Century-Crofts.
6. Holaday, B. (1980). Implementing the Johnson model for nursing practice. In J.P. Riehl, & C. Roy (Eds.), *Conceptual models for nursing practice* (2d ed.). New York: Appleton-Century-Crofts.
7. Johnson, D.E. (1954). Collegiate nursing education. *Coll. Publ. Rel. Quarterly, 5:*32-35.
8. Johnson, D.E. (1959, April). A philosophy of nursing. *Nursing Outlook, 7:*198-200.
9. Johnson, D.E. (1959, May). The nature of a science of nursing. *Nursing Outlook, 7:*291-294.
10. Johnson, D.E. (1961, Jan.). Nursing's specific goal in patient care. Faculty Colloquium, School of Nursing, University of California, Los Angeles (unpublished lecture).
11. Johnson, D.E. (1961, June). A conceptual basis for nursing care. Third Conference, C.E. Program, University of California, Los Angeles. (Unpublished lecture).
12. Johnson, D.E. (1961, Nov.). The significance of nursing care. *American Journal of Nursing, 61:*63-66.
13. Johnson, D.E. (1964, Dec.). Nursing and higher education. *International Journal of Nursing Studies, 1:*219-225.
14. Johnson, D.E. (1965, April). Is nursing meeting the challenge of family needs? Wisconsin League for Nursing. Madison, Wisconsin (Unpublished lecture).
15. Johnson, D.E. (1968, April). One conceptual model of nursing. Vanderbilt University, Nashville, Tennessee (Unpublished lecture).
16. Johnson, D.E. (1968, May-June). Theory in

nursing: Borrowed and unique. *Nursing Research, 17:*206-209.
17. Johnson, D.E. (1974, Sept.-Oct.). Development of theory: A requisite for nursing as a primary health profession. *Nursing Research, 23:*372-377.
18. Johnson, D.E. (1978). State of the art of theory development in nursing. In *Theory development: What, why, how?* New York: National League for Nursing. NLN publication 15-1708.
19. Johnson, D.E. (1980). The behavioral system model for nursing. In J.P. Riehl & C. Roy (Eds.), *Conceptual models for nursing practice* (2d ed.). New York: Appleton-Century-Crofts.
20. Johnson, D.E. (1984). Personal correspondence.
21. Johnson, D.E. (1984). Curriculum vitae.
22. Johnson, D.E. (1988). Personal correspondence.
23. Lorenz, K. (1966). *On aggression.* New York: Harcourt.
24. Loveland-Cherry, C., & Wilkerson, S. (1983). Dorothy Johnson's behavioral systems model. In J. Fitzpatrick & A. Whall (Eds.), *Conceptual models of nursing: Analysis and application.* Bowie, Md.: Robert J. Brady.
25. Majesky, S.J., Brester, M.H., & Nishio, K.T. (1978). Development of a research tool: Patient indicators of nursing care. *Nursing Research, 27(6):*365-371.
26. Rawls, A. (1980). Evaluation of the Johnson behavioral model in clinical practice: Report of a test and evaluation of the Johnson theory. *Image, 12:*13-16.
27. Rapoport, A. (1968, Feb.). *Foreword to modern systems research for the behavioral scientist.* Chicago: Aldine.
28. Small, B. (1980). Nursing visually impaired children with Johnson's model as a conceptual framework. In J.P. Riehl and C. Roy (Eds.), *Conceptual models for nursing practice* (2d ed.). New York: Appleton-Century-Crofts.
29. Stamler, C. (1971). Dependency and repetitive visits to nurses' office in elementary school children. *Nursing Research, 20(3):*254-255.

BIBLIOGRAPHY
Primary Sources
Book Chapters

Johnson, D.E. (1964, June 19-26). Is there an identifiable body of knowledge essential to the development of a generic professional nursing program? In M. Maker (Ed.), *Proceedings of the first inter-university faculty work conference.* Stowe, Vt.: New England Board of Higher Education.

Johnson, D.E. (1973). Medical-surgical nursing: Cardiovascular care in the first person. In ANA Clinical Sessions: New York: Appleton-Century-Crofts, pp. 127-134.

Johnson, D.E. (1976). Foreword. In J.R. Auger, *Behavioral systems and nursing.* Englewood Cliffs, N.J.: Prentice-Hall.

Johnson, D.E. (1980). The behavioral system model for nursing. In J.P. Riehl & C. Roy (Eds.), *Conceptual models for nursing practice* (2d ed.). New York: Appleton-Century-Crofts.

Johnson, D.E., et al. (1978). State of the art of theory development in nursing. In *Theory development: What, why, how?* New York, National League for Nursing. NLN publication 15-1708.

Articles

Johnson, D.E. (1943, March). Learning to know people. *American Journal of Nursing, 43:*248-252.

Johnson, D.E. (1954). Collegiate nursing education. *Coll. Publ. Rel. Quarterly, 5:*32-35.

Johnson, D.E. (1959, April). A philosophy of nursing. *Nursing Outlook, 7:*198-200.

Johnson, D.E. (1959, May). The nature of a science of nursing. *Nursing Outlook, 7:*291-294.

Johnson, D.E. (1961, Oct.). Patterns in professional nursing education. *Nursing Outlook, 9:*608-611.

Johnson, D.E. (1961, Nov.). The significance of nursing care. *American Journal of Nursing, 61:*63-66.

Johnson, D.E. (1962, July-Aug.). Professional education for pediatric nursing. *Children, 9:*153-156.

Johnson, D.E. (1964, Dec.). Nursing and higher education. *International Journal of Nursing Studies, 1:*219-225.

Johnson, D.E. (1965, Sept.). Today's action will determine tomorrow's nursing. *Nursing Outlook, 13:*38-41.

Johnson, D.E. (1965, Oct.). Crying in the newborn infant. *Nursing Science, 3:*339-355.

Johnson, D.E. (1966, Jan. 16). Year round programs set the pace in health careers promotion. *Hospitals, 40:*57-60.

Johnson, D.E. (1966, Oct.). Competence in practice: Technical and professional. *Nursing Outlook, 14:*30-33.

Johnson, D.E. (1967, April). Powerlessness: A sig-

nificant determinant in patient behavior? *Journal of Nursing Educators, 6:*39-44.
Johnson, D.E. (1967). Professional practice in nursing. *NLN Convention Papers, 23:*26-33.
Johnson, D.E. (1968, April). Toward a science in nursing. *So. Medical Bulletin, 56:*13-23.
Johnson, D.E. (1968, May-June). Theory in nursing: Borrowed and unique. *Nursing Research, 17:*206-209.
Johnson, D.E. (1968). Critique: Social influences on student nurses in their choice of ideal and practiced solutions to nursing problems. *Communicating Nursing Research, 1:*150-155.
Johnson, D.E. (1974, Sept. & Oct.). Development of theory: A requisite for nursing as a primary health profession. *Nursing Research, 23:* 372-377.
Johnson, D.E., Wilcox, J.A., & Moidel, H.C. (1967, Nov.). The clinical specialist as a practitioner. *American Journal of Nursing, 67:*2298-2303.
Johnson, D.E., & McCaffery, M. (1967, Fall). Effect of parent group discussion upon epistemic responses. *Nursing Research, 16:*352-358.

Audiotape

Johnson, D.E. (1978, Dec.). Paper presented at the Second Annual Nurse Educator Conference, New York. Audiotape available from Teach 'em Inc., 160 E. Illinois Street, Chicago, Ill. 60611.

Videotape

The Nurse Theorists: Portraits of Excellence: Dorothy Johnson. 1988, Oakland, California: Studio III. Videotape available from Fuld Video Project, 370 Hawthorne Avenue, Oakland, Cal. 94609.

Unpublished Lectures

Johnson, D.E. (1961). Nursing's specific goal in patient care. Presentation given at a Faculty Colloquium, University of California, Los Angeles.
Johnson, D.E. (1961). A conceptual basis for nursing care. Presentation given at the Third Conference, C.E. Program, at the University of California, Los Angeles.
Johnson, D.E. (1965). Is nursing meeting the challenge of family needs? Presentation given to the Wisconsin League for Nursing at Madison, Wisconsin.
Johnson, D.E. (1968). One conceptual model of nursing. Lecture given at Vanderbilt University.

Correspondence

Johnson, D.E. (1984, Feb.). Curriculum vitae.
Johnson, D.E. (1984, Feb.). Personal correspondence.
Johnson, D.E. (1988, Mar.). Personal correspondence.

Secondary Sources

Books

Auger, J.R. (1976). *Behavioral systems and nursing.* Englewood Cliffs, N.J.: Prentice-Hall.
Chinn, P.L. (1983). *Advances in nursing theory development.* Rockville, Md.: Aspen Systems.
Chinn, P.L., & Jacobs, M.K. (1987). *Theory and nursing: A systematic approach.* St. Louis: C.V. Mosby.
Feshbach, S. (1970). Aggression. In P. Mussen (Ed.), *Carmichael's manual of child psychology* (3d ed.). New York: John Wiley & Sons.
Fitzpatrick, J.J., & Whall, A.L. (1983). *Conceptual models of nursing: Analysis and application.* Bowie, Md.: Robert J. Brady.
Fitzpatrick, J.J., et al. (1982). *Nursing models and their psychiatric mental health applications.* Bowie, Md.: Robert J. Brady.
Infante, M.S. (1982). *Crisis theory: A framework for nursing practice.* Reston, Va.: Reston Publishing.
Kim, H.S. (1983). *The nature of theoretical thinking in nursing.* Norwalk, Conn.: Appleton-Century-Crofts.
Riehl, J.P., & Roy, C. (1980). *Conceptual models for nursing practice.* New York: Appleton-Century-Crofts.
Walker, L.O., & Avant, K.C. (1983). *Strategies for theory construction in nursing.* Norwalk, Conn.: Appleton-Century-Crofts.

Dissertation

Lovejoy, N.C. (1981). *An empirical verification of the Johnson behavioral system model for nursing.* Doctoral dissertation. University of Alabama in Birmingham.

Book Chapters

Damus, K. (1974). An application of the Johnson behavioral system model for nursing practice. In J.P. Riehl & C. Roy (Eds.), *Conceptual models for nursing practice.* New York: Appleton-Century-Crofts, pp. 218-233.

Damus, K. (1980). An application of the Johnson behavioral system model for nursing practice. In J.P. Riehl & C. Roy (Eds.), *Conceptual models for nursing practice* (2d ed.). New York: Appleton-Century-Crofts, pp. 274-289.

Fawcett, J. (1984). Johnson's behavioral systems model. In J. Fawcett, *Analysis and evaluation of conceptual models of nursing*. Philadelphia: F.A. Davis, pp. 53-84.

Glennin, C.G. (1980). Formulation of standards of nursing practice using a nursing model. In J.P. Riehl & C. Roy (Eds.), *Conceptual models for nursing practice* (2d ed.). New York: Appleton-Century-Crofts, pp. 290-301.

Grubbs, J. (1974). An interpretation of the Johnson behavioral systems model for nursing practice. In J.P. Riehl & C. Roy (Eds.), *Conceptual models for nursing practice*. New York: Appleton-Century-Crofts, pp. 160-194.

Grubbs, J. (1980). An interpretation of the Johnson behavioral system model for nursing practice. In J.P. Riehl & C. Roy (Eds.), *Conceptual models for nursing practice* (2d ed.). New York: Appleton-Century-Crofts, pp. 217-249.

Holaday, B. (1974). Implementing the Johnson model for nursing practice. In J.P. Riehl & C. Roy (Eds.), *Conceptual models for nursing practice* (2d ed.). New York: Appleton-Century-Crofts, pp. 197-206.

Holaday, B. (1980). Implementing the Johnson model for nursing practice. In J.P. Riehl & C. Roy (Eds.), *Conceptual models for nursing practice* (2d ed.). New York: Appleton-Century-Crofts, pp. 255-263.

Loveland-Cherry, C., & Wilkerson, S.A. (1983). Dorothy Johnson's behavioral systems model. In J.P. Fitzpatrick & A.L. Whall (Eds.), *Conceptual models of nursing: Analysis and application*. Bowie, Md.: Robert J. Brady, pp. 117-135.

Meleis, A.I. (1985). Dorothy Johnson. In A.I. Meleis, *Theoretical nursing: Development and progress*. Philadelphia: J.B. Lippincott, pp. 195-205.

Riehl, J.P., & Roy, C. (1980). Appendix. Nursing assessment tool using Johnson model. In J.P. Riehl & C. Roy (Eds.), *Conceptual models for nursing practice* (2d ed.). New York: Appleton-Century-Crofts, pp. 250-254.

Skolny, M.S., & Riehl, J.P. (1974). Hope: Solving patient and family problems by using a theoretical framework. In J.P. Riehl & C. Roy (Eds.), *Conceptual models for nursing practice*. New York: Appleton-Century-Crofts, pp. 206-218.

Small, B. (1980). Nursing visually impaired children with Johnson's model as a conceptual framework. In J.P. Riehl & C. Roy (Eds.), *Conceptual models for nursing practice* (2d ed.). New York: Appleton-Century-Crofts, pp. 264-273.

Steven, B.J. (1979). Criteria for evaluating theories. In B.J. Stevens, *Nursing theory: Analysis, application, evaluation*. Boston: Little, Brown, pp. 49-67.

Directional and Biographical Sources

Henderson, J. (1957-1959). *Nursing studies index* (Vol. IV). Philadelphia: J.B. Lippincott.

Articles

Abdellah, F.G. (1969). Dept. HEW-Health administration center of health services research and development health services. *Nursing Research, 18(5)*:390-393.

Adam, E. (1983). Frontiers of nursing in the 21st century: Development of models and theories on the concept of nursing. *Journal of Advanced Nursing, 8*:41-45.

Ainsworth, M. (1964). Patterns of attachment behavior shown by the infant in interaction with mother. *Merrill Palmer Quarterly, 10(1)*:51-58.

Arndt, C. (1970). Role sharing in diversified role set director of nursing service. *Nursing Research, 19(3)*:253-259.

Bates, B. (1970). Doctor and nurse, changing nurse, and relations. *New England Journal of Medicine, 283*:129-130.

Brandt, E.M. (1967). Comparison of on job performance of graduates with school of nursing objectives. *Nursing Research, 16(1)*:50-60.

Brester, M.H., Majesky, S.J., & Nishio, K.T. (1978, Nov.-Dec.). Development of a research tool: Patient indicators of nursing care. *Nursing Research, 27*:365-371.

Broncatello, K.F. (1980). Anger in action: Application of the model. *Advances in Nursing Science, 2(2)*:13-24.

Bullough, B. (1976). Influences on role expansion. *American Journal of Nursing, 76*(9):1476-1481.

Chance, K.S. (1982). Nursing models: A requisite for professional accountability. *Advances in Nursing Science, 4(2)*:57-65.

Conway, B. (1971). Effects of hospitalization on adolescence. *Adolescence, 6(21)*:77-92.

Crawford, G. (1982). The concept of pattern in nursing conceptual development and measurement. *Advances in Nursing Science, 5(1):*1-6.

Craig, S.L. (1980). Theory development and its relevance for nursing. *Journal of Advanced Nursing, 5(4):*349-355.

Darnell, R.E. (1973). Promotion of interest in role of physician association as a potential career opportunity for nurses alternative strategy. *Social Science and Medicine, 7(7):*495.

Dee, U., & Auger, J.A. (1983, May). A patient classification system based on behavioral system model of nursing. Part 2. *Journal of Nursing Administration, 13:*18-23.

Derdiarian, A.K. (1983, July-Aug.). An instrument for theory and research development using the behavioral systems model for nursing: The cancer patient. Part I. *Nursing Research, 32:*196-201.

Derdiarian, A.K., & Forsythe, A.B. (1983, Sept.-Oct.). An instrument for theory and research development using the behavioral systems model for nursing: The cancer patient. Part II. *Nursing Research, 32:*260-266.

Evans, R.T. (1969). Exploration of factors involved in maternal adaption to breastfeeding. *Nursing Research, 18(1):*28-33.

Flint, R.T. (1969). Recent issues in nursing manpower review. *Nursing Research, 18(3):*217-222.

Fritz, E. (1966). Baccalaureate nursing education: What is its job? *American Journal of Nursing, 66(6):*1312-1316.

Georgopo, B.S. (1970). Nursing kardex behavior in an experimental study of patient units with and without clinical nurse specialists. *Nursing Research, 19(3):*196-218.

Godley, S.T. (1976). Community based orientation and mobility programs. *Nursing Outlook, 70(10):*429-432.

Gortner, S.R. (1977). Overview of nursing research in United States. *Nursing Research, 26*(1):16-23.

Gray, S.E. (1977). Do graduates of technical and professional nursing programs differ in practice? *Nursing Research, 26(5):*368-373.

Greaves, F. (1980). Objectively toward curriculum improvement in nursing education in England and Wales. *Journal of Advanced Nursing, 5:*591-599.

Hadley B.J. (1969). Evolution of a conception of nursing. *Nursing Research, 18(5):*400-405.

Hall, B.P. (1981). The change paradigm in nursing: Growth versus persistence. *Advances in Nursing Science, 3(4):*1-6.

Hogstel, M.O. (1977). Associate degree and baccalaureate graduates: Do they function differently. *American Journal of Nursing, 77(10):*1598-1600.

Holaday, B. (1974). Achievement behavior in chronically ill children. *Nursing Research, 23:*25-30.

Holaday, B. (1981). Maternal response to their chronically ill infants' attachment behavior of crying. *Nursing Research, 30:*343-348.

Holaday, B. (1982). Maternal conceptual set development: Identifying patterns of maternal response to chronically ill infant crying. *Maternal-Child Nursing Journal, 11(1):*47-58.

Iveson-Iveson, J. (1982). Standards of behavior . . . theories of nursing practice . . . the Johnson model. *Nursing Mirror, 155(20):*38.

Ketefian, S. (1981). Critical thinking: Educational preparation and development of moral judgment among selected groups of practicing nurses. *Nursing Research, 30(2):*98-103.

Kohnk, M.F. (1973). Do nursing educators practice what is preached? *American Journal of Nursing, 73(9):*1571.

Lovejoy, N. (1983). The leukemic child's perceptions of family behaviors. *Oncology Nursing Forum, 10(4):*20-25.

Majesky, S.J. (1978). Development of a research tool: Patient indicators of nursing care. *Nursing Research, 27(6):*365-371.

Mauksch, I.G. (1972). Prescription for survival. *American Journal of Nursing, 72*(12):2189-2193.

McCain, R.F. (1965, April). Systematic investigation of medical-surgical nursing content. *Journal of Nursing Education, 4:*23-31.

McFarlane, E.A. (1980). Nursing theory: Comparison of four theoretical proposals. *Journal of Advanced Nursing, 5:*3-19.

McQuaid, E.A. (1979). How do graduates of different types of programs perform on state boards? *American Journal of Nursing, 79(2):*305-308.

Rawls, A.C. (1980, Feb.). Evaluation of the Johnson behavioral model in clinical practice. *Image, 12*: 13-16.

Rickelma, B.L. (1971). Bio-psych-social linguistics conceptual approach to nurse-patient interaction. *Nursing Research, 20(5):*398-403.

Rogers, C.G. (1973). Conceptual models as guides

to clinical nursing specialization. *Journal of Nursing Education, 12(4)*:2-6.

Rogers, J.C. (1982, Jan.). Order and disorder in medicine and occupational therapy. *American Journal of Occupational Therapy, 36*:29-35.

Scher, M.E. (1975). Stereotyping and role conflicts between medical students and psychiatric nurses. *Hospital and Community Psychiatry, 26(4)*: 219-221.

Secrest, H.P. (1968). Nurses and collaborative peritonatal research project. *Nursing Research, 17*:292.

Smith, M.C. (1974). Perceptions of head nurses, clinical nurse specialists, nursing educators and nursing office personnel re: performance of selected nursing activities. *Nursing Research, 23(6)*:505-510.

Smith, M.C. (1976). Patient responses to being transferred during hospitalization. *Nursing Research, 25(3)*:192-196.

Smithern, C. (1969). Vocal behavior of infants as related to nursing procedures of rocking. *Nursing Research, 18(3)*:256-258.

Stamler, C. (1971). Dependency and repetitive visits to nurses' offices in elementary school children. *Nursing Research, 20(3)*:254-255.

Stevens, B.J. (1971). Analysis of structural forms used in nursing curricula. *Nursing Research, 20(5)*:388-397.

Taylor, S.D. (1975). Bibliography on nursing research 1950-1975. *Nursing Research, 24(3)*: 207-225.

Vaillot, M.C. (1970). Hope; restoration of being. *American Journal of Nursing, 10(2)*:268.

Waltz, C.F. (1978). Faculty influence on nursing students' preference in practice. *Nursing Research, 27(2)*:89-97.

Waters, V.H. (1972). Nursing practice: Implemental and supplemental. *Nursing Research, 21(2)*: 124-131.

White, M.B. (1972). Importance of selected nursing activities. *Nursing Research, 21(1)*:4-14.

Zbilut, J.P. (1978). Epistemologic constraints to development of a theory of nursing. *Nursing Research, 27(2)*:128-129.

Other Sources

Ainsworth, M. (1964). Patterns of attachment behavior shown by the infant in interaction with mother. *Merrill-Palmer Quarterly, 10(1)*:51-58.

Ainsworth, M. (1972). Attachment and dependency: A comparison. In J. Gewirtz (Ed.), *Attachment and dependency*. Englewood Cliffs, N.J.: Prentice-Hall.

Atkinson, J.W. (1966). *Feather NT: A theory of achievement maturation*. New York: John Wiley & Sons.

Buckley, W. (Ed). (1968). *Modern systems research for the behavioral scientist*. Chicago: Aldine.

Chin, R. (1961). The utility of system models and developmental models for practitioners. In K. Benne, W. Bennis, & R. Chin (Eds.), *The planning of change*. New York: Holt, Rinehart, & Winston.

Crandal, V. (1963). Achievement. In H.W. Stevenson (Ed.), *Child psychology*. Chicago: University of Chicago Press.

Feshbach, S. (1970). Aggression. In P. Mussen (Ed.), *Carmichael's manual of child psychology* (3d ed., Vol. 2). New York: John Wiley & Sons.

Gerwitz, J. (Ed.). (1972). *Attachment and dependency*, Englewood Cliffs, N.J.: Prentice-Hall.

Grinker, R.R. (Ed.). (1956). *Toward a unified theory of human behavior*. New York: Basic Books.

Heathers, G. (1955). Acquiring dependence and independence: A theoretical orientation. *Journal of General Psychology, 87*:277-291.

Kagan, J. (1964). Acquisition and significance of sex typing and sex role identity. In Hoffman M.L. & Hoffman L.W., (Eds.), *Review of child development research*. New York: Russell Sage Foundation.

Leitch, M., & Escalona, E. (1949). The reaction of infants to stress. In *Psychoanalytic study of the child* (Vols. 3-4). New York: International Universities Press.

Lorenz, K. (1966). *On aggression*. New York: Harcourt.

Mead, M. (1953). *Cultural patterns and technical change*. World Federation for Mental Health, UNESCO.

Rapoport, A. (1968). Foreword. In W. Buckley (Ed.), *Modern systems research for the behavioral scientist*. Chicago: Aldine.

Resnik, H.L.P. (1972). *Sexual behaviors*. Boston: Little, Brown.

Robson, K.S. (1967). Patterns and determinants of maternal attachment. *Journal of Pediatrics 77*: 976-985.

Rosenthal, M. (1967). The generalization of dependency from mother to a stranger. *Journal of Child Psychology and Psychiatry, 8:*177-183.

Sears, R., Maccoby, E., & Levin, H. (1954). *Patterns of child rearing.* White Plains, N.Y.: Row, Peterson.

Selye, H. (1956). *The stress of life.* New York: McGraw-Hill.

Simmons, L.W., & Wolff, H.G. (1954). *Social science in medicine.* New York: Russell Sage Foundation.

Walike, B., Jordan, H.A., & Stellar, E. (1969). Studies of eating behavior. *Nursing Research, 18:* 108-113.

26

Sister Callista Roy

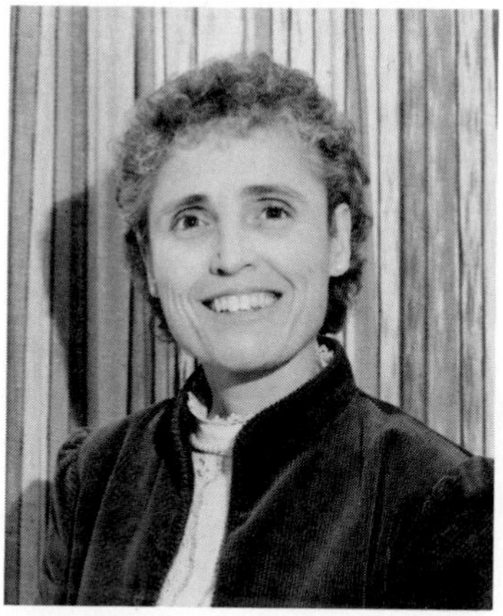

Adaptation Model

Carolyn L. Blue, Karen M. Brubaker, Julia M. Fine, Martha J. Kirsch, Katherine R. Papazian, Cynthia M. Riester

CREDENTIALS AND BACKGROUND OF THE THEORIST

Sister Callista Roy, a member of the Sisters of Saint Joseph of Carondelet, was born October 14, 1939, in Los Angeles, California. She received a Bachelor of Arts in Nursing in 1963 from Mount Saint Mary's College in Los Angeles and a Master of Science in Nursing from the University of California at Los Angeles in 1966. After earning her nursing degrees, Roy began her education in sociology, receiving both an M.A. in Sociology in 1973 and a Ph.D. in Sociology in 1977 from the University of California.

While working toward her master's degree, Roy was challenged in a seminar with Dorothy E. Johnson to develop a conceptual model for nursing. Roy had worked as a pediatric staff nurse and had noticed the great resiliency of children and their ability to adapt in response to major physical and psychological changes. Roy was impressed by adaptation as an appropriate conceptual framework for nursing. The

The authors wish to express their appreciation to Sister Callista Roy for critiquing the chapter.

basic concepts of the model were developed while Roy was a graduate student at UCLA from 1964 to 1966.

Roy began operationalizing her model in 1968 when Mount Saint Mary's College adopted the adaptation framework as the philosophical foundation of the nursing curriculum. Roy was an associate professor and chairperson of the Department of Nursing at Mount Saint Mary's College until 1982. From 1983 to 1985, she was a Robert Wood Johnson Post Doctoral Fellow at the University of California in San Francisco as a clinical nurse scholar in neuroscience. During this time she conducted research on nursing interventions for cognitive recovery in head injuries and on the influence of nursing models on clinical decision making. In 1988 Roy began the newly created position of graduate faculty nurse theorist at Boston College School of Nursing.[42]

Roy has published many books, chapters, and periodical articles and has presented numerous lectures and workshops focusing on her nursing adaptation theory. She is a member of Sigma Theta Tau, having received the National Founder's Award for Excellence in Fostering Professional Nursing Standards in 1981. Her achievements include a 1984 Honorary Doctorate of Humane Letters by Alverno College, a 1985 Honorary Doctorate from Eastern Michigan University, and a 1986 A.J.N. Book of the Year Award for *Essentials of the Roy Adaptation Model.* Roy has been recognized in the *World Who's Who of Women, Personalities of America,* and as a Fellow of the American Academy of Nursing.

THEORETICAL SOURCES

Roy's Adaptation Model for Nursing was derived in 1964 from Harry Helson's work in psychophysics. In Helson's Adaptation Theory, adaptive responses are a function of the incoming stimulus and the adaptive level. The adaptation level is made up of the pooled effect of three classes of stimuli: (1) focal stimuli, which immediately confront the individual; (2) contextual stimuli, which are all other stimuli present; and (3) residual stimuli, those factors that are relevant but that cannot be validated. Helson's work developed the concept of the adaptation level zone, which determines whether a stimuli will elicit a positive or negative response. According to Helson's theory, adaptation is a process of responding positively to environmental changes.[34]

Roy[34] combines Helson's work with Rapoport's definition of *system* and views the person as an adaptive system. With Helson's Adaptation Theory as a foundation, Roy[34] developed and further refined the model using concepts and theory from B.P. Dohrenwend, R.S. Lazarus, N. Malaznik, D. Mechanic, and H. Selye. Roy gave special credit to coauthors Driever, for outlining subdivisions of self-integrity, and Martinez and Sato, for identifying both common and primary stimuli affecting the modes. Other coworkers also elaborated the concepts: M. Pousch and J. Van Landingham for the interdependence mode and B. Randall for the role function mode.

In the years following the development of her theory, Roy developed the model as a framework for nursing practice, research, and education.[41] According to Roy,[21] more than 1500 faculty and students have contributed to the theoretical development of the Adaptation Model.

In *Introduction to Nursing: An Adaptation Model,* Roy discussed self-concept. She and her collaborators used the work of A. Coombs and D. Snygg regarding self-consistency and major influencing factors of self-concept. Social interaction theories provided a theoretical basis. Cooley indicates in Epstein's publication that self-perception is influenced by one's perceptions of other's responses. Mead expanded the idea by hypothesizing that self-appraisal uses the "generalized other." Sullivan suggests that self arises from social interaction. Gardner and Erickson provide developmental approaches.[30:263-265] The other modes—physiological, role functioning, and interdependence—were drawn similarly from biological and behavioral sciences for an understanding of the person.

Roy is developing the humanism value base of her model. The model uses concepts from A.H. Maslow to explore beliefs and values of persons. According to Roy, humanism in nursing is the belief in the person's own creative power or the belief that the person's own coping abilities will enhance wellness. Roy's holistic approach[30] to nursing is grounded in humanism.

USE OF EMPIRICAL EVIDENCE

The use of Roy's Adaptation Model in nursing practice led to further clarification and refinement. A 1971 pilot research study and a survey research study from 1976 to 1977 led to some tentative confirmations of the model.[28]

From this beginning, the adaptation model has been supported through research in practice and in education.* B. Rambo[16] and B. Randell[17] have expanded Roy's model for nursing implementation. According to Roy[30] there is increasing testing through research related to the model.

Tiedeman[39] assesses Roy's assumptions for soundness by classifying them into three levels according to their foundation in: (1) previous research, (2) accepted theory, particularly theory with empirical substantiating data, or (3) personal experience. The first level is the strongest base; the third, the weakest. Roy's assumptions from systems theory and from stress-adaptation theories can be classified into the second level. However, Roy's assumption, which conceptualizes the person as having four modes of adaptation—physiological needs, self-concept, role function, and interdependence relations—is based on experience of Roy and others.[39] Roy[20,26,28] admits the assumption needs empirical data for support. In a 1983 address, she noted that these categories have been refined and established as useful and valid for nursing assessment.

*References 2, 7, 13, 14, 33, 40.

MAJOR CONCEPTS AND DEFINITIONS

SYSTEM. A system is "a set of units so related or connected as to form a unity or whole and characterized by inputs, outputs, and control and feedback processes."[30:27]

ADAPTATION LEVEL. A person's adaptation level is "a constantly changing point, made up of focal, contextual, and residual stimuli, which represent the person's own standard of the range of stimuli to which one can respond with ordinary adaptive responses."[30:27-28]

ADAPTATION PROBLEMS. Adaptation problems are "the occurrences of situations of inadequate response to need deficits or excesses."[25:4] In the second edition of *Introduction to Nursing,* Roy goes on to say "It can be noted at this point that the distinction being made between adaptation problems and nursing diagnosis is based on the developing work in both of these fields. At this point, adaptation problems are seen not as nursing diagnosis, but as areas of concern for the nurse related to adapting person or group (within each adaptive mode)."[30:89-90]

FOCAL STIMULUS. A focal stimulus is "the degree of change or stimulus most immediately confronting the person and the one to which the person must make an adaptive response, that is, the factor that precipitates the behavior."[30:43]

CONTEXTUAL STIMULI. Contextual stimuli are "all other stimuli present that contribute to the behavior caused or precipitated by the focal stimuli."[30:43]

RESIDUAL STIMULI. Residual stimuli are "factors that may be affecting behavior but whose effects are not validated."[30:43]

REGULATOR. A regulator is a "subsystem coping mechanism which responds automatically through neural-chemical-endocrine processes."[30:28]

COGNATOR. A cognator is a "subsystem coping mechanism which responds through complex processes of perception and information processing, learning, judgment, and emotion."[30:28]

ADAPTIVE (EFFECTOR) MODES. Adaptive, or effector, modes are a "classification of ways of coping that manifest regulator and cognator activity, that is, physiologic, self-concept, role function, and interdependence."[30:28]

ADAPTIVE RESPONSES. Adaptive responses are "responses that promote integrity of the person in terms of the goals of survival, growth, reproduction, and mastery."[30:28]

INEFFECTIVE RESPONSES. Ineffective responses are "responses that do not contribute to adaptive goals, that is, survival, growth, reproduction, and mastery."[30:28]

PHYSIOLOGICAL MODE. "Physiological needs involve the body's basic needs and ways of dealing with adaptation in regard to fluid and electrolytes; exercise and rest; elimination; nutrition; circulation and oxygen; and regulation, which includes the senses, temperature, and endocrine regulation."[34:43]

SELF-CONCEPT MODE. "Self-concept is the composite of beliefs and feelings that one holds about oneself at a given time. It is formed from perceptions, particularly of other's reactions, and directs one's behavior. Its components include: (1) the physical self, which involves sensation and body image; and (2) the personal self, which is made up of self-consistency, self-ideal or expectancy, and the moral, ethical self (Driever, 1976)."[34:43-44]

ROLE PERFORMANCE MODE. "Role function is the performance of duties based on given positions in society. The way one performs a role is dependent on one's interaction with the other in the given situation. The major roles that one plays can be analyzed by imagining a tree formation. The trunk of the tree is one's primary role, that is, one's developmental level—for example, generative adult female. Secondary roles branch off from this—for example, wife, mother, and teacher. Finally, tertiary roles branch off from secondary roles—for example, the mother role might involve the role of P.T.A. president for a given period of time (Malaznik, 1976). Each of these roles is seen as occurring in a dyadic relationship, that is, with a reciprocal role."[34:44]

INTERDEPENDENCE MODE. "The interdependence mode involves one's relations with significant others and support systems. In this mode one maintains psychic integrity by meeting needs for nurturance and affection (Poush and Van Landingham, 1977)."[34:44]

MAJOR ASSUMPTIONS

Roy has discussed her scientific and philosophical assumptions at the International Nursing Theory Conferences in Edmonton, Alberta, May 2-3, 1984, and at other conferences. She outlines scientific assumptions from systems theory and Helson's Adaptation Level Theory and philosophical assumptions from humanistic values.

Assumptions from Systems Theory:

1. A system is a set of units so related or connected as to form a unity or whole.
2. A system is a whole that functions as a whole by virtue of the interdependence of its parts.

3. Systems have inputs, outputs, and control and feedback processes.
4. Input, in the form of a standard or feedback, often is referred to as *information*.
5. Living systems are more complex than mechanical systems and have standards and feedback to direct their functioning as a whole.

Assumptions from Helson's Theory:

1. Human behavior represents adaptation to environmental and organismic forces.
2. Adaptive behavior is a function of the stimulus and adaptation level, that is, the pooled effect of the focal, contextual, and residual stimuli.
3. Adaptation is a process of responding positively to environmental changes. This positive response decreases the response necessary to cope with the stimuli and increases sensitivity to respond to other stimuli.
4. Responses reflect the state of the organism as well as the properties of stimuli and hence are regarded as active processes.

Assumptions from Humanism:

1. Persons have their own creative power.
2. A person's behavior is purposeful and not merely a chain of cause and effect.
3. Person is holistic.
4. A person's opinions and viewpoints are of value.
5. The interpersonal relationship is significant.

Nursing

Nursing is defined broadly as a "theoretical system of knowledge which prescribes a process of analysis and action related to the care of the ill or potentially ill person."[25:4] Roy[30:3-4] differentiates nursing as a science from nursing as a practice discipline. Nursing science is "a developing system of knowledge about persons that observes, classifies, and relates the processes by which persons positively affect their health status."[30:3-4] Nursing as a practice discipline is "nursing's scientific body of knowledge used for the purpose of providing an essential service to people, that is, promoting ability to affect health positively."[30:3-4]

Roy's goal[1,30] of nursing is to help man adapt to changes in his physiological needs, his self-concept, his role function, and his interdependence relations during health and illness. Nursing fills a unique role as a facilitator of adaptation by assessing behavior in each of these four adaptive modes and intervening by managing the influencing stimuli.[1,30]

Person

According to Roy,[25:7] a person is a "biopsychosocial being in constant interaction with a changing environment." Roy[1,30,32] defined the person, the recipient of nursing care, as a living, complex, adaptive system with internal processes (the cognator and regulator) acting to maintain adaptation in the four adaptive modes (physiological needs, self-concept, role function, and interdependence). The person as a living system is "a whole made up of parts or subsystems that function as a unity for some purpose."[32:53]

Health

Health is "a state and a process of being and becoming an integrated and whole person. Lack of integration represents lack of health."[1:50] Roy[30:24] derived this definition from the thought that adaptation is a process of promoting physiological, psychological, and social integrity, and that integrity implies an unimpaired condition leading to completeness or unity. In her earlier work, Roy viewed health along a continuum flowing from death and extreme poor health to high-level wellness and peak wellness. As man moves along the health-illness continuum, he will encounter problems to which he must adapt.[2] However, Roy's more recent writings have focused more on health as a process.

Health and illness are one inevitable dimension of the person's total life experience.[19] Nursing is concerned with this dimension. When mechanisms for coping are ineffective, illness results. Health ensues when man continually adapts. As people adapt to stimuli, they are free to respond to other stimuli. The freeing of energy from ineffective coping attempts can promote healing and enhance health.[30:26]

Environment

According to Roy,[30:22] environment is "all the conditions, circumstances, and influences surrounding and affecting the development and behavior of persons or groups." Environment is the input into the person as an adaptive system involving both internal and external factors. These factors may be slight or large, negative or positive. However, any environmental change demands increasing energy to adapt to the situation. Factors in the environment that affect the person are categorized as focal, contextual, and residual stimuli.

THEORETICAL ASSERTIONS

Roy's model focuses on the concept of adaptation of man. Her concepts of nursing, person, health, and environment are all interrelated to this central concept. The person continually scans the environment for stimuli so he can respond and ultimately adapt. Nursing has a unique goal to assist the person in his adaptation effort by managing the environment. The result is attainment of an optimum level of wellness by the person.*

As an open, living system, the person receives inputs or stimuli from both the environment and the self. The adaptation level is determined by the combined effect of the focal, contextual, and residual stimuli. Adaptation occurs when the person responds positively to environmental changes. This adaptive response promotes the integrity of the person, which leads to health. Ineffective responses to stimuli leads to disruption of the integrity of the person.†

There are two interrelated subsystems in Roy's model (Figure 26-1). The primary, functional, or control processes subsystem consists of the regulator and the cognator. The secondary, effector subsystem consists of four adaptive modes: physiological needs, self-concept, role-function, and interdependence.‡

Roy views the regulator and cognator as methods of coping. Perception of the person links the regulator with the cognator in that "input into the regulator is transformed into perceptions. Perception is a process of the cognator. The responses following perception are feedback into both the cognator and the regulator."[9:67]

The four adaptive modes of the second sub-

*References 1, 17, 20, 21, 28, 30, 32, 34.
†References 1, 17, 20, 21, 28, 30, 32
‡References 1, 17, 20, 21, 28, 30, 32.

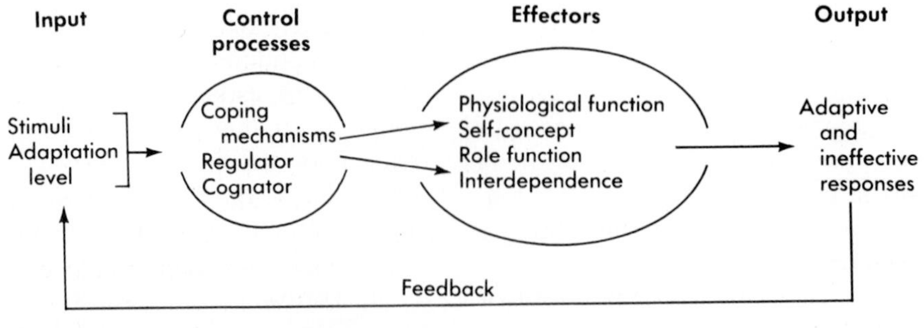

Figure 26-1. Person as an adaptive system.
From Sister Callista Roy (1984), *Introduction to Nursing: An Adaptation Model* (2d ed.), p. 30. Reprinted by permission of Prentice-Hall, Inc., Englewood Cliffs, N.J.

system in Roy's model provide form or manifestations of cognator and regulator activity. Responses to stimuli are carried out through these four modes. The mode's purpose is to achieve physiological, psychological, and social integrity. Interrelated propositions of the cognator and regulator subsystems link the systems of the adaptive modes.[7]

Man as a whole is made up of six subsystems. These subsystems—the regulator, cognator, and the four adaptive modes—are interrelated to form a complex system for the purpose of the adaptation of man. Relationships between the four adaptive modes occur when internal and external stimuli affect more than one mode; when disruptive behavior occurs in more than one mode; or when one mode becomes the focal, contextual, or residual stimulus for another mode.[2,4,13]

LOGICAL FORM

Roy's Adaptation Model for Nursing is both deductive and inductive. It is deductive in that much of Roy's theory is derived from Helson's psychophysics theory. Helson developed the concepts of focal, contextual, and residual stimuli, which Roy redefined within nursing to form a typology of factors related to adaptation levels of persons. Roy also uses other concepts and theory outside the discipline of nursing and relates these to her adaptation theory.

Roy's adaptation theory is inductive in that she developed the four adaptive modes from research and the practice experiences of herself, her colleagues, and her students. Roy[25,28,30] built on the conceptual framework of adaptation and as a result developed a step-by-step model by which nurses use the nursing process to administer nursing care to promote adaptation in situations of health and illness.

ACCEPTANCE BY THE NURSING COMMUNITY

Practice

Using Roy's six-step nursing process, the nurse assesses first the behaviors and second the stimuli affecting those behaviors. In a third step the nurse makes a statement or nursing diagnosis of the person's adaptive state and, fourth, sets goals to promote adaptation. Fifth, nursing interventions are aimed at managing the stimuli to promote adaptation. The last step in the nursing process is evaluation.[1] By manipulating the stimuli and not the patient, the nurse enhances "the interaction of the person with their environment, thereby promoting health."[1:51]

H.T.F. Brower and B.J. Baker[2] consider Roy's model useful for nursing practice because it outlines the features of the discipline and provides direction for practice as well as for education and research. The model considers goals, values, the client, and practitioner interventions. These authors view Roy's nursing process as well developed: the two-level assessment assisted in identification of nursing goals and diagnoses. They also note the need for continued work on a typology of nursing and on organizing categories of nursing interventions.

It is a valuable theory for nursing practice because it includes a goal that is specified as the aim for activity and prescriptions for activities to realize the goal.[5] The goal of the model is the person's adaptation in four adaptive modes in situations of health and illness. The prescriptions or interventions are the management of stimuli by removing, increasing, decreasing, or altering them. These prescriptions can be obtained by listing practice-related hypotheses generated by the model.[1,30]

The nursing process is well suited for use in a practice setting. The two-level assessment is unique to this model and leads to the identification of adaptation problems or nursing diagnosis. Beginning work is being done on a typology of nursing diagnoses.[30,34] Intervention is based specifically on the model, but there is a need to develop an organization of categories of nursing interventions.[34]

The model was used in practice by graduate nursing students as cited by Wagner[40] in 1976. They found some blurring in the categories of self-concept, role function, and interdependence when deciding where a given behavior belonged. They also found the nursing process lengthy and repetitive, taking much time to complete. The model was useful in inpatient settings, except in intensive care units where there were rapid changes in the patient's condition. The students also found it easier to use the model in outpatient settings such as clinics and physician's offices.[40] The model provided a system that accounted for physical needs as well as psychosocial needs. It was particularly useful in the pediatric setting, because it allowed for assessment of covert psychological needs of children.

Galligan[9] in 1979 reported the model had been been used by nurses who cared for young, hospitalized children. Schmitz in 1980 used the model in a community setting for patients receiving care in the home. The model enabled needs assessment, goal setting, and prioritization of goals. Interventions and evaluations were reported to be more efficient and effective.

In May 1979 three nursing administrators initiated a pilot study using the model in an 18-bed unit in Arlington, Virginia. Evaluation and revision of the nursing assessment tools were conducted. By April 1980, the model was in practice. Early research suggests that it enhanced patient satisfaction and improved health outcomes. Consistent with the model, the nurses began to enhance their professionalism by writing complete care plans and phrasing patient problems in terms of nursing diagnosis. A year after initiation, the model was still supported by the staff. The group directors admitted that the model's abstractness required diligence in applying it to practice. They also contended that further validation of the theory was needed.

In September 1981 a research study was published that dealt with problems associated with nursing home applications for elderly persons. The research was done within the framework of the adaptation model. The research design was used to identify adaptation problems, and hypotheses were formulated. The study concluded that, "As a broad conceptual framework, the Roy Adaptation Nursing Model served as a useful tool for systematically gathering responses regarding adaptation problems experienced by the elderly persons and their significant others."[7]

Fitzpatrick and others[8] also found Roy's model useful in the psychological assessment of the family. These authors utilized the model to analyze role function needs and interdependence needs, which may lead to maladaption in a troubled family system. The authors asserted that the nurse, as the environmental change agent, could thus improve a maladaptive family system.

Another research study, published in August 1983, used the model to analyze the content of 20 interviews of parents whose children had been recently diagnosed as having cancer. Although operational definitions of Roy's adaptation modes were used in the study, the origins of the definitions remain unclear. The authors of the study found the framework applicable as a result of its ability to treat multiple patient variables.[38]

In 1986 Logan[12] described the practical use of the model and explored its appropriateness for palliative care nursing and its applicability in improving care of the dying patient. Logan noted that basic assumptions to the Roy Model seemed to correlate with the palliative care philosophy, except that terminology relating to goals differed. A utility index was used to assess the usefulness of the model based on the criteria of: feasibility, practicality, compatibility, social benefit, and completeness. The Roy nursing process is well illustrated by Logan's application of the model with an oncology case study. The nursing care plan is described and includes analysis of diagnosis and behaviors. Logan suggests the need to perfect the model's language in the use of like words when describing like things.

During the 1980s a number of health care agencies have begun implementing the Roy Adaptation Model as a basis for nursing practice. Roy has compiled a list of experienced resource persons who can assist with this work in the United States and Canada (see Appendix A).

Education

The Adaptation Model has also been useful in the educational setting and is currently in use at Mount Saint Mary's College, Department of Nursing.[30] Mount Saint Mary's program demonstrates the relationship of nursing theory to nursing education. Three vertical strands run throughout the curriculum. These include two theory strands (the adapting person and health-illness) and one practice strand (nursing management). There are two horizontal strands in the curriculum—nursing process and student adaptation/leadership. The horizontal strands enhance the theory and practice of the vertical strands. All strands within the curriculum build in complexity from one level to the next.[27] In addition, the model allows for increasing knowledge in both the areas of theory and practice.[22]

Roy[22,27] states that the model defines for students the distinct purpose of nursing, which is to promote man's adaptation in each of the adaptive modes in situations of health and illness. The model also distinguishes nursing science and medical science by having the content of these areas taught in separate courses. She stresses collaboration but delineates separate goals for nurses and physicians. The nurse's goal, according to Roy,[21:167] "is to help the patient put his energy into getting well," while the medical student focuses on "the patient's position on the health-illness continuum with the goal of causing movement along the continuum." She views the model as a valuable tool to analyze overlap and distinctions between the professions of nursing and medicine. Roy[27] believes that curriculum based on this model helps in theory development by the students, who also learn how to test theories and develop new theoretical insights. Roy[21:167] states that the model is advantageous for an integrated curriculum and that "it leads to objectives, points out content to be used, and specifies patterns for learning and teaching."

In 1976 the model was used for curriculum development of a practitioner program at the University of Miami in Florida. Organization of curriculum content and selections of student learning experiences were derived from the model. Course objectives included identifying adaptive problems and distinguishing between effective and noneffective coping mechanisms. Application of the model resulted in decreased anxiety in the students and provided a framework to give direction to the education of practitioners.[2] Carveth[3] proposed the use of conceptual models as one means of improving the scientific knowledge base in nurse-midwifery. This author asserted that the use of Roy's model will assist nurse-midwives to systematically study, communicate, define, and describe their interdependent role.

Throughout the 1970s and 1980s, the Roy model has been implemented as a basis for curriculum development in associate degree, diploma, baccalaureate, and higher degree programs in many countries. Articles and books on Roy's model have been published in several languages, including Portuguese, Japanese, and French. Roy and her colleagues have provided consultation for this work in more than 30 schools in the United States, Canada, and abroad.

Research

If research is to affect practitioners' behavior, it must be directed at testing and retesting conceptual models for nursing practice. Roy[30] has stated that theory development and the testing of developed theories are nursing's highest priorities. The model must be able to generate testable hypotheses for it to be researchable.

As previously stated, Roy's theory has generated a number of general propositions. From these general propositions, specific hypotheses can be developed and tested. B.J. Hill and C.S. Roberts[10] have demonstrated the development of testable hypotheses from the model, as has

Roy. Data to validate or support the model would be created by the testing of such hypotheses, but to date there has been little research in this area.[39]

Roy[20] has identified a set of concepts forming a model from which the process of observation and classification of facts would lead to postulates. The postulates concern the occurrence of adaptation problems, coping mechanisms, and interventions based on laws derived from factors making up the response potential of the focal, contextual, and residual stimuli. Roy[22-24] is in the early stages of outlining a typology of adaptation problems or nursing diagnoses. Research and testing are needed in the areas of typology and categories of interventions that fit into the model. General propositions have been developed that need to be tested.[32]

A group of graduate students at DePaul University tested the model in a number of practice situations. The students adapted an assessment tool and tested the model in episodic settings in a variety of units in different hospitals. They also used distributive settings in physicians' offices, industrial health settings, and outpatient clinics. The students concluded that the model provided a good framework for ordering a variety of observations and was flexible enough to be used in both episodic and distributive settings.[38] The study provided empirical support for the model only in the area of the process of assessment within the four adaptive modes.

Limadri[11] studied the model as a conceptual framework in her descriptive research study and in her practice with abused women in an outpatient setting. She identified patterns of help-seeking behaviors in a group of 40 abused women. From her experiences in practice, Limadri analyzed the model's construct interrelationships and expanded Roy's original model to illustrate a conceptualization of the abused women's adaptive response in help-seeking behaviors. Limadri[11:58] did report difficulty with mode overlap, but found "the model provides a useful framework to identify the complex needs of the client."

Silva[37] in 1987 used the Roy Model to structure the perceived needs of family members of patients undergoing surgery. The four modes were reflected in responses to a questionnaire, but the patterning of relationships was somewhat different than that suggested by the model. Some needs classified in the psychosocial modes were found to be interrelated, whereas other needs, theoretically related to these modes, appeared independent. Silva also found the physiological mode relatively independent of the psychosocial modes. She suggests further refinement of the modes to clarify the interdependent and interrelated areas of each. Roy[31] in her response to this article states that Silva's use of factor analysis in exploring and testing the model contributes to the basic science of adaptation nursing.

Silva[36] points out that using the conceptual framework of a theory for a research study is not in itself a test of the theory. Most of the researchers using Roy's model have not actually tested the assumptions, propositions, or hypotheses of her model, but have provided much face validity for its usefulness.[15]

Some research has been done on the model, but more is needed for further validation. The model does generate many testable hypotheses related to practice and theory.[39]

FURTHER DEVELOPMENT

The Roy Adaptation Model is an approach to nursing that has made and can continue to make a significant contribution to nursing's body of knowledge, but a few needs remain in the development of the theory. Some assumptions about the model should be validated, such as the assumption that the person has four modes of adaptation. A more thoroughly defined typology of nursing diagnosis and an organization of categories of interventions are needed. There is some overlapping of the categories of self-concept, role function, and interdependence. Roy has sought to define health more clearly by deemphasizing the concept of a health-illness continuum and conceptualizing health as integration and wholeness of the person. This more clearly incorporates the adaptive mechanisms of the comatose patient in response to tactile and verbal stimuli.

There appear to be problems involved in using the model in an intensive care unit where situations change rapidly. Roy notes that it is helpful to use a system for setting priorities with the model. When a priority-setting system is used in conjunction with the model, it might be better suited for use in a critical care setting.[26:690] A chapter regarding life closure was added to the 1984 edition of *Introduction to Nursing: An Adaptation Model.* Support and encouragement of adaptation to the dying process is an integral component of nursing.

Of great significance is the use by Roy and Roberts[34] of elements of the model to construct for each subsystem and mode a series of propositions. They acknowledge that the propositions are too simplistic, implying linear bivariate relationships, and state that further work must be done. This work gives starting points for theory-testing research to validate the subsystems of the model. Roy sees a possibility of combining these propositions into interrelated systems and thus building actual theory. Note that Roy classifies her model as a conceptualization of nursing, not as a theory, and calls for more middle range theory development in nursing.[29]

Limadri[11] concluded that Roy and Roberts[34] obscured the regulator mechanism and the physiological mode by superimposing one on the other in forming propositions. She further suggested a rather sweeping modification: grouping the physiologiccal mode into a category of the biological self and grouping the other three modes into the psychosocial self. Fitzpatrick and others[8] reformulated the model to include the alternate nursing intervention strategy of increasing the adaptation range as well as that of manipulating stimuli. Roy's model is useful and contributes to the science and practice of nursing.

EVALUATION OF THE THEORY

Clarity

According to Chinn and Jacobs,[4:140] "clarity requires the semantic and structural organization of goals, assumptions, concepts, definitions, relationships, and structure into a logically coherent whole." Duldt and Giffin[6] state that Roy's arrangement of concepts is logical, but that the development of definitions is inadequate related to her original format. Terms and concepts borrowed from other disciplines are not redefined for nursing. Roy's theory examples tend to use a biopsychosocial set as the principle for organizing, instead of the adaptive modes and the internal processors. One limitation these authors cite is that Roy claims to follow a holistic view, but leaves out "spiritual, humanistic, and existential aspects of being a person." Instead "man is defined as a survival-oriented, behaviorist (condition-response), amoral, living system."[6:246]

Mastel and Hammond[14:75] discussed difficulties with Roy's model in classifying certain behaviors due to overlapping of concept definitions. The problem identified dealt with theory conceptualization and the need for mutually exclusive categories to classify human behavior. Their problem with the person's position on the health-illness continuum has been clarified by Roy in the redefining of health as personal integration. However, other researchers[11:37] have also referred to difficulty in classifying behavior exclusively in one adaptive mode.

A part of the structural inconsistency of the model occurs because a series of assumptions borrowed from behavioristic thought and systems theory are difficult to reconcile with the assumptions of humanism. This combination of such divergent theoretical roots may be a basis for a part of the internal tension of the Roy model, but these assumptions of humanism are what makes the model applicable to nursing.

Simplicity

The Roy model includes the concepts of nursing, person, health-illness, environment, adaptation, and nursing activities. It also includes the subconcepts of regulator, cognator, and the four effector modes of physiological, self-concept, role function, and interdependence. Because this theory has several major concepts and subconcepts and numerous relational statements, it is complex.

Generality

Roy[30] defines her model as drawn from multiple middle range theories and advocates multiple middle range theories for use in nursing. Middle range theories are testable, but have sufficient generality to be scientifically interesting.[41] Roy's model has been classified as a grand theory. The broad scope is an advantage because the model may be used for other theory building and testing in studying smaller ranges of phenomena. Roy's model is generalizable to all settings in nursing practice, but is limited in scope because it primarily addresses the concept of person-environment adaptation and focuses primarily on the client; information on the nurse is implied.

Empirical Precision

Increasing complexity within theories often helps increase empirical precision. When subcomponents are designated within the theory, the empirical precision increases, assuming the broad concepts are based in reality.[4]

Because Roy's broad concepts stem from theory in physiological psychology, psychology, sociology, and nursing, empirical data indicate that this general theory base has substance.

Roy[20,28] studied and analyzed 500 samples of patient behaviors collected by nursing students. From this analysis, Roy proposed her four adaptive modes in man. This is the least supported of Roy's concepts.[39]

Roy's assumptions can also be analyzed to determine what type of statements they are. The eight assumptions of the Adaptation Model of Nursing follow:

1. The person is a biopsychosocial being.
2. The person is in constant interaction with a changing environment.
3. To cope with a changing world, the person uses both innate and acquired mechanisms, which are biological, psychological, and sociological in origin.
4. Health and illness are one inevitable dimension of the person's life.
5. To respond positively to environmental changes, the person must adapt.
6. The person's adaptation is a function of the stimulus he is exposed to and his adaptation level.
7. The person's adaptation level is such that it comprises a zone indicating the range of stimulation that will lead to a positive response.
8. The person is conceptualized as having four modes of adaptation: physiological needs, self-concept, role function, and interdependence relations.[28:180-182]

Of the eight basic assumptions presented in the model, assumptions 1 through 5 are existence statements. Assumptions 6 and 7 are associational statements. As defined by Reynolds,[18] relational statements can be either associational or causal. The relational statements are the relations that may be tested.

Roy[32,34] identifies many propositions in relation to the regulator and cognator mechanisms and the self-concept, role function, and interdependence modes. These propositions have varying degrees of support from general theory and empirical data. The majority of the propositions are relational statements and can also be tested.[39] Testable hypotheses have been derived from the model.[10]

Derivable Consequences

Derivable consequences refer to how practically useful, important, and generally sufficient the theory is in relation to achieving valued nursing outcomes. The theory needs to guide research and practice, generate ideas, and differentiate the focus of nursing from other service professions.[4]

The Roy adaptation model has a clearly defined nursing process and can be useful in guiding clinical practice. The model is also capable of generating new information through the testing of the hypotheses that have been derived from it.[39]

CONCLUSION

Meleis[15:180] asserts that there are three types of nursing theorists: those who focus on needs, those who focus on interaction, and those who focus on outcome. Roy's Adaptation Model is classified as an outcome theory, defined by this author as "a well-articulated conception of man as a nursing client and of nursing as an external regulatory mechanism." Roy, in applying the concepts of system and adaptation to man as a client of nursing, has presented her articulation of man for nurses to use as a tool in practice, education, and research. Her conceptions of person and of the nursing process contribute to the science and the art of nursing. The Roy Adaptation Model deserves further study and development by nursing educators, researchers, and practitioners.

REFERENCES

1. Andrews, H., & Roy, C. (1986). *Essentials of the Roy Adaptation Model.* Norwalk, Conn.: Appleton-Century-Crofts.
2. Brower, H.T.F., & Baker, B.J. (1976, Nov.). The Roy adaptation model: Using the adaptation model in a practitioner curriculum. *Nursing Outlook, 24:*686-689.
3. Carveth, J.A. (1987). Conceptual models in nurse-midwifery. *Journal of Nurse-Midwifery, 32(1):*20-25.
4. Chinn, P., & Jacobs, M.K. (1987). *Theory and nursing: A systematic approach.* St. Louis: C.V. Mosby.
5. Dickoff, J., James, P., & Wiedenbach, E. (1968, May). Theory in practice discipline, part I, practice oriented theory. *Nursing Research, 17:*413-415.
6. Duldt, B., & Giffin, K. (1985). *Theoretical perspectives for nursing.* Boston: Little, Brown, & Co., pp. 242-247.
7. Farkas, L. (1981, March). Adaptation problems with nursing home application for elderly persons: An application of the Roy adaptation nursing model. *Journal of Advanced Nursing, 6:*363-368.
8. Fitzpatrick, J., Whall, A., Johnston, R., & Floyd, J. (1982). *Nursing models and their psychiatric mental health applications.* Bowie, Md.: Robert J. Brady Co.
9. Galligan, A.C. (1979, Jan.). Using Roy's concept of adaptation to care for young children. *The American Journal of Maternal Child Nursing, 4:*24-28.
10. Hill, B.J., & Roberts, C.S. (1981). Formal theory construction: An example of the process. In C. Roberts & S.L. Roberts (Eds.), *Theory construction in nursing: An adaptation model.* Englewood Cliffs, N.J.: Prentice-Hall.
11. Limadri, B.J. (1986). Research and practice with abused women, use of the Roy model as an explanatory framework. *Advanced Nursing Science, 8(4):*52-61.
12. Logan, M. (1986). Palliative care nursing: Applicability of the Roy model. *Journal of Palliative Care, 1(2):*18-24.
13. Mastal, M., & Hammond, H. (1980, July). Analysis and expansion of the Roy model: A contribution to holistic nursing. *Advances in Nursing Science, 3:*7-78.
14. Mastal, M., Hammond, H., & Roberts, M. (1982, June). Theory into hospital practice: A pilot implementation. *The Journal of Nursing Administration, 12:*9-15.
15. Meleis, A.I. (1986). *Theoretical nursing development and process.* Philadelphia: J..B. Lippincott, pp. 206-218.
16. Rambo, B. (1983). *Adaptation nursing: Assessment and intervention.* Philadelphia: W.B. Saunders.
17. Randell, B., Tedrow, M.P., & Van Landing-

ham, J. (1982). *Adaptation nursing: The Roy conceptual model applied.* St. Louis: C.V. Mosby.
18. Reynolds, P.D. (1971). *A primer in theory construction.* Indianapolis: Ind.: Bobbs-Merrill.
19. Riehl, J.P., & Roy, C. (Eds.). (1980). *Conceptual models for nursing practice* (2d ed.). New York: Appleton-Century-Crofts.
20. Roy, C. (1970, March). Adaptation: A conceptual framework in nursing. *Nursing Outlook, 18:*42-45.
21. Roy, C. (1971, April). Adaptation: A basis for nursing practice. *Nursing Outlook, 19:*254-257.
22. Roy, C. (1973, March). Adaptation: Implications for curriculum change. *Nursing Outlook, 21:*163-168.
23. Roy, C. (1975, Feb.). A diagnostic classification system for nursing. *Nursing Outlook, 23:*90-94.
24. Roy, C. (1976, Summer). The impact of nursing diagnosis. *Nursing Digest,* 4:67-69.
25. Roy, C. (1976). *Introduction to nursing: An adaptation model.* Englewood Cliffs, N.J.: Prentice-Hall.
26. Roy, C. (1976, Nov.). The Roy adaptation model: Comment. *Nursing Outlook, 24:*690-691.
27. Roy, C. (1979, Feb.). Relating nursing theory to nursing education: A new era. *Nurse Educator, 4:*16-21.
28. Roy, C. (1980). The Roy adaptation model. In J.P. Riehl & C. Roy (Eds.), *Conceptual models for nursing practice* (2d ed.). New York: Appleton-Century-Crofts, pp. 179-188.
29. Roy, C. (1983). Theory development in nursing: A proposal for direction. In N. Chaska (Ed.), *The nursing profession: A time to speak.* New York: McGraw-Hill, pp. 453-467.
30. Roy, C. (1984). *Introduction to nursing: An adaptation model* (2d ed.). Englewood Cliffs, N.J.: Prentice-Hall.
31. Roy, C. (1987). Response to "Needs of spouses of surgical patients, a conceptualization within the Roy adaptation model." *Scholarly Journal for Nursing Practice, 1(1):*45-50.
32. Roy, C., & McLeod, D. (1981). Theory of the person as an adaptive system. In C. Roy & S.L. Roberts (Eds.), *Theory construction in nursing: An adaptation model.* Englewood Cliffs, N.J.: Prentice-Hall.
33. Roy, C., & Obloy, M. (1978, Oct.). The practitioner movement. *American Journal of Nursing, 78:*1698-1702.
34. Roy, C., & Roberts, S. (1981). *Theory construction in nursing: An adaptation model.* Englewood Cliffs, N.J.: Prentice-Hall.
35. Schmitz, M. (1980). The Roy adaptation model: Application in a community setting. In J.P. Riehl & C. Roy (Eds.), *Conceptual models for nursing practice* (2d ed.). New York: Appleton-Century-Crofts.
36. Silva, M.C. (1986). Research testing theory, state of the art. *Advanced Nursing Science, 9(1):*1-11.
37. Silva, M.C. (1987). Needs of spouses of surgical patients, a conceptualization within the Roy adaptation model. *Scholarly Inquiry for Nursing Practice, 1(1):*29-44.
38. Smith, C.E., et al. (1983, Aug.). Content analyses of interviews using a nursing model: A look at parents adapting to the impact of childhood cancer. *Cancer Nursing, 6:*269-275.
39. Tiedeman, M.E. (1983). The Roy Adaptation Model. In J. Fitzpatrick & A. Whall, *Conceptual models of nursing: Analysis and application.* Bowie, Md.: Robert J. Brady, 157-180.
40. Wagner, P. (1976, Nov.). The Roy adaptation model: Testing the adaptation model in practice. *Nursing Outlook, 24:*682-685.
41. Walker, L.O., & Avant, K.C. (1983). *Strategies for theory construction in nursing.* Norwalk, Conn.: Appleton-Century-Crofts.
42. Sr. Callista Roy to assume nurse theorist post at Boston College. (1987). *Nursing & Health Care, 8(9):*536.

BIBLIOGRAPHY

Primary Sources

Books

Andrews, H., & Roy, C. (1986). *Essentials of the Roy adaptation model.* Norwalk, Conn.: Appleton-Century-Crofts.

Riehl, J.P., & Roy, C. (Eds.). (1974). *Conceptual models for nursing practice.* Englewood Cliffs, N.J.: Prentice-Hall.

Riehl, J.P., & Roy, C. (Eds.). (1980). *Conceptual models for nursing practice* (2d. ed.). New York: Appleton-Century-Crofts.

Roy, C. (1976). *Introduction to nursing: An adaptation model:* Englewood Cliffs, N.J.: Prentice-Hall.

Roy, C. (1982). *Introduction to nursing: An adaptation model.* Japanese translation by Yuriko Kanematsu. Japan: UNI Agency.

Roy, C. (1984). *Introduction to nursing: An adaptation model* (2d ed.). Englewood Cliffs, N.J.: Prentice-Hall.

Roy, C., & Roberts, S. (1981). Theory construction in nursing: An adaptation model, Englewood Cliffs, N.J.: Prentice-Hall, Inc.

Book Chapters

Roy, C. (1974). The Roy adaptation model. In J.P. Riehl & C. Roy (Eds.), *Conceptual models for nursing practice.* New York: Appleton-Century-Crofts.

Roy, C. (1975, June). Adaptation framework. In *Curriculum innovation through framework application.* Loma Linda, Calif.: Loma Linda University.

Roy, C. (1978). The stress of hospital events: Measuring changes in level of stress. In M.V. Batey (Ed.), *Symposium on stress.* In Conference on Communicating Nursing Research. Boulder, Colo: Western Interstate Commission on Higher Education (WICHE), Vol. 11.

Roy, C. (1978, Jan. 12-13). Conceptual framework for primary care in baccalaureate programs. In *Primary Care Conference,* U.S. Department of Health, Education, and Welfare. Denver, Col.

Roy, C. (1979). Health-illness (powerlessness) questionnaire and hospitalized patient decision-making. In M.J. Ward & C.A. Lindeman (Eds.), *Instruments for measuring nursing practice and other health care variables* (Vol. 1). Hyattsville, Md.: U.S. Department of Health, Education, and Welfare.

Roy, C. (1980). Expose de Callista Roy sur theorie. Expose de Callista Roy sur l'utilisation de sa theorie au neveau de la recherche. In Acta Nursological 3, Ecole Genevoise D. Infirmieres Le Bon Secours, Geneve.

Roy, C. (1980). The Roy adaptation model. In J.P. Riehl & C. Roy (Eds.), *Conceptual models for nursing practice.* (2nd ed.). New York: Appleton-Century-Crofts.

Roy, C. (1981). A systems model of nursing care and its effect on the quality of human life. *Proceedings of the International Congress on Applied Systems Research and Cybernetics.* London: Pergamon Press.

Roy, C., & McLeod, D. (1981). Theory of the person as an adaptive system. In C. Roy, & S.L. Roberts (Eds.). *Theory construction in nursing: An adaptation model.* Englewood Cliffs, N.J.: Prentice-Hall.

Roy, S.C. (1983). Theory development in nursing: A proposal for direction. In N. Chaska (Ed.), *The nursing profession: A time to speak.* New York: McGraw-Hill.

Roy, S.C. (1983). Roy's adaptation model and application to family case studies. In I. Clements, & F. Roberts (Eds.), *Theoretical approaches to family health.* New York: John Wiley & Sons.

Roy, C. (1983). Roy adaptation model, the expectant family—analysis and application of the Roy adaptation model, and the family in primary care—analysis and application of the Roy adaptation model. In I. Clements, & F. Roberts (Eds.), *Family health: A theoretical approach to nursing care.* New York: John Wiley & Sons.

Roy, S.C. (1983). A conceptual framework for clinical specialist practice. In A. Harris, & J. Sproos (Eds.), *The clinical nurse specialist in theory and practice.* New York: Grune & Stratton.

Roy, C. (1983). Foreword. In B.J. Rambo, *Adaptation nursing: Assessment and intervention..* Philadelphia: Saunders.

Roy, C. (1984, May 20-23). The Roy adaptation model: Applications in community health nursing. In *Proceedings of the Annual Community Health Nursing Conference.* University of North Carolina, Chapel Hill, N.C:

Roy, C. (1984). Framework for classification systems development: Progress and issues. *Proceedings of the fifth national conference on the classification of nursing diagnosis.* St. Louis: C.V. Mosby.

Roy, C. (1984). The Roy adaptation model: Applications in community health nursing. *Proceedings of the eighth annual ccommunity health nursing conference.* Chapel Hill, N.C.: University of North Carolina:

Roy, S.C. (1985). Practice in action: Clinical research. In K.E. Barnard & G.R. Smith (Eds.). *Faculty practice in action: Annual symposium on nursing faculty practice, 2.* New York: American Academy of Nursing, pp.. 192-200.

Roy, C. (1985). The future of the nursing science: Response of the Academy, at Scientific Session of the American Academy of Nursing. Kansas City, Mo: American Academy of Nursing.

Roy, Sr.C. (1988). Sister Callista Roy. In T.M. Schorr and A. Zimmerman (eds). Making choices: Taking chances. St. Louis: C.V. Mosby Co.

Roy C. and Anivay, J. (1988). Roy's Adaptation Model: Theories for nursing administration. In B. Henry, C. Arndt, M. DiVincenti, A. Marriner-Tomey (Eds.), *Dimensions of nursing administration.* Boston; Blackwell Scientific.

Roy, C. (1987). Roy's adaptation model. In Parse, R.R., *Nursing science: Major paradigms, theories, and critiques*. Philadelphia: Saunders.

Roy, C. (1988) Human information processing and nursing research. In J. Fitzpatrick & R.L. Tauton (Eds.), *Annual Review of Nursing Research, 6*. New York: Springer.

Articles

Roy, C. (1967, Feb.). Role cues and mothers of hospitalized children. *Nursing Research, 16:*178-182.

Roy, C. (1970, March). Adaptation: A conceptual framework in nursing. *Nursing Outlook, 18:*42-45.

Roy, C. (1971, April). Adaptation: A basis for nursing practice. *Nursing Outlook, 19:*254-257.

Roy, C. (1973). Adaptation: Implications for curriculum change. *Nursing Outlook, 21:*163-168.

Roy, C. (1975, Feb.). Adaptation: Implications for curriculum change. *Nursing Outlook, 23:*90-94.

Roy, C. (1975, Feb.). A diagnostic classification system for nursing. *Nursing Outlook, 23:*90-94.

Roy, S.C. (1975, May). The impact of nursing diagnosis. *AORN Journal, 21:*1023-1030.

Roy, C. (1976). Comment. *Nursing Outlook, 24:*690-691.

Roy, C. (1976, Summer). The impact of nursing diagnosis. *Nursing Digest,* 4:67-69.

Roy, C. (1976, Nov.). The Roy adaptation model: Comment. *Nursing Outlook, 24:*690-691.

Roy, C., & Obloy, M. (1978, Oct.). The practitioner movement. *American Journal of Nursing, 78:* 1698-1702.

Roy, C. (1979, Feb.). Relating nursing theory to nursing education: A new era. *Nurse Educator, 4:*16-21.

Roy, C. (1979, Dec.). Nursing diagnosis from the perspective of a nursing model. *Nursing Diagnosis Newsletter,* Vol. 6. St. Louis School of Nursing.

Roy, C. (1983). To the Editor. *Nursing Research, 23:*320.

Gortner, S., Ellis, R., Roy, C., Williams, C., Benner, P., & Mercer, R. (1984). Explanation in nursing science. *Symposium Abstract in Community Nursing Research, 17:*101-103.

Roy, C. (1985). Nursing research makes a difference. *Newsletter of Nurses Educational Fund, Inc, 4(1):*2-3.

Roy, C. (1985). Acoustic Neuroma, Notes. *Accoustic Neuroma Association, 13:*8-9.

Roy, C. (1987). Response to "Needs of spouses of surgical patients, a conceptualization within the Roy adaptation model." *Scholarly Journal for Nursing Practice, 1(1):*45-50.

Roy, C. (1988). An explication of the philosophical assumptions of the Roy adaptation model. *Nursing Science Quarterly, 1(1).*

Dissertation

Roy, C. (1977). *Decision-making by the physically ill and adaptation during illness.* Doctoral dissertation. University of California, Los Angeles.

Booklet

Roy, S.C., et al. (1979). *Getting our act together.* New York, National League of Nursing. Publication No. 52-1805.

Audiotape

Roy, C. (1978, Dec.). Paper presented at the second Annual Nurse Educator Conference. Audiotape available from Teach 'em Inc., 160 E. Illinois Street, Chicago, Ill. 60611.

Roy, C. (1984, May). Nurses' Theorist Conference at Edmonton, Alberta. Audiotape available from Kennedy Recordings, R.R. 5, Edmonton, Alberta TSP 4B7.

Correspondence

Roy, S.C. (1984, March 26). Curriculum vitae.

Roy, S.C. (1988, March 8). Curriculum vitae.

Interview

Roy, S.C. (1984, March 25). Telephone interview.

Professional Profile: "Sister Callista Roy: Influencing the direction of nursing." (1985). *Focus on Critical Care Nursing, 12(3):*45-46.

Secondary Sources

Book Reviews

Riehl, J.P., & Roy, S.C. (1974). *Conceptual models for nursing practice.*
*Nursing Outlook, 23:*457, July 1975.
*Nursing Research, 24:*306-307, July-August 1975.

Roy, S.C. (1976). *Introduction to nursing: An adaptation model.*
*American Journal of Nursing, 77:*1359, August 1977.
*Nursing Outlook, 25:*658, October 1977.

Roy, S.C., & Roberts, S. (1981). *Theory construction in nursing.*
*Nursing Outlook, 30:*141, February 1982.

Books

Chinn, P.L., & Jacobs, M.K. (1987). *Theory and nursing: A systematic approach.* St. Louis: C.V. Mosby.

Fitzpatrick, J.J., & Whall, A.L., (1983). *Conceptual models of nursing: Analysis and application.* Bowie, Md.: Robert J. Brady.

Fitzpatrick, J.J., et al. (1982). *Nursing models: Applications to psychiatric mental health nursing.* Bowie, Md.: Robert J. Brady.

Kim, H.S. (1983). *The nature of theoretical thinking in nursing.* Norwalk, Conn.: Appleton-Century-Crofts.

Nicoll, L.H. (1986). *Perspectives on Nursing Theory.* Boston, Mass.: Little, Brown, & Co.

Potter, D.O. (Ed.). (1984). *Practices nurses' reference library.* Springhouse, Pa.: Nursing 84 Books Springhouse Corporation.

Rambo, B. (1983). *Adaptation nursing: Assessment and intervention.* Philadelphia: W.B. Saunders.

Randell, B., Tedrow, M.P., & Van Landingham, J. (1982). *Adaptation nursing: The Roy conceptual model applied.* St. Louis: C.V. Mosby.

Reynolds, P.D. (1971). *A primer in theory construction.* Indianapolis, Ind.: Bobbs-Merrill.

Torres, G. (1986). *Theoretical Foundations of Nursing.* Norwalk, Conn.: Appleton-Century-Crofts, pp. 151-165.

Walker, L.O., & Avant, K.C. (1983). *Strategies for theory construction in nursing.* Norwalk, Conn.: Appleton-Century-Crofts.

Book Chapters

Blue, C.L., Brubaker, K.M., Papazian, K.R., & Riester, C.M. (1986). "Sister Callista Roy: Adaptation Model." In Marriner, A. (Ed.), *Nursing theorists and their work.* St. Louis, Mo.: C.V. Mosby, pp. 297-312.

Downey, C. (1974). Adaptation nursing applied to an obstetric patient. In J.P. Riehl & C. Roy (Eds.), *Conceptual models for nursing practice,* New York: Appleton-Century-Crofts.

Fawcett, J. (1984). Roy's adaptation model. In Fawcett, J., *Analysis and evaluation of conceptual models of nursing.* Philadelphia: F.A. Davis, pp. 247-285.

Fawcett, J. (1981). Assessing and understanding the cesarean father. In C.F. Kehoe (Ed.), *The cesarean experience: Theoretical and clinical perspectives for nurses.* New York: Appleton-Century-Crofts, pp. 371-376.

Fitzpatrick, J.J., et al. (1982). *Nursing models: Applications to psychiatric mental health nursing.* Bowie, Md.: Robert J. Brady.

Galbreath, J.G. (1980). Sister Callista Roy. In Nursing Theories Conference Group, J.B. George, Chairperson, *Nursing theories: The base for professional nursing practice.* Englewood Cliffs, N.J.: Prentice-Hall, pp. 199-212.

Galbreath, J.G. (1985). Sister Callista Roy. In J.B. George (Ed.), *Nursing Theories* (2d ed.). Englewood Cliffs, N.J.: Prentice-Hall, pp. 300-318.

Germain, C.P. (1984). Power and powerlessness in the adult hospitalized cancer patient. In *Cancer Nursing in the 80's: Proceedings of the 3d International Conference of Cancer Nursing.* Melbourne, Australia: The Cancer Institute/Peter MacCallum Hospital and the Royal Melbourne Hospital, pp. 158-162.

Gordon, J. (1974). Nursing assessment and care plan for a cardiac patient. In J.P. Riehl & C. Roy (Eds.), *Conceptual models for nursing practice.* New York: Appleton-Century-Crofts.

Hill, B.J., & Roberts, C.S. (1981). Formal theory construction: An example of the process. In C. Roy & S.L. Roberts (Eds.), *Theory construction in nursing: An adaptation model.* Englewood Cliffs, N.J.: Prentice-Hall, pp. 30-39.

Idle, B.A. (1978). SPAL: A tool for measuring self-perceived adaptation level appropriate for an elderly population. In Sigma Theta Tau, *Clinical nursing research: Its strategies and findings. Proceedings from the Fifth Annual Nursing Research Conference, Tucson, Arizona, Sept. 15-16, 1977.* Indianapolis: Sigma Theta Tau. Monograph, Series 79-Two. University of Arizona.

Kehoe, C.F. (1981). Identifying the nursing needs of the postpartum cesarean mother. In C.F. Kehoe (Ed.), *The cesarean experience: Theoretical and clinical perspective for nurses.* New York: Appleton-Century-Crofts, pp. 85-141.

Kehoe, C.F., & Fawcett, J. (1981). An overview of the Roy adaptation model. In C.F. Kehoe (Ed.), *The cesarean experience: Theoretical and clinical perspectives for nurses.* New York: Appleton-Century-Crofts, pp. 79-84.

Leddy, S. & Pepper, J.M. (1985). Sister Callista Roy's adaptation model. In S. Leddy & J.M. Pepper, *Conceptual Bases of Professional Nursing*. Philadelphia: J.B. Lippincott, pp. 142-144.

Levesque, L. (1980, Oct. 22-24). Rehabilitation of the chronically ill elderly: A method of operationalizing a conceptual model for nursing. In R.C. MacKay & E.G. Zilm (Eds.), *Research for practice: Proceedings of the National Nursing Research Conference*, Halifax, Nova-Scotia.

Lewis, F., et al. (1978). Measuring adaptation of chemotherapy patients. In J.C. Krueger, A.H. Nelson, & M. Opal, *Nursing Research: Development, collaboration, utilization*. Rockville, Md.: Aspen Systems.

Meleis, A.I. (1985). Sister Callista Roy. In A.I. Meleis, *Theoretical nursing: Development and progress*. Philadelphia: J.B. Lippincott, pp. 206-218.

Sato, M. (1986). The Roy Adaptation Model. In P. Winsted-Fry, (Ed.), *Case Studies in Nursing Theory*. New York: National League for Nursing, 103-125.

Schmitz, M: (1980). The Roy adaptation model: Application in a community setting. In J.P. Riehl & C. Roy (Eds.), *Conceptual models for nursing practice* (2d ed.). New York: Appleton-Century-Crofts, pp. 193-206.

Starr, S.L. (1980). Adaptation applied to the dying patient. In J.P. Riehl & C. Roy (Eds.), *Conceptual models for nursing practice* (2d ed.). New York: Appleton-Century-Crofts, pp. 189-192.

Tiedeman, M.E. (1983). The Roy adaptation model. In J. Fitzpatrick & A. Whall, (Eds.), *Conceptual models of nursing: Analysis and application*. Bowie, Md.: Robert J. Brady, pp. 157-180.

Articles

Aggleton, P., & Chalmers, H. (1984, Oct.). The Roy Adaptation Model. *Nursing Times, 80:*45-48.

Andreoli, K.G., & Thompson, C.E. (1977, June). The nature of science in nursing. *Image, 9(2):*33-37.

Beckstrand, J. (1980). A critique of several conceptions of practice theory in nursing. *Research in Nursing and Health, 3:*69-79.

Brower, H.T.F., & Baker, B.J. (1976, Nov.). The Roy adaptation model: Using the adaptation model in a practitioner curriculum. *Nursing Outlook, 24:*686-689.

Camooso, C., Green, M., & Reilly, P. (1981). Students' adaptation according to Roy. *Nursing Outlook, 29:*108-109.

Carveth, J.A. (1987). Conceptual models in nurse-midwifery. *Journal of Nurse-Midwifery, 32(1):*20-25.

Chance, K.S. (1982). Nursing models: A requisite for professional accountability. *Advances in Nursing Science, 4(2):*57-65.

Cottrell, B.H., & Shannaha, M.D. (1987). Effect of the birth chair in duration of 2d stage labor and maternal outcome. *Nursing Research, 35(6):*364-367.

Dickoff, J., James, P., & Wiedenbach, E. (1968, May). Theory in a practice discipline. Part I. Practice oriented theory. *Nursing Research, 17:*413-435.

Farkas, L. (1981, March). Adaptation problems with nursing home application for elderly persons: An application of the Roy adaptation nursing model. *Journal of Advanced Nursing, 6:*363-368.

Fawcett, J. (1981). Needs of cesarean birth parents. *Journal of Obstetric, Gynecologic, and Neonatal Nursing, 10:*371-376.

Fawcett, J. & Buritt, J. (1985). An exploratory study of antenatal preparation for cesarean birth. *Journal of Obstetric, Gynecologic, and Neonatal Nursing, 14:*224-230.

Galligan, A.C. (1979, Jan.). Using Roy's concept of adaptation to care for young children. *The American Journal of Maternal Child Nursing, 4:*24-28.

Gamble, N., & S. Devaney. (1985). Application of the adaptation framework in an LPN program, a project. *Missouri Nurse, 54(6):*10-13.

Gartner, S.R., & Nahm, H. (1977, Jan.-Feb.). An overview of nursing research in the United States. *Nursing Research, 26:*10-29.

Germain, C.P. (1984). Sheltering abused women: A nursing perspective. *Journal of Psychological Nursing, 22(9):*24-31.

Glasper, A. (1986). Spotlight on children. Scaling down a model. *Nursing Times, 82(43):*53-58.

Goodwin, J.O. (1980). A cross-cultural approach to integrating nursing theory and practice. *Nurse Educator, 5(6):*15-20.

Gunderson, L.P., & Kenner, C. (1987, Aug.). Neonatal Stress: Physiologic adaptation and nursing implications. *Neonatal Network*. 37-42.

Hammong, E., Roberts, M.P., & Silva, M.C. (1983, Spring). The effect of Roy's first level and second level assessment of nurses; determination of accurate nursing diagnoses. *Virginia Nurse*. 14-17.

Hoon, E. (1986). Game playing, a way to look at nursing models. *Journal of Advanced Nursing, 11(4)*:421-427.

Janelli, L.M. (1980). Utilizing Roy's adaptation model from a gerontological perspective. *Journal of Gerontological Nursing, 6(3)*:140-150.

Johnson, D.E. (1974), Sept.-Oct.). Development of theory: A requisite for nursing as a primary health profession. *Nursing Research, 23*:372-377.

Kasemwatana, S. (1982). An application of Roy's adaptation model. *Thai Journal of Nursing, 31(1)*:25-46.

Limadri, B.J. (1986). Research and practice with abused women, use of the Roy model as an explanatory framework. *Advanced Nursing Science 8(4)*:52-61.

Laros, J. (1977). Deriving outcome criteria from a conceptual model. *Nursing Outlook, 25*:333-336.

Lewis, F.M., Firsich, S.C., & Parsell, S. (1979). Clinical tool development for adult chemotherapy patients: Process and content. *Cancer Nursing, 2*:99-108.

Mastal, M., & Hammond, H. (1980, July). Analysis and expansion of the Roy adaptation model: A contribution to holistic nursing. *Advances in Nursing Science, 2*:71-81.

Mastal, M., Hammond, H., & Roberts, M. (1982, June). Theory into hospital practice: A pilot implementation. *The Journal of Nursing Administration, 12*:9-15.

Norris, S., Campbell, L., & Brenkert, S. (1982). Nursing procedures and alternations in transcutaneous oxygen tension in premature infants. *Nursing Research, 31*:330-336.

Park, K.O. (1982). Study of Roy's adaptation model. *Trehan Kanho, 21(3)*:49-58 (Japan).

Porth, C.M. (1977). Physiological coping: A model for teaching pathophysiology. *Nursing Outlook, 25*:781-784.

Richard, L. (1982). Roy's adaptation model, *Infirmiere Canadienne (Montreal), 24(9)*:12-13.

Robitaille-Tremblay, M. (1983). Les soins infirmiers en psychiatrie a l'ere d'un modele conceptual. *L'infirmiere Canadienne, 6*:37-40.

Robitaille-Tremblay, M. (1984, Aug.). A data collection tool for the psychiatric nurse. *The Canadian Nurse, 31(7)*:26-31.

Silva, M.C. (1977, Oct.). Philosophy science theory: Interrelationships and implications for nursing research. *Image, 9(3)*:59-63.

Silva, M.C. (1986). Research testing nursing theory, state of the art. [published erratum appears in *ANS* 1987, Jan., *9(2)*:ix.] *Advanced Nursing Science, 9(1)*:1-11.

Silva, M.C. (1987). Needs of spouses of surgical patients, a conceptualization within the Roy adaptation model. *Scholarly Inquiry for Nursing Practice, 1(1)*:29-44.

Smith, C.E., Garvis, M.S., & Martinson, I.M (1983, Aug.). Content analysis of interviews using a nursing model: A look at parents adapting to the impact of childhood cancer. *Cancer Nursing, 6*:269-275.

Torosian, L.C., DeStefano, M., & Dietrick-Gallager, M. (1985). Day gynecologic chemotherapy unit: An innovative approach to changing health care systems. *Cancer Nursing, 8*:221-227.

Wagner, P. (1976, Nov.). The Roy adaptation model: Testing the adaptation model in practice. *Nursing Outlook, 24(11)*:682-685.

Other Sources

Coombs, A., & Snygg, D. (1959). *Individual behavior: A perceptual approach to behavior.* New York: Harper Brothers.

Dohrenwend, B.P. (1961). The social psychological nature of stress. A framework for causal inquiry. *Journal of Abnormal and Social Psychology, 62(2)*:294-302.

Driever, M.J. (1976). Theory of self-concept. In C. Roy (Ed.), *Introduction to nursing: An adaptation model.* Englewood Cliffs, N.J.: Prentice-Hall.

Ellis, R. (1968, May-June). Characteristics of significant theories. *Nursing Research, 17*:217-223.

Epstein, S. (1973, May). The self-concept revisited or a theory of a theory. *American Psychologist, 28:(5)*:404-416.

Erickson, E.H. (1963). *Childhood and society* (2d ed.). New York: W.W. Norton.

Gardner, B.D. (1964). *Development in early childhood.* New York: Harper & Row.

Helson, H. (1964). *Adaptation-level theory: An experimental and systematic approach to behavior.* New York: Harper & Row.

Lazarus, R.S. (1966). *Psychological stress and the coping process.* New York: McGraw-Hill.

Lazarus, R.S., Averill, J.R., & Opton, E.M., Jr. (1974). The psychology of coping: Issues of research and assessment. In G.V. Coelho, D.A. Hamburg, & J.E. Adams (Eds.), *Coping and adaptation*. New York: Basic Books.

Malaznik, N. (1976). Theory of role function. In C. Roy (Ed.), *Introduction to nursing: An adaptation model*. Englewood Cliffs, N.J.: Prentice-Hall.

Maslow, A.H. (1968). *Toward a psychology of being* (2d ed.). New York: Van Nostrand Reinhold.

Mead, G.H. (1934). *Mind, self, and society*. Chicago: University of Chicago.

Mechanic, D. (1974). Social structure and personal adaptation: Some neglected dimensions. In G.V. Coelho, D.A. Hamburg, & J.E. Adams (Eds.), *Coping and adaptation*. New York: Basic Books.

Mechanic, D. (1970). Some problems in developing a social psychology of adaptation to stress. In J. McGrath (Ed.), *Social and psychological factors in stress*. New York: Holt, Rinehart, & Winston.

Miller, J.G. (1965, July). Living systems: Basic concepts. *Behavioral Science, 10*:193-237.

Pousch, M., & Van Landingham, J. (1977). *Interdependence mode module*. Class handout, Mount St. Mary's College, Los Angeles.

Randell, B. (1976). Development of role function. In C. Roy (Ed.), *Introduction to nursing: An adaptation model*. Englewood Cliffs, N.J.: Prentice-Hall.

Reynolds, P.D. (1971). *A primer in theory construction*. Indianapolis, Ind.: Bobbs-Merrill.

Selye, H. (1978). *The stress of life*. New York: McGraw-Hill.

Sullivan, H.S. (1953). *The interpersonal theory of psychiatry*. New York: W.W. Norton.

APPENDIX A: RESOURCES FOR IMPLEMENTING ROY ADAPTATION MODEL IN CLINICAL PRACTICE

Maureen T. Jakocko, R.N., M.N.
Director of Inservice Education
Childrens Hospital of Orange County
P.O. Box 5700
Orange, California 92613-5700

Linda Sowden, R.N., M.N.
Clinical Nurse Specialist
USCD Medical Center
225 W. Dickinson St.
San Diego, California 92103-1990

Martha R. Tremblay, R.N., M.A.
Nurse Clinical Specialist
Assistant Professor, School of Nursing
University of Ottawa,
451 Smyth Road,
Ottawa, Ontario, Canada K1H 8M5

Imogene King

27

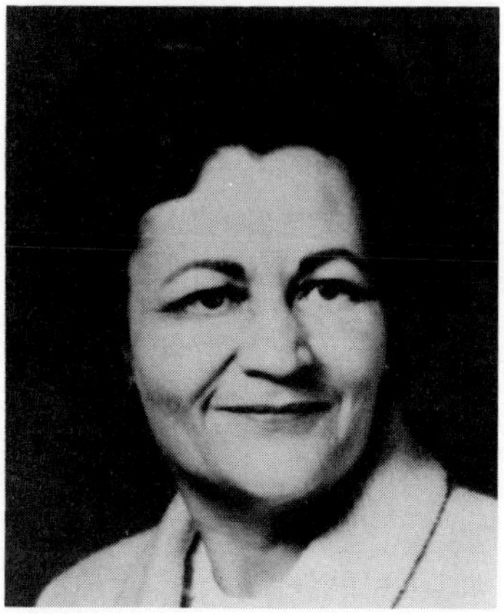

Theory of Goal Attainment

Mary Lee Ackermann, Sallie Anne Brink, Jo Anne Clanton, Cathy Greenwell Jones, Sandra L. Moody, Gwynn Lee Perlich, Debra L. Price, Beth Bruns Prusinski

CREDENTIALS AND BACKGROUND OF THE THEORIST

Imogene King earned a diploma in nursing from St. John's Hospital School of Nursing in St. Louis in 1945. She then worked as an office nurse, school nurse, staff nurse, and private duty nurse to support herself while studying for a baccalaureate degree. In 1948 she received a Bachelor of Science in Nursing Education from St. Louis University. From 1947 to 1958 King worked as an instructor in medical-surgical nursing and then as an assistant director at St. John's Hospital School of Nursing. She went on to earn an M.S.N. in 1957 from St. Louis University and a Doctor of Education degree from Teachers College, Columbia University, New York, in 1961. King was awarded an honorary Ph.D. from Southern Illinois University in 1980.

From 1961 to 1966, King was an associate professor of nursing at Loyola University in Chicago, where she developed a master's degree program in nursing using a conceptual frame-

The authors wish to express appreciation to Dr. Imogene King for critiquing the chapter.

work. During this time her book, *Toward a Theory for Nursing: General Concepts of Human Behavior,* was conceptualized, the literature reviewed, and a contract from a publishing company signed. Between 1966 and 1968 King served as Assistant Chief of Research Grants Branch, Division of Nursing in the Department of Health, Education, and Welfare. While she was in Washington, D.C., her article "A Conceptual Framework for Nursing" was published in *Nursing Research.* From 1968 to 1972 King was the director of the School of Nursing at The Ohio State University in Columbus. The manuscript for her book had been submitted to the publisher by the time she accepted this administrative position, and it was subsequently published in 1971. In *Toward a Theory for Nursing* King concludes, "A systematic representation of nursing is required ultimately for developing a science to accompany a century or more of art in the everyday world of nursing."[7:129]

King returned to Chicago in 1972 as a professor in the Loyola University graduate program. From 1978 to 1980 she also served as the Coordinator of Research in Clinical Nursing at the Loyola Medical Center, Department of Nursing. From 1972 to 1975 she was a member of the Defense Advisory Committee on Women in the Services for the Department of Defense. In 1980 King moved to Tampa, Florida, where she is currently a professor at the University of South Florida College of Nursing. The manuscript for her second book, *A Theory for Nursing: Systems, Concepts, Process,* was submitted to the publisher in June 1980 and published in 1981.

King is a member of the American Nurses' Association, the Florida Nurses' Association, National League for Nursing, and several honorary and professional societies. In addition to her books, she has authored several book chapters and multiple articles in professional journals. A third book, *Curriculum and Instruction in Nursing,* was published in 1986.

THEORETICAL SOURCES

King[7:ix] states in the preface of *Toward a Theory for Nursing* that the book's purpose "is to propose a conceptual frame of reference for nursing . . . to be utilized . . . by students and teachers, and also by researchers and practitioners to identify and analyze events in specific nursing situations. The framework suggests that the essential characteristics of nursing are those properties that have persisted in spite of environmental changes." King[7:125] proposed that her first book was "a way of thinking about the real world of nursing," that it suggested "an approach for selecting concepts perceived to be fundamental for the practice of professional nursing," and that it showed "a process for developing concepts that symbolize experiences within the physical, psychological, and social environment in nursing." "A search of the literature in nursing and other behavioral science fields, discussion with colleagues, attendance at numerous conferences, inductive and deductive reasoning, and some critical thinking about the information gathered, lead me to formulate my own theoretical framework."[8:37] King[7:124] wrote in 1971 that although nurses were individuals and professionals, nursing was "not yet a science."

When in a telephone interview King[13] was asked who influenced her work, she said the sources were "too numerous to mention." However, at a conference of nursing theorists she stated the General Systems Theory from the behavioral sciences led to the development of her "dynamic interacting systems."[10] She identified in this system three distinct levels of functions: (1) individuals, (2) groups, and (3) society (Figure 27-1). King[5:10] states in her second book that "if the goal of nursing is concern for the health of individuals and the health care of groups, and if one accepts the premise that human beings are open systems interacting with the environment, then a conceptual framework for nursing must be organized to incorporate these ideas." King's concepts and definitions of

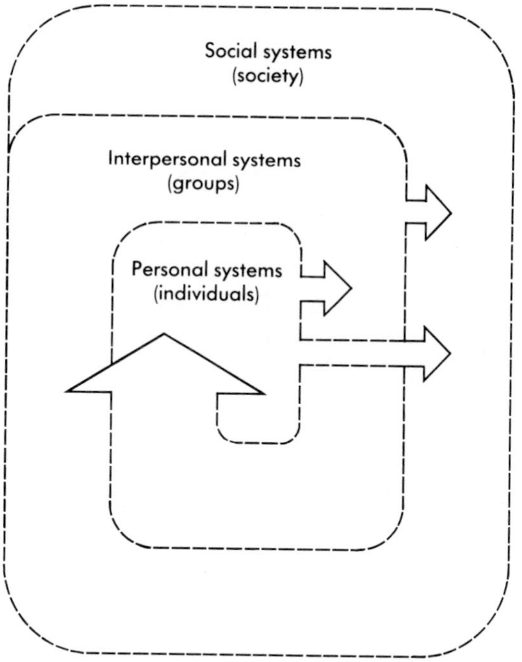

Figure 27-1. Dynamic interacting systems.
Used with permission from King, I.M. (1971). *Toward a Theory for Nursing*. New York: John Wiley & Sons, p. 20. Revised in I.M. King (1981). *A theory for nursing: Systems, concepts, process*. New York: John Wiley & Sons, p. 11.

those concepts were derived from theories and research.

USE OF EMPIRICAL EVIDENCE

King[12:11] defines theory as "a set of concepts, which, when defined, are interrelated and observable in the world of nursing practice." "Concepts are abstract ideas that give meaning to our sense perceptions, . . . mental images formed by generalizations from these particular impressions."[7:11-12] For King,[10] theory serves to "build scientific knowledge for nursing," and she has identified two methods for cultivating theory. First, a theory can be developed and then tested with research. But the procedure can also be reversed and enable research to initiate the development of theory. King[10] states, "It is my opinion that in today's world of building knowledge for a complex profession such as nursing, one must consider a composite of these two strategies."

Many research studies are cited in King's books, especially with regard to the development of the concepts relating to her theory, but only a few of those studies are briefly mentioned here. With regard to "perception" King examined studies by F.H. Allport, K.J. Kelley and K.R. Hammond, W.H. Ittleson and H. Cantril, and others. In her development of definitions for "space," R. Sommer and R. Ardrey's studies were used and B.B. Minkley's research was noted. For "time," J. E. Orme's work was acknowledged. In the examination of "communication," theories and models were presented and the studies of P. Watzlawick, J.H. Beavin, and D.D. Jackson; and D. Krieger were noted. Studies by J.F. Whiting, I. Orlando, and J. Bruner were examined for information on "interaction" and "transaction."[8] J. Dewey's theory of knowledge, which dealt with self-action, interaction, and transaction in knowing and the known, and A. Kuhn's work on transactions were also used.[14]

With regard to research, in 1975 King[8:9] noted, "Most studies have centered on technical aspects of patient care and of the health care systems rather than on patient aspects directly. . . . Few problems have been stated that begin with what the patient's condition demands or what the patient wants." In her 1981 book King[11:151-152] states, "Several theoretical formulations about interpersonal relations and nursing process have been described in nursing situations," citing studies by H. Peplau, I. Orlando, H. Yura and M. Walsh, and herself. However, "Few nursing studies have provided empirical data about nursing process phenomena related to human interaction."

King[11:152] notes that Orlando's study "supports the idea that nursing process is reciprocal" because goal identifications exists for nurses and patients. She adds that this study varies from others in that it "described the nurse-patient interaction process that leads to goal attainment."[11:153] King also discusses her own descriptive study, which tested goal attainment and operationally defined a concept of transaction as an integral component of the theory. A method of nonparticipant observation was used to collect information on nurse-patient interactions in a patient care hospital setting. Volunteer patients and graduate nursing students participated, and the students were specifically trained before the study. Multiple interactions were examined with both verbal and nonverbal communication activities recorded as raw data, including whether goals and the means to achieve them were explored and mutually agreed upon. The study provided a classification system useful in nurse-patient interactions.[11:150-156]

A systems approach is used in the development of the theory of goal attainment. King[11:4-10] notes that for about the last two decades, systems have been used to comprehend and respond to "changes and complexity in health care organizations." She adds, "Some scientists who have been studying systems have noted that the only way to study human beings interacting with the environment is to design a conceptual framework of interdependent variables and interrelated concepts."[11:10] In 1971 King[7:91] called the nursing act a process, stating, "The nursing process is a series of acts which connote action, reaction, interaction. Transaction follows when a reciprocal relationship is established by the nurse and patient" and both mutually set the goal to be achieved.

In her second book King[11:144] stated, "A theory of goal attainment was derived from the conceptual framework of interpersonal systems. The dyad, nurse and client, is one type of interpersonal system." In noting the intricate nature of nursing, King developed a conceptual framework consisting of an open system encompassing three parts. "An awareness of the complex dynamics of human behavior in nursing situations prompted the formulation of a conceptual framework that represents personal, interpersonal and social systems as the domain of nursing."[11:13]

Each of the three components uses human beings as the basic element because as individuals, human beings exchange matter, energy, and information with other individuals and the environment. Individuals exist within personal systems, and King provides an example of a "total system" as being a patient or a nurse. King believes that it is necessary to understand the concepts of perception, self, body image, growth and development, and time and space in order to comprehend human beings as persons. Interpersonal systems, or groups, are formed when two or more individuals interact, for example, forming dyads (two people) or triads (three people). Families, when acting as small groups, would be considered in this area of the system. Comprehension of this system requires the concepts of role, interaction, communication, transaction, and stress.[11:10-11]

The final interacting system consists of groups with similar concerns or interests in a society, and is referred to as a *social system.* A religious, educational or health care system exists here. The influential behavior of a family on an individual's growth and development in the society is another example. Within the health care system, the concepts of organization, power, authority, decision making, and role are essential for comprehension of this dynamic system.[11:11-12]

MAJOR CONCEPTS AND DEFINITIONS

"The major concepts in the theory of goal attainment are interaction, perception, communication, transaction, role, stress, growth and development, and time and space."[11:145]

INTERACTION. King[11:145] defines *interaction* as "a process of perception and communication between person and environment and between person and person, represented by verbal and nonverbal behaviors that are goal directed." Each individual in an interaction (nurse and client) "brings different knowledge, needs, goals, past experiences, and perceptions, which influence the interactions."[11:145]

PERCEPTION. *Perception* was defined as "each person's representation of reality."[11:146] According to King, this concept includes the import and transformation of energy, and processing, storing, and exporting information. "Perceptions are related to past experiences, concept of self, socioeconomic groups, biological inheritance, and educational background."[11:146]

COMMUNICATION. Communication was defined as "a process whereby information is given from one person to another either directly . . . or indirectly. . . . Communication is the information component of the interactions."[11:146] The exchange of verbal and nonverbal signs and symbols between nurse and client, or client and environment, is communication.[11:146-147]

TRANSACTION. "Transactions are defined as purposeful interactions that lead to goal attainment."[11:1] King goes on to subsequently expand the definition of transactions to include "observable behavior of human beings interacting with their environment . . . the valuation component of human interactions."[11:147]

ROLE. Role was defined as "a set of behaviors expected of persons occupying a position in a social system; rules that define rights and obligations in a position."[11:147] If expectations of a role differ, then role conflict and confusion exists. This may lead to decreased effectiveness of the nursing care provided.

STRESS. Stress is "a dynamic state whereby a human being interacts with the environment."[11:147] Stress "involves an exchange of energy and information between the person and the environment for regulation and control of stressors . . . an energy response of an individual to persons, objects, and events."[11:147] An increase in the stress of individuals interacting can narrow the perceptual field and decrease rationality. An increase in stress may also affect nursing care.

GROWTH AND DEVELOPMENT. King[11:148] defined growth and development as "continuous changes in individuals at the cellular, molecular, and behavioral levels of activities . . . conducive to helping individuals move toward maturity."

TIME. "Time is defined as a sequence of events moving onward to the future. . . . Time is a duration between one event and another as uniquely experienced by each human being."[11:148]

SPACE. "Space is defined as existing in all directions and is the same everywhere."[11:148] Space "is the immediate environment in which nurse and client interact."[11:149]

MAJOR ASSUMPTIONS

King's personal philosophy about human beings and life influenced her assumptions. Her conceptual framework and theory of goal attainment "are based on an overall assumption that the focus of nursing is human beings interacting with their environment leading to a state of health for individuals, which is an ability to function in social roles."[11:143]

Nursing

"Nursing is an observable behavior found in the health care systems in society."[7:125] The goal of nursing "is to help individuals maintain their health so they can function in their roles."[11:3-4] Nursing is viewed as an interpersonal process of action, reaction, interaction, and transaction. Perception of nurse and client also influences the interaction process.

Person

Specific assumptions relating to person follow:

> Individuals are social beings.
> Individuals are sentient beings.
> Individuals are rational beings.
> Individuals are perceiving beings.
> Individuals are controlling beings.
> Individuals are purposeful beings.
> Individuals are action-oriented beings.
> Individuals are time-oriented beings.[11:143]

King wrote, "Individuals have a right to knowledge about themselves, . . . a right to participate in decisions that influence their life, their health, and community service [and] . . . a right to accept or reject health care."[11:143]

Health

Health is viewed as a dynamic state in the life cycle; illness is an interference in the life cycle. Health implies continuous adaptation to stress "in the internal and external environment through optimum use of one's resources to achieve maximum potential for daily living."[11:5] "Health is the function of nurse, patient, physician, family and other interactions."[7:126]

Environment

King states, "An understanding of the ways that human beings interact with their environment to maintain health is essential for nurses."[11:2] Open systems imply interactions occur between the system and its environment, inferring that the environment is constantly changing. "Adjustments to life and health are influenced by [an] individual's interactions with environment. . . . Each human being perceives the world as a total person in making transactions with individuals and things in the environment."[11:141]

PROPOSITIONS

1. If perceptual accuracy (PA) is present in nurse-client interactions (I), transactions (T) will occur.

$$PA(I) \xrightarrow{+} T$$

2. If nurse and client make transactions (T), goals will be attained (GA).

$$T \xrightarrow{+} GA$$

3. If goals are attained (GA), satisfactions (S) will occur.

$$GA \xrightarrow{+} S$$

4. If goals are attained (GA), effective nursing care (NC_e) will occur.

$$GA \xrightarrow{+} NC_e$$

5. If transactions (T) are made in nurse-client interactions (I), growth and development (GD) will be enhanced.

$$(I)T \xrightarrow{+} GD$$

6. If role expectations and role performance as perceived by nurse and client are congruent (RCN), transactions (T) will occur.

$$RCN \xrightarrow{+} T$$

7. If role conflict (RC) is experienced by nurse and client or both, stress (ST) in nurse-client interactions (I) will occur.

$$RC(I) \xrightarrow{+} ST$$

8. If nurses with special knowledge and skills communicate (CM) appropriate information to clients, mutual goal setting (T) and goal attainment (GA) will occur. [Mutual goal setting is a step in transaction and thus has been diagrammed as transaction.]

$$CM \xrightarrow{+} T \xrightarrow{+} GA$$

From Austin, J.K., & Champion, V.L. (1983). King's theory for nursing: Explication and evaluation. In P.L. Chinn (Ed.), *Advances in nursing theory development*. Rockville, Md.: Aspen Systems. Used with permission by Aspen Systems Corporation.

THEORETICAL ASSERTIONS

The propositions shown in the following box describe the relationships between King's concepts. Diagrams follow each proposition. When the propositions are analyzed, 23 relationships are not specified, none are negative, and 22 are positive (Figure 27-2).

King's theory of goal attainment focuses on the interpersonal system and the interactions that take place between individuals, specifically in the nurse-client association, the dyadic phase. The relationships between King's major concepts that are important to this aspect of the interaction process can be explained through Figure 27-3. In this nursing process, each member of the dyad perceives the other and makes judgments; action results, and together these activities culminate in reaction. Interaction results, and if "perceptual accuracy" exists and any disturbances are conquered, transaction is the outcome. The system is open in order to permit feedback, because perception is potentially influenced by each phase of the activity.[7:90-93;11:145-146]

As previously noted, King's descriptive study relating to the theory of goal attainment resulted in a means for analyzing interactions, as presented in the box on p. 352.

King derived the following seven hypotheses from Goal Attainment Theory.

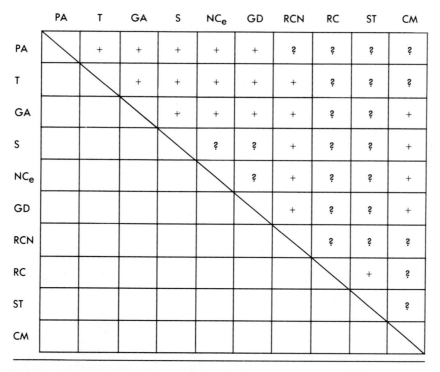

	PA	T	GA	S	NC_e	GD	RCN	RC	ST	CM
PA		+	+	+	+	+	?	?	?	?
T			+	+	+	+	+	?	?	?
GA				+	+	+	+	?	?	+
S					?	?	+	?	?	+
NC_e						?	+	?	?	+
GD							+	?	?	+
RCN								?	?	?
RC									+	?
ST										?
CM										

Figure 27-2. Relationship table. *PA,* perceptional accuracy; *T,* transactions; *GA,* goals attained; *S,* satisfactions; *NC_e,* effective nursing care; *GD,* growth and development; *RCN,* role congruency; *RC,* role conflict; *ST,* stress; *CM,* communicate.

Used with permission from Austin J.K., & Champion, V.L. (1983). King's theory for nursing: Explication and evaluation. In P.L. Chinn (Ed.), *Advances in nursing theory development.* Rockville, Md.: Aspen Systems, p. 58.

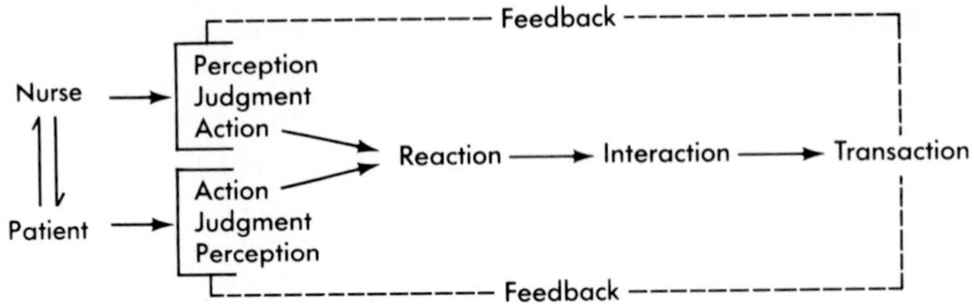

Figure 27-3. A process of human interactions.
Used with permission from King, I.M. (1971). *Toward a theory for nursing*. New York: John Wiley & Sons, p. 92.

1. Perceptual congruence in nurse-patient interactions increases mutual goal setting.
2. Communication increases mutual goal setting between nurses and patients and leads to satisfactions.
3. Satisfactions in nurses and patients increase goal attainment.
4. Goal attainment decreases stress and anxiety in nursing situations.
5. Goal attainment increases patient learning and coping ability in nursing situations.
6. Role conflict experienced by patients, nurses, or both decreases transactions in nurse-patient interactions.
7. Congruence in role expectations and role performance increases transactions in nurse-patient interactions.[11:156]

CLASSIFICATION SYSTEM OF NURSE-PATIENT INTERACTIONS THAT LEAD TO TRANSACTIONS

ELEMENTS IN INTERACTIONS

Action
Reaction
Disturbance
Mutual goal setting
Explore means to achieve goal
Agree on means to achieve goal
Transaction
Goal(s) achieved

From King, I.M. (1981). *A theory for nursing*. Used with permission from John Wiley & Sons, New York, p. 156.

Figure 27-4 combines some factors from the classification system and the process of human interaction. Both client and nurse perceive throughout the process; they communicate, thus creating action. Actions result in reactions, and, if there is a disturbance, goals may be set. At this point, means for goal achievement are explored and agreed upon, transactions are made, and goal attainment results.

LOGICAL FORM

King[10] indicated at the second annual Nurse Educators' Conference in December 1978 that theory development is composed of inductive and deductive reasoning. She believes theory's primary purpose is to generate new knowledge through research.

King[9:36] wrote in 1975 that her "personal approach to synthesizing knowledge for nursing was to use data and information available from research in nursing and related fields and from my 25 years in active practice, teaching, and research. From all the knowledge available, a theoretical framework relevant for nursing was formulated." In this framework King placed four major concepts that centered around man. She believed that man was an open system, but that energy exchange took place within and external to human organism, and that this led to behavioral responses. The four concepts were social systems, interpersonal relationships, perceptions, and health.[9:37] King proposed her theory of goal attainment in *A Theory for Nursing:* "This theory describes the

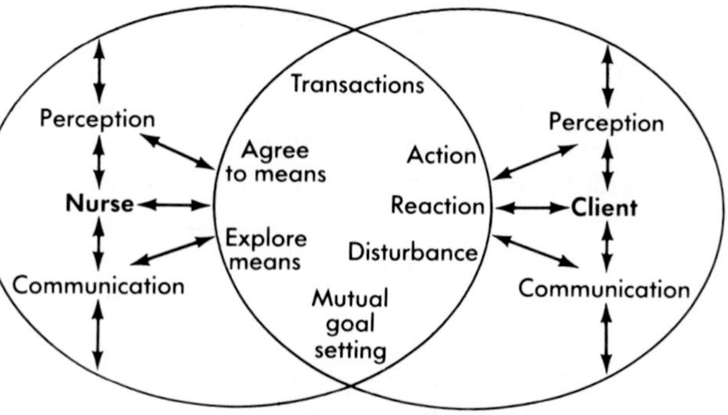

Figure 27-4. Schematic diagram of a theory of goal attainment.
From King, I.M. (1981). *A theory for nursing*. Used with permission from John Wiley & Sons, New York, p. 157.

nature of nurse-client interactions that lead to achievement of goals."[9:142]

> Nurses purposefully interact with clients mutually to establish goals and to explore and agree on means to achieve goals. Mutual goal setting is based on nurses' assessment of client's concerns, problems, and disturbances in health, their perceptions of problems, and their sharing information to move toward goal attainment.[11:142-143]

In the 1981 publication there is less dichotomy between health and illness. Illness is referred to as an interference in the life cycle.[11:5] King also reformulated to provide a more open system relationship between person and environment. In the second book King[11] uses adjustment instead of adaptation, and the terms *person, human being,* and *individual* rather than *man.*

Although King's original framework was very abstract and dealt with "only a few elements of concrete situations,"[7:128] she believed her four concepts were "relevant in every nursing situation."[7:128]

There was logical progression of development in the theory from 1971 to 1981. King derived her theory from the conceptual framework available in 1971. Her theory "organizes elements in the process of nurse-client interactions that result in outcomes, that is, goals attained."[11:143]

King[7:128] stated in her first book, "The discovery of knowledge must be disseminated continuously to the practitioners in such a way that they are able to use it in their practice. . . . Descriptive data collected systematically provide cues for generating hypotheses for research in human behavior in nursing situations." During the 1978 nursing theorist conference, King[10] indicated that if nurses were taught this process they could begin to predict outcomes in nursing. "This theory should serve as a standard of practice related to nurse-patient interactions, and is in this sense a normative theory."[11:145] These ideas have been expanded to show the process of the theory in relation to family health.[4:182-183]

ACCEPTANCE BY THE NURSING COMMUNITY

Practice

Although Goal Attainment Theory is relatively new to nursing, it appears to have been accepted for practice. Its relationship to practice is obvious because the profession of nursing is one that functions through interactions with individuals and groups within the environment. Before King's theory was published, Brown[2:469] stated, "This proposed intrasystems model provides an approach for stimulating continued learning, for establishing innovative foundations for nursing practice, and for generating inquiry through research." King[11:157] states, "Theory, because it is abstract, cannot be immediately applied to nursing practice or to concrete nursing education programs. When empirical referents are identified, defined, and described . . . theory is useful and can be applied in concrete situations."

King derived the Goal Oriented Nursing Record (GONR), based on L.L. Weed's Problem Oriented Medical Record (POMR), from Goal Attainment Theory. A method of collecting data, identifying problems and implementing and evaluating care, it has been used effectively in patient settings. King[12:12] states, "Nurses who have knowledge of the concepts of this theory of Goal Attainment are able to accurately perceive what is happening to patients and family members and are able to suggest approaches for coping with the situations." "The theory and the GONR are useful in practice as nurses have the ability to provide individualized plans of care while encouraging active participation from clients in the decision making phase."[12:11,17] The GONR is one approach to document effectiveness of nursing care.

Education

King's[13] conceptual framework was recently used at Ohio State University for curriculum design in the nursing program, and presently the graduate program at the University of Texas at Houston is doing the same. The Department of Medical-Surgical Nursing at Loyola University in Chicago was using portions of King's steps of nursing process at the graduate level. In 1980, Brown and Lee[2:468] noted that King's concepts were useful in developing a framework "for use in nursing education, nursing practice, and for generating hypotheses for research. . . . [It] provides a systematic means of viewing the nursing profession, organizing a body of knowledge for nursing, and clarifying nursing as a discipline." Shirley Steel used King's framework as the framework for her book, *Child Health and the Family*.

Research

"Research can be designed and conducted to implement this system in a hospital unit, in ambulatory care, in community nursing and home care. This information system can be designed for any patient population and for current and future computerization of records in health care systems."[11:17] In a telephone interview King[13] provided more examples of how her conceptual framework and her GONR are presently being or will soon be used in nursing practice and research. King has said that she would be happy to assist students in testing her theory and working with faculty developing curriculum from her conceptual framework. D. Polit and B. Hunger[15] cite her theory in giving examples and discussing different aspects of the research process.

FURTHER DEVELOPMENT

Because this theory was published only in 1981, there has been little time for digesting, testing, and evaluating. King[13] is coinvestigator with a colleague, Dr. Ross, in a study of goal attainment related to functional abilities in residents in two nursing homes.

While maintaining her position as a professor at the University of South Florida, King serves as a consultant and continues to expand her GONR in diverse situations. She states, "Any profession that has its primary mission in the delivery of social services requires continuous research to discover new knowledge that can be applied to improve practice. . . . The basis for the practice of nursing is knowledge; its activity is guided by the intellect, and applied in the practical realm."[7:112-113]

CRITIQUE

Simplicity

King's theory presents nine major concepts, thus making the theory complex. The concepts are easily understood because they are defined to show interrelations in nursing practice.

Some of the definitions of the basic concepts are derived from research literature. King's definition of *stress* states that stress has positive consequences. She gives examples of the negative effects of stress on patients with sensory deprivation and sensory overload.

King maintains that her definitions are clear and conceptually derived from the identified characteristics.

Generality

King's theory has been criticized for having limited application in areas of nursing where patients are unable to interact competently with the nurse. However, King maintains that she has made transactions with comatose patients; nurse midwives have made transactions with newborns; and psychiatric nurses have applied the knowledge of her theory to make transactions with psychiatric patients. Its use with groups has not been clarified.

King responds that 80% of communication is nonverbal. She says,

> Try observing a really good nurse interact with a baby or a child who has not yet learned the language. If you systematically recorded your observations, you would be able to analyze the behaviors and find many transactions at a nonverbal level. I have a beautiful example of that when I was working side by side with a graduate student in a neuro unit with a comatose patient. I was talking to the patient, explaining everything that was happening and showing the graduate student what I believe to be important in nursing care. When the patient regained consciousness a few days later, she asked the nurse in the unit to find that wonderful nurse who was the only one who explained what was happening to her. She wanted to thank her. I made transactions. I could observe her muscle movement. She was trying to help us as a physician poked a tube down her throat. A nurse midwife reports observing transactions between mothers and newborns. Psychiatric nurses have reported to me the value of my theory in their practice. So the need in nursing is to broaden nurses' knowledge of communication and that is what my theory is all about.[14]

King believes critics are assuming that a theory will address every person, event, and situation, which is impossible. She reminds critics that even Einstein's theory of relativity could not be tested completely until space travel made testing possible.[14]

Empirical Precision

King has gathered empirical data on the nurse-patient interaction process that leads to goal attainment. A descriptive study was conducted to test the goal attainment theory. From a sample of 17 patients, goals were attained in 12 cases (70% of the sample). If nursing students were taught the goal attainment theory, and if it were used in nursing practice, goal attainment could be measured along with the effectiveness of nursing care.

Because King's theory is relatively new, empirical testing is in the beginning stages, and it remains to be seen if relationships exist between the concepts. The 27th Annual Research Conference at the University of South Florida College of Nursing in February of 1988 was titled "Building Knowledge for Nursing: Testing King's Theory." This was truly an international conference with presentations by nurses from Canada, Sweden, the United States, and Japan.

King is presently acting as a consultant to researchers testing hypotheses derived from her theory, in addition to conducting her research to test her theory. She hopes researchers will continue to do more testing of the theory.

Derivable Consequences

For a theory to be useful in nursing practice, it should focus on at least one aspect of the nursing process. King's theory focuses on the planning and implementation phases of the nursing process. The nurse-patient dyad interact, devise mutually agreed-on goals, explore means to achieve goals, transact, and attain goals.

King maintains that her theory focuses on all aspects of the nursing process (APIE), but her process is the theoretical basis for the Yura and Walsh process as method. King compares her process model, the Yura and Walsh nursing process model, and the scientific method by identifying the elements of each of the four processes and their similarities. She believes one must assess to set mutual goals, plan to provide alternate means to achieve goals, and evaluate to determine if the goal was attained. King[14] says she is "the only one who has provided a theory that deals with choices, alternatives, participation of all individuals in decision making and specifically deals with outcomes of nursing care." Her theory is being used to implement theory-based practice in several areas of nursing practice in Canada and the United States. King is presently working with a colleague to derive a theory of administration for nursing from her conceptual systems model.

REFERENCES

1. Austin, J.K., & Champion, V.L. (1983). King theory for nursing: Explication and evaluation. In P. Chinn, *Advances in nursing theory development.* Rockville, Md.: Aspen Publications.
2. Brown, S.T., & Lee, B.T. (1980). Imogene King's conceptual framework: A proposed model for continuing nursing education. *Journal of Advanced Nursing, 5(5)*:467-473.
3. Chinn, P.L., (1983). *Advances in nursing theory development.* Rockville, Md.: Aspen Systems.
4. Clements, I.W., & Roberts, F.B. (1983). *Family Health: A theoretical approach to nursing care.* New York: John Wiley & Sons.
5. Daubenmier, M.J., & King, I.M. (1973). Nursing process models: A systems approach. *Nursing Outlook, 21*:512-517.
6. Gonat, P.J. (1983). Imogene M. King: A theory for nursing. In J. Fitzpatrick, & A. Whall, *Conceptual models of nursing: Analysis and application.* Bowie, Md.: Robert J. Brady.
7. King, I.M. (1971). *Toward a theory for nursing: General concepts of human behavior.* New York: John Wiley & Sons.
8. King, I.M. (1975). Patient aspects. In L.J. Schumann, R.D. Spears, Jr. & J.P. Young (Eds.), *Operations research in health care: A critical analysis.* Baltimore: Johns Hopkins University Press.
9. King, I.M. (1975). A process for developing concepts for nursing through research. In P. Verhonick, *Nursing research.* Boston: Little, Brown.
10. King, I.M. (1978, Dec.). Speech presented at Second Annual Nurse Educators' Conference, New York. Audiotape available from Teach 'Em, Inc., Chicago.
11. King, I.M. (1981). *A theory for nursing: Systems, concepts, process.* New York: John Wiley & Sons.
12. King, I.M. (1984). Effectiveness of nursing care: Use of a goal oriented nursing record in end stage renal disease. *American Association of Nephrology Nurses and Technicians Journal, 11(2)*:11-17, 60.
13. King, I.M. (1984). Telephone interview.
14. King, I.M. (1985). Personal correspondence.
15. Polit, D. and Hunger, B. (1983). Nursing Research: Principles and Methods. Philadelphia: J.B. Lippincott.

BIBLIOGRAPHY

Primary Sources

Books

King, I.M. (1971). *Toward a theory for nursing: General concepts of human behavior.* New York: John Wiley & Sons.

King, I.M. (1981). *A theory for nursing: Systems, concepts, process.* New York: John Wiley & Sons.

King, I.M. (1986). *Curriculum and Instruction in Nursing: Concepts and Process.* Norwalk, Conn.: Appleton-Century-Crofts.

Book Chapters

King, I.M. (1975). A process for developing concepts for nursing through research. In P.J. Verhonick (Ed.), *Nursing research* (Vol. I). Boston: Little, Brown.

King, I.M. (1975). Patient aspects. In L.J. Schuman, R.D. Speas, Jr., & J.P. Young (Eds.), *Operations research in health care: A critical analysis.* Baltimore: The Johns Hopkins University Press.

King, I.M. (1976). The health care systems: Nursing intervention subsystem. In H.H. Werley, et al. (Eds.), *Health research: The systems approach.* New York: Springer.

King, I.M. (1983). King's theory of nursing. In I.W. Clements & F.B. Roberts (Eds.), *Family health: A theoretical approach to nursing care.* New York: John Wiley & Sons.

King, I.M. (1984). A theory for nursing: King's conceptual model applied in community health nursing. In M.K. Asay & C.C. Ossler (Eds.), *Proceedings of the Eighth Annual Community Health Nursing Conference: Conceptual models of nursing applications in community health nursing.* Chapel Hill: University of North Carolina.

King, I.M. (1988). Imogene M. King. In T.A. Schorr & A. Zimmerman (Eds.), *Making Choices, Taking Chances.* St. Louis: C.V. Mosby Co.

King, I. (1988). King's System framework for nursing administration. In B. Henry, C. Arndt, M. DiVincenti, A. Marriner-Tomey (Ed.). *Dimensions of nursing administration.* Boston Blackwell Scientific.

Portions of Chapters

King, I.M. (1983). Analysis and application of King's theory of goal attainment. In "The family coping with a medical illness." In I.W. Clements & F.B. Roberts (Eds.), *Family health: A theoretical approach to nursing care.* New York: John Wiley & Sons.

Articles

Daubenmire, M.J., & King, I.M. (1973). Nursing process models: A systems approach. *Nursing Outlook, 21(8):*512-517.

King, I.M. (1964, Oct.). Nursing theory: Problems and prospects. *Nursing Science,* pp. 394-403.

King, I.M. (1968). A conceptual frame of reference for nursing. *Nursing Research, 17(1):*27-31.

King, I.M. (1970). A conceptual frame of reference for nursing. *Japanese Journal of Nursing Research, 3:*199-204.

King, I.M. (1970). Planning for change. *Ohio Nurses Review, 45:*4-7.

King, I.M. (1978). U.S.A.: Loyola University of Chicago school of nursing. *Journal of Advanced Nursing,* 3(4):390.

King, I.M. (1984). Effectiveness of nursing care: Use of a goal-oriented nursing record in end-stage renal disease. *American Association of Nephrology Nurses and Technicians Journal, 11(2):*11-17, 60.

King, I.M., & Tarsitano, B. (1982). The effect of structured and unstructured preop teaching: A replication. *Nursing Research, 31(6):*324-329.

King, I.M. (1987). Translating nursing research into practice. *Journal of Neuroscience Nursing, 19(1).*

King, I.M. (1985). Collaborative relationship in nursing research. *Florida Nurse, 33(2):*3,15.

King, I.M. (1985). Patient education: Barriers and gateways. *Florida Nurse, 33(5):* 4, 15.

King, I.M. (1984). Philosophy of nursing education: A national survey. *Western Journal of Nursing Research, 6(4):*387-406.

King, I.M. (1988). Concepts: Essential elements of theories. *Nursing Science Quarterly, 1(1):*22-24.

Samples, J., Vancott, M.L., Long, C., King, I.M., & Kersenbrock, A. (1985). Circadian rhythms: Basis for screening for fever. *Nursing Research, 34(6):*377-379.

NLN Publications

King, I.M. (1978). *How does the conceptual framework provide structure for the curriculum? Curriculum process for developing or revising baccalaureate nursing programs.* New York: NLN Publication 15-1700, pp. 23-34.

King, I.M. (1978). The "why" of theory development. In *Theory development: What, why, how?* New York: NLN Publication 15-1708, pp. 11-16.

King, I.M. (1986). *King's Theory of Goal Attainment.* New York: NLN Publication 15-2152, pp. 197-213.

Letters to the Editor

King, I.M. (1975). Reaction to "The patient rights advocate," by G.J. Annas, & J. Healey. *Journal of Nursing Administration, 5(1):*40-41.

Forewords

King, I.M. (1969). Symposium on neurologic and neurosurgical nursing. *Nursing Clinics of North America, 4(2):*199-200.

Audio Tapes

King, I.M. (1978, Dec. 4-6). *Nursing theory.* Nursing Resources, Inc., Wakefield, Mass.

King, I.M. (1978) *Second Annual Nurse Educators' Conference,* held in New York City. Audiotape available from Teach 'em, Inc. 160 E. Illinois Street, Chicago, Ill. 60611.

King, I.M. (1984, 1986). *Nurse Theorist Conference* held at Edmonton, Alberta. Audio tapes available from Kennedy Recording, R.R. 5, Edmonton, Alberta, T5P 487.

King, I.M. (1985, 1987). King's Theory. *Nurse Theorist Conference* held in Pittsburgh, Pa. Audio tape available from Meetings International, 1200 Delor Ave., Louisville, Ky. 40217

Video Tapes

King, I.M. (1987). King's Theory. *Nurse Theorist Conference* held in Pittsburgh, Pa. Videotape available from Meetings International, 1200 Delor Ave., Louisville, Ky. 40217.

The Nurse Theorist: Portraits of Excellence: Imogene King. (1989) Oakland: Studio III from Fuld Video Project, 370 Hawthorne Avenue, Oakland, CA 94609.

Presented Papers

King, I.M. (1980, April 21). *Theory development in nursing*. Paper presented at Georgia State University, Atlanta.

Personal Communication

King, I.M. (1984, Oct. 22). Telephone interview.
King, I.M. (1988, Mar. 8). Telephone interview.

Secondary Sources
Book Reviews

King, I.M. (1971). *Toward a theory for nursing: General concepts of human behavior*.
*Association of Operating Room Nurses' Journal, 14:*126, 1971.
*Canadian Nurse, 67:*40, 1971.
*Nursing Outlook, 19:*513, 1971.
*Nursing Research, 20:*462, 1971.
*American Journal of Nursing, 72:*1153, 1972.
*Journal of Nursing Administration, 2:*63, 1972.
*South African Nursing Journal, 40:*32, 1973.

King, I.M. (1981). *A theory for nursing: Systems, concepts, process*.
*American Association of Nurses and Nephrology Technicians Journal, 3:*39-40, 1981.
*Nursing Mirror, 154:*32, 1982.
*Nursing Outlook, 30:*414, 1982.
*Nursing Times, 78:*331, 1982.
*Research in Nursing and Health, 5:*166-167, 1982.
*Today's OR Nurse, 4:*62, 1982.
*Western Journal of Nursing Research, 4:*103-104, 1982.
Australian Nurses Journal, 12(7):33-34, 1983.

Books

Bevis, E.O. (1982). *Curriculum building in nursing: A process*. St. Louis: C.V. Mosby.

Chaska, N.L. (Ed.). (1983). *The nursing profession: A time to speak*. New York: McGraw-Hill.

Chinn, P.L. (Ed.). (1983). *Advances in nursing theory development*. Rockville, Md.: Aspen Systems.

Chinn, P.L., & Jacobs, M.K. (1983). *Theory and nursing: A systematic approach*. St. Louis: C.V. Mosby.

Fitzpatrick, J.J., & Whall, A.L. (1983). *Conceptual models of nursing: Analysis and application*. Bowie, Md.: Robert J. Brady.

Fitzpatrick, J.J., et al. (1982). *Nursing models and their psychiatric mental health applications*, Bowie, Md.: Robert J. Brady.

Kim, H.S. (1983). *The nature of theoretical thinking in nursing*. Norwalk, Conn.: Appleton-Century-Crofts.

Nursing Theories Conference Group, J.B. George, Chairperson. (1980). *Nursing theories: The base for professional nursing practice*. Englewood Cliffs, N.J.: Prentice-Hall.

Polit, D., & Hungler, B. (1983). *Nursing research: Principles and methods*. Philadelphia: J.B. Lippincott.

Steele, S., (1981). *Child health and the family: Nursing concepts and management*. New York: Masson.

Stevens, B.J. (1984). *Nursing theory: Analysis, application, evaluation* (2d. ed.). Boston: Little, Brown.

Thibodeau, J.A. (1983). *Nursing models: Analysis and evaluation*. Monterey, Cal.: Wadsworth.

Walker, L.O., & Avant, K.C. (1983). *Strategies for theory construction in nursing*. Norwalk, Conn.: Appleton-Century-Crofts.

Who's Who in America (43d. ed.) (1984). Chicago: Marquis.

Who's Who in the Midwest. (1984). Chicago: Marquis.

Who's Who in American Women. (1986).

Who's Who in American Nursing. (1987, 1988).

Book Chapters

Austin, J.K., & Champion, V.L. (1983). King theory for nursing: Explication and evaluation. In P. Chinn, *Advances in nursing theory development*. Rockville, Md.: Aspen Publication, pp. 49-61.

Chinn, P.L., & Jacobs, M.K. (1983). Theory in nursing: A current overview. In *Theory and nursing: A systematic approach*. St. Louis: C.V. Mosby, pp. 190-191.

Fawcett, J. (1984). King's open systems model. In *Analysis and evaluation of conceptual models of nursing*. Philadelphia: F.A. Davis, pp. 83-113.

Fitzpatrick, J., et al. (1982). Nursing models. In *Nursing models and their psychiatric mental health application*. Bowie, Md.: Robert J. Brady, pp. 62-64.

George, J.B. (1980). Imogene M. King. In Nursing Theories Conference Group, J.B. George, Chairperson, *Nursing theories: The base for professional nursing practice*. Englewood Cliffs, N.J.: Prentice-Hall, pp. 184-198.

Gonot, P.J. (1983). Imogene M. King: A theory for nursing. In J. Fitzpatrick & A. Whall, *Conceptual models of nursing: Analysis and application*. Bowie, Md.: Robert J. Brady, pp. 221-243.

Meleis, A.I. (1985). Imogene King. In *Theoretical nursing: Development and progress*. Philadelphia: J.B. Lippincott, pp. 230-237.

Thibodeau, J.A. (1983). History of the development of nursing models. In *Nursing models: Analysis and evaluation*. Monterey, Cal.: Wadsworth, pp. 37-38.

Articles

Brown, S.T., & Lee, B.T. (1980). Imogene King's conceptual framework: A proposed model for continuing nursing education. *Journal of Advanced Nursing, 5(5)*:467-473.

Chance, K.S. (1982). Nursing models: A requisite for professional accountability. *Advances in Nursing Science, 4(2)*:46-65.

Connelly, C.E. (1986). Replication research in nursing. *AORN, 23(1):71-77.*

Craig, S.L. (1980). Theory development and its relevance for nursing. *Journal of Advanced Nursing, 5(4)*:349-355.

Daubenmier, M.J., & King, I.M. (1973). Nursing process models: A systems approach. *Nursing Outlook, 21*:512-517.

Flaskeru, J.H. (1986). On "Toward a Theory of Nursing Action: Skills and Competency in Nurse-Patient Interaction." *Nursing Research, 35(7)*:250-252.

Gortner, S.R., & Nahm, H. (1977). An overview of nursing research in the U.S. *Nursing Research, 26(1)*:10-33.

Jones, P.S. (1978, Nov.) An adaptation model for nursing practice. *American Journal of Nursing, 78*:1900-1906.

Kasch, C.R. (1986). Toward a Theory of Nursing Action: Skills and Competency in Nurse-Patient Interaction. *Nursing Research, 35(4)*:226-229.

Luker, K.A. (1979). Measuring life satisfaction in an elderly female population. *Journal of Advanced Nursing, 4(5)*:503-511.

McFarlane, E.A. (1980). Nursing theory: The comparison of four theoretical proposals. *Journal of Advanced Nursing, 5(1)*:3-19.

Reed, P.G. (1986). A Model for Constructing a Conceptual Framework for Education in Clinical Speciality. *Journal of Nursing Education, 25(9)*:295-329.

Schwirian, P.M., & Kisker, K.L. (1977). Perceptions of health among baccalaureate nursing students. *Journal of Nursing Education, 16(6)*:2-9.

Weikel, C. (1986). Informed consent: Ethical dilemma. *Today's O R Nurse, 9(1)*:11-15.

Whall, A.L. (1980). Congruence between existing theories of family functioning and nursing theories. *Advances in Nursing Science, 3(1)*:59-67.

Other Sources

Allport, F.H. (1955). *Theories of perception and the concept of structure,* New York: John Wiley & Sons.

Bruner, J.S., & Krech, W. (Eds.). (1968). *Perception and personality*. New York: Greenwood.

Bruner, J., Goodnow, J., & Austin, G. (1962). *A study in thinking*. New York: John Wiley & Sons.

Buber, M. (1958). *I and thou*. New York: Charles Scribner's Sons.

Churchman, C.W. (1968). *The systems approach*. New York: Dell.

Churchman, C.W., Ackoff, R., & Wilson, R. (1957). *Introduction to operations research*. New York: John Wiley & Sons.

Counte, M.A., & Christman, I.P. (1981). *Interpersonal behavior and health care*. Boulder, Colo.: Westview.

Dewey, J., & Bentley, A.F. (1949). *Knowing and the known*. Westport, Conn.: Greenwood.

Dubin, R. (1978). *Theory building*. New York: Free Press.

Dubos, R. (1961). *Mirage of health*. New York: Doubleday.

Dubos, R. (1963). *The torch of life*. New York: Pocket Books.

Dubos, R. (1973). *Man adapting*. New Haven: Yale University Press.

Erikson, E. (1964). *Childhood and society*. New York: Norton.

Fawcett, J. (1978). The "what" of theory development. In *Theory development: What, why, how?* New York: NLN Publication 15-1708.

Feigl, H., & Brodbeck, M. (Eds.). (1953). *Readings in the philosophy of science.* New York: Appleton-Century-Crofts.

Freud, S. (1965). *New introductory lectures on psychoanalysis.* New York: W.W. Norton.

Gesell, A.L. (1946). *The child from five to ten.* New York: Harper & Sons.

Gesell, A.L. (1952). *Infant development,* New York: Harper & Row.

Hall, J.E., & Weaver, B.R. (1977). *Distributive nursing: A system approach to community health.* Philadelphia: J.B. Lippincott.

Ittleson, W.H., & Cantril, H. (1954). *Perception: A transactional approach.* Garden City, N.Y.: Doubleday.

Jersild, A.T. (1954). *Child psychology.* New York: Prentice Hall.

Jersild, A.T. (1963). *The psychology of adolescence.* London: Macmillan.

Kelley, K.J., & Hammond, K.R. (1964). An approach to the study of clinical inference. *Nursing Research, 13(4)*:314-322.

Kerlinger, F. (1973). *Foundations of behavioral research* (2nd ed.). New York: Holt, Rinehart, & Winston.

Krieger, D. (1975, May). The therapeutic touch: The imprimatur of nursing. *American Journal of Nursing, 75*:784-787.

Knutson, A. (1965). *The individual, society, and health behavior.* New York: Russell Sage Foundation.

Kuhn, A. (1975). *Unified social science.* Homewood, Ill.: Dorsey Press.

Linton, R. (1936). *The study of man.* New York: Appleton-Century-Crofts.

Merton, R. (1957). *Social theory and social structure.* New York: Macmillan.

Minckley, B.B. (1968, March). Space and place in patient care. *American Journal of nursing, 68*:510-516.

Nagel, E. (1961). *The structure of science.* New York: Harcourt Brace & World.

Orlando, I.J. (1961). *The dynamic nurse-patient relationship.* New York: G.P. Putnam's Sons.

Orlando, I.J. (1972). *The discipline and teaching of nursing process.* New York: G.P. Putnam's Sons.

Orem, D.E. (1971). *Nursing: Concepts of practice.* Scarborough, Ontario: McGraw-Hill.

Orem, D.E. (1979). *Concept formalization in nursing-process and product.* Boston: Little, Brown.

Orem, D.E. (1969). *Time, experience and behavior.* New York: American Elsevier.

Parsons, T. (1951). *The social system.* New York: The Free Press.

Peplau, H. (1952). *Interpersonal relations in nursing.* New York: Putnam's.

Piaget, J. (1962). *Judgment and reasoning in the child.* New York: Humanities. (Reproduction of 1928 ed.).

Seyle, H. (1974). *Stress without distress.* Philadelphia: J.B. Lippincott.

Spiegel, J. (1971). *Transactions: The interplay between individual, family, and society.* New York: Science House.

Thibaut, J., & Jones, E. (1958). Interaction goals as bases of inference in interpersonal perception. In R. Tagiuri, & L. Petrullo (Eds.), *Persons, perception, and interpersonal behavior.* Palo Alto, Calif.: Stanford University Press.

von Bertalanffy, L. (1968). *General systems theory.* New York: Braziller.

Watzlawick, P., Beavin, J.H., & Jackson, D.D. (1967). *Pragmatics of human communication.* New York: Norton.

Weed, L.L. (1969). *Medical records, medical education, and patient care.* Cleveland: Case Western Reserve University Press.

Wiener, N. (1967). *The human use of human beings.* New York: Avon.

Whiting, J.F. (1955, Oct. 5). Q-sort: A technique for evaluating perceptions of interpersonal relationships. *Nursing Research, 4*:70-75.

Wilson, R.N. (1965). The social structure of a general hospital. In J. Skipper and R. Leonard (Eds.), *Social interaction and patient care.* Philadelphia: J.B. Lippincott.

Wooldridge, P.J., et al (1983). *Behavioral science and nursing theory.* St. Louis: C.V. Mosby.

Yura, H., & Walsh, M. (1978). *The nursing process.* New York: Appleton-Century-Crofts.

28

Betty Neuman

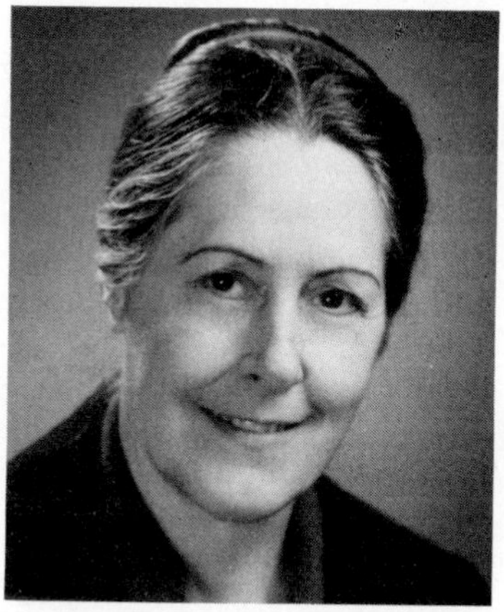

Systems Model

Susan Matthews Harris, Mary E. Hermiz, Mary Meininger, Sandra E. Steinkeler

CREDENTIALS AND BACKGROUND OF THE THEORIST

Betty Neuman was born in 1924 on a farm near Lowell, Ohio. Her father was a farmer and her mother a homemaker. She developed a sense of love for the land while growing up in rural Ohio, and it was because of this rural background that her compassion for people in need evolved. Neuman's first nursing education was completed at Peoples Hospital School of Nursing (now General Hospital) in Akron, Ohio, in 1947. She then moved to Los Angeles to live with relatives. In California she held various positions, including head and hospital staff nurse and school and industrial nurse. She was also involved in clinical teaching in the medical-surgical, communicable disease, and critical care areas. Because she had always had an interest in people's behavior and reaction to struggles, she attended the University of California at Los Angeles with a focus on public health and psychology. She completed her baccalaureate degree in nursing in 1957 and then helped estab-

The authors wish to express appreciation to Judy K. Cowling, Margaret Louis, Rosalie Mirenda, and Betty Neuman for assistance with data collection.

lish and manage her husband's obstetrical and gynecological practice. In 1966 she received her master's degree in Mental Health, Public Health Consultation from UCLA.[26,27] She received a doctoral degree in Clinical Psychology from Pacific Western University in 1985.[30]

Neuman was a pioneer in nursing involvement in mental health. She developed a post-masters community mental health program for nurses at UCLA and was one of the first two nurses to pioneer development of the nurse counselor role in Los Angeles–based community crisis centers. She developed her first explicit teaching and practice model for mental health consultation in the late 1960s, before the creation of her systems model. Neuman designed a conceptual model for nursing in 1970 in response to requests from UCLA graduate students who wanted a course that emphasized breadth rather than depth in understanding human variables in nursing problems. The model initially was developed to integrate student learning of client variables and extended beyond the medical model.[33:265] It included such behavioral science concepts as problem-finding and prevention. Neuman first published her model in 1972. She spent the following decade defining and refining various aspects of the model in preparation for her first book, *The Neuman Systems Model: Application to Nursing Education and Practice*, in 1982. A second edition (1989) contains further development and revision of the model.[28]

Since developing her model, Neuman has been involved in various professional activities, including professional publications and paper presentations, consultations, and conferences, and has served as a group facilitator, lecturer, and instructor. She has remained an active private practice therapist as a licensed clinical member of the American Association of Marriage and Family Therapists since 1970. Neuman maintains her role as consultant internationally for nursing schools and practice agencies adopting the model.[30]

THEORETICAL SOURCES

The model has some similarity to Gestalt theory.[25:14] Gestalt theory maintains that the homeostatic process is the process by which an organism maintains its equilibrium, and consequently its health, under varying conditions. Neuman describes adjustment as the process by which the organism satisfies its needs. Because many needs exist and each may upset client balance or stability, the adjustment process is dynamic and continuous. All life is characterized by this ongoing interplay of balance and imbalance within the organism. When the stabilizing process fails to some degree, or when the organism remains in a state of disharmony for too long and is consequently unable to satisfy its needs, illness may develop. When this compensatory process fails completely, the organism may die.[34:4] The Gestalt approach, then, considers the individual as a function of the organism-environmental field and considers behavior a reflection of relatedness within that field.[34:25]

The model is also derived from philosophical views of deChardin and Bernard Marx.[25:14] Marxist philosophy suggests that the properties of parts are determined partly by the larger wholes within dynamically organized systems. Along with this, Neuman[25:14] confirmed that the patterns of the whole influence awareness of the part, which is drawn from deChardin's philosophy of the wholeness of life. She used H. Selye's definition of *stress,* which is the nonspecific response of the body to any demand made on it.[39:14] Stress increases the demand for readjustment. This demand is nonspecific; it requires adaptation to a problem, irrespective of what the problem is. The essence of stress is therefore the nonspecific demand for activity.[39:15] Stressors are tension-producing stimuli with the potential for causing disequilibrium, such as situational or maturational crises.[32:14]

Neuman's model also reflects general systems theory, that is, the nature of living open systems. This theory states that all the elements are in interaction in a complex organization.[25:3] From G. Caplan's conceptual model for levels of prevention, Neuman relates these prevention levels to nursing in the following manner: Primary prevention involves counteracting harmful environmental stressors before occurrence of illness.[7:26] Secondary prevention attempts to reduce the effect or possible effect of stressors through early diagnostic and effective treatment of illness symptoms. Tertiary prevention attempts to reduce the residual effects following treatment.[7:113] Neuman's model stems from a synthesis of knowledge from several science disciplines and also incorporates her philosophic beliefs and earlier clinical experience, particularly in mental health nursing.[11:36]

USE OF EMPIRICAL EVIDENCE

Neuman conceptualized the model from sound theories rather than from nursing research. She evaluated the model by submitting a tool to her nursing students who were beginning their master's program. The outcome data was published in the 1972 issue of *Nursing Research*. Because the tool was for student evaluation rather than statistical evidence, the model originally lacked empirical support. However, recent research has produced considerable empirical evidence in support of the Neuman Systems Model.

MAJOR CONCEPTS AND DEFINITIONS

The major concepts identified in the model (see Figure 28-1) are: wholistic client approach, open system, basic structure, environment, stressors, lines of defense and resistance, degree of reaction, prevention as intervention, and reconstitution.[25] Neuman's second edition included further development of the concepts of wholistic approach, content, process, input and output, feedback, negentropy, entropy, stability, wellness, and illness.[29]

WHOLISTIC CLIENT APPROACH. The Neuman Systems Model is a dynamic, open, systemic approach to client care originally developed to provide a unifying focus for nursing problem definition and for best understanding the client in interaction with the environment. The model is also considered appropriate for use by other health care providers. The client as a system may be defined as a person, family, group, community, or issue.[29]

WHOLISTIC CONCEPT. Clients are viewed as wholes whose parts are in dynamic interaction. The model considers all variables simultaneously affecting the client system: physiological, psychological, sociocultural, developmental, and spiritual. Neuman included the spiritual variable in the second book edition.[29] She has changed the spelling of the term *holistic* to *wholistic* in the second edition to enhance understanding of the term as referring to the whole person.[30]

OPEN SYSTEM. A system is open when its elements are exchanging information energy within its complex organization. Stress and reaction to stress are basic components of an open system.[29]

ENVIRONMENT. Internal and external forces affecting and being affected by the client at any time comprise the environment.[29]

CONTENT. The five variables (physiological, psychological, sociocultural, developmental, and spiritual) of man in interaction with the environment comprise the whole system of the client.[29]

BASIC STRUCTURE. "The basic structure consists of all variables as survival factors common to man, as well as, unique individual characteristics."[29] The inner circle of the diagram (Figure 28-1) represents the basic survival factors or energy resources of the client.

PROCESS OR FUNCTION. "The exchange of matter, energy, and information with the envi-

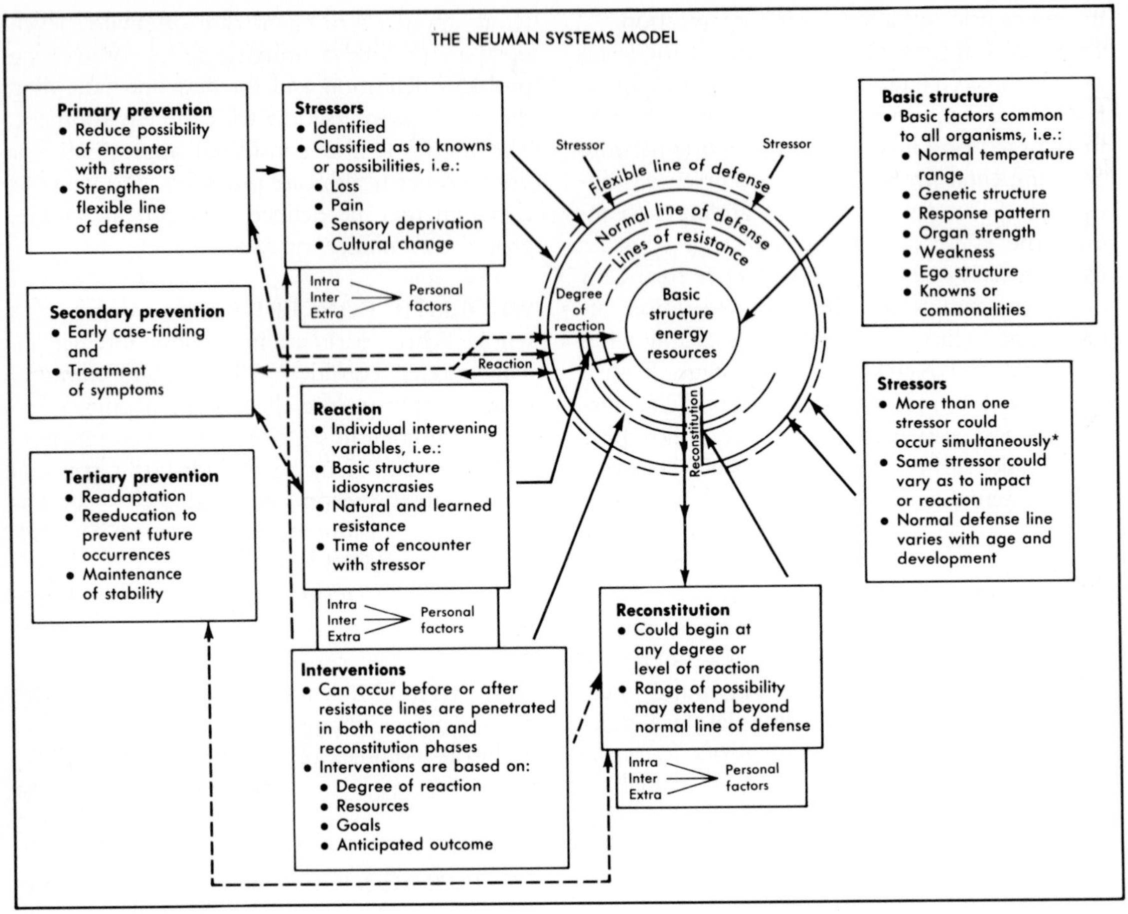

Figure 28-1. The Neuman Systems Model.

ronment and the interaction of the parts and subparts of the system of man. A living system tends to move toward wholeness, stability, wellness, and negentropy."[29]

INPUT AND OUTPUT. "The matter, energy, and information exchanged between man and environment which is entering or leaving the system at any point in time."[29]

FEEDBACK. "The process within which the matter, energy, and information, as system output, provides feedback for corrective action to change, enhance, or stablize the system."[29]

NEGENTROPY. A process of energy absorption that assists the system's progression toward stability or wellness.[29]

ENTROPY. A process of energy depletion that moves the system to illness or death.[29]

STABILITY. As man copes with stressors, he is able to maintain an adequate level of health.

Functional harmony or balance preserves the integrity of the system.[29]

STRESSORS. Stressors are environmental forces that may alter system stability. Neuman[25:14] views stressors as:

1. Intrapersonal—forces occurring within the individual, e.g., conditioned responses.
2. Interpersonal—forces occurring between one or more individuals, e.g., role expectations.
3. Extrapersonal—forces occurring outside the individual, e.g., financial circumstances.

Stressors are "stimuli which might penetrate both the client's flexible and normal lines of defense resulting in either a positive or negative outcome."[29]

WELLNESS. Wellness exists when the parts of the client system are interacting in harmony.[29]

ILLNESS. Disharmony among the parts of the system is considered illness in varying degrees.[29]

NORMAL LINE OF DEFENSE. The normal line of defense is the outer solid circle. It represents a state of equilibrium of the individual, or the state of adaptation the individual has maintained over time that is considered normal for him.

> This is a result or composite of several variables and behaviors such as the individual's usual coping patterns, lifestyle, developmental stage, and so forth; it is basically the way in which an individual deals with stressors while functioning within the cultural pattern in which he was born and to which he attempts to conform.[25:15]

FLEXIBLE LINES OF DEFENSE. The outer broken ring is called the flexible line of defense. It is dynamic and can be rapidly altered over a short period of time. It is perceived as a protective buffer for preventing stressors from breaking through the solid line of defense. The relationship of the variables (physiological, psychological, sociocultural, developmental, and spiritual)[29] can affect the degree to which an individual is able to use his flexible line of defense against possible reaction to a stressor or stressors, such as loss of sleep. It is important to strengthen this flexible line of defense to prevent a possible reaction.[25:15]

LINES OF RESISTANCE. The series of broken rings surrounding the core vary in size and distance from the center and are called the *flexible lines of resistance.* These represent the internal factors that help the client defend against a stressor. An example of this is the body's immune response system.[25:15]

DEGREE OF REACTION. "The degree of reaction is the amount of system instability resulting from stressor invasion of the normal line of defense."[29]

PREVENTION AS INTERVENTION. Interventions are purposeful actions to help the client retain and/or maintain system stability. They can occur before or after resistance lines are penetrated in both reaction and reconstitution phases. Neuman supports beginning intervention when a stressor is either suspected or identified.[25:15] Interventions are based on possible or actual degree of reaction, resources, goals, and the anticipated outcome. Neuman identifies three levels of intervention—primary, secondary, and tertiary, as follows:

Primary prevention. Primary prevention is carried out when a stressor is suspected or identified. A reaction has not yet occurred, but the degree of risk is known. Neuman[25:15] states, "The actor or intervener would perhaps attempt to reduce the possibility of the individual's encounter with the stressor or in some way attempt to strengthen the individual's flexible line of defense to decrease the possibility of a reaction."

Secondary prevention. Secondary prevention involves interventions or treatment initiated after symptoms have occurred. Both the client's internal and external resources would be used toward system stabilization in order to strengthen internal lines of resistance, reduce the reaction, and increase resistance factors.[25:15]

Tertiary prevention. Tertiary prevention is intervention following the active treatment or secondary prevention stage. It focuses on readaptation and stability. A primary goal is to strengthen resistance to stressors by reeducation to help prevent recurrence of reaction or regression. This leads back in a circular fashion toward primary prevention. An example would be avoidance of stressors known to be hazardous to the client.[25:16]

RECONSTITUTION. Reconstitution is the state of adaptation to stressors in the internal and external environment.[25:17] Reconstitution can begin at any degree or level of reaction and may progress beyond, or stabilize somewhat below the client's previous normal line of defense. Included in reconstitution are interpersonal, intrapersonal, extrapersonal, and environmental factors interrelated with physiological, psychological, sociocultural, developmental, and spiritual variables.[25:13;29]

MAJOR ASSUMPTIONS

Nursing

Neuman believes nursing is concerned with the whole person. She views nursing as a "unique profession in that it is concerned with all of the variables affecting an individual's response to stress."[25:14] Because the nurse's perception influences the care given, Neuman states that the caregiver's perceptual field must be assessed as well as the client's. She has developed an assessment and intervention tool to help with this task.

Person

The Neuman Systems Model presents the client as a whole person, that is, as a dynamic composite of interrelationships between physiological, sociocultural, developmental, and spiritual factors. The client is viewed as being in constant change or motion, "in reciprocal action with the environment."[25:9]

Health

Neuman[32:9] defines *health* or *wellness* as "the condition in which all parts and subparts (variables) are in harmony with the whole of the client. Disharmony reduces the wellness state." Man then is an interacting open system with the environment and is either in a dynamic state of wellness or is experiencing some degree of ill health. Health is reflected in the level of wellness. "If man's total needs are met, he is in a state of optimal wellness. Conversely, a reduced state of wellness is the result of needs not met."[25:9]

Environment

Environment is critical to Neuman's model. She states that both internal and external environments exist. The person maintains varying degrees of harmony and balance between the internal and external environment. "Environment has been conceptualized as all factors affecting and affected by the system."[25:9] Thus stressors, which are an important part of the model, comprise the environment. Emphasis is on all stressors—intrapersonal, interpersonal, extrapersonal—that might disturb the person's normal line of defense. Created environment has been added to complete the environmental typology.

THEORETICAL ASSERTIONS

Theoretical assertions are the relationships among the essential concepts of the model. The Neuman model depicts the nurse as an active participant with the client and as "concerned with all the variables affecting an individual's response to stressors."[17:14] The client is in a reciprocal relationship with the environment in that "he interacts with this environment by adjusting himself to it or adjusting it to himself."[17:14] Neuman links the four essential concepts of person, environment, health, and nursing in her statements regarding primary, secondary, and tertiary prevention.

LOGICAL FORM

Neuman used both deductive and inductive logic in developing her model. As previously discussed, Neuman derived her model from other theories and disciplines. The model is also a product of Neuman's philosophy and observations made in mental health nursing and clinical counseling.[12:36]

ACCEPTANCE BY THE NURSING COMMUNITY

Neuman's model has been described as a grand nursing theory by Walker and Avant. A grand theory consists of a global conceptual framework that defines broad perspectives for practice, and includes diverse ways of viewing nursing phenomena based on these perspectives.[42:4] As a grand theory the Neuman Systems Model provides a comprehensive foundation for scientific nursing practice, education, and research.

The Neuman model is being utilized throughout the United States and in Canada, England, Denmark, Portugal, Ghana, Australia, Costa Rica, The Republic of China, Taiwan, Korea, Sweden, and Wales. As an example, following the use of the model with students in public health nursing at the Danish School of Advanced Nursing Education at Aarhus University and the subsequent publication describing its application to care of the elderly, 400 visiting nurse organizations utilized the Neuman model to evaluate nursing interventions. Neuman states that the Danish Health Ministry is currently funding a program to develop national primary preventive health care services to the elderly using her model.[23:140;30]

The model has been adapted equally well to all levels of nursing education and a wide variety of practice areas. It has been adapted transculturally and is used extensively for public health nursing in other countries.

Universal appeal for the model is also reflected in the development of the First International Symposium on the Neuman Systems Model, which was held in Philadelphia in 1986.[22;28] As a result of the positive response from the nursing community, a biannual symposium has evolved. The second symposium was hosted in Kansas City, Missouri, in October 1988.[20;22;28;38]

Practice

Mirenda states that the Neuman model has broad relevance for current and future nursing practice. Use of the model by nurses facilitates goal-directed, unified, wholistic approaches to client care, yet it is also appropriate for interdisciplinary use to prevent fragmentation of client care. The model delineates a client system and classification of stressors that can be understood and utilized by all members of the health care team.[23:140]

Neuman has developed the Neuman Nursing Process Format to implement the model. It is comprised of the following three steps: nursing diagnosis, nursing goals, and nursing outcomes (see Figure 28-2). Nursing diagnosis consists of obtaining a broad, comprehensive data base from which variances from wellness can be determined. Goals are then established by negotiation with the client for desired prescriptive changes to correct variances from wellness. Nursing outcomes are determined by nursing intervention through use of one or more of the three prevention as intervention modes. Evaluation then takes place either to confirm the desired outcome goals or to reformulate subsequent nursing goals.

Neuman has developed several instruments to facilitate the utilization of the systems model. The assessment/intervention tool (see Appendix A) can assist the nurse in synthesizing client data (Figure 28-4, p. 382). An intermediate step, now developed as an intervention typology, facilitates operationalization of the conceptual model (Figure 28-5, p. 383). Guidelines to establish nursing goals, nursing interventions,

Figure 28-2. Nursing Process Format for the Neuman Model.

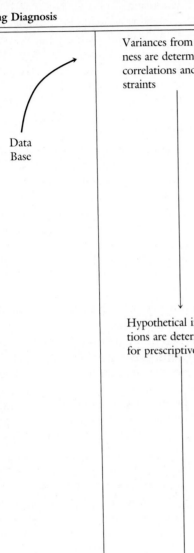

Nursing Diagnosis

Data Base

Variances from wellness are determined by correlations and constraints

Hypothetical interventions are determined for prescriptive change

I. Nursing Diagnosis
   A. Data Base: Determined by:
      1. Identification and evaluation of potential or actual stressors which pose a threat to the stability of the client and/or client system.
      2. Assessment of condition and strength of basic structure factors and energy resources.
      3. Assessment of characteristics of the flexible and normal lines of defense, lines of resistance, degree of potential reaction, reaction, and/or potential for reconstitution following a reaction.
      4. Identification, classification, and evaluation of potential and/or actual intra-, inter-, and extrapersonal interactions between the client and environment, considering all five variables.
      5. Evaluation of past, present, and possible future life-process and coping patterns influence on client system stability.
      6. Identification and evaluation of actual and potential internal and external resources for optimal state of wellness.
      7. Identification and resolution of perceptual differences between care givers and client/client system.

   NOTE: In all the above areas of consideration the care giver simultaneously considers (dynamic interactions in the client/client system) all five variables: physiological, psychological, sociocultural, developmental and spiritual.

   B. Variances from Wellness: Determined by:
      1. Synthesis of theory with client data identifies the condition from which a comprehensive diagnostic statement can be made. Goal prioritization is determined by client/client system wellness level, system stability needs, and total available resources to accomplish desired goal outcomes.
      2. Hypothetical goals and interventions are postulated to reach the desired client stability or wellness level, i.e., to maintain the normal line of defense and retain the flexible line of defense thus protecting the basic structure.

Figure 28-2. Nursing Process Format for the Neuman Model, cont'd.

Nursing Goals

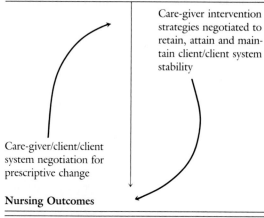

Care-giver intervention strategies negotiated to retain, attain and maintain client/client system stability

Care-giver/client/client system negotiation for prescriptive change

II. Nursing Goals: Determined by:

1. Negotiations with the client for desired prescriptive change or goal outcomes to correct variances from wellness, based on classified needs and resources identified in the nursing diagnosis.
2. Appropriate prevention as intervention strategies are negotiated with the client for retention, attainment and/or maintenance of client system stability as desired outcome goals. Theoretical perspectives used for assessment and client data synthesis are analogous to those used for intervention.

Nursing Outcomes

Confirmation of prescriptive change or reformulation of nursing goals

Nursing intervention using one or more prevention modes.

Short term goal outcomes influence intermediate/long-range goal determination

Client outcome validates nursing process, and acts as feedback for further system input as required.

III. Nursing Outcomes: Determined by:

1. Nursing intervention accomplished through use of one or more of the following three prevention modes: (1) primary prevention (action to retain system stability). (2) secondary prevention (action to attain system stability). (3) tertiary prevention (action to maintain system stability), usually following secondary prevention/intervention.
2. Evaluation of outcome goals following intervention either confirms outcome goals or serves as a basis for reformulation of subsequent goals based on systemic feedback principals.
3. Intermediate and long-range goals for subsequent nursing action are structured in relation to short-term goal outcomes.
4. Client goal outcome validates the nursing process.

Figure 28-3. Format for prevention as intervention.
Copyright 1980 by Betty Neuman. Revised 1987 by Betty Neuman. Used with permission.

Primary Prevention	Secondary Prevention	Teritary Prevention
Nursing Action* to: 1. Classify stressors† as to client/client system threat to stability. Prevent stressor invasion. 2. Provide information to maintain or strengthen existing client/client system strengths. 3. Support positive coping and functioning. 4. Desensitize existing or possible noxious stressors. 5. Motivate toward wellness. 6. Coordinate/integrate interdisciplinary theories and epidemiologic input. 7. Educate/reeducate. 8. Use stress as a positive intervention strategy.	Nursing Action to: 1. Following stressor invasion, protect basic structure. 2. Mobilize and optimize internal/external resources toward stability and energy conservation. 3. Facilitate purposeful manipulation of stressors and reactions to stressors. 4. Motivate, educate, and involve client and client system in health care goals. 5. Facilitate appropriate treatment/intervention measures. 6. Support positive factors toward wellness. 7. Promote advocacy by coordination/integration. 8. Provide primary prevention/intervention as required.	Nursing Action to: 1. During reconstitution, attain/maintain maximum level of wellness and stability following treatment. 2. Educate, reeducate, and/or reorient as needed. 3. Support client/client system toward appropriate goal directedness. 4. Coordinate and integrate health service resouces 5. Provide primary and/or secondary prevention/intervention as needed.

*A first priority for nursing action, in each of the areas of prevention as intervention, is to determine the nature of stressors and their threat to the client/client system.
Some general categorical functions for nursing action are initiation, planning, organization, monitoring, coordinating, implementing, integrating, advocating, supporting and evaluating. An example of a limited classification system for stressors is illustrated by the following four categories: 1) deprivation, 2) excess, 3) change, and 4) intolerance.

and nursing outcomes are all presented by Neuman in her nursing process format (Figures 28-6 and 28-7, pp. 385–386).

The breadth of the Neuman model has resulted in its application and adaptation in a variety of nursing practice settings with individuals, families, groups, and communities. Numerous examples are described in Neuman's books.[25;28]

The model was used in the Hospice of Windsor in Ontario to organize multidisciplinary assessments and interventions for individuals and families dealing with life-threatening and terminal illnesses.[10:257] Baker used the model in planning for the psychological needs of individuals with respiratory diseases.[3:241] Sullivan has applied Neuman's model to nursing assessment and intervention in the acute phase of spinal cord injury.[40:34] Kiernan and Scoloveno have used the model in the assessment of neonates and their families.[17:2] Darland selected the Neuman model as a basis for purposeful nursing intervention to assist individuals and families affected by congenital adrenocortical hyperplasia.[9:120]

Adaptations of the Neuman Systems Model in nursing practice are diverse. Goldblum-Graff and Graff adapted the model to family therapy[13:217]; Bowman utilized it in the assessment of child day-care centers[5:324]; Babcock adapted and applied Neuman's model in a cardiac stepdown unit and found that the use of the assessment tool created an open rapport with the client, thereby enhancing overall communication.[2] A case study approach was selected by Ross and Bourbannais to demonstrate application of the model to home nursing care of a post-myocardial infarction client.[36:200]

Anderson, McFarlane, and Helton adapted the model to develop a community health needs assessment in which the authors identified violence toward women as a major community health concern. Funding from the March of Dimes was subsequently obtained for a community wide program to prevent battering of pregnant women by their spouses and to promote violence-free relationships.[1:220]

The Neuman Systems Model is utilized equally well with clients as individuals, groups, or communities. Its comprehensive, systemic nature allows for a wide variety of clinical practice, research, and administrative applications.

Education

The model has also been well accepted in academic circles. It is widely utilized as a curriculum guide oriented toward wellness and is used at all levels of nursing education throughout the United States. For example, in the associate degree program at Indiana University/Purdue University at Ft. Wayne, Indiana, one of the objectives for nursing graduates is to demonstrate ability to use the Neuman Systems Model in nursing practice.[16] Achievement of this objective prepares students to use or develop a wholistic framework for nursing practice.

Neuman's model has been selected for baccalaureate programs on the basis of its theoretical and comprehensive perspectives for a wholistic curriculum.[19:128] For example, the University of Pittsburgh became the first baccalaureate nursing program to implement the model in an integrated curriculum.[18:117;30] Saint Anselm College School of Nursing in Manchester, New Hampshire, and Neumann College School of Nursing in Aston, Pennsylvania, have also incorporated the model into baccalaureate curriculum design.[22;29]

Ross, Bourbannais, and Carroll describe the selection and application of the Neuman model at the University of Ottawa for the final year of a generic baccalaureate program that incorporates a curriculum design of theoretical pluralism. An emphasis on collaboration with clients, an interdisciplinary approach to care, and Neuman's focus on prevention as intervention with a wholistic approach to client conditions were identified by the faculty as important areas of concern for beginning professional nurses.[37:76-79]

At Northwestern State University in Shreveport, Louisiana, the faculty determined that a systems model approach was preferred for their master's program because of the universality of its application. They chose to adapt the Neuman model in their program for their master's clinician, the role being one of mediator between stressors and the various lines of defense and resistance of the client or client system.[24:168-169] Many universities have adopted this model and use its conceptual framework. Acceptance by the nursing community for education therefore is clearly evident.

Research

For nursing to advance as a scientific discipline, testing the efficacy and usefulness of nursing models through controlled research is imperative. Research of components of the model for additional explication and generation of testable nursing theories through research are examples of the Neuman model's potential contribution to research activity and nursing knowledge.[23:139]

Increasing empirical utilization of the Neuman Systems Model is evident in the nursing community. Craddock and Stanhope tested the usefulness of the model in a home health-care agency, obtaining results suggestive of the model's utility in categorization of data for nursing assessment and planning for the client's care.[8:163] Ziemer investigated the effects of primary prevention and lines of defense upon the impact of stressors in clients undergoing abdominal surgery. Empirical indicators in Ziemer's study included preoperative information, client coping behaviors, postoperative pain intensity, distress, and symptoms of surgical complications.[11:164-165]

Ziegler has derived a taxonomy for nursing diagnosis from the Neuman model at Texas Woman's University that is being validated. Ziegler states that a nursing diagnosis taxonomy could provide a more systematized method for organizing nursing research and for developing nursing theory.[43:55]

Hoch conducted research with the Neuman Systems Model while searching for appropriate frameworks for the organization of geriatric nursing practice.[14:10] The results of the study with elderly adults in the community setting support the use of the model in the planning and delivery of nursing care.[14:17] Louis and Koertvelyessy conducted a 1987 international survey study of the Neuman model in student nursing research projects, reporting a total of 42 studies completed or in process. The authors utilized the steps of the research process to analyze the identified studies and to make recommendations for further testing and theory development.[20;21] Abstracts of these studies are presented in the second edition of Neuman's book.

Neuman reports that her model is one of the three most frequently utilized models for nursing research. She has also identified additional topics for further research using her model. She suggests that evaluation of primary preventive health education programs for school children, availability of alternative health-care delivery services to clients, development of primary prevention programs for adults in the middle years of 40 to 60, and evaluation of multidisciplinary health promotion programs are appropriate contemporary issues for exploration and research with the Neuman model.[27,28,30]

FURTHER DEVELOPMENT

A conceptual model identifies relevant phenomena and describes the interrelationships in general and abstract terms, representing the initial step in the development of theoretical statements.[12:31] Walker and Avant have previously described the Neuman model as being at a very early stage of theory development.[42:142] However, findings from Louis and Koertvelyessy's recent international study suggest support for the utility of the model for theory development in nursing. A systematized format has been developed by Louis for use of the model in nursing research.[21]

Although Craddock and Stanhope have recommended simplification of the model's schematic, the diagram has remained unchanged due to continuous positive feedback to Neuman on its completeness. The authors also suggest clarification of the nurse's role in the health-care system and identification of intervention techniques at the various levels of prevention as additional areas of further development for the Neuman model.[8:166]

Several critics have identified a need for further development of Neuman's derivation of systems theory, as well as a more dynamic conceptualization of stress.[12:40;41:146] Although her original model describes both mechanistic (stimulus-response) and organismic (wholistic) views of the relationship between the individual and the environment, Neuman reports that her refined model's primary focus is an organismic view of stress with an emphasis on the reciprocal interaction between the client and the environment.[31] Torres also recommends further specification and integration of the multidimensional variables within the individual and the environment.[41:150]

Buchanan has used the concepts of the Neuman Systems Model in community health nursing to develop a "macro systems" nursing view (1) to facilitate a community approach to relationships between the client and the environment and (2) to intervene with preventive, corrective, and rehabilitative measures.[6:52-53]

Neuman and Koertvelyessy have identified as a major theory for the model the theory of optimal client system stability. Neuman views the prevention as intervention concept as having potential for theoretical formulation and states that several other theories are inherent within the model.[29] Nursing research is needed to validate the Neuman Systems Model and the newly defined theory of optimal client system stability.

A Neuman Systems Model Trustee Group has been established by Neuman to preserve, protect, and perpetuate the integrity of the model for the future of nursing. Its international members, personally selected by Neuman, are dedicated professionals using the model.[29]

CRITIQUE

Neuman developed a comprehensive nursing conceptual model that operationalizes systems concepts for nursing relevant to the breadth of nursing phenomena. It should remain relevant as well to future nursing needs such as the ANA and WHO concerns for primary prevention. Its lack of specificity allows for a wide range of nurse creativity in its use.

Clarity

Neuman presents abstract concepts that are familiar to nursing. Although additional definitions could be helpful, the model's concepts of client, environment, health, and nursing are all inherent and congruent with traditional values. Concepts defined by Neuman and those borrowed from other disciplines are used consistently throughout the model.

Simplicity

Multiple interactions and interrelationships comprise this broad systemic model; they are organized in a complex yet logical manner, and variables tend to overlap to some degree. The concepts coalesce, but a loss of theoretical meaning would occur if they were completely separated. Neuman states that the concepts can be separated for analysis, specific goal setting, and interventions.[31] The model can be used to delineate further the systems concept for nursing and describe various other health-care systems as well. It can be used to explain the client's dynamic state of equilibrium and the reaction or possible reaction of stressors as a result of environmental conflict. Using the prevention concept within the framework, one can predict the origin of stressors. The model can be used to describe, explain, or predict nursing phenomena. Because of the complex nature of the model, it cannot be described as a simple framework, yet nurses using the model describe it as easy to understand and adapt within a variety of cross-cultural groups.

Generality

The Neuman nursing framework has been used in various nursing situations and is general and comprehensive enough to be useful in all health-care settings, including administration and research. Other related health fields can use this framework because of its systemic nature and emphasis on the client as a whole. The social goals and utility of the framework, for example, wholistic care, prevention, and systems concepts, are congruent with present social values.

Some concepts are broad and represent the phenomenon of the person or client, and others are more definitive and identify specific modes of action, such as primary prevention. The subgoals can be identified as broad nursing actions. Because of the broad scope of this framework, it can be considered general in nature yet inclusive of all nursing phenomena under consideration.

Empirical Precision

Although the framework has not been completely tested to date, nursing scientists are demonstrating increasing interest in and utilization of the model to guide nursing research. Hoffman has described a list of variables and selected operational definitions that have been derived from the Neuman model.[15:49-53] Ziegler's nursing diagnosis taxonomy is a useful contribution to further research and theory development. Findings by Hoch suggest that planned nursing interventions based on the Neuman model are more effective in decreasing dysphasia and increasing life satisfaction among elderly retirees than the absence of planned intervention.[14:17] Louis and Koertvelyessy's 1987 survey on the utilization of the model in nursing research provides further documentation of increasing empiricism with the model. Additional testing and refinement will increase the model's empirical precision, including use of the steps of the research process, analysis, and synthesis of findings from multiple studies as they are completed.[21]

Derivable Consequences

Neuman's conceptual framework provides the professional nurse with important guidelines for assessment of the whole person, utilization of the nursing process, and implementation of preventive intervention. The focus on primary prevention and interdisciplinary care facilitates improved quality of care and is futuristic. Active client participation and negotiation of nursing goals may facilitate improved communication and compliance with the nursing plan of care.

Another derivable consequence of the model is its proven ability to generate nursing theory. With continued theory development through research with the model, nursing can expand its scientific knowledge.

The Neuman Systems Model provides an appropriate nursing framework and comprehensive approach to contemporary and future global phenomena and concerns facing nursing in the twenty-first century.[23:155] The role of the nurse in the future can become dominant if the nursing profession accepts the challenge to assume leadership in the unification of health-care delivery using the broad systems perspectives of the Neuman Systems Model.[8:168]

REFERENCES

1. Anderson, E., McFarland, J., & Helton, A. (1986). Community-as-client: A model for practice. *Nursing Outlook, 34(5)*:220-224.
2. Babcock, P. (1984, June 10). Telephone interview.
3. Baker, N.A. (1982). Use of the Neuman model in planning for the psychological needs of the respiratory disease patient. In B. Neuman, *The Neuman systems model: Application to nursing education and practice*. Norwalk, Conn.: Appleton-Century-Crofts, pp. 241-256.
4. Bertalanffy, L. von. (1968). *General systems theory*. New York: George Braziller.
5. Bowman, G. (1982). The Neuman assessment tool adapted for child day-care centers. In B. Neuman, *The Neuman systems model: Application to nursing education and practice*. Norwalk, Conn.: Appleton-Century-Crofts, pp. 324-334.
6. Buchanan, B.F. (1987). Human-environment interaction: A modification of the Neuman systems model for aggregates, families, and the community. *Public Health Nursing, 4(1)*:52-64.
7. Caplan, G. (1964). *Principles of preventive psychiatry*. New York: Basic Books.
8. Craddock, R.B., & Stanhope, M.K. (1980). The Neuman health care systems model: Recommended adaptation. In J.P. Riehl & C. Roy, *Conceptual models for nursing practice*. New York: Appleton-Century-Crofts, pp. 159-169.
9. Darland, N.W. (1986). Congenital adrenocortical hyperplasia: Supportive nursing interventions. *Journal of Pediatric Nursing, 1(2)*:117-123.
10. Echlin, J.D. (1982). Palliative care and the Neuman model. In B. Neuman, *The Neuman systems model: Application to nursing education and practice*. Norwalk, Conn.: Appleton-Century-Crofts.
11. Fawcett, J. (1984). *Analysis and evaluation of conceptual models of nursing*. Philadelphia: F.A. Davis Co.
12. Fawcett, J., Carpenito, L.J., Efinger, J., Goldblum-Graff, D., Groesbeck, M., Lowry, L.W., McCreary, C.S., & Wolf, Z.R. (1982). A framework for analysis and evaluation of conceptual models of nursing with an analysis of the Neuman systems model. In B. Neuman, *The Neuman systems model: Application to education and practice*. Norwalk, Conn.: Appleton-Century-Crofts, pp. 30-43.
13. Goldblum-Graff, D., & Graff, H. (1982). The Neuman model adapted to family therapy. In B. Neuman, *The Neuman systems model: Application to nursing education and practice*. Norwalk, Conn.: Appleton-Century-Crofts, pp. 217-222.
14. Hoch, C.C. (1987). Assessing delivery of nurs-

ing care. *Journal of Gerontological Nursing, 13(11)*:10-17.
15. Hoffman, M.K. (1982). From model to theory construction: An analysis of the Neuman health-care system model. In B. Neuman, *The Neuman systems model: Application to nursing education and practice*. Norwalk, Conn.: Appleton-Century-Crofts, pp. 44-54.
16. Indiana University, Purdue University at Ft. Wayne. (1983). *Behavioral objectives for the associate degree program.*
17. Kiernan, B.S., & Scoloveno, M.A. (1986). Assessment of the neonate. *Topics in Clinical Nursing, 8(1)*:1-10.
18. Knox, J.E., Kilchenstein, L., & Yakulis, I.M. (1982). Utilization of the Neuman model in an integrated baccalaureate program: University of Pittsburgh. In B. Neuman, *The Neuman systems model: Application to nursing education and practice*. Norwalk, Conn.: Appleton-Century-Crofts.
19. Lebold, M.M., & Davis, L.H. (1982). A baccalaureate nursing curriculum based on the Neuman systems model: Saint Xavier College. In B. Neuman, *The Neuman systems model: Application to nursing education and practice*. Norwalk, Conn.: Appleton-Century-Crofts.
20. Louis, M. (1988, January 10). Telephone interview.
21. Louis, M., & Koertvelyessy, A. (In press). Neuman model: Use in research. In B. Neuman (Ed.), *The Neuman systems model: Applications in nursing education and practice* (2d ed.). Norwalk, Conn.: Appleton-Lange.
22. Mirenda, R. (1988, January 10). Telephone interview.
23. Mirenda, R.M. (1986). The Neuman systems model: Description and application. In P. Winstead-Fry (Ed.), *Case studies in nursing theory*. New York: National League of Nursing, pp. 127-167.
24. Moxley, P.A., & Allen, M.H. (1982). The Neuman systems model approach in a master's degree program: Northwestern State University. In B. Neuman, *The Neuman systems model: Application to nursing education and practice*. Norwalk, Conn.: Appleton-Century-Crofts.
25. Neuman, B. (1982). *The Neuman systems model: Application to nursing education and practice.* Norwalk, Conn.: Appleton-Century-Crofts.
26. Neuman, B. (1983). Curriculum vitae.
27. Neuman B. (1984, June 3). Telephone interview.
28. Neuman, B. (1988, Jan. 10). Telephone interview.
29. Neuman, B. (1988, Jan. 20). Personal correspondence.
30. Neuman, B. (1988, Feb. 11). Telephone interview.
31. Neuman, B. (1988, Feb. 18). Personal correspondence.
32. Neuman, B.M. (1977, Jan. 17). An explanation of the Betty Neuman Nursing Model. Paper presented to Indiana University-Purdue University at Fort Wayne, Indiana.
33. Neuman, B.M., & Young, R.J. (1972, May-June). A model for teaching total person approach to patient problems. *Nursing Research, 21*:264-269.
34. Perls, F. (1973). *The Gestalt approach: Eye witness to therapy*. Palo Alto, Cal.: Science and Behavior Books.
35. Reynolds, P.D. (1971). *A primer in theory construction*. Indianapolis, Ind.: Bobbs-Merrill.
36. Ross, M.M., & Bourbannais, F.F. (1985). The Neuman systems model in nursing practice: A case study approach. *Journal of Advanced Nursing, 10*:199-207.
37. Ross, M.M., Bourbannais, F.F., & Carroll, G. (1987). Curriculum design and the Betty Neuman systems model: A new approach to learning. *International Nursing Review, 34(3)*:75-79.
38. Russell, J. (1988, Jan. 10). Telephone interview.
39. Selye, H. (1974). *Stress without distress.* Philadelphia: J.B. Lippincott.
40. Sullivan, J. (1986). Using Neuman's model in the acute phase of spinal cord injury. *Focus on Critical Care, 13(5)*:34-41.
41. Torres, G. (1986). *Theoretical foundations of nursing*. Norwalk, Conn.: Appleton-Century-Crofts.
42. Walker, L.O., & Avant, K. (1983). *Strategies for theory construction in nursing*. Norwalk, Conn.: Appleton-Century-Crofts.
43. Ziegler, S.M. (1982). Taxonomy for nursing diagnosis derived from the Neuman systems model. In B. Neuman, *The Neuman systems model: Application to nursing education and practice*. Norwalk, Conn.: Appleton-Century-Crofts, pp. 55-68.

BIBLIOGRAPHY

Primary Sources

Books

Neuman, B. (1989). *The Neuman systems model: Applications in nursing education and practice* (2d ed.). Norwalk, Conn.: Appleton-Lange.

Neuman, B. (1982). *The Neuman systems model: Application to nursing education and practice.* Norwalk, Conn.: Appleton-Century-Crofts.

Neuman, B., Deloughery, G.W., & Gebbie, M. (1971). *Consultation and community organization in community mental health nursing.* Baltimore: Williams & Williams.

Book Chapters

Neuman, B. (1983). Analysis and application of Neuman's health care model. In I.W. Clements & F.B. Roberts, *Family health: A theoretical approach to nursing care.* New York: John Wiley & Sons, pp. 353-367.

Neuman, B. (1983). Family interaction using the Betty Neuman health care systems model. In I.W. Clements & F.B. Roberts, *Family health: A theoretical approach to nursing care.* New York: John Wiley & Sons, pp. 239-254.

Neuman, B. (1980). The Betty Neuman health care systems model: A total person approach to patient problems. In J.P. Riehl & C. Roy (Eds.), *Conceptual models for nursing practice* (2d ed.). New York: Appleton-Century-Crofts, pp. 119-134.

Neuman, B. (1974). The Betty Neuman health care systems model: A total person approach to patient problems. In J.P. Riehl & C. Roy, (Eds.), *Conceptual models for nursing practice.* New York: Appleton-Century-Crofts, pp. 94-104.

Neuman, B., & Wyatt, M. (1980). The Neuman stress/adaptation systems approach to education for nurse administrators. In J.P. Riehl & C. Roy (Eds.), *Conceptual models for nursing practice* (2d ed.). New York: Appleton-Century-Crofts, pp. 142-150.

Articles

Neuman, B., Deloughery, G.W. and Gebbie, K.M. (1974, Jan.). Teaching organizational concepts to nurses in community mental health. *Journal of Nursing Education, 13:1.*

Neuman, B.M., Deloughery, G.W., & Gebbie, K.M. (1970, Jan.-Feb.). Levels of utilization: Nursing specialists in community mental health. *Journal of Psychiatric Nursing and Mental Health Services, 8(1)*:37-39.

Neuman, B.M., Deloughery, G.W., & Gebbie, K.M. (1970). Changes in problem solving ability among nurses receiving mental health consultation: A pilot study. *Communicating Nursing Research, 3*:41-52.

Neuman, B.M., Deloughery, G.W., & Gebbie, K.M. (1971, Oct.). Nurses in community mental health: An informative interpretation for employees of professional nurses. *Public Personnel Review, 32(4).*

Neuman, B.M., Deloughery, G.W., & Gebbie, K.M. (1972, Feb.). Mental health consultation as a means of improving problem solving ability in work groups: A pilot study. *Comparative Group Studies, 3(1)*:81-97.

Neuman, B., & Wyatt, M.A. (1981, Jan.). Prospects for change: Some evaluative reflections by faculty members from one articulated baccalaureate program. *Journal of Nursing Education, 20*:40-46.

Neuman, B.M., & Young, R.J. (1972, May-June). A model for teaching total person approach to patient problems. *Nursing Research, 21*:264-269.

Professional Papers

Neuman, B. (1970, Nov.). *Emerging leadership in mental health: Preparation of community mental health specialists.* Presented at the World Mental Health Assembly, Washington, D.C.

Neuman, B. (1970, Nov.). *Improved utilization of nurses in community mental health.* Position paper presented to the Task Force for Development of the California State Plan for Health, Sacramento.

Neuman, B. (1970, April, May). *A pilot study to measure change in problem solving ability among nurses receiving mental health consultation.* Paper presented at the Western Interstate Commission for Higher Education Conference on Communicating Research in Nursing, Salt Lake City, and at the State Department of Mental Health Center for Training in Community Psychiatry, Los Angeles.

Neuman, B. (1971, March). *Toward healthy, productive group interaction.* Paper presented to the Psychiatric Mental Health Conference Group, California Nurses' Association Convention, Anaheim.

Neuman, B. (1980, Dec.). *A systems approach to the integrity of the client/client system based on the Neuman model.* Paper presented at the International Congress on Applied Systems Research and Cybernetics, Acapulco, Mexico.

Neuman, B. (1985, April). *The Neuman systems model for nursing.* Paper presented for the Royal College of Nursing and *Senior Nurse Magazine,* jointly sponsored, Models for Nursing Conference, University of Manchester, Manchester, England.

Neuman, B. (1985, April). *The Neuman systems model: Its relevance to nursing education, practice and research.* Paper presented to The Post Graduate School of Nursing, Aarhus and Copenhagen, Denmark, and to the Danish Institute for Health and Nursing Research, Copenhagen, Denmark.

Neuman, B. (1985, Aug.). *The Neuman systems model: Application to nursing education, practice and research.* Paper presented for the Nursing Theory in Action Conference, sponsored by Boyle, Letourneau & Associates, Inc., Edmonton, Alberta.

Neuman, B. (1986, Aug.). *The Neuman systems model: Usage in nursing education, practice and research.* Paper presented to the Nursing Theory Congress on Theoretical Pluralism: Direction for a Practice Discipline, sponsored by the Ryerson School of Nursing, Toronto, Ontario, Canada.

Correspondence

Neuman, B. (1984, June 4). Personal correspondence.

Neuman, B. (1988, Jan. 20). Personal correspondence.

Neuman, B. (1988, Feb. 18). Personal correspondence.

Interviews

Neuman, B. (1984, June 3). Telephone interview.

Neuman, B. (1988, Jan. 10). Telephone interview.

Neuman, B. (1988, Feb. 11). Telephone interview.

Neuman, B. (1988, May). Telephone interview.

Secondary Sources

Book Reviews

Hawkins, J. (1983). [Review of *The Neuman systems model: Application to nursing education and practice.*] *Western Journal of Nursing Research, 5:*182-183.

Varricchio, C.G. (1983). [Review of *The Neuman systems model: Application to nursing education and practice*]. *American Journal of Nursing, 83:*963-964.

Book Chapters

Arndt, C. (1982). Systems theory and educational programs for nursing service administration. In B. Neuman, *The Neuman systems model: Application to nursing education and practice.* Norwalk, Conn.: Appleton-Century-Crofts, pp. 182-187.

Arndt, C. (1982). Systems concepts for management of stress in complex health-care organizations. In B. Neuman, *The Neuman systems model: Application to nursing education and practice.* Norwalk, Conn.: Appleton-Century-Crofts, pp. 107-116.

Baker, N.A. (1982). The Neuman systems model as a conceptual framework for continuing education in the work place. In B. Neuman, *The Neuman systems model: Application to nursing education and practice.* Norwalk, Conn.: Appleton-Century-Crofts, pp. 260-266.

Baker, N.A. (1982). Use of the Neuman model in planning for the psychological needs of the respiratory disease patient. In B. Neuman, *The Neuman systems model: Application to nursing education and practice.* Norwalk, Conn.: Appleton-Century-Crofts, pp. 241-256.

Balch, C. (1974). Breaking the lines of resistance. In J.P. Riehl & C. Roy, *Conceptual models for nursing practice.* New York: Appleton-Century-Crofts, pp. 130-134.

Beitler, B., Tkachuck, B., & Aamodt, D. (1980). The Neuman model applied to mental health, community health, and medical-surgical nursing. In J.P. Riehl and C. Roy (Eds.), *Conceptual models for nursing practice* (2d ed.). New York: Appleton-Century-Crofts, pp. 170-178.

Benedict, M.B., & Sproles, J.B. (1982). Application of the Neuman model to public health nursing practice. In B. Neuman, *The Neuman systems model: Application to nursing education and practice.* Norwalk, Conn.: Appleton-Century-Crofts, pp. 223-240.

Bower, F.L. (1982). Curriculum development and the Neuman Model. In B. Neuman, *The Neuman systems model: Application to nursing education and practice.* Norwalk, Conn.: Appleton-Century-Crofts, pp. 94-99.

Bowman, G.E. (1982). The Neuman assessment tool adapted for child day-care centers. In Neuman, B., *The Neuman systems model: Application to nursing education and practice.* Norwalk, Conn.: Appleton-Century-Crofts, pp. 324-334.

Breckenridge, D.M. (1982). Adaptation of the Neuman systems model for the renal client. In B. Neuman, *The Neuman systems model: Application to nursing education and practice.* Norwalk, Conn.: Appleton-Century-Crofts, pp. 267-277.

Cardona, V.D. (1982). Client rehabilitation and the Neuman model. In B. Neuman, *The Neuman systems model: Application to nursing education and practice.* Norwalk, Conn.: Appleton-Century-Crofts, pp. 278-290.

Clark, F. (1982). The Neuman systems model: A clinical application for psychiatric nurse practitioners. In B. Neuman, *The Neuman systems model: Application to nursing education and practice.* Norwalk, Conn.: Appleton-Century-Crofts, pp. 335-354.

Conners, V.L. (1982). Teaching the Neuman systems model: An approach to student and faculty development. In B. Neuman, *The Neuman systems model: Application to nursing education and practice.* Norwalk, Conn.: Appleton-Century-Crofts, pp. 176-181.

Conners, V., Harmon, V.M., & Langford, R.W. (1982). Course development and implementation using the Neuman systems model as a framework: Texas Woman's University (Houston Campus). In B. Neuman, *The Neuman systems model: Application to nursing education and practice.* Norwalk, Conn.: Appleton-Century-Crofts, pp. 153-158.

Craddock, R.B., & Stanhope, M.K. (1980). The Neuman health care systems model: Recommended adaptation. In J.P. Riehl & C. Roy, (Eds.), *Conceptual models for nursing practice* (2d ed.). New York: Appleton-Century-Crofts, pp. 159-169.

Cross, J. (1985). Betty Neuman. In J. George (Ed.), *Nursing theories: The base for professional nursing practice.* Englewood Cliffs, N.J.: Prentice-Hall, pp. 258-285.

Cunningham, S.G. (1982). The Neuman model applied to an acute care setting: Pain. In B. Neuman, *The Neuman systems model: Application to nursing education and practice.* Norwalk, Conn.: Appleton-Century-Crofts, pp. 291-296.

Davis, L.H. (1982). Aging: A social and preventive perspective. In B. Neuman, *The Neuman systems model: Application to nursing education and practice.* Norwalk, Conn.: Appleton-Century-Crofts, pp. 211-216.

Dunbar, S.B. (1982). Critical care and the Neuman model. In B. Neuman, *The Neuman systems model: Application to nursing education and practice.* Norwalk, Conn.: Appleton-Century-Crofts, pp. 297-307.

Echlin, D.J. (1982). Palliative care and the Neuman model. In B. Neuman, *The Neuman systems model: Application to nursing education and practice.* Norwalk, Conn.: Appleton-Century-Crofts, pp. 257-259.

Fawcett, J. (1984). Neuman systems model. In J. Fawcett, *Analysis and evaluation of conceptual models of nursing.* Philadelphia: F.A. Davis, pp. 154-174.

Fawcett, J., Carpenito, L., Epinger, J., Goldblum-Graff, D., Groesbeck, M., Lowry, L., McCreary, C., & Wolf, Z. (1982). A framework for analysis and evaluation of conceptual models of nursing with an analysis and evaluation of the Neuman systems model. In B. Neuman, *The Neuman systems model: Application to nursing education and practice.* Norwalk, Conn.: Appleton-Century-Crofts, pp. 30-43.

Goldblum-Graff, D., & Graff, H. (1982). The Neuman model adapted to family therapy. In B. Neuman, *The Neuman systems model: Application to nursing education and practice,* Norwalk, Conn.: Appleton-Century-Crofts, pp. 217-222.

Gunter, L.M. (1982). Application of the Neuman systems model to grontic nursing. In B. Neuman, *The Neuman systems model: Application to nursing education and practice,* Norwalk, Conn.: Appleton-Century-Crofts, pp. 196-210.

Harty, M.B. (1982). Continuing education in nursing and the Neuman model. In B. Neuman, *The Neuman systems model: Application to nursing education and practice.* Norwalk, Conn.: Appleton-Century-Crofts, pp. 100-106.

Hermiz, M.E., & Meininger, M. (1986). Betty Neuman: Systems model. In A. Marriner (Ed.), *Nursing theorists and their work.* St. Louis: C.V. Mosby, pp. 313-331.

Hoffman, M.K. (1982). From model to theory construction: An analysis of the Neuman health-care systems model. In B. Neuman, *The Neuman systems model: Application to nursing education and practice.* Norwalk, Conn.: Appleton-Century-Crofts, pp. 44-54.

Johnson, N., Vaughn-Wrobel, B., Ziegler, S.M., Hugh, L., Bush, H.A., & Kurtz, P. (1982). Use of the Neuman health-care systems model in the master's curriculum: Texas Woman's University. In B. Neuman, *The Neuman systems model: Application to nursing education and practice.* Norwalk, Conn.: Appleton-Century-Crofts, pp. 130-152.

Knox, J.E., Kilchenstein, L., & Yakulis, I.M. (1982). Utilization of the Neuman model in an integrated baccalaureate program: University of Pittsburgh.

In B. Neuman, *The Neuman systems model: Application to nursing education and practice.* Norwalk, Conn.: Appleton-Century-Crofts, pp. 117-123.

Lebold, M., & Davis, L. (1980). A baccalaureate nursing curriculum based on the Neuman health systems model. In J.P. Riehl & C. Roy (Eds.), *Conceptual models for nursing practice* (2d ed.). New York: Appleton-Century-Crofts, pp. 151-158.

Lebold, M.M., & Davis, L.H. (1982). A baccalaureate nursing curriculum based on the Neuman systems model: Saint Xavier College. In B. Neuman, *The Neuman systems model: Application to nursing education and practice.* Norwalk, Conn.: Appleton-Century-Crofts, pp. 124-129.

Leddy, S., & Pepper, J.M. (1985). Models of nursing. In S. Leddy, & J.M. Pepper, *Conceptual bases of professional nursing.* Philadelphia: J.B. Lippincott Co., pp. 135-149.

Louis, M., & Koertvelyessy, A. (In press). Neuman model: Use in research. In B. Neuman (Ed.), *The Neuman systems model: Applications in nursing education and practice* (2d ed.). Norwalk, Conn.: Appleton-Lange.

McInerey, K.A. (1982). The Neuman systems model applied to critical care nursing of cardiac surgery clients. In B. Neuman, *The Neuman systems model: Application to nursing education and practice.* Norwalk, Conn.: Appleton-Century-Crofts, pp. 308-315.

Mayers, M.A., & Watson, A.B. (1982). Nursing care plans and the Neuman systems model. In B. Neuman, *The Neuman systems model: Application to nursing education and practice.* Norwalk, Conn.: Appleton-Century-Crofts, pp. 69-84.

Mirenda, R.M. (1986). The Neuman systems model: Description and application. In P. Winstead-Fry (Ed.), *Case studies in nursing theory.* New York: National League of Nursing, pp. 127-167.

Moxley, P.A., & Allen, L.M.H. (1982). The Neuman systems model approach in a master's degree program: Northwestern State University. In B. Neuman, *The Neuman systems model. Application to nursing education and practice.* Norwalk, Conn.: Appleton-Century-Crofts, pp. 168-175.

Neal, M.C. (1982). Nursing care plans and the Neuman systems model: II. In B. Neuman, *The Neuman systems model: Application to nursing education and practice.* Norwalk, Conn.: Appleton-Century-Crofts, pp. 85-93.

Pinkerton, A. (1974). Use of the Neuman model in a home health-care agency. In J.P. Riehl & C. Roy (Eds.), *Conceptual models for nursing practice.* New York: Appleton-Century-Crofts, pp. 122-129.

Reed, K. (1982). The Neuman systems model: A basis for family psychosocial assessment and intervention. In B. Neuman, *The Neuman systems model: Application to nursing education and practice.* Norwalk, Conn.: Appleton-Century-Crofts, pp. 188-195.

Rice, M.J. (1982). The Neuman systems model applied in a hospital medical unit. In B. Neuman, *The Neuman systems model: Application to nursing education and practice.* Norwalk, Conn.: Appleton-Century-Crofts, pp. 310-323.

Thibodeau, J.A. (1983). A systems model: The Neuman model. In J.A. Thibodeau, *Nursing models: Analysis and evaluation.* Monterey, Cal.: Wadsworth, pp. 105-123.

Tollett, S.M. (1982). Teaching geriatrics and gerontology: Use of the Neuman systems model. In B. Neuman, *The Neuman systems model: Application to nursing education and practice.* Norwalk, Conn.: Appleton-Century-Crofts, pp. 157-164.

Torres, G. (1986). Systems-oriented theories. In G. Torres, *Theoretical foundations of nursing.* Norwalk, Conn.: Appleton-Century-Crofts, pp. 112-165.

Venable, J. (1974). The Neuman health-care systems model: An analysis. In J.P. Riehl & C. Roy (Eds.), *Conceptual models for nursing practice.* New York: Appleton-Century-Crofts, pp. 115-121.

Venable, J.F. (1980). The Neuman health-care systems model: An analysis. In J.P. Riehl & C. Roy (Eds.), *Conceptual models for nursing practice* (2d ed.), New York: Appleton-Century-Crofts, pp. 135-141.

Vokaty, D.A. (1982). The Neuman systems model applied to the clinical nurse specialist role. In B. Neuman, *The Neuman systems model: Application to nursing education and practice.* Norwalk, Conn.: Appleton-Century-Crofts, pp. 165-167.

Whall, A. (1983). The Betty Neuman health care systems model. In J. Fitzpatrick & A.L. Whall (Eds.), *Conceptual models of nursing analysis and application.* Bowie, Md.: Robert J. Brady, pp. 204-219.

Walker, L.O., & Avant, K.C. (1983). Theory analysis: The Betty Neuman health care systems model: A total person approach to patient problems. In L.A. Walker & K.C. Avant, *Strategies for theory construction in nursing.* Norwalk, Conn.: Appleton-Century-Crofts, pp. 133-143.

Ziegler, S.M. (1982). Taxonomy for nursing diagnosis derived from the Neuman systems model. In B. Neuman, *The Neuman systems model: Application to nursing education and practice*. Norwalk, Conn.: Appleton-Century-Crofts, pp. 55-68.

Articles

Anderson, E., McFarlane, J., & Helton, A. (1986). Community-as-client: A model for practice. *Nursing Outlook, 34(5)*:220-224.

Buchanan, B.F. (1987). Human-environment interaction: A modification of the Neuman systems model for aggregates, families, and the community. *Public Health Nursing, 4(1)*:52-64.

Darland, N.W. (1986). Congenital adrenocortical hyperplasia: Supportive nursing interventions. *Journal of Pediatric Nursing, 1(2)*:117-123.

Hoch, C.C. (1987). Assessing delivery of nursing care. *Journal of Gerontological Nursing, 13(1)*:10-17.

Johnson, P.T. (1983). Black hypertension: A transcultural case study using the Betty Neuman model of nursing care. *Issues in Health Care, 4*:191-210.

Kiernan, B.S., & Scoloveno, M.A. (1986). Assessment of the neonate. *Topics in clinical nursing, 8(1)*:1-10.

Ross, M., & Bourbonnais, F. (1985). The Neuman systems model in nursing practice: A case study approach. *Journal of Advanced Nursing, 10*:199-207.

Ross, M.M. Bourbonnais, F.F., & Carroll, G. (1987). Curriculum design and the Betty Neuman systems model: A new approach to learning. *International Nursing Review, 34(3)*:75-79.

Sullivan, J. (1986). Using Neuman's model in the acute phase of spinal cord injury. *Focus on Critical Care, 13(5)*:34-41.

Tlaskund, J.H. (1980). Areas in theory development. *Advances in Nursing Science, 3*:1-7.

Utz, S.W. (1980). Applying the Neuman model to nursing practice with hypertensive clients. *Cardiovascular Nursing, 16*:29-34.

Dissertations

Capers, C.F. (1986). *Perceptions of problematic behavior as held by lay black adults and registered nurses.* Doctoral dissertation. University of Pennsylvania.

Dunbar, S.B. (1983). *The effect of formal patient education on selected psychological and physiological variables of adaptation after acute myocardial infarction.* Doctoral dissertation. University of Alabama.

Glazer, G.L. (1984). *The relationship between pregnant women's anxiety levels and stressors and their partners' anxiety levels and stressors.* Doctoral dissertation. Case Western Reserve University.

Schlosser, S.P. (1985). *The effect of anticipatory guidance on mood state in primiparas experiencing unplanned cesarean delivery (metropolitan area, southeast).* Doctoral dissertation. University of Alabama.

Schmidt, C.C. (1982). *A comparison of the effectiveness of two nursing models in decreasing depression and increasing life satisfaction of retired individuals.* Doctoral dissertation. University of Pittsburgh.

Thornbill, B.E. (1985). *A Q-analysis of stressors in the primipara during the immediate postpartal period.* Doctoral dissertation. University of Alabama.

Underwood, P.W. (1986). *Psychosocial variables: Their prediction of birth complications and relation to perception of childbirth (life stress, social support, coping, commitment).* Doctoral dissertation. University of Michigan.

Ziemer, M.M. (1982). *Providing patients with information prior to surgery and the reported frequency of coping behaviors and development of symptoms following surgery.* Doctoral dissertation. University of Pennsylvania.

Interviews

Babcock, P. (1984, June 10). Telephone interview.

Louis, M. (1988, Jan. 10). Telephone interview.

Mirenda, R. (1988, Jan. 10). Telephone interview.

Russell, J. (1988, Jan. 10). Telephone interview.

Unpublished papers

Babcock, B. *Euthanasia and the Neuman model.*

Beaman, C. *The leukemia client and the Neuman model.*

Burton, C. *The Neuman systems model: Application with black clients and their families.*

Crow, S. *Client advocacy using the Neuman total person approach: A nursing art.*

Edwards, B. *The Neuman model applied in a community mental health partial hospitalization program.*

Green, P. *A modified assessment-intervention tool for the Neuman systems model used with colostomy patients.*

Lassan, R. *Use of the Neuman systems model in the care of the high-risk newborn.*

Lowry, L. *Application of the Neuman systems model to a clinical study: Ego functions in normal pregnant women.*

Vanore, N. *Application of the Neuman systems model to an acute drug psychosis in a psychiatric clinical situation.*
Wardian, J. *Child abuse and the Neuman model.*

*Appendix A**

For nurses who wish to develop their *own* assessment-intervention tools for use with the Neuman Systems Model, the following considerations should be made: (1) that proper assessment would include all knowledge of factors influencing the client's perceptual field and (2) that the meaning of a stressor would be validated by both the client and caregiver; thus, distortions become apparent for resolution toward relevant nursing action.

Figure 28-4, now entitled An Assessment/Intervention Tool Development Guide, is a revision of the former Intermediate Step in the Neuman Model, in Riehl and Roy (1974 and 1980) publications. Because of its wide usage, it is carried forward for those who may continue to benefit from its use in development of their own "tools." This guide should facilitate linkage of the Neuman Systems Model concepts to an operational assessment and intervention tool by identifying some facts and conditions from which client goals are established and modified. Its utility for care continuity and clarification of caregiver role relationships needs exploration.

THE ASSESSMENT/INTERVENTION TOOL

The assessment/intervention tool (Figure 28-4) is designed to include the various aspects of the Neuman Systems Model while allowing for inclusion of other areas of information, such as individual specific client or larger client system needs, for example, age, situational differences, or special requirements for financial aid.

The assessment/intervention tool is readily adaptable for use by nursing to determine limited needs of individual clients as well as broadly based concerns of the client system, such as entire communities or social issues. A unique feature is that the kind of data obtained from the clients' own perceptions of their conditions influences the overall goals for nursing action. Hence, the form itself is not to be submitted to the client but should be used as a question for obtaining comprehensive data.

The following format should offer a progressive total view of facts and conditions from which client goals are developed and modified as needed. Because all caregivers can relate to this assessment/intervention format, continuity of care should be facilitated through its use and role relationships clarified.

AN EXPLANATION OF THE ASSESSMENT/INTERVENTION TOOL

Category A—Biographic Data (see Figure 28-5)

A-1. This section includes general biographic data. However, certain agencies may require additional data in this area.

A-2. Referral source and related information are important. They provide a background history about the client and make possible any contacts with those who interviewed the client earlier. Requests from agencies for reciprocal relationships might be recorded in this area.

Category B—Stressors as Perceived by Clients

B-1. It is important to find out from the clients how they perceive or experience their particular situation or condition. By clarifying clients' perceptions, data are obtained for optimal care planning.

B-2. Clients should be allowed to discuss how their present lifestyles are related to past, or usual, lifestyle patterns. A marked change may be significantly related to the course of an illness or possible illness.

*Used with permission from Reihl, J.P. and Roy, C. (1974). Conceptual models for Nursing Practice. New York: Appleton-Century Crofts, pp. 108-114.

Figure 28-4 An assessment/intervention tool development guide.

Primary Prevention	Secondary Prevention	Tertiary Prevention
*Stressors** Covert or potential	*Stressors** Overt, actual or known	*Stressors** Overt, or residual—possible covert
Reaction Hypothetical or possible based on available knowledge	*Reaction* Identified symptoms or known stress factors	*Reaction* Hypothetical or known—residual symptoms or known stress factors
Assessment† Based on client assessment, experience, and theory Risk or possible hazard based on client/nurse perception Meaning of experience to client Lifestyle factors Coping patterns (past, present, possible) Individual differences identified	*Assessment†* Determined by nature and degree of reaction Determine internal/external available resources to resist the reaction Rationale for goals—collaborative goal setting with client	*Assessment†* Determined by degree of stability following treatment and further potential reconstitution for possible regression factors
Intervention Strengthen client flexible line of defense Client education Desensitization to stressors Stressor avoidance Strengthen individual resistance factors	*Intervention as treatment* Wellness variance—overt symptoms—nursing diagnosis Need priority and related goals Client strengths and weaknesses related to the five client variables Shift of need priorities as client responds to treatment (primary prevention needs and tertiary prevention may occur simultaneously with treatment or secondary prevention) Intervention in maladaptive processes Optimal use of internal/external resources such as energy conservation, noise reduction, and financial aid	*Intervention as reconstitution following treatment* Motivation Education-reeducation Behavior modification Reality orientation Progressive goal setting Optimal use of available internal/external resources Maintenance of client optimal functional level

*Environmental stressors include intra-, inter-, and extrapersonal factors.
†Assessment/intervention, based on the Neuman Systems Model, ideally would consider simultaneously the interrelationship of the five interacting and interdependent client variables: physiological, psychological, sociocultural, developmental, and spiritual.

B-3. This area relates to coping patterns. It is important to learn what similar conditions may have existed in the past and how the client has dealt with them. Such data provide insight about the type of resources available that were mobilized to deal with the situation. Past coping patterns may be significantly related to the present situation, making possible certain predictions as to what a client may or may not be able to accomplish. For example, symptoms of present loss might be exaggerated following unresolved past losses.

Figure 28-5. An assessment/intervention tool based on the Neuman Systems Model.

CLIENT

A. *Intake Summary*
   1. Name ______________________
      Age ______________________
      Sex ______________________
      Marital Status ______________________
   2. Referral source and related information.

B. *Stressors as Perceived by Client* (If client is incapacitated, secure data from family or other resources.)
   1. What do you consider your major stress area, or areas of health concern? (Identify these areas)
   2. How do present circumstances differ from your usual pattern of living? (Identify life-style patterns)
   3. Have you ever experienced a similar problem? If so, what was that problem and how did you handle it? Were you successful? (Identify past coping patterns)
   4. What do you anticipate for yourself in the future as a consequence of your present situation? (Identify perceptual factors, i.e., reality versus distortions-expectations, present and possible future coping patterns)
   5. What are you doing and what can you do to help yourself? (Identify perceptual factors, i.e., reality versus distortions-expectations, present and possible future coping patterns)
   6. What do you expect care givers, family, friends, or others to do for you? (Identify perceptual factors, i.e., reality versus distortions-expectations, present and possible future coping patterns)

C. *Stressors as Perceived by Care Giver*
   1. What do you consider to be the major stress area, or areas of health concern? (Identify these areas)
   2. How do present circumstances seem to differ from the client's usual pattern of living? (Identify life-style patterns)
   3. Has the client ever experienced a similar situation? If so, how would you evaluate what the client did? How successful do you think it was? (Identify past coping patterns)
   4. What do you anticipate for the future as a consequence of the client's present situation? (Identify perceptual factors, i.e., reality versus distortions-expectations, present and possible future coping patterns)
   5. What can the client do to help himself? (Identify perceptual factors, i.e., reality versus distortions-expectations, present and possible future coping patterns)
   6. What do you think the client expects from care givers, family, friends or other resources? (Identify perceptual factors, i.e., reality versus distortions-expectations, present and possible future coping patterns)

SUMMARY OF IMPRESSIONS

Note any discrepancies or distortions between the client perception and that of the care giver related to the situation.

D. *Intrapersonal Factors*
   1. Physical (Examples: degree of mobility; range of body function)
   2. Psycho-sociocultural (Examples: attitudes, values, expectations, behavior patterns and nature of coping patterns)
   3. Developmental (Examples: age, degree of normalcy, factors related to present situation)
   4. Spiritual belief system (Examples: hope and sustaining factors)

E. *Interpersonal Factors*
   Examples are resources and relationship of family, friends, or care givers that either influence or could influence Area D.

F. *Extrapersonal Factors*
   Examples are resources and relationship of community facilities, finances, employment, or other areas which either influence or could influence Areas D and E.

Continued.

Figure 28-5. An assessment/intervention tool based on the Neuman Systems Model, cont'd.

G. *Formulation of a comprehensive nursing diagnosis*
Is accomplished by identifying and ranking the priority of needs based on total data obtained from the client's perception, the care giver's perception, and/or other resources, i.e., laboratory reports, other care givers or agencies. Appropriate theory is related to the above data.

With this format, reassessment is a continuous process and is related to the effectiveness of intervention based upon the prior stated goals. Effective reassessment would include the following as they relate to the total client situation:

1. Changes in nature of stressors and priority assignments.
2. Changes in intrapersonal factors.
3. Changes in interpersonal factors.
4. Changes in extrapersonal factors.

In reassessment it is important to note the change of priority of goals in relation to the primary, secondary, and tertiary prevention as intervention categories. An assessment tool of this nature should offer a current, progressive, and comprehensive analysis of the client's total circumstances and relationship of the five client variables (physiologic, psychologic, sociocultural, developmental and spiritual) to environmental influences.

B-4. The area of client expectations is important in planning health-care interventions. Goals for care could be inappropriate if not based on clarification of how clients perceive their situations or conditions. For example, a client might erroneously think his situation is terminal all the while that the caregiver attempts to prepare the client for living.

B-5. If the extent of client motivation to help themselves can be learned, available internal and external resources can be more wisely used in their behalf.

B-6. The health-care cost factor can often be a source of stress for the client. Sufficient data should be obtained from the clients about health-care services they feel are needed. However, the practitioner should bear in mind that the client frequently requires help in determining what services are realistic.

Category C—Stressors as Perceived by Caregiver

The fact that caregivers have a perspective different from that of the client is considered a positive factor. Yet, education, past experiences, values, personal biases, and unresolved personal conflicts can distort the caregiver's clear conception of the client's actual condition. Category C was included to reduce this possibility. Questions one through six are essentially the same as those in Category B so that the client's own perception can be compared with the caregiver's. The interviewer should know the basis for his own perceptions as well as the client's so that the reality of the client's situation or condition can be fairly accurately described in a summary of impressions.

Categories D, E, and F—as Perceived by Both Caregiver and Client

These categories deal with the intra-, inter-, and extrapersonal factors illustrated on the model diagram. In order to assess an individual's total situation or condition at any point, it is necessary to know the relationship among internal environmental factors, factors occurring between the individual and his environment, as well as external environmental factors that are or could affect the individual. This set of questions attempts to clarify these relationships so that it is possible to establish goal priorities.

Category G—Nursing Diagnosis

A clear comprehensive statement of the client condition requires the reconciliation of perceptual differences between client and caregiver. All pertinent aspects of client data must be ordered according to need priority before appropriate client goals can be determined.

Summary of Goals with Rationale

Once the major problem has been defined in relation to all factors affecting the client situation or condition, further classification is needed. A decision must be made as to what form of intervention should take priority. For example, if a reaction has not yet occurred and the client has been assessed as being in a high-risk category, intervention should begin at the primary prevention intervention level. Moreover, one should be able to state the logic or rationale for the intervention. If a reaction is noted on assessment (that is, symptoms are obvious), intervention should begin at the secondary prevention level (treatment). When assessment is made following treatment, intervention

Primary Prevention (Prevention of Treatment)	Secondary Prevention (Treatment)	Tertiary Prevention (Follow up after Treatment)
Immediate Goals: 1. 2. 3. Rationale:		
Intermediate Goals: 1. 2. 3. Rationale:		
Future Goals: 1. 2. 3. Rationale:		

Figure 28-6. Summary of Goals with Rationale.

should begin at the tertiary prevention level (follow-up after treatment).

By relating all factors affecting the client, it is possible to determine fairly accurately what type of intervention is needed (primary, secondary, or tertiary) as well as the rationale to support the stated goals. At whatever point interventions are begun, it is important to attempt to project possible future health care requirements. This data may not be readily available on initial assessment, but should be noted when possible to provide a comprehensive and progressive view of the client's total condition. It is important to relate this section of the assessment/intervention tool to the intervention (worksheet) plan (Figure 28-6).

Intervention Plan to Support Stated Goals

This portion of the assessment/intervention tool is a form of worksheet (Figure 28-7) that provides progressive data as to the type of intervention given by goal as listed and ranked by priority. The type of interventions, and their outcomes, are noted. The comment section might include data useful for future planning, such as new goal priorities based upon changes in the client's condition or responses, and success or failure of past and/or present interventions. This format classifies each intervention in a consistent, progressive, and comprehensive manner to which any caregiver can meaningfully relate. This system of classifying data over

Primary Prevention	**Secondary Prevention**	**Tertiary Prevention**
Date		
Goals*	Goals*	Goals*
1.	1.	1.
2.	2.	2.
3.	3.	3.
Intervention:	Intervention:	Intervention:
Outcome:	Outcome:	Outcome:
Comments:	Comments:	Comments:

*Goals are stated in order of priority.

Figure 28-7. Intervention plan to support stated goals.

Reproduced with revision from Neuman, B. (1974). The Betty Neuman Health Care Systems Model: A Total Approach to Patient Problems. In J.P. Riehl and C. Roy (Eds.), *Conceptual Models for Nursing Practice*. New York, Appleton-Century-Crofts.

time allows one to see the relationship of the part to the whole, that is, to view the client in total perspective, thereby reducing the possibility of fragmentation of care and possibly reducing cost factors.

Appendix B

The following is an incomplete listing of schools and agencies using the Neuman Systems Model or selected concepts from it.

EDUCATIONAL PROGRAMS

Aarhus University, Advanced School of Nursing, Aarhus, Denmark.

Aarhus University, Advanced School of Nursing, Brands Campus, Copenhagen, Denmark.

Altoona Hospital, School of Nursing, Altoona, Pennsylvania. Diploma program.

Anne Marie College, Paxton, Massachusetts. Baccalaureate program.

Bob Jones University, School of Nursing, Greenville, South Carolina. Baccalaureate program.

California State University, Fresno, California. Baccalaureate and master's program.

Concordia College, Milwaukee, Wisconsin. Baccalaureate program.

Delta State College, Cleveland, Mississippi. Baccalaureate program.

Esoola De Enfermagen De Saude Publica, Lisbon, Portugal. Public Health Nurse Education.

Heritage Community College, Hull, Quebec, Canada. Associate degree program.

Indiana University–Purdue University at Fort Wayne, Indiana, School of Nursing. Associate degree program.

Lander College, Greenwood, South Carolina. Baccalaureate program.

Marshall University, School of Nursing, Huntington, West Virginia. Baccalaureate program.

Medical University of South Carolina, Charleston, South Carolina.

Methodist Central Hospitals of Memphis, Nursing Diploma School, Memphis, Tennessee.

Minnesota Intercollegiate Nursing Consortium, St. Paul, Minnesota. Baccalaureate program.

Neumann College, Aston, Pennsylvania. Baccalaureate program.

North Dakota State University, Tri-County, Fargo, North Dakota. Baccalaureate program.

Northwestern State University of Louisiana, Shreveport, Louisiana. Graduate program.

Queens University, School of Nursing, Kingston, Ontario, Canada. Baccalaureate program.

Rutgers State University of New Jersey, School of Nursing, Newark, New Jersey. Baccalaureate program.

Saint Anselm College, School of Nursing, Manchester, New Hampshire. Baccalaureate program.

Saint Xavier College, School of Nursing, Chicago, Illinois. Baccalaureate and graduate programs.

Santa Fe Community College, School of Nursing, Gainesville, Florida. Associate degree program.

Seattle Pacific University, School of Nursing, Seattle, Washington. Baccalaureate program.

Simmons College, Boston, Massachusetts. Baccalaureate program.

Southern College, Southern, West Virginia. Associate degree program.

Southern Oregon State College, Ashland, Oregon. Baccalaureate program.

Syracuse University, School of Nursing, Syracuse, New York. Baccalaureate program.

Texas Women's University at Dallas and Houston, Denton, Texas. Graduate program.

Union College, School of Nursing, Lincoln, Nebraska. Baccalaureate program.

University of British Columbia, Vancouver, Canada.

University of Kuwait, Kuwait City, Kuwait. Associate degree and baccalaureate programs.

University of London, Diploma in Nursing School, Colchester Institute, London, England.

University of Missouri, School of Nursing, Kansas City, Missouri. Master's program.

University of Nevada at Las Vegas, School of Nursing, Las Vegas, Nevada. Associate degree, baccalaureate, and master's programs.

University of Ottawa, Public Health and Perinatal Nursing, Ottawa, Canada. Master's program.

University of Pittsburgh, School of Nursing, Pittsburgh, Pennsylvania. Baccalaureate program.

University of Portland, School of Nursing, Portland, Oregon. Master's program.

University of Puerto Rico, School of Nursing, San Juan, Puerto Rico. Baccalaureate and master's programs.

University of Saskatchewan, School of Nursing, Saskatoon, Saskatchewan, Canada. Baccalaureate program.

University of Southern Colorado, Colorado. Baccalaureate program.

University of Texas, Tyler, Texas. Baccalaureate program.

University of Wyoming, School of Nursing, Laramie, Wyoming. Baccalaureate program.

Yakima Valley Community College, Yakima, Washington. Associate degree program.

Yan Ming Medical College, Nursing Program, Taipei, Taiwan.

CLINICAL AGENCIES

Albert Einstein Medical Center, Hospice Program, Philadelphia, Pennsylvania.

Bernadotte Gaarden Nursing Home, Hadsund, Denmark.

Bolton Road Community Mental Health Centre, Yorkshire, England.

Boston City Health Department, Community Health Nursing, Health and Hospitals, Boston, Massachusetts.

Colchester Institute, Community Educational Studies for Nursing, Colchester, Essex, England.

Community Nursing Service, County of Moldrup, Denmark.

Community Psychiatric Nurse Practice, Breconshire, Powys, Wales.

Friends Hospital (Psychiatric Hospital), Nursing Service, Philadelphia, Pennsylvania.

High Roads Hospital (Peter McGinnis, Unit Nursing Advisor), Yorkshire, England.

Jefferson Davis Memorial Hospital, Nursing Service, Natchez, Mississippi.

John Astor House, Department of Continuing Nurse Education, London, England.

Juan de Fuca Hospitals, Victoria, British Columbia, Canada.

Mercy Catholic Medical Center, Fitzgerald Mercy Division, Nursing Service Department, Darby, Pennsylvania.

Metropolitan General Hospital, Hospice Program, Windsor, Ontario, Canada.

Middlesex-London Health Unit, Community Health Nursing, London, Ontario, Canada.

Mount Sinai Hospital, Nursing Service Department, Hartford, Connecticut.

Pembury Hospital (Sue Torkington, Community Tutor), Pembury, Tunbridge Wells, Kent, England.

Peterborough Civic Hospital, Nursing Service, Peterborough, Ontario, Canada.

Regional Perinatal Education Program of Eastern Ontario, Nursing Department, Ottawa, Ontario, Canada.

Rehabilitation Institute of the South, Nursing Department, Shreveport, Louisiana.

Roblealtor Child Care Center, Latino American Missions, Costa Rica.

St. Elizabeth, Visiting Nurse Association, Willowdale, Ontario, Canada.

St. Vincent Hospital, Nursing Service, Melbourne, Australia.

University Hospital, Nursing Service, Saskatoon, Saskatchewan, Canada.

University of Maryland, Maryland Institute of Emergency Medical Services, Critical Care Unit, Baltimore, Maryland.

Veteran's Administration, Nursing Service, Roseburg, Oregon.

Veteran's Hospital, Nursing Program, Taipei, Taiwan.

Victoria Hospital, Toronto, Ontario, Canada.

Visiting Nurse Agencies, Denmark.

UNIT V

Energy Fields

29

Myra Estrin Levine

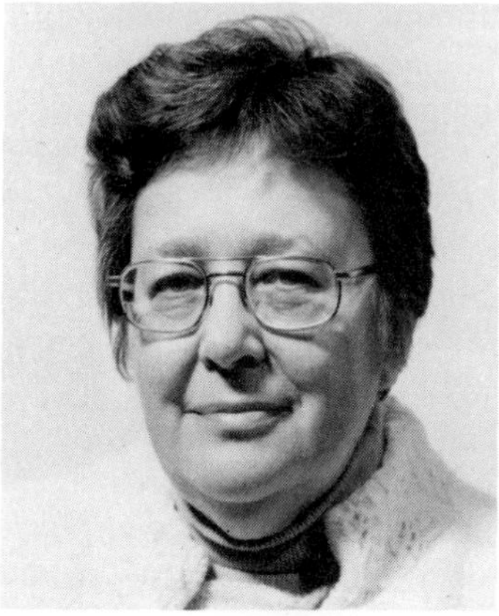

Four Conservation Principles

Karen J. Foli, Tamara Johnson, Ann Marriner-Tomey, Mary Carolyn Poat, LaDema Poppa, Roberta Woeste, Susan T. Zoretich

CREDENTIALS AND BACKGROUND OF THE THEORIST

Myra Estrin Levine obtained a diploma from Cook County School of Nursing in 1944, an S.B. from the University of Chicago in 1949, and an M.S.N. from Wayne State University in 1962, and has taken postgraduate courses at the University of Chicago.[29] Hutchins' curriculum was being taught to undergraduate students at that time. All students took a year-long survey in the biological, physical, and social sciences and the humanities. The students read and analyzed primary work under the guidance of distinguished professors. Irene Beland became Levine's mentor while she was a graduate student at Wayne State and directed her attention to many of the authors who greatly influenced her thinking.[31,32]

Levine has enjoyed a varied career. She has been a private duty nurse (1944), a civilian nurse in the U.S. Army (1945), a preclinical instructor in the physical sciences at Cook County (1947-1950), the director of Nursing

The authors wish to express appreciation to Myra Levine for critiquing the chapter.

at Drexel Home in Chicago (1950-1951), and a surgical supervisor at the University of Chicago Clinics (1951-1952) and at Henry Ford Hospital in Detroit (1956-1962). She worked her way up the academic ranks at Bryan Memorial Hospital in Lincoln, Nebraska (1951), Cook County School of Nursing (1963-1967), Loyola University (1967-1973), Rush University (1974-1977), and the University of Illinois (1962-1963, 1977-1987). She chaired the Department of Clinical Nursing at Cook County School of Nursing (1963-1967) and coordinated the graduate nursing program in oncology at Rush University (1974-1977). Levine was the director of the Department of Continuing Education at Evanston Hospital (March-June 1974) and a consultant to the department (July 1974-1976). She was an adjunct associate professor of Humanistic Studies at the University of Illinois 1981-1987. She is now a Professor Emerita, Medical Surgical Nursing, University of Illinois at Chicago. In 1974 Levine went to Tel-Aviv University, Israel, as visiting associate professor and returned as a visiting professor in 1982. She was also a visiting professor at Recanati School of Nursing, Ben Gurion University of the Negev, Beer Sheva, Israel (March-April, 1982).

Levine has received numerous honors, including being a charter fellow of the American Academy of Nursing (1973), honorary membership in the American Mental Health Aid to Israel (1976), and honorary recognition from the Illinois Nurses' Association. She was the first recipient of the Elizabeth Russell Belford Award for excellence in teaching from Sigma Theta Tau (1977). Both the first and second editions in her book *Introduction to Clinical Nursing* received AJN Book of the Year awards and her 1971 book, *Renewal for Nursing,* was translated into Hebrew.[29] Levine was listed in *Who's Who in American Women* (1977-1988) and in *Who's Who in American Nursing* (1987).[29,30] Levine was an active leader in the American Nurses' Association and the Illinois Nurses' Association. After her retirement in 1987, she remained active in theory development and encouraged questions and research about her theory.[28]

A dynamic speaker, she is a frequent presentor on programs, workshops, seminars, and panels, and a prolific writer regarding nursing and education. Although she never intended to develop theory, she provided an organizational structure for teaching medical-surgical nursing and a stimulus for theory development. "The Four Conservation Principles of Nursing"[20] was the first statement of the conservation principles. Other preliminary work included "Adaptation and Assessment: A Rationale for Nursing Intervention,"[19] "For Lack of Love Alone,"[21] and "The Pursuit of Wholeness."[22] The first edition of her book using the conservation principles, *Introduction to Clinical Nursing,* was published in 1969. She addressed the consequences of the four conservation principles in "Holistic Nursing."[23] The second edition of the book was published in 1973. Since then, Levine[25,26] has presented about the conservation principles at nurse theory conferences, some of which have been audiotaped,[25] and at the Allentown College of St. Francis de Sales Conferences[26] in April 1984.

In 1988 substantial change and clarification about her theory were published in her chapter "Four Conservation Principles: Twenty Years Later" in Riehl's book *Conceptual Models for Nursing Practice.* She elaborates on how redundancy characterizes availability of adaptive responses when stability is threatened. Adaptation processes establish a body economy to safeguard the individual's stability. Adaptation is the essence of conservation.[27]

THEORETICAL SOURCES

Levine learned historical viewpoints of diseases and that the way people think about disease changes over time from Beland's presentation of the theory of specific causation and multiple factors. Beland directed Levine's attention to numerous authors who became influential in her thinking, including Kurt Goldstein,[12] Sir

Arthur Sherrington,[40] and Rene Dubos.[5,6] Levine uses James E. Gibson's definition[11] of perceptual systems, Erik Erikson's differentiation[8,9] between total and whole, Hans Selye's stress theory,[34] and M. Bates' models[1] of external environment. Levine is proud that Martha Rogers was her first editor.[31,32]

USE OF EMPIRICAL EVIDENCE

Levine believes that specific nursing activities can be deduced from scientific principles. The scientific theoretical sources have been well researched. She based much of her work on accepted science principles and a natural law, conservation of energy.[35,36]

MAJOR CONCEPTS AND DEFINITIONS

HOLISTIC. "Whole, health, hale are all derivations of the Anglo-Saxon word, Hal."[26] Levine[8:92;22:94;26] quotes Erikson, who says, "Wholeness emphasizes a sound, organic, progressive, mutuality between diversified functions and parts within an entirety, the boundaries of which are open and fluent."

HOLISM. *Holism* means that "human beings are more than and different from the sum of their parts."[23:253;38:146] "Perceiving the 'wholes' depends upon recognizing the organization and interdependence of observable phenomena."[4:255]

INTEGRITY. Integrity is from the Latin *integer,* meaning one.[25]

CONSERVATION. Conservation is from the Latin word *conservatio,* meaning to keep together.[15,24,25]

Levine's model[24,33] stresses nursing interactions and interventions that are intended "to keep together the unique and individual resources that each individual brings to his predicament." Those interactions are based on the scientific background of the conservation principles. Nursing care is based on scientific knowledge and nursing skills. There are four conservation principles.

CONSERVATION PRINCIPLES

Conservation of energy. The individual requires a balance of energy and a constant renewal of energy in order to maintain life activities. That energy is challenged by processes such as healing and aging. This second law of thermodynamics applies to everything in the universe, including people.

Conservation of structural integrity. Healing is a process of restoring structural integrity. Nurses should limit the amount of tissue involved in disease by early recognition of functional changes and by nursing interventions.

Conservation of personal integrity. Self-worth and a sense of identity are important. Nurses can show patients respect by calling them by name, respecting their wishes, valuing personal possessions, providing privacy during procedures, supporting their defenses, and teaching them.

Conservation of social integrity. Life gains meaning through social communities, and health is socially determined. Nurses fulfill professional roles, provide for family members, assist with religious needs, and use interpersonal relationships to conserve social integrity.[21;22:13-18;32]

ADAPTATION. "Adaptation is a process of change whereby the individual retains his integrity within the realities of his environment."[24:11;32] Some adaptations are successful. Some are not. Adaptation is a matter of degree, not an all-or-nothing process.[24:11;32] Change is selective, not random. The outcomes of the change can sometimes be predicted; when it is, it can be observed and measured.

ENVIRONMENT. Environment is "where we are constantly and actively involved."[33] The person and his relationship to the environment is what counts.[33]

Levine also views each individual as having his own environment, both internally and externally. The internal environment can be related by nurses as the physiological and pathophysiological aspects of the patient. Levine uses a definition of the external environment from Bates, who suggests three levels: perceptual, operational, and conceptual. The perceptual level includes the aspects of the world about us that we are able to intercept and interpret with our sense organs. The operational level contains things that affect us physically even though we cannot directly perceive them, such as microorganisms. At the conceptual level, the environment is constructed from cultural patterns, characterized by a spiritual existence, and mediated by the symbols of language, thought, and history.[24:12] There are four levels of integration that safeguard the end and help a person maintain his integrity or wholeness.[24:9]

ORGANISMIC RESPONSE. The capacity of the individual to adapt to his environmental condition has been called the organismic response. It can be divided into four levels of integration: fight or flight, inflammatory response, response to stress, and perceptual response.

Fight or flight. The most primitive response is the flight or fight syndrome. The individual perceives that he is threatened, whether or not a threat does actually exist. Hospitalization, illness, and new experiences elicit a response. The individual responds by being on the alert to find more information and to assure his safety and well-being.

Inflammatory response. This is a defense mechanism to protect the self from insult in a hostile environment. It is a way of healing. This response uses available energy to remove or keep out unwanted irritants or pathogens. But it is limited in time because it drains the individual's energy reserves. Environmental control is important.

Response to stress. Selye described the stress response syndrome as predictable, nonspecifically induced organismic changes. The wear and tear of life is recorded on the tissues and reflects long-term hormonal responses to life experiences that cause structural changes. It is characterized by irreversibility and influences the way patients respond to nursing care.

Sensory response. This response is based on the individual's perceptual awareness. It occurs only as the individual experiences the world around him. This response is used by the individual to seek and maintain safety for himself. It is information seeking.[20:95-96;21;32]

TROPHICOGNOSIS. Levine recommended trophicognosis as an alternative to nursing diagnosis. It is a scientific method to reach a nursing care judgment.[18]

MAJOR ASSUMPTIONS

Introduction to Clinical Nursing is a text for beginning nursing students that uses the conservation principles as an organizing framework. Therefore Levine does not specifically identify her assumptions.

Nursing

"Nursing is a human interaction."[24:1] "Professional nursing should be reserved for those few who can complete a graduate program as demanding as that expected of professionals in any other discipline. . . . There will be very few professional nurses."[17:214] "Nursing practice—and this includes the teaching of nurses—has always mirrored prevailing theories of health and disease."[19:2450] "It is the nurse's task to bring a body of scientific principles on which decisions depend into the precise situation which she shares with the patient. Sensitive observation and the selection of relevant data form the basis for her assessment of his nursing requirements."[19:2452] "The nurse participates actively in every patient's environment, and much of what she does supports his adjustments as he struggles in the predicament of illness."[19:2452] The essence of Levine's theory is that "When nursing intervention influences adaptation favorably, or toward renewed social well-being, then the nurse is acting in a therapeutic sense; when the response is unfavorable, the nurse adds supportive care."[24:13;19:2452;32] The goal of nursing is to promote wholeness.[23:258]

Person

Person is "who we know ourself to be: a sense of identity."

Health

Health is socially determined. It is predetermined by social groups and is not just an absence of pathological conditions.[32] "Change is characteristic of life, and adaptation is the method of change. The organism retains its integrity in both the internal and external environment through its adaptive capability."[24:10]

Environment

Environment is the "context in which we live our lives."[31] It is not a passive backdrop. We are active participants in it.[31]

THEORETICAL ASSERTIONS

Because Levine's work was intended to provide an organizational structure for teaching medical-surgical nursing rather than to develop theory, she did not explicitly identify theoretical assertions. Although many theoretical assertions can be generated from her work, the four major ones are:

1. "Nursing intervention is based on the conservation of the individual patient's energy."[24:13;20:47]
2. "Nursing intervention is based on the conservation of the individual patient's structural integrity."[24:13;20:53]
3. "Nursing intervention is based on the conservation of the individual patient's personal integrity."[24:13;20:53]
4. "Nursing intervention is based on the conservation of the individual patient's social integrity."[24:14;20:56]

LOGICAL FORM

Levine primarily uses deductive logic. In developing her model, Levine integrates theories and concepts from the humanities and the sciences of nursing, physiology, psychology, and sociology. She uses the information to analyze nursing practice situations and describe nursing skills and activities.

ACCEPTANCE BY THE NURSING COMMUNITY

Practice

Levine helps define what nursing is by identifying the activities it encompasses while giving the scientific principles behind them. Conservation principles, levels of integration, and other concepts can be used in numerous contexts. Hirschfield[15] has used the principles of conservation in care of the older adult. Taylor[41,42] used them to measure outcomes of nursing care and then again in her textbook.

Education

Levine wrote a textbook for beginning students that introduced material into curricula that had not been taught before. She presented an early discussion of death and dying and believed that women should be awakened after a breast biopsy and consulted about the next step.[24:356-359;31;32]

Introduction to Clinical Nursing provides an organizational structure for teaching medical-surgical nursing. In both the 1969 and 1973 editions, Levine presents a model at the end of each of the first nine chapters. Each model contains objectives, essential science concepts, and nursing process to give nurses a foundation for nursing activities. The nine models are:

1. "Vital signs," including temperature, pulse, and respirations.[24:34-42]
2. "Body movement and positioning," in-

cluding body posture, body mechanics, bed rest, and ambulation.[24:86-92]

3. "Ministration of personal hygiene needs," including personal and environmental hygiene.[24:131-139]
4. "Pressure gradient systems in nursing intervention," specifically fluids.[24:198-208]
5. "Nursing determinants in provision for nutritional needs," including psychological, cultural, religious, socioeconomic, and therapeutic needs for fluids and nourishment.[24:245-253]
6. "Pressure gradient systems in nursing," specifically gases and pulmonary ventilation.[24:292-303]
7. "Local application of heat and cold," stressing patient's safety and comfort.[24:332-339]
8. "The administration of medications."[24:381-393]
9. "Establishing an aseptic environment," including teaching patients principles of asepsis.[24:435-440]

Critics argue that although the text is labeled introductory, a beginning student would need a fairly extensive background in physical and social science to use it.[3] Another critic suggests a definite strength is the emphasis of scientific principles, but a weakness of the text is that it does not present adequate examples of pathological profiles when disturbances are discussed. For this reason, one reviewer recommends the text as supplementary or complementary, rather than as a primary text.[4] Levine wrote a teacher's manual to assist in the use of her book.[31]

Hall[14] indicates Levine's model is one used as a curriculum model. Several graduate students are using Levine's model for theses and dissertations.[31]

Research

Fitzpatrick and Whall[10:115] state, "All in all, Levine's model served as an excellent beginning. Its contribution has added a great deal to the overall development of nursing knowledge." Many research questions can be generated from Levine's model. Several graduate students are using the conservation principles as a framework for their research.[31,32]

FURTHER DEVELOPMENT

Levine and others are working to use the conservation principles as the basis of a taxonomy of nursing diagnosis. Levine is also working on a theory of redundancy that still requires much discussion and critique because it is not definitive yet. Much related research is still needed.[31,32]

CRITIQUE

Clarity

Levine's model possesses clarity. Fitzpatrick and Whall[10] believe Levine's work to be both internally and externally consistent. Esposito and Leonard[7:160] state that Levine's ideas are, "organized in such a way as to be sequential and logical." They add that there are no apparent contradictions in the model.

Simplicity

Although the four conservation principles initially appear simple, they contain subconcepts and multiple variables. However, this remains one of the simpler models.

Generality

The four conservation principles can be used in all nursing contexts.

Empirical Precision

Levine used deductive logic to develop her model, which can be used to generate research questions.

Derivable Consequences

Various authors disagree as to the level of contributions provided by Levine's model. The four conservation principles was one of the earliest models and seems to be receiving increasing recognition.

REFERENCES

1. Bates, M. (1967). A naturalist at large. *Natural History, 76(6)*:8-16.

2. Beland, I. (1971). *Clinical nursing: Pathophysiological and psychosocial implications* (2d ed.). New York: Macmillan.
3. Book Review. (1970, Jan.). *Canadian Nurse, 66:*42.
4. Book Review. (1974, May). *Canadian Nurse, 70:*39.
5. Dubos, R. (1961). *Mirage of health.* Garden City, N.Y.: Doubleday.
6. Dubos, R. (1965). *Man adapting.* New Haven, Conn.: Yale University Press.
7. Esposito, C.H., & Leonard, M.K. (1980). Myra Estrin Levine. In Nursing Theories Conference Group, J.B. George, Chairperson, *Nursing theories: The base for professional nursing practice.* Englewood Cliffs, N.J.: Prentice-Hall.
8. Erikson, E.H. (1964). *Insight and responsibility.* New York: W.W. Norton.
9. Erikson, E.H. (1968). *Identity: Youth and crisis.* New York: W.W. Norton.
10. Fitzpatrick, J.J., & Whall, A.L. (1983). *Conceptual models of nursing: Analysis and application.* Bowie, Md.: Robert J. Brady.
11. Gibson, J.E. (1966). *The senses considered as perceptual systems.* Boston: Houghton Mifflin.
12. Goldstein, K. (1963). *The organism.* Boston: Beacon Press.
13. Hall, E.T. (1966). *The hidden dimension.* Garden City, N.Y.: Doubleday.
14. Hall, K.V. (1979). Current trends in the use of conceptual frameworks in nursing education. *Journal of Nursing Education, 18(4):*26-29.
15. Hirschfeld, M.J. (1976). The cognitively impaired older adult. *American Journal of Nursing, 76:*1981-1984.
16. Levine, M.E. (1963). Florence Nightingale: The legend that lives. *Nursing Forum, 2(4):*24-35.
17. Levine, M.E. (1965, June). The professional nurse and graduate education. *Nursing Science, 3:*206.
18. Levine, M.E. (1966). Trophicognosis: An alternative to nursing diagnosis. In *Exploring progress in medical-surgical nursing practice.* New York: American Nurses' Association.
19. Levine, M.E. (1966, Nov.). Adaptation and assessment: A rationale for nursing intervention. *American Journal of Nursing, 66:*2450.
20. Levine, M.E. (1967). The four conservation principles of nursing. *Nursing Forum, 6:*45.
21. Levine, M.E. (1967, Dec.). For lack of love alone. *Minnesota Nursing Accent, 39:*179.
22. Levine, M.E. (1969, Jan.). The pursuit of wholeness. *American Journal of Nursing, 69:*93.
23. Levine, M.E. (1971, June). Holistic nursing. *Nursing Clinics of North America, 6:*253.
24. Levine, M.E. (1973). *Introduction to clinical nursing* (2d ed.). Philadelphia: F.A. Davis.
25. Levine, M.E. (1978). Paper presented at the Second Annual Nurse Educators' Conference, New York. (Audiotape).
26. Levine, M.E. (1984, April). *A conceptual model for nursing: The four conservative principles.* In the proceedings from Allentown College of St. Francis Conference.
27. Levine, M.E. (1988). The four conservation principles: Twenty years later. In Riehl (Ed.), *Conceptual models for nursing practice* (3d Ed.). New York: Appleton-Century-Crofts.
28. The nursing theorist: Portraits of excellence: Myra Levine. (1988). Oakland: Studio III. Videotape available from Fuld Video Project, 370 Hawthorne Avenue, Oakland, CA 94609.
29. Levine, M.E. (1984). Curriculum vitae.
30. Levine, M. (1988). Curriculum Vitae.
31. Levine, M.E. (1984). Telephone interviews.
32. Levine, M.E. (1985). Telephone interviews.
33. Levine, M. (1988). Telephone interviews.
34. Levine, M.E. (1984). Personal correspondence.
35. Levine, M.E. (1985). Personal correspondence.
36. Levine, M. (1988). Personal correspondence.
37. Levine, M.E., & Levine, E.B. (1965, Dec.). Hippocrates: Father of nursing too. *American Journal of Nursing, 65:*86.
38. Rogers, M.E. (1970). *An introduction to the theoretical basis of nursing.* Philadelphia: F.A. Davis.
39. Selye, H. (1956). *The stress of life.* New York: McGraw-Hill.
40. Sherrington, A. (1906). *Integrative function of the nervous system.* New York: Charles Scribner's Sons.
41. Taylor, J.W. (1974). Measuring the outcomes of nursing care. *Nursing Clinics of North America, 9:*337-348.
42. Taylor, J., & Ballenger, S. (1980). *Neurological dysfunction and nursing interventions.* New York: McGraw-Hill.
43. Tillich, P. (1961). The meaning of health. *Perspectives in Biology and Medicine, 5:*92-100.

BIBLIOGRAPHY

Primary Sources

Books

Levine, M.E. (1969). *Introduction to clinical nursing.* Philadelphia: F.A. Davis.

Levine, M.E. (1971). *Renewal for nursing.* Philadelphia: F.A. Davis.

Levine, M.E. (1973). *Introduction to clinical nursing* (2d ed.). Philadelphia: F.A. Davis.

Book Chapters

Levine, M.E. (1964). Nursing Service. In M. Leeds & H. Shore, *Geriatric institutional management.* New York: J.P. Putnam & Sons.

Levine, M.E. (1966). Trophicognosis: An alternative to nursing diagnosis. In *ANA regional conference papers* (Vol. 2: Medical-Surgical Nursing).

Levine, M.E. (1972). Benoni. In *Comprehensive clinical papers* (Vol. 6: The nurse and the dying patient). American Journal of Nursing Company.

Levine, M.E. (1973). Adaptation and assessment: A rationale for nursing intervention. In M.E. Hardy (Ed.), *Theoretical foundations for nursing.* New York: Irvington.

Levine, M.E. (1988). Myra Levine. In T.M. Schorr & A. Zimmerman (Eds)., *Making choices taking chances: Nursing leaders tell their stories.* St. Louis: C.V. Mosby Company.

Levine, M.E. (1988). The four conservation principles: Twenty years later. In J. Riehl (Ed.), *Conceptual models for nursing practice* (3d Ed.). New York: Appleton-Century-Crofts.

Articles

Levine, M.E. (1963). Florence Nightingale: The legend that lives. *Nursing Forum, 2(4):*24-35.

Levine, M.E. (1964, Feb.). Not to startle, though the way were steep. *Nursing Science, 2:*58-67.

Levine, M.E. (1964, Dec.). There need be no anonymity. *First, 18(9):*4.

Levine, M.E. (1965, June). The professional nurse and graduate education. *Nursing Science, 3:* 206-214.

Levine, M.E. (1965). Trophicognosis: An alternative to nursing diagnosis. *ANA Regional Clinical Conferences, 2:*55-70.

Levine, M.E. (1966, Nov.). Adaptation and assessment: A rationale for nursing intervention. *American Journal of Nursing, 66(11):*2450-2453.

Levine, M.E. (1967). The four conservation principles of nursing. *Nursing Forum, 6:*45-59.

Levine, M.E. (1967, May). Medicine-nursing dialogue belongs at patient's bedside. *Chart, 64(5):*136-137.

Levine, M.E. (1967, July). This I believe: About patient-centered care. *Nursing Outlook, 15:*53-55.

Levine, M.E. (1967, Dec.). For lack of love alone. *Accent, 39(7):*179-202.

Levine, M.E. (1968, Feb.). Knock before entering personal space bubbles (Part 1). *Chart, 65(2):* 58-62.

Levine, M.E. (1968, March). Knock before entering personal space bubbles (Part 2). *Chart, 65(3):* 82-84.

Levine, M.E. (1968, April). The pharmacist in the clinical setting: A nurse's viewpoint. *American Journal of Hospital Pharmacy, 25(4):*168-171. (Also translated into Japanese and published in *Kyushu National Hospital Magazine for Western Japan*).

Levine, M.E. (1969). Nursing for the 21st century. *National Student Association.*

Levine, M.E. (1969, Jan.). The pursuit of wholeness. *American Journal of Nursing, 69:*93-98.

Levine, M.E. (1969, Feb.). Constructive student power. *Chart, 66(2):*42FF.

Levine, M.E. (1969, Oct.). Small hospital—big nursing. *Chart, 66:*265-269.

Levine, M.E. (1969, Nov.). Small hospital—big nursing. *Chart, 66:*310-315.

Levine, M.E. (1970). Dilemma. *ANA Clinical Conferences,* pp. 338-342.

Levine. M.E. (1970, April). Breaking through the medications mystique. Published simultaneously in *American Journal of Nursing, 70(4):*799-803, and *American Journal of Hospital Pharmacy, 27(4):* 294-299.

Levine, M.E. (1970, Oct.) The intransient patient. *American Journal of Nursing, 70:*2106-2111.

Levine, M.E. (1971, May). Considers implications for nursing in the use of physician's assistants. *Hospital Topics, 49:*60-63.

Levine, M.E. (1971, June). Holistic nursing. *Nursing Clinics of North America, 6:*253-264.

Levine, M.E. (1970, July-Dec.). Symposium on a drug compendium: View of a nursing educator. *Drug Information Bulletin,* pp. 133-135.

Levine, M.E. (1971, June). The time has come to speak of health care. *AORN Journal, 13:*37-43.

Levine, M.E. (1972, February). Nursing educators—An alientating elite? *Chart, 69(2)*:56-61.

Levine, M.E. (1972, March.). Benoni. *American Journal of Nursing, 72(3)*:466-468.

Levine, M.E. (1972, March.). Nursing grand rounds: Complicated case of CVA. *Nursing '72, 2(3)*:3-34. (With P. Moschel, J. Taylor, & G. Ferguson).

Levine, M.E. (1972, May). Nursing grand rounds: Insulin reactions in a brittle diabetic, *Nursing '72, 2(5)*:6-11 (with L. Line, A. Boyle, E. Kopacewski).

Levine, M.E. (1972, June). Issues in rehabilitation: The quadriplegic adolescent. *Nursing '72, 2*:6 (with M. Scanlon, P. Gregor, R. King, & N. Martin).

Levine, M.E. (1972, Sept.). Nursing grand rounds: Severe trauma, *Nursing '72, 2*:9:33-38 (with J. Zoellner, B. Ozmon, & E. Simunek).

Levine, M.E. (1972, Oct.). Nursing grand rounds: Congestive failure. *Nursing '72, 2:10*:18-23. (with C. Hallberg, M. Kathrein, & R. Cox).

Levine, M.E. (1973). On creativity in nursing. *Image, 3(3)*:15-19.

Levine, M.E. (1973, Nov.). A letter from Myra, *Chart, 70(9)*. (Also in *Israel Nurses' Journal*, December 1973, in English and Hebrew).

Levine, M.E. (1974, Oct.). The pharmacist's clinical role in interdisciplinary care: A nurse's viewpoint. *Hospital Formulary Management, 9*:47.

Levine, M.E. (1975, Jan.-Feb.). On creativity in nursing. *Nursing Digest, 3*:38-40.

Levine, M.E. (1977, May). Nursing ethics and the ethical nurse. *American Journal of Nursing, 77*:845-849.

Levine, M.E. (1978, June). Cancer chemotherapy: A nursing model. *Nursing Clinics of North America, 13(2)*:271-280.

Levine, M.E. (1978, July). Kapklvoo and nursing, too. *Research in Nursing and Health, 1(2)*:51 (Editorial).

Levine, M.E. (1978, Nov.). Does continuing education improve nursing practice? *Hospitals, 52(21)*:138-140.

Levine, M.E. (1979). Knowledge base required by generalized and specialized nursing practice. *ANA Publications (G-127)*:57-69.

Levine, M.E. (1980). The ethics of computer technology in health care. *Nursing Forum, 19(2)*:193-198.

Levine, M.E. (1982, March-April). Bioethics of cancer nursing. *Rehabilitation Nursing, 7*:27-31, 41.

Levine, M.E. (1982, March-April). The bioethics of cancer nursing. *Journal of Enterostomal Therapy, 9*:11-13.

Levine, M.E. (1984, April). A conceptual model for nursing: The four conservative principles. In the proceedings from Allentown College of St. Francis Conference.

Levine, M.E. (1988, Feb.). Antecedents from adjunctive disciplines: Creation of nursing theory. *Nursing Science Quarterly*, Inaugural Issue.

Levine, M.E. & Levine, E.B. (1965, Dec.). Hippocrates: Father of nursing, too. *American Journal of Nursing, 65(12)*:86-88.

Levine, M.E., Porter, A.L., & McDonald, A. (1973, Sept.). Giving diabetics control of their own lives. *Nursing '73, 3*:44-49.

Levine, M.E., & Rayder, M. (1979, Nov.). Problem: A new nurse asks why preoperative teaching isn't done . . . three answers from experience. *American Journal of Nursing, 77*:10.

Book Reviews

Levine, M.E. (1985, March). Review of B. Stevens, nursing theory, (2d Ed.). *Research in Nursing and Health, 8(1)*.

Levine, M.E. (1985, May). Book review, G. Fjermedal, *Magic Bullets. Oncology Nursing Forum 12(3):101-102.*

Audiotapes

Levine, M.E. (1978, Dec.). Paper presented at the Second Annual Nurse Educator Conference, New York: Audiotape available from Teach 'em Inc., 160 E. Illinois Street, Chicago, Ill. 60611.

Levine, M.E. (1979). Paper presented at nursing theory conference. Audiotapes (2 reels) available from Teach 'em Inc., 160 E. Illinois Street, Chicago, Ill. 60611.

Levine, M.E. (1984, May). Paper presented at Nursing Theory Conference, Boyle, Letoueneau Conference, Edmonton, Canada. Audiotapes available from Ed Kennedy, Kennedy Recording, R.R.5, Edmonton, Alberta, Canada TSP4B7 (403-470-0013).

Videotape

The Nursing theorist: Portraits of Excellence: Myra Levine. (1988). Oakland: Studio III. Videotape available from Fuld Video Project, 370 Hawthorne Avenue, Oakland, Cal. 94609.

Proceedings

Levine, M.E. (1976, Jan.). On the nursing ethnic and the negative command. *Proceedings of the Intensive Conference* (Faculty of the University of Illinois Medical Center.) Philadelphia: Society for Health and Human Values.

Levine, M.E. (1977). History of nursing in Illinois. *Proceedings of the Bicentennial Workshop of the University of Illinois College of Nursing.* University of Illinois Press.

Levine, M.E. (1977). Primary nursing: Generalist and specialist education. *Proceedings of the American Academy of Nursing.* Kansas City, Mo.

Levine, M.E. (In press). What's wrong about rights? *Proceedings of the 1st International Congress on Nursing Law and Ethics.* Berlin: Springer.

Interviews

Levine, M. (1984). Telephone interviews.
Levine, M. (1985). Telephone interviews.
Levine, M. (1988). Telephone interviews.

Correspondence

Levine, M. (1984). Curriculum vitae.
Levine, M. (1984). Personal correspondence.
Levine, M. (1985). Personal correspondence.
Levine, M. (1988). Personal correspondence.

Secondary Sources

Book Reviews

Levine, M.E. (1969). *Introduction to clinical nursing.*
*Bedside Nurse, 2:*4, September-October 1969.
*Canadian Nurse, 66:*42, January 1970.
*American Journal of Nursing, 70:*99+ January 1970.
*Nursing Outlook, 18:*20, February 1970.
*American Journal of Nursing, 70:*2220+ October 1970.
*Nursing Mirror, 132:*43, April 2, 1971.
*Bedside Nurse, 4:*2, November 1971.
*Canadian Nurse, 76:*47, December 1971.
*Nursing Mirror, 133:*16, December 17, 1971.
*American Journal of Nursing, 74:*347, February 1974.
*Canadian Nurse, 70:*39, May 1974.
*Nursing Outlook, 22:*301, May 1974.

Levine, M.E. (1969). *Renewal for nursing.*
*Supervisor Nurse, 2:*68, August 1971.
*Bedside Nurse, 4:*2, November 1971.
*AANA Journal, 49:*495, December 1971.
*Canadian Nurse, 67:*47, December 1971.
*Nursing Mirror, 133:*16, December 1971.

Book Chapters

Chinn, P.L., & Jacobs, M.K. (1983). *Theory in nursing: A systematic approach.* St. Louis: C.V. Mosby, p. 188.

Esposito, C.H., & Leonard, M.K. (1980) Myra Estrin Levine. In Nursing Theories Conference Group. J.B. George, Chairperson, *Nursing theories: The base for professional nursing practice.* Englewood Cliffs, N.J.: Prentice-Hall, pp. 150-163.

Fawcett, J. (1984). Levine's conservation model. In J. Fawcett, *Analysis and evaluation of conceptual models of nursing.* Philadelphia: F.A. Davis, pp. 115-144.

Griffith, J.W. & Christensen, P. (1982). *Nursing process: Application of theories, frameworks, and models.* St. Louis: C.V. Mosby, pp. 12, 193-226.

Griffith-Kenney, J.W., & Christensen, P. (1986). *Nursing process: Application of theories, frameworks, and models.* St. Louis: C.V. Mosby, pp. 6, 24-25.

McLane, A. (1987). Taxonomy and nursing diagnosis, a critical view. In A. McLane (Ed.). *Classification proceedings of the Seventh Annual Conference of Nursing of North America.* St. Louis: C.V. Mosby.

Meleis, A.I. (1985). Myra Levine. In A.I. Meleis, *Theoretical nursing: Development and progress.* Philadelphia: J.B. Lippincott, pp. 275-283.

Pieper, B.A. (1983). Levine's nursing model. In J.J. Fitzpatrick & A.L. Whall, *Conceptual models of nursing: Analysis and application.* Bowie, Md.: Robert J. Brady, pp. 101-115.

Stevens, B. (1979). *Nursing theory: Analysis, application, evaluation.* Boston: Little, Brown (14 citations in the text).

Books

Dubos, R. (1961). *Mirage of health.* Garden City, N.Y.: Doubleday.

Dubos, R. (1965). *Man adapting.* New Haven, Conn.: Yale University Press.

Erikson, E.H. (1964). *Insight and responsibility.* New York: W.W. Norton.

Erikson, E.H. (1968). *Identity: Youth and crisis.* New York: W.W. Norton.

Gibson, J.E. (1966). *The senses considered as perceptual systems.* Boston: Houghton Mifflin.

Goldstein, K. (1963). *The organism.* Boston: Beacon Press.

Rogers, M.E. (1970). *An introduction to the theoretical basis of nursing.* Philadelphia: F.A. Davis.

Selye, H. (1956). *The stress of life.* New York: McGraw-Hill.

Sherrington, A. (1906). *Integrative function of the nervous system.* New York: Charles Scribner & Sons.

Taylor, J., & Ballenger, S. (1980). *Neurological dysfunction and nursing interventions.* New York: McGraw-Hill.

Articles

Bates, M. (1967). A naturalist at large. *Natural History, 76(6):*8-16.

Hall, K.V. (1979). Current trends in the use of conceptual frameworks in nursing education. *Journal of Nursing Education, 18(4):*26-29.

Flaskerud, J.H., & Halloran, E.J. (1980). Areas of agreement in nursing theory development. *Advances in Nursing Science, 3(1):*1-7.

Hirschfeld, M.J. (1976). The cognitively impaired older adult. *American Journal of Nursing, 76:*1981-1984.

Taylor, J.W. (1974). Measuring the outcomes of nursing care. *Nursing Clinics of North America, 9:*337-348.

Tillich, P. (1961). The meaning of health. *Perspectives in Biology and Medicine, 5:*92-100.

Tompkins, E.S. (1980). Effect of restricted mobility and dominance on perceived duration. *Nursing Research, 29(6):*333-338.

30

Martha E. Rogers

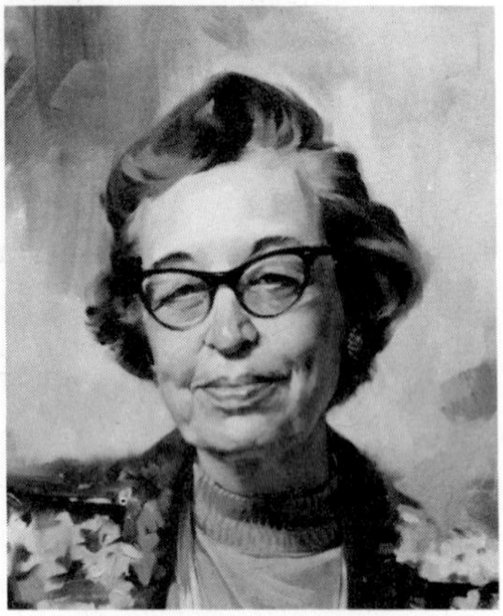

Unitary Human Beings

Joann Sebastian Daily, Judy Sporleder Maupin, Martha Carole Satterly, Denise L. Schnell, Therese L. Wallace

CREDENTIALS AND BACKGROUND OF THE THEORIST

Martha E. Rogers was born May 12, 1914, in Dallas, Texas, the eldest of four children. She began her collegiate education at the University of Tennessee in Knoxville, where she studied science from 1931 to 1933. She received her nursing diploma from Knoxville General Hospital School of Nursing in 1936. In 1937 she received a B.S. from George Peabody College in Nashville, Tennessee. Her other degrees include an M.A. in public health nursing supervision from Teacher's College, Columbia University, New York, in 1945 and an M.P.H. in 1952 and a Sc.D. in 1954, both from Johns Hopkins University in Baltimore.

For 21 years, from 1954 to 1975, she was Professor and Head of the Division of Nursing at New York University. Since 1975, she has been Professor, and in 1979 she became Professor Emerita.

Rogers' early nursing practice was in rural public health nursing in Michigan and in visit-

The authors wish to express appreciation to Dr. Lois Meier for her assistance and to Dr. Martha Rogers for critiquing the chapter.

ing nurse supervision, education, and practice in Connecticut. She then established the Visiting Nurse Service of Phoenix, Arizona. Her publications include three books and over 200 articles; she continues to write and publish extensively. She has lectured in 46 states, the District of Columbia, Puerto Rico, Mexico, Holland, China, Newfoundland, Columbia, Brazil, and other countries.[20]

Rogers has received honorary doctorates in Science, Letters, and Humane Letters from 1978 to the present from such renowned institutions as Duquesne University, University of San Diego, Iona College, Fairfield University, Emory University, Adelphi University, Mercy College, and Washburn University of Topeka. In addition, she has received numerous awards and citations for her contributions and leadership in nursing. She has received citations for "Inspiring Leadership in the Field of Intergroup Relations" by Chi Eta Phi Sorority, "In Recognition of Your Outstanding Contribution to Nursing" by New York University, "For Distinguished Service to Nursing" by Teachers College, and many others. She has also been honored by the many awards, funds, and scholarships that have been established in her name.[20]

A verbal portrait of Rogers might include such descriptive terms as stimulating, challenging, controversial, idealistic, visionary, prophetic, philosophic, academic, outspoken, humorous, blunt, and ethical. She has been widely recognized and honored for her contributions and leadership in nursing. Her colleagues consider her one of the most original thinkers in nursing.[7:245]

THEORETICAL SOURCES

Rogers' early grounding in the liberal arts and sciences is apparent in the origin of her conceptual system and its ongoing development. Though introduced in earlier publications, the abstract system was first formally published in 1970 as *An Introduction to the Theoretical Basis of Nursing*. Rogers has continued to clarify and define her concepts in later publications and presentations such as her chapter in *Explorations on Martha Rogers' Science of Unitary Human Beings*, by Violet Malinski.[8]

Rogers draws on a knowledge base gained from anthropology, psychology, sociology, astronomy, religion, philosophy, history, biology, physics, mathematics, literature, and other sources to create her model of unitary human beings and the environment as energy fields integral to the life process.[6:166] A statement frequently repeated in her writings is, "Man is a unified whole possessing his own integrity and manifesting characteristics that are more than and different from the sum of his parts."[15:47] Furthermore, human behavior is described as synergystic, defining *synergy* as "the unique behavior of whole systems, unpredicted by any behaviors of their component functions taken separately."[2:19] In the prologue of *An Introduction to the Theoretical Basis of Nursing* she states, "Man's biological, physical, social, psychological, and spiritual heritages become an indivisible whole as scientific facts are merged with human warmth."[15:xii]

Several sources influenced Rogers' theorizations. During the mid-nineteenth century, Florence Nightingale's proposals and statistical data placed man within the framework of the natural world, and "the foundation for the scope of modern nursing was laid."[15:30]

As the nineteenth century moved into the twentieth, classical physics gave way to field physics, and events of the physical world had a new unity. In 1905 Einstein's theory of relativity introduced the four coordinates of space-time.[15:31]

In 1935 Burr and Northrop's "The Electro-Dynamic Theory of Life" stated the concepts of the pattern and organization of the electrodynamic field, the outcome of whose activity is wholeness, organization, and continuity. Rogers[15:32] says, "An electrical field was replacing the cell as the fundamental unit of biological systems."

In the 1950s von Bertalanffy introduced

general systems theory, which presented a general science of wholeness. The term *negentropy* was brought into use to signify increasing order, complexity, and heterogeneity.[15:51]

A theme of Rogers' writings and discussions may be paraphrased, "You cannot understand the *whole* by studying the parts, and the *whole* is more than and different from the sum of its parts."

USE OF EMPIRICAL EVIDENCE

"The conceptual system that underwrites a Science of Unitary Human Beings does not derive from one or more of the basic sciences. . . . A multiplicity of knowledges from many sources flows in novel ways to create a kaleidoscope of potentialities."[8:4] As supporting evidence for her conceptual model, Malinski cites nurse researcher M. Rawnsley of Boston University, who in 1977 framed her research solely within the Rogerian framework. This was a turning point for the Science of Unitary Human Beings research. Hypotheses were derived from the Rogerian conceptual framework for the first time.[8]

MAJOR CONCEPTS AND DEFINITIONS

In 1970 Rogers' conceptual model of nursing rested upon a set of basic assumptions that described the life process in man. The life process was characterized by wholeness, openness, unidirectionality, pattern and organization, sentience, and thought.[15:90]

Since 1970 Rogers has revised and updated this conceptual model, and she correlates this need for change with accelerating scientific and technological advances. In 1983 Rogers changed her wording from that of "Unitary Man" to "Unitary Human Beings" in an effort to remove the concept of gender. It was also at this time that she stressed "unitary human beings are not to be confused with current popular usage of the term 'holistic'. . ." but that "a science of unitary human beings is unique to nursing as well as having relevance for other fields."[18]

Rogers postulates that human beings are dynamic energy fields integral with environmental fields. Both human and environmental fields are identified by pattern and characterized by a universe of open systems. From these concepts, in her 1983 paradigm, four building blocks for her model are postulated. These are energy field, a universe of open systems, pattern, and four-dimensionality.[17:222]

ENERGY FIELD. An energy field constitutes the fundamental unit of both the living and the nonliving. Field is a unifying concept, and energy signifies the dynamic nature of the field. Energy fields are infinite. Two fields are identified: the human field and the environmental field.[17] "Specifically human beings and environment *are* energy fields."[19:2]

"The *unitary human being* (human field) is defined as an irreducible, four-dimensional energy field identified by pattern and manifesting characteristics different from those of the parts and which cannot be predicted from knowledge of the parts. The *environmental field* is defined as an irreducible, four-dimensional energy field identified by pattern and manifesting characteristics different from those of the parts. Each environmental field is specific to its given human field. Both change continuously and creatively."[19:2] They are irreducible.

UNIVERSE OF OPEN SYSTEMS. The concept of the universe of open systems holds that energy fields are infinite, open, and integral with one another.[17] The human and the environmental field are in continuous process and are open systems.

PATTERN

Pattern identifies energy fields. It is the distinguishing characteristic of a field and is perceived as a single wave. The nature of the pattern changes continuously and innovatively. Each human field pattern is unique and is integral with its own environmental field.[17]

"Manifestations of pattern have been described as unique and refer to behaviors, qualities, and characteristics of the field"; a sense of self is a field manifestation, the nature of which is unique to each individual.[4:30] The human field pattern is integral with the environmental field. The pattern is constantly changing and may manifest disease, illness, or pain.[23]

FOUR-DIMENSIONALITY. *Four dimensionality* is defined as a nonlinear domain without spatial or temporal attributes. All reality is postulated to be four dimensional.[17]

From this conceptual system, Rogers derives the Principles of Homeodynamics, which pos-

Table 30-1. Evolution of principles of homeodynamics—1970, 1980, 1983, 1986

An Introduction to the Theoretical Basis of Nursing 1970	Nursing: A Science of Unitary Man 1980	Science of Unitary Human Beings: A Paradigm for Nursing 1983	Dimensions of Health: A View From Space 1986
Resonancy—continuously propagating series of waves between man and environment	*Resonancy*—the continuous change from lower to higher frequency wave patterns in the human and environmental fields	*Resonancy*—the continuous change from lower to higher frequency wave patterns in human and environmental fields	*Resonancy*—the continuous change from lower to higher frequency wave patterns in human and environmental fields
Helicy—continuous, innovative change growing out of mutual interaction of man and environment along a spiralling longitudinal axis bound in space-time	*Helicy*—nature of change between human and environmental fields is continuously innovative, probabilistic, and increasingly diverse, manifesting nonrepeating rhythmicities	*Helicy*—the continuous, innovative, probabilistic, increasing diversity of human and environmental field patterns, characterized by nonrepeating rhythmicities	*Helicy*—the continuous innovative, probabilistic, increasing diversity of human and environmental field patterns, characterized by nonrepeating rhythmicities
Reciprocy—continuous mutual interaction between the human field and environmental field	*Complementarity*—the continuous, mutual, simultaneous interaction between human and environmental fields	*Integrality*—the continuous mutual human field and environmental field process	*Integrality*—the continuous mutual human field and environmental field process
Synchrony—change in the human field and simultaneous state of environmental field at any given point in space-time.			

Conceptualized by Joann Daily from the following sources: Rogers, M.E. (1970). *An introduction to the theoretical basis of nursing.* Philadelphia: F.A. Davis; Riehl, J.P., & Roy, C. (Eds.). (1980). *Conceptual models for nursing practice* (2d ed.). New York: Appleton-Century-Crofts; Rogers, M.E. (1983). Science of unitary human beings: A paradigm for nursing. In I.W. Clements, & F.B. Roberts, *Family health: A theoretical approach to nursing care.* New York: John Wiley & Sons. Revised by Denise Schnell and Therese Wallace in 1988 to include: Rogers, M.E. (1986). *Dimensions of Health: A View From Space,* obtained through correspondence with Martha Rogers, March 1988.

tulate a way of perceiving unitary human beings. Table 30-1 depicts the evolution of these principles from 1970 to 1986. Rogers says, "The life process is homeodynamic. . . . These principles postulate the way the life process is and predict the nature of its evolving."[15:96]

Reed extrapolates the principles of resonancy, helicy, and integrality to increase our understanding. The helicy principle describes spiral development rather than a cyclical motion. This motion is continuous, nonrepeating, and always innovative patterning. According to the principle of resonancy, this patterning becomes more resonant over development, changing from lower to higher frequency. Resonancy is an enrichment process that accompanies the life span's increasing complexity. The third principle of homeodynamics, integrality, stresses the continuous mutual process of person and environment.[11]

Rogers repeatedly states that change is probabilistic. According to *Webster's Ninth New Collegiate Dictionary, probabilism* is a theory that certainty is impossible, especially in the sciences, and that probability suffices to govern action and belief.[21] Rogers[15:57] goes on to say, "Probability statistics provide a basis for practical operations. Prediction is a fundamental necessity for knowledgeable intervention that has as its goal the betterment of man."

MAJOR ASSUMPTIONS

Nursing

"Historically the term *nursing* most often has been used as a verb signifying 'to do.' When nursing is perceived as a science, the term *nursing* becomes a noun signifying 'a body of abstract knowledge.'"[17:1] Rogers describes nursing as a learned profession that is both a science and an art. "Nursing is a humanistic science dedicated to compassionate concern for maintaining and promoting health, preventing illness, and caring for and rehabilitating the sick and disabled."[15:vii] Nursing seeks to promote symphonic interaction between the environment and man, to strengthen the coherence and integrity of the human beings, and to direct and redirect patterns of interaction between man and his environment for the realization of maximum health potential.[15:122]

Rogers states, "Maintenance and promotion of health, prevention of disease, nursing diagnosis, intervention and rehabilitation encompass the scope of nursing's goals. Nursing is concerned with people—all people—well and sick, rich and poor, young and old. The arena of nursing's services extend into all areas where there are people; at home, at school, at work, at play; in hospitals, nursing homes, and clinics; on this planet and now moving into outer space."[2:19]

The professional practice of nursing is creative and imaginative and exists to serve people. It is rooted in intellectual judgment, abstract knowledge, and human compassion. Professional nursing practice has no dependent functions, but collaborative ones.[15:122] Professional practitioners participate "in the coordination of their knowledges and skills with those of professional personnel in other health disciplines."[15:128]

> Nursing intervention is predicated upon the wholeness of man and derives its safety and effectiveness from a unified concept of human functioning. Nursing is concerned with evaluating the simultaneous state of the individual (or group) and the environment, and the preceding configurations leading up to the present. Intervention is dependent on evaluation and adds a conscious dimension to enhancing probabilistic outcomes toward a predetermined goal.[15:124]

The safe practice of nursing intervention depends on the nature and amount of scientific knowledge the individual brings to practice and the imaginative, intellectual judgment that puts such knowledge to use in the service to mankind. Nursing is a "science of unitary human being" and is therefore unique because it is the only science that deals with the whole person.[17:1]

Person

Rogers' unitary human being is a unified being integral with the environment. Man is in continuous mutual process with his environment in his totality and "the whole cannot be understood when it is reduced to particulars."[15:44] Human beings "are not disembodied entities, nor are they mechanical aggregates. . . . They behave as a totality. . . . Man is a unified whole possessing his own integrity and manifesting characteristics that are more than and different from the sum of his parts."[15:46-47] A science of unitary human beings is basic to nursing and requires a new view and a conceptual system specific to nursing's concern. People and their environment are perceived as irreducible energy fields integral with one another and continuous and creative in their evolution.

Rogers defines *person* as an open system in continuous process with the open system that is environment. She defines *unitary man* as "an irreducible four dimensional energy field identified by pattern and manifesting characteristics that are specific to the whole and which cannot be predicted from knowledge of the parts" (Appendix A).

Rogers' primary concern is that nursing view the person as an irreducible whole. This is not to be confused with *holistic,* which is often used to mean the sum of all the parts. An irreducible whole is different from the sum of the parts. She also conceptualizes the person as a sentient being able to participate creatively in change.

Environment

Rogers[17:2] defines *environment* as "an irreducible, four dimensional energy field identified by pattern and manifesting characteristics different from those of the parts. Each environmental field is specific to its given human field. Both change continuously and creatively."

Environmental fields are infinite, and change is continuously innovative, probabilistic, and characterized by increasing diversity. Environmental and human fields are identified by wave patterns manifesting continuous change. Environmental and human fields are in continuous and mutual process.

Health

Rogers uses *health* in many of her earlier writings, but never really defines the term. She uses the term *positive health* to symbolize wellness and the absence of disease and major illness.[15] Her promotion of positive health connotes direction in helping people with opportunities for rhythmic consistency.[15]

Health is used by Rogers as a value term defined by the culture or individual. Health and illness are manifestations of pattern and are considered "to denote behaviors that are of high value and low value."[7:248] Events manifested in the life process indicate the extent to which man achieves maximum health according to some value systems.

THEORETICAL ASSERTIONS

In 1970 Rogers identified five assumptions that are also theoretical assertions supporting her model derived from literature on man, physics, mathematics, and behavioral science:

1. Man is a unified whole possessing his own integrity and manifesting characteristics more than and different from the sum of his parts (energy field).[15:47]
2. Man and environment are continuously exchanging matter and energy with one another (openness).[15:54]
3. The life process evolves irreversibly and unidirectionally along the space-time continuum (helicy).[15:59]
4. Pattern and organization identify man and reflect his innovative wholeness (pattern and organization).[15:65]
5. Man is characterized by the capacity for abstraction and imagery, language and thought, sensation, and emotion (sentient, thinking being).[15:73]

Ten years later Rogers had further developed "Nursing: A Science of Unitary Man." The science of nursing seeks to study the nature and direction of unitary human development integral with the environment. Rogers[15:47] believes "man lives in a probabilistic universe" and therefore is subject to the laws of probability. Probability statistics provide a basis for prediction that is a fundamental necessity for knowledgeable intervention with the goal of the betterment of man.[15:57] Professional practice of nursing flows from the application of knowledge.

Rogers sees the need for predictive principles that guide nursing practice. These principles emerge from nursing's conceptual system. Nursing science seeks to make intelligible knowledge about man and his world that has significance for nursing practice. The phenomenon central to nursing's conceptual system is man's life process. "The life process in man is a phenomenon of wholeness, of continuity, of dynamic and creative change."[15:84] Nursing is an empirical science that seeks to describe, explain, and predict the life process in man. If the life process in man is to be studied and understood, the normal and the pathological must be treated equally. The life process has its own unity, inseparable from environment, and is characterized as the whole.[15:85]

Rogers' prerequisite to the practice of nursing is the development of the science of nursing with the goal of providing a body of knowledge that stems from scientific research and logical analysis and is capable of being translated into nursing practice. Rogers' conceptual model of unitary man is a clear, direct statement about the unique focus of nursing: a flexible and creative, individualized, and socially oriented compassionate and skillful use of nursing science.

In "Dimensions of Health: A View from Space," Rogers continues these theoretical assertions but adds a new dimension. She states, "People struggle to extricate themselves from no longer tenable world views. Utopian dreams of disease control flounder amidst out-dated concepts of homeostasis, adaptation, and causality."[19:1] She lists iatrogenesis, nosocomial conditions, and hypochondriasis as the major health problems in the United States today. Rogers quotes Fritz Capra, from his book *The Turning Point,* "We are trying to apply concepts of an out-dated world view to a reality that can no longer be understood in terms of these concepts."[19:2] Rogers stresses that a new world view focusing on people and their environments is necessary. "A new world view compatible with the most progressive knowledge available is a necessary prelude to studying human health and to determining modalities for its promotion whether on this planet or in the outer reaches of space."[19:2]

LOGICAL FORM

Rogers uses a dialectic method as opposed to a logistic, problematic, or operational method. In this type of method, Rogers explains nursing by referring to broader principles that explain mankind. She then explains mankind through principles that characterize the universe. The method is based on the perspective of a whole that organizes the parts.[9:21-22]

Rogers' model of unitary man is clearly deductive and logical. The Theory of Relativity, General Systems Theory, Electro-Dynamic Theory of Life, and many other theories contributed ideas for Rogers' model. The central components of the model, unitary man and environment, are integral with one another. The basic building blocks of her model are energy field, openness, pattern, and four dimensionality and when synthesized with other facts and ideas provide for a new conceptual system—a new world view. These concepts form the basis of nursing's abstract conceptual system, which relates to nursing and health. From the abstract conceptual system, Rogers derives the principles of helicy, resonancy, and integrality. These broad generalizations postulate the nature and direction of unitary man's development. Other theories have been derived from the abstract conceptual system, such as the theory of accelerating evolution, paranormal events, and rhythmical correlates of change. The derived theories are intended to explain, predict, and describe phenomena related to the life process of man.

ACCEPTANCE BY NURSING COMMUNITY

Practice

Rogers' conceptual model views nursing as a body of knowledge specific to nursing to be used with the primary goal the betterment of man. This view implies that nursing has great social significance.

Rogers believes the theories derived from her conceptual model are translatable to practice. An example of this is seen in her quote, "A theory of accelerating evolution deriving from this conceptual system puts in different perspective today's rapidly changing norms in blood pressure levels, children's behavior, longer waking periods, and other events."[19:3] She begins to extrapolate these ideas in her papers "The Science of Unitary Human Beings: A Paradigm for Nursing" and "Dimensions of Health: A View from Space."[17,19] She envisions changes in nursing practice based on theories evolving from her model.

The abstract conceptual model is a necessary prelude to practice. It provides a base for research and theory development, which provide the knowledge base for practice. The model has served as a basis for explication of other nursing conceptualizations by Newman, Parse, and Fitzpatrick. "Rogers' model does not require that one discard all previous knowledge, but it does require that such knowledge be viewed differently."[10:21] This knowledge must then be discarded as it becomes absolute or contradicts new knowledge.

A specific example of the use of the "energy fields" application to research is seen in the use of therapeutic touch. Rogers' postulations regarding energy fields are supported in the literature. Burr and Northrop "emphasize the field as basic to all living systems and pattern and organization as basic to all that exists in the universe. . . . Life fields are described as similar in nature to the fields in physics, with laws regarding their organization and direction that imply purpose."[4:30]

In relation to therapeutic touch, Rogers describes man as being an energy field. Man "as" an energy field is called the *human field.* This field is identified by pattern.

The field is infinite but realistically is most clearly "felt" within several feet of the body. To the trained person the energy field can be assessed. By focusing attention on the person, it is possible for the therapist to "feel" the energy field of another person. "The field has qualities of strength, differentiation, and integrity. These qualities vary from person to person and are affected by pain and illness."[23:708]

Education

Rogers repeatedly discusses structuring the nursing education programs to teach nursing as a science and as a learned profession. The education of nurses is based on nursing science and committed to human service.

In the early 1960s Rogers proposed that the preparation for learned practice in nursing requires the baccalaureate degree. At that time her goal seemed idealistic, but today her assertions are becoming the standard rather than the exception. In 1987, North Dakota was the first state to mandate the baccalaureate level as the entry level for professional nursing.

She said, "The only people competent to teach nursing or to teach what nurses are supposed to do are qualified nurses."[16:65] Her advocacies are evidenced in nursing education today as more nurses have been prepared to teach nurses at all levels of nursing education.

Research

Rogers' conceptual model is directly related to research and theory development in nursing science. The conceptual model provides a stimulus and direction for scientific activity. Principles of homeodynamics are being studied. Investigation into the nature of field patterning and the search for indices of patterning have begun. The integral nature of the man-environment relationship and the growing complexity of life have been used in recent studies using Rogers' model. Hypotheses are being developed and theories are being devised from the systems studied.[7:6]

Recent studies using Rogers' conceptual model as a base are numerous.

> Human field motion has been investigated with the variables of sensation seeking (Lindley), imposed motion of the elderly (Gueldner), meditation (MacCrae), power (Barrett), and red and blue light and blindness (Ludomirski-Kalmanson).[8:39]

FURTHER DEVELOPMENT

TYPOLOGY. A typology is "a method of organizing and categorizing."[12:4] Whatever method of categorizing is used should include the criteria of exhaustiveness, mutual exclusiveness, and consistency with the concepts used in the theory.[12:5] Rogers' consistency of concepts has greatly increased as her Principles of Homeodynamics have been refined and the terms and definitions have remained the same. Exhaustiveness and mutual exclusiveness are criteria that Rogers, as well as most other nursing theorists, is continually striving to achieve.

OPERATIONAL DEFINITIONS. Operational definitions are missing. See the enclosed glossary in Appendix A for list of conceptual definitions.

COMPLEXITY. The complexity of Rogers' work has made the concepts and relationships difficult to understand. Current studies have been able to simplify and clarify some of the concepts and relationships, but, looking at the conceptual model in total perspective, it still must be categorized as complex.

MEASUREMENT TOOLS. Tools should "not become the focus of nursing practice because they are time limited and can detract from the patient."[23:19] The lack of precise instrumentation to measure the concepts and relationships of Rogers' conceptual model has been noted by several authors, but new tools have been and are being developed and are in use.

Rogers[10,11,13] has frequently identified the need for adequate measuring instruments. She states, "New tools of measurement are necessary adjuncts to studying questions arising out of a world view that is different from the prevalent view."[17:4]

The development of adequate and precise instruments to measure concepts and relationships remains a real need. It should be a high priority of nurse researchers.

STYLE. Anderson[1:541] wrote that Rogers' "style may discourage readers from seeking out the germinal concepts in the book which are worthy of consideration." Rogers' style is philosophical, but it is the complexity of her conceptual model that makes reading the material slow and laborious.

CRITIQUE

Simplicity

Rogers' conceptual model is not simple. It is complex. She uses multiple concepts that are not easily understood. She relates these concepts in her Principles of Homeodynamics.

Generality

Rogers' conceptual model is abstract and is therefore generalizable and powerful. It is usually considered a grand theory or a macro theory. It is broad in scope and attempts to explain everything.

Empirical Precision

Rogers' conceptual model is abstract. Many would have difficulty understanding the concepts and relationships without a strong knowledge of other fields of study. Rogers' conceptual model is deductive in logic and "the major criticism of deductive theories is the lack of empirical support."[3:443] "The difficulty in understanding the principles, the lack of operational definitions, and inadequate tools for measurement are the major limitations to the effective utilization of this theory."[6:180-181] Rogers' early model lacked empirical precision, yet empirical precision has greatly increased as Rogers' conceptual model has been further developed. The abstract system generates theories that are testable.

Derivable Consequences

Besides the previously mentioned recent studies, many other research studies have been done (See Appendix B). All these studies have implications for guiding nursing practice and education and suggest further research.

Rogers sees the nurse as an integral part of the client's environment. She also sees nursing as a unique science that deals with "unitary human beings" who are different from the sum of their parts.[15:13] This differentiates nursing from other professions and basic sciences.

Many ideas for future study have been suggested by Rogers.[15:103-120] Based on this, it can be said that Rogers' conceptual model is useful.

CONCLUSION

Rogers is a brilliant nursing theorist. She is years ahead of her time. Understanding of her concepts and principles requires a foundation in general education, a willingness to let go of the traditional, and an ability to perceive the world in a new and creative way.

Rogers has many pertinent views for the future. She states, "Only as the science of nursing takes on form and substance can the art of nursing achieve new dimensions of artistry."[2:22] She continues to emphasize nursing services as indispensable to public safety and health.

The goal of health workers and of the public focuses properly on the promotion of health. In a dynamic continuously innovative world, one does not, for example, prevent disease. Rather, in the process of change there are many potentialities, only some of which will be actualized. Therapeutic modalities will increasingly emphasize the noninvasive. Diversity will be accorded high value. Human health will not be measured by adding up parameters of biological, physical, social, psychological, and like phenomena.[2:22]

Again, Rogers[17:1] said it well when she quoted Capra as saying, "we are trying to apply concepts of an out-dated world view to a reality that can no longer be understood in terms of these concepts." She continued:

> A science of unitary human beings basic to nursing requires a new world view and a conceptual system specific to nursing's phenomenon of concern. . . . Seeing the world from this viewpoint requires a new synthesis, a creative leap, and the inculcation of new attitudes and values. . . . A science of unitary human beings identifies nursing's uniqueness and signifies the potential of nurses to fulfill their social responsibility in human service.[13:1,4]

REFERENCES

1. Anderson, E.H. (1979, Nov.-Dec.). Researchers' bookshelf. *Nursing Research, 19(6)*:541.
2. Butterfield, S.E. (1983). In search of commonalities: Analysis of two theoretical frameworks. *International Journal of Nursing Studies, 20(1)*:15-22.
3. Chaska, N.L. (Ed.). (1983). *The nursing profession: A time to speak.* New York: McGraw-Hill.
4. Clarke, P.N. (1986). Theoretical and measurement issues in the study of field phenomena. *Advances in Nursing Science, 9(1)*:29-39.
5. Chinn, P.L., & Jacobs, M.K. (1983). *Theory and nursing: A systematic approach.* St. Louis: C.V. Mosby.
6. Falco, S.M., & Lobo, M.L. (1980). Martha Rogers. In Nursing Theories Conference Group, J.B. George, Chairperson, *Nursing theories: The base for professional practice.* Englewood Cliffs, N.J.: Prentice-Hall.
7. Fitzpatrick, J.J., & Whall, A.L. (1983). *Concep-*

tual models of nursing: Analysis and application. Bowie, Md.: Robert J. Brady.

8. Malinski, V.M. (1986). *Explorations on Martha Rogers' Science of Unitary Human Beings.* New York: Appleton-Century-Crofts.
9. McHugh, M. (1986). Nursing process: Musings on the method. *Holistic Nursing Practice, 1(1):*21-28.
10. Newman, M.A. (1979). *Theory development in nursing.* Philadelphia: F.A. Davis.
11. Reed, P.G. (1987, Feb.). Constructing a conceptual framework for psychosocial nursing. *Journal of Psychosocial Nursing and Mental Health Services, 25(2):*24-28.
12. Reynolds, P.D. (1971). *A primer in theory construction.* Indianapolis, Ind.: Bobbs-Merrill.
13. Riehl, J.P., and Roy, C. (Eds.). (1980). *Conceptual models for nursing practice* (2d ed.). New York: Appleton-Century-Crofts.
14. Rogers, M.E. (1961). *Educational revolution in nursing.* New York: Macmillan.
15. Rogers, M.E. (1970). *An introduction to the theoretical basis of nursing.* Philadelphia: F.A. Davis.
16. Rogers, M.E. (1972). *Challenge to nursing . . . professional nursing practice . . . evaluation.* NLN Publication #15-1456. Dept. Baccalaureate Higher Education Degree Programs, pp. 62-65.
17. Rogers, M.E. (1983). Science of unitary human beings: A paradigm for nursing. In I.W. Clements & F.B. Roberts, *Family health: A theoretical approach to nursing care.* New York: John Wiley & Sons.
18. Rogers, M.E. (1984, Oct.). The science of unitary man: An interview with Martha Rogers with E. Donnelly at Indiana University School of Nursing.
19. Rogers, M.E. (1986, September). *Dimensions of health: A view from space.* Paper presented at the conference on "Law and Life in Space," September 12, 1986. Center for Aerospace Sciences, University of North Dakota.
20. Rogers, M.E. (1988, March). Personal Correspondence.
21. *Webster's Ninth New Collegiate Dictionary.* (1983). Springfield, Mass.: Merriam-Webster.
22. Whelton, B.J. (1979). An operationalization of Martha Rogers' theory throughout the nursing process. *International Journal of Nursing Studies, 16(1):*7-20.
23. Wright, S.M. (1987, Sept.). The use of therapeutic touch in the management of pain. *The Nursing Clinics of North America, 22(3):*705-713.

BIBLIOGRAPHY

Primary Sources

Books

Rogers, M.E. (1961). *Educational revolution in nursing.* New York: Macmillan.

Rogers, M.E. (1964). *Reveille in nursing.* Philadelphia: F.A. Davis.

Rogers, M.E. (1970). *An introduction to the theoretical basis of nursing.* Philadelphia: F.A. Davis.

Book Chapters

Rogers, M.E. (1983). Beyond the horizon. In N.L. Chaska, *The nursing profession: A time to speak.* New York: McGraw-Hill.

Rogers, M.E. (1983). Science of unitary human beings: A paradigm for nursing. In Imelda W. Clements & Florence B. Roberts, *Family health: A theoretical approach to nursing care.* New York: John Wiley & Sons.

Articles

Fulp, E.M., & Rogers, M.E. (1982, Nov.-Dec.). N.C. Nurses visit China health services for a billion people. *Tar Heel Nurse, 44(6):* 5, 8.

Keddy, B., et al. (1986, Nov.). The doctor-nurse relationship: An historical perspective. Canada in the 1920s and/or 1930s. *Journal of Advanced Nursing, 11(6):*745-753.

Lambertsen, E., et al. (1966, May). Action, reaction: Four New York State Nurses Association members react to the American Nurses Association position paper on education. *New York State Nurse, 38(3):*6-8.

Rogers, M.E. (1953, May). Responses to talks on menstrual health. *Nursing Outlook, 1(5):*272-274.

Rogers, M.E. (1959, Spring). Responses to talks on menstrual health. *Nursing Research, 8:*114-115 (Abstract).

Rogers, M.E. (1963). Building a strong educational foundation. *American Journal of Nursing, 63:*94-95.

Rogers, M.E. (1963, June-July). The clarion call. *Nursing Science,* 1:134-135.

Rogers, M.E. (1963). Some comments on the theoretical basis of nursing practice. *Nursing Science, 1:*11-13, 60-61.

Rogers, M.E. (1964, Feb.). Professional standards: Whose responsibility? *Nursing Science, 2:*71-73.

Rogers, M.E. (1965, Jan.). What the public demands of nursing today. *RN, 28:*80.

Rogers, M.E. (1965). Legislative and licensing problems in health care. *Nursing Administration Quarterly, 2:*71-78.

Rogers, M.E. (1965, Oct.). Editorial: Collegiate education in nursing. *Nursing Science, 3(5):*362-365.

Rogers, M.E. (1965, Dec.). Editorial: Higher education in nursing. *Nursing Science, 3(6):*443-445.

Rogers, M.E. (1966). Doctoral education in nursing. *Nursing Forum, 5(2):*75-82.

Rogers, M.E. (1966). New designs—experiments in action. *National League Nursing Conference Paper, 20:*23-26.

Rogers, M.E. (1966, Winter). Quality nursing—cliche or challenge? *Maine Nurse, 9(1):*2-4.

Rogers, M.E. (1967, March). Teacher preparation. *NLN Department of Associate Degree Programs, 2:*20-36.

Rogers, M.E. (1968, Feb.). Nursing science: Research and researchers, *Record, 69:*469.

Rogers, M.E. (1969, March). Nursing research: Relevant to Practice? *Nursing Research Conference, 5:*352-359.

Rogers, M.E. (1969, Sept.). Nursing education for professional practice. *Catholic Nurse, 18(1):*28-37, 63-64.

Rogers, M.E. (1969, Nov.-Dec.). Preparation of the baccalaureate degree graduate. *New Jersey State Nurses Association Newsletter, 25(5):*32-37.

Rogers, M.E. (1970, Spring). Yesterday a nurse, tomorrow a manager; what now? *Journal of New York State Nurses Association, 1(1):*15-21.

Rogers, M.E. (1972). *Challenge to nursing . . . professional nursing practice . . . evaluation.* NLN Publication #15-1456. Dept. Baccalaureate Higher Education Degree Programs, pp. 62-65.

Rogers, M.E. (1972, Jan.). Nursing: To be or not to be? *Nursing Outlook, 20(1):*42-46.

Rogers, M.E. (1972, Dec.). Nursing's expanded role . . . and other euphemisms. *Journal of New York State Nurses Association, 3(4):*5-10.

Rogers, M.E. (1975). Yesterday a nurse, today a manager: What now? *Image, 2:*12-13.

Rogers, M.E. (1975). Forum: Professional commitment in nursing. *Image, 2:*12-13.

Rogers, M.E. (1975). Euphemisms in nursing's future. *Image, 7:*3-9.

Rogers, M.E. (1975, Aug.). Reactions to the two foregoing presentations, in challenge to nursing . . . professional nursing practice . . . evaluation. NLN Publication #15-1456. *Nursing Outlook, 20:*436.

Rogers, M.E. (1975, Aug.). Research is a growing word. *Nursing Science, 31:*283-294.

Rogers, M.E. (1975, October). Nursing is coming of age . . . Through the practitioner movement. *American Journal of Nursing, 75(10):*1834-43, 1859.

Rogers, M.E. (1977). Legislative and licensing problems in health care. *Nursing Administration Quarterly, 2:*71-78.

Rogers, M.E. (1978, Jan.-Feb.). Peer Review: A 1985 dissent. *Health PAC Bulletin, 80:*32-35.

Rogers, M.E. (1979, Dec.). Contemporary American leaders in nursing: An oral history. An interview with Martha E. Rogers. *Kango-Tenbo, 4(12):*1126-1138.

Rogers, M.E. (1985, April). *Nursing education: Preparing for the future.* NLN Publication #15-1974, pp. 11-14.

Rogers, M.E. (1985, Aug.). Euphemisms in nursing's future. *Kango, 37(9):*101-113.

Rogers, M.E. (1985, Sept.). *High touch in a high-tech future.* Perspectives in nursing—1985-1987: Based on presentations at the seventeenth NLN biennial convention. NLN Publication #41-1985, pp. 25-31.

Rogers, M.E. (1985, Nov.-Dec.). Classics from our heritage. The nature and characteristics of professional education for nursing. *Journal of Professional Nursing, 1(6):*381-383.

Rogers, M.E. (1985, Nov.-Dec.). Classics from our heritage. The need for legislation for licensure to practice professional nursing. *Journal of Professional Nursing, 1(6):*384.

Rogers, M.E. (1987, May). *Nursing research in the future.* NLN Publication #14-2203, pp. 121-123.

Sanford, R., & Rogers, M. (1978, July). The SAIN alternative: An interview with Martha Rogers. *Journal of Nursing Care, 11(7):*20-23.

Audiotape

Rogers, M.E. (1978, Oct. 20). *Nursing science: A science of unitary man.* Distinguished Lecture Series, Wright State University, Dayton, Ohio.

Rogers, M.E. (1978, Dec.). Paper presented at the Second Annual Nurse Educator Conference, New

York. Audiotape available from Teach 'em Inc., 160 E. Illinois Street, Chicago, Ill. 60611.

Rogers, M.E. (1980). *The science of unitary man.* Media For Nursing. New York.

Rogers, M.E. (1984, May). Paper presented at Nurses Theorist Conference, Edmonton, Alberta, Canada. Audiotape available from Kennedy Recordings, R.R. 5, Edmonton, Alberta, Canada TSP 4B7. (403-470-0013).

Rogers, M.E. (1987, May). *Rogers' framework.* Nurse Theorist Conference held in Pittsburgh, Pa. Audiotape available from Meetings International, 1200 Delor Avenue, Louisville, Ky. 40217.

Videotape

Distinguished Leaders in Nursing—Martha Rogers. (1982). Capitol Heights, Md: The National Audiovisual Center. Video tape available from National Institutes of Health, National Library of Medicine, Bethesda, Md. 20894 and from Sigma Theta Tau International, 1200 Washerway Blvd., Indianapolis, Ind. 46209.

Nursing Theory: A Circle of Knowledge. (1987). New York: National League for Nursing. Available from author, 10 Columbus Circle, New York, N.Y. 10019.

Rogers, M.E. (1984, Oct.). *The science of unitary man:* An interview with Martha Rogers with E. Donnelly at Indiana University School of Nursing.

Rogers, M.E. (1987, May). *Rogers' framework.* Nurse Theorist Conference held in Pittsburgh, Pa. Videotape available from Meetings International, 1200 Delor Avenue, Louisville, Ky. 40217.

The Nurse Theorist: Portraits of Excellence—Martha Rogers. (1988). Oakland, Cal.: Studio III. Videotape available from Fuld Video Project, Studio III, 370 Hawthorne Avenue, Oakland, Cal. 94609.

Lectures

Rogers, M.E. (1962, March). *Viewpoints—critical areas for nursing education in baccalaureate and higher degree programs.* An address given at the meeting of the Council of Member Agencies of the Department of Baccalaureate and Higher Degree Programs, Williamsburg, Virginia, March 26, 1962. New York, National League for Nursing, Department of Baccalaureate and Higher Degree Programs.

Rogers, M.E., et al. (1955). *Prenatal and paranatal factors in the development of behavior problems among the elementary school children.* Doctoral of Science dissertation, Baltimore, Johns Hopkins University.

Rogers, M.E. (1984, Sept. 28.). *Current issues for nursing in the next decade.* Indiana Central University, Indianapolis.

Rogers, M.E. (1986, Sept.). *Dimensions of health: A view from space.* Paper presented at the Conference on Law and Life in Space, September 12, 1986. Center for Aerospace Sciences, University of North Dakota.

Dissertation

Rogers, M.E. (1954). *The association of maternal and fetal factors with the development of behavior problems among elementary school children.* Doctor of Science dissertation, Baltimore, Johns Hopkins University.

Correspondence

Rogers, M.E. (1988, March). Personal correspondence.

Secondary Sources

Book Review

Anderson, E.H. (1970, Nov.-Dec.). Researchers' bookshelf. *Nursing Research, 19(6)*:541.

Books

Argyris, C., & Schon, D. (1974). *Theory in practice.* San Francisco: Jossey-Bass.

Bertalanffy, L. von (1960). *Problems of life.* New York: Harper Torch.

Bertalanffy, L. von (1960). *General systems theory: Foundations, developments, application.* New York: George Braziller.

Chardin, T. (1961). *The phenomenon of man.* New York: Harper Torch.

Chaska, N.L. (1983). *The nursing profession: A time to speak.* New York: McGraw-Hill.

Chinn, P.L., & Jacobs, M.K. (1983). *Theory and nursing: A systematic approach.* St. Louis: C.V. Mosby.

Directory of Nurses with Doctoral Degrees. (1984). Kansas City, Mo.: American Nurses' Association.

Dossey, L. (1982). *Space, time, and medicine.* Boulder, Col.: Shambhala Publications.

Einstein, A. (1961). *Relativity.* New York: Crown.

Fitzpatrick, J.J., & Whall, A.L. (1983). *Conceptual models of nursing: Analysis and application.* Bowie, Md.: Robert J. Brady.

George, J.B. (1985). Nursing Theories: The Base for Professional Nursing Practice (2d ed.). Englewood Cliffs, N.J.: Prentice-Hall.

Goldstein, K. (1939). *The organism.* New York: American Book.

Hanchett, E.S. (1979). *Community health assessment: A conceptual tool kit.* New York: John Wiley & Sons.

Herrick, C.J. (1956). *The evolution of human nature.* Austin: University of Texas Press.

King, I.M. (1971). *Toward a theory for nursing.* New York: John Wiley & Sons.

Lewin, K. (1964). *Field theory in the social sciences.* New York: Harper Torch.

Malinski, V.M. (Ed.). (1986). *Explorations on Martha Rogers' science of unitary human beings.* Norwalk, Conn.: Appleton-Century-Crofts.

Marriner, A. (1986). *Nursing theorists and their work.* St. Louis: C.V. Mosby.

Newman, M.A. (1979). *Theory development in nursing.* Philadelphia: F.A. Davis.

Parse, R.R. (1981). *Man-living-health. A theory of nursing.* New York: John Wiley & Sons.

Polanyi, M. (1958). *Personal knowledge.* Chicago: University of Chicago Press.

Reynolds, P.D. (1971). *A primer in theory construction.* Indianapolis, Ind.: Bobbs-Merrill.

Riehl, J.P., & Roy, C. (Eds.). (1980). *Conceptual models for nursing practice* (2d ed.). New York: Appleton-Century-Crofts.

Safier, G. (1977). *Contemporary American leaders: An oral history.* New York: McGraw-Hill.

Sarter, B. (1988). *The stream of becoming: A study of Martha Rogers' theory.* New York: NLN.

Sigma Theta Tau Directory of Nurse Researchers. (1983). Indianapolis, Ind.: Sigma Theta Tau.

Stevens, B.J. (1979). *Nursing theory: Analysis, application, evaluation.* Boston: Little, Brown.

Toffler, A. (1970). *Future shock.* New York: Random House.

Toffler, A. (1980). *The third wave.* New York: William Morrow.

Walker, L.O., and Avant, K.C. (1983). *Strategies for theory construction in nursing.* Norwalk, Conn.: Appleton-Century-Crofts.

Webster's Ninth New Collegiate Dictionary. (1983). Springfield, Mass.: Merriam-Webster.

Who's Who in American Nursing. (1986-1987). Washington, D.C.: Society of Nursing Professionals.

Book Chapters

Falco, S.M., & Lobo, M.L. (1980). Martha Rogers. In Nursing Theories Conference Group, J.B. George, Chairperson, *Nursing theories: The base for professional practice.* Englewood Cliffs, N.J.: Prentice-Hall.

Fawcett, J. (1984). Rogers life process model. In J. Fawcett, *Analysis and evaluation of conceptual models of nursing.* Philadelphia, F.A. Davis.

Field, L., & Newman, M. (1982). Clinical application of the unitary man framework: Case study analysis (1980). In M.J. Kim, & D.A. Moritz (Eds.), *Classification of nursing diagnosis: Proceedings of the third and fourth national conference.* New York: McGraw-Hill.

Madrid, M., & Winstead-Fry, P. (1986). Rogers' conceptual model. In P. Winstead-Fry (Ed.), *Case studies in nursing theory.* New York: National League for Nursing.

Meleis, A.I. (1985). Martha Rogers. In A.I. Meleis, *Theoretical nursing: Development and progress.* Philadelphia: J.B. Lippincott.

Articles

Aggleton, P., & Chalmers, H. (1984, Dec.). Models and theories: Rogers' unitary field model. Within the bounds of the nursing process—part 4. *Nursing Times, 80(50)*:35-39.

Anderson, M. (1980). A psychosocial screening tool for ambulatory health-care clients: A pilot study of validity. *Nursing Research, 29(6)*:347-351.

A science of unitary human beings—a paradigm for nursing. (1984, Oct.). *Kango, 36(11)*:18-47.

Atwood, J.R., & Gill-Rogers, B.P. (1984). Metatheory, methodology, and practicality: Issues in research uses of Rogers' science of unitary man. *Nursing Research, 33(2)*:88-91.

Barnard, K.E. (1977). Maternal-child nursing research: Review of past and strategies for future. *Nursing Research, 26(3)*:193-200.

Barnard, K.E. (1980). Knowledge for practice: Directions for the future. *Nursing Research, 29(4)*:208-212.

Barrett, E.A. Manhart. (1988, May). Using Rogers' science of unitary human beings in nursing practice. *Nursing Science Quarterly. 1(2)*:50-51.

Bateau, J. (1985, May-June). Case study in family therapy: A Rogers/Minuchin reformation. *Michigan Nurse, 58(3)*:7-9.

Blair, C. (1979). Hyperactivity in children: Viewed within the framework of synergistic man. *Nursing Forum, 18*:293-303.

Boyd, C. (1985). Toward an understanding of

mother-daughter identification using concept analysis. *Advances in Nursing Science, 7(3)*:78-86.

Brouse, S.H. (1985). Effect of gender role identity on patterns of feminine and self concept scores from late pregnancy to early postpartum. *Advances in Nursing Science, 7(3)*:32-48.

Bullough, B. (1975). Barriers to nurse practitioner movement: Problems of women in a womens field. *International Journal of Health Services, 5(2)*:225-233.

Bullough, B. (1976). Influences on role expansion. *American Journal of Nursing, 76(9)*:1476-1481.

Burr, H.S., & Northrop, F.S.E. (1935). The electrodynamic theory of life. *Quarterly Review of Biology, 10*:322-333.

Butterfield, S.E. (1983). In search of commonalities: Analysis of two theoretical frameworks. *International Journal of Nursing Studies, 20(1)*:15-22.

Change through environmental interaction makes aging exciting: An interview with Martha Rogers. (1985, Feb.). *Journal of Gerontological Nursing, 11(2)*:35-36.

Clarke, P.N. (1986). Theoretical and measurement issues in the study of field phenomena. *Advances in Nursing Science, 9(1)*:29-39.

Conway, M.E. (1985). Toward greater specificity in defining nursing's metaparadigm. *Advances in Nursing Science, 7(4)*:73-81.

Cooperative nursing investigations: Role for everyone. (1974). *Nursing Research, 23(6)*:452-456.

Craig, S.L. (1980). Theory development and its relevance for nursing. *Journal of Advanced Nursing, 5(4)*:349-355.

Crawford, G. (1985). A theoretical model of support network conflict experienced by new mothers. *Nursing Research, 34(2)*:100-102.

Cronenwett, L.R. (1983). Helping and nursing models. *Nursing Research, 32(6)*:342-346.

Donnelly, G.F. (1986). Nursing theory: Evolution of a sacred cow. *Holistic Nursing Practice, 1(1)*:1-7.

Duffey, M., & Muhlenkamp, A.F. (1974, Sept.). Framework for theory analysis. *Nursing Outlook, 22*:570-574.

Ellis, R. (1968, May-June). Characteristics of significant theories. *Nursing Research, 17*:217-222.

Fawcett, J. (1975). Family as a living open system: Emerging conceptual framework for nursing. *International Nursing Review, 22(4)*:113-116.

Fawcett, J. (1977). Relationship between identification and patterns of change in spouses body images during and after pregnancy. *International Journal of Nursing Studies, 14(4)*:199-213.

Fawcett, J. (1984). The metaparadigm of nursing: Present status and future refinements. *Image, 16(3)*:84-87.

Flaskerud, J.H. (1986). On toward a theory of nursing action: Skills and competency in nurse-patient interaction. *Nursing Research, 35(4)*:250-252.

Floyd, J.A. (1983). Research using Rogers' conceptual system: Development of a testable theorem. *Advances in Nursing Science, 5(2)*:37-38.

Floyd, J.A. (1984). Interaction between personal sleep-wake rhythms and psychiatric hospital rest-activity schedule. *Nursing Research, 33(5)*:255-259.

Gill, B.P., & Atwood, J.R. (1981). Reciprocy and helicy used to relate MEGF and wound healing. *Nursing Research, 30(2)*:68-72.

Goldberg, W.G., & Fitzpatrick, J.J. (1980). Movement therapy with the aged. *Nursing Research, 29(6)*:339-346.

Greaves, F. (1980). Objectively toward curriculum improvement in nursing: Education in England and Wales. *Journal of Advanced Nursing, 5(6)*:591-599.

Gresham, F.M. (1981). Assessment of children's social skills. *Journal of School Psychology, 19(2)*:120-133.

Gunter, L.M., & Miller, J.C. (1977). Toward a nursing gerontology. *Nursing Research, 26(3)*:208-221.

Hardy, M.F. (1974, March-April). Theories: Components, development, evaluation. *Nursing Research, 23*:100-107.

Hardy, M.F. (1978). Perspectives on nursing theory. *Advance in Nursing Science, 1*:37-48.

Heidt, P. (1981). Effect of therapeutic touch on anxiety level of hospitalized patients. *Nursing Research, 30(1)*:32-37.

Impact of physical-physiological activity on infants growth and development. (1972). *Nursing Research, 21(3)*:210-219.

Interview with Dr. Rogers. (1984, Oct.). *Kango, 36(11)*:48-51.

Iveson, J. (1982, Dec.). The four dimensional nurse. The Rogers' model of nursing. *Nursing Mirror, 155(22)*:52.

Johnson, D.E. (1974). Development of a theory: A requisite for nursing as a primary health profession. *Nursing Research, 23(5)*:372-377.

Johnson, M. (1983). Some aspects of the relation between theory and research in nursing. *Journal of Advanced Nursing, 8(1)*:21-28.

Johnson, R.L., Fitzpatrick, J.J., & Donovan, M.D. (1982). Developmental stage: Relationship to temporal dimensions. *Nursing Research, 31*:120 (Abstract).

Jones, P.S. (1978). Adaptation model for nursing practice. *American Journal of Nursing, 78(11)*: 1900-1906.

Katz, V. (1971) Auditory stimulation and developmental behavior of the premature infant. *Nursing Research, 20(3)*:196-201.

Keller, E., & Bzdek, V.M. (1986). Effects of therapeutic touch on tension headache pain. *Nursing Research, 35(2)*:101-106.

Ketefian, S. (1976). Curriculum change in nursing-education: Sources of knowledge utilized. *International Nursing Review, 23(4)*:107-115.

Ketefian, S. (1981). Critical thinking, educational preparation, and development of moral judgment among selected groups of practicing nurses. *Nursing Research, 30(2)*:98-103.

Ketefian, S. (1981). Moral reasoning and moral behavior among selected groups of practicing nurses. *Nursing Research, 30(3)*:171-176.

Kim, H.S. (1983). Use of Rogers' conceptual system in research: Comments. *Nursing Research, 32(2)*: 89-91.

Krieger, D. (1976). Healing by laying on of hands as a facilitator of bioenergetic change: The response of in vivo human hemoglobin. *International Journal of Psychoenergetic Systems, 1*:121-129.

Lanara, V.A. (1976). Philosophy of nursing and current nursing problems. *International Nursing Review, 23(2)*:48-54.

Levine, N.H. (1976). A conceptual model for obstetric nursing. *Journal of Obstetrics, Gynecologic, and Neonatal Nursing, 5(2)*:9-15.

McCrae, J. (1979). Therapeutic touch in practice. *American Journal of Nursing, 79*:664-665.

Majesky, S.J., Brester, M.H., & Nishio, K.T. (1978). Development of a research tool: Patient indicators of nursing care. *Nursing Research, 27(6)*:365-371.

McFarlane, E.A. (1980). Nursing theory: Compassion of four theoretical proposals. *Journal of Advanced Nursing, 5(1)*:3-19.

McHugh, M. (1986). Nursing process: Musings on the method. *Holistic Nursing Practice, 1(1)*:21-28.

Miller, L.A. (1979). An explanation of therapeutic touch using the science of unitary man. *Nursing Forum, 18*:278-287.

Moccia, P. (1985). A further investigation of "dialectical thinking as a means of understanding systems-in-development: Relevance to Rogers's principles." *Advances in Nursing Science, 7(4)*:33-38.

Moore, G. (1982). Perceptual complexity, memory and human duration experience. *Nursing Research, 31(3)*:189 (Abstract).

Nicoll, L.H., Meyer, P.A., & Abraham, I.L. (1985). Critique: External comparison of conceptual nursing models. *Advances in Nursing Science, 7(4)*:1-9.

Papowitz, L. (1986, April). During resuscitation, some patients face a life-or-death choice that no one else will know about—unless they ask. *American Journal of Nursing, 86*:416-418.

Peterson, M. (1987). Time and nursing process. *Holistic Nursing Practice, 1(3)*:72-80.

Porter, L.S. (1972). The impact of physical-physiological activity on infant growth and development. *Nursing Research, 21(3)*:210-219.

Porter, L.S. (1985). Is nursing ready for the year 2000? *Nursing Forum, 22(2)*:53-57.

Reed, P.G. (1986). Developmental resources and depression in the elderly. *Nursing Research, 35(6)*:368-374.

Reed, P.G. (1987, February). Constructing a conceptual framework for psychosocial nursing. *Journal of Psychosocial Nursing and Mental Health Services, 25(2)*:24-28.

Reed, P.G., et al. (1982). Suicidal crises: Relationship to the experience of time. *Nursing Research, 31*:122 (Abstract).

Rehabilitation workshops: Change in attitudes of nurses. (1972). *Nursing Research, 21(2)*:132-137.

Reiner, D.K. (1977). Persons in process: Model for professional education. *Archives of the Foundation of Thanatology, 6(3)*:24.

Rejoinder to commentary: Toward a clearer understanding of concept of nursing theory. (1972). *Nursing Research, 21(1)*:59-62.

Roberts, K.L. (1985). Theory of nursing as curriculum content. *Journal of Advanced Nursing, 10*:209-215.

Roy, C., & Obloy, M. (1978). Practitioner movement: Toward a science of nursing. *American Journal of Nursing, 78(10)*:1698-1702.

Sarter, B. (1987). Evolutionary idealism: A philo-

sophical foundation for holistic nursing theory. *Advances in Nursing Science, 9(2)*:1-9.
Sarter, B. (1988). Philosophical sources of nursing theory. *Nursing Science Quarterly, 1(2)*:52-59.
Schoen, D.C. (1975). Comparing body systems and conceptual approaches to nursing education. *Nursing Research, 24(5)*:383-387.
Sheahan, J. (1980). Some aspects of the teaching and learning in nursing. *Journal of Advanced Nursing, 5(5)*:491-511.
Silva, M.C. (1986). Research testing nursing theory: State of the art. *Advances in Nursing Science, 9(1)*:1-11.
Silva, M.C., & Rothbart, D. (1984). An analysis of changing trends in philosophies of science on nursing theory development and testing. *Advances in Nursing Science, 6(2)*:1-13.
Smith, C.S. (1988, May). Testing propositions derived from Rogers' conceptual system. *Nursing Science Quarterly, 1(2)*:60-67.
Smith, M.J. (1986, Oct.). Human-environment process: A test of Rogers' principle of integrality. *Advances in Nursing Science, 9(1)*:21-28.
Taylor, S.D. (1975). Bibliography on nursing research: 1950-1974. *Nursing Research, 24(3)*:207-255.
Theiss, B.E. (1976). Investigation of perceived role functions and attitudes of nurse practitioner role in a primary care clinic. *Military Medicine, 141(2)*:85-89.
Uys, L.R. (1987, May). Foundational studies in nursing. Orem, King and Rogers. *Journal of Advanced Nursing, 12(3)*:275-280.
Walker, L.O., & Nicholson, R. (1980). Criteria for evaluating nursing process models. *Nurse Educator, 5(5)*:8-9.
Whall, A.L. (1981). Nursing theory and the assessment of families. *Journal of Psychiatric Nursing and Mental Health Services, 19(1)*:30-36.
Whelton, B.J. (1979). An operationalization of Martha Rogers' theory throughout the nursing process. *International Journal of Nursing Studies, 16(1)*:7-20.
White, E.J. (1986, May-June). Appraising the need for altered sexuality information. *Rehabilitation Nurse, 11(3)*:6-9.
Wright, S.M. (1987, Sept.). The use of therapeutic touch in the management of pain. *The Nursing Clinics of North America, 22(3)*:705-713.
Yano, M., Onodera, T., & Higuchi, Y. (1980, Summer). Discussion on "An Introduction to the Theoretical Basis of Nursing" by Martha E. Rogers. *Kango-Kenkyu, 13(3)*:228-239.
Young, A.A., & Keil, C. (1981, April). The Washburn nursing curriculum: Interpreting Martha Rogers in the Land of Oz. *Kansas Nurse, 56(4)*:7-8.

Dissertation

Rawnsley, M.M. (1977). *Perception of the speed of time in aging and in dying: An empirical investigation of holistic theory of nursing proposed by Martha Rogers.* Doctoral dissertation. Boston University.

Other

Burr, H.S. (1962). *The nature of man and the meaning of existence.* Springfield, Ill.: Charles C Thomas.
Capra, F. (1982). *The turning point: Science, society, and the rising culture.* New York: Simon and Schuster.
Laszlo, E. (Ed.). (1972). *The relevance of general systems theory.* New York: George Braziller.

Appendix A

GLOSSARY

Learned Profession:	A science and an art.
Science:	An organized body of abstract knowledge arrived at by scientific research and logical analysis.
Art:	The imaginative and creative use of knowledge.
Negentropy:	Increasing heterogeneity, differentiation, diversity, complexity of pattern.
Energy Field:	The fundamental unit of the living and the non-living. Field is a unifying concept. Energy signifies the dynamic nature of the field. Energy fields are infinite.
Pattern:	The distinguishing characteristic of an energy field perceived as a single wave.

Four Dimensional:	A non-linear domain without spatial or temporal attributes.
Conceptual System:	An abstraction. A representation of the universe or some portion thereof.
Unitary Man: (Human field)	An irreducible, four dimensional energy field identified by pattern and manifesting characteristics that are specific to the whole and which cannot be predicted from knowledge of the parts.
Environment:	An irreducible, four dimensional energy field identified by pattern and integral with the human field.

Appendix B

SELECTED DOCTORAL DISSERTATIONS BASED ON *NURSING: SCIENCE OF UNITARY HUMAN BEINGS*

Barrett, Elizabeth Ann. (1983). *An Empirical Investigation of Rogers' Principle of Helicy: The Relationship of Human Field Complexity, Human Field Motion, and Power.* New York University.

Cowling, W. Richard. (1982). *The Relationship of Mystical Experience, Differentiation, and Creativity in College Students: An Empirical Investigation of the Principle of Helicy in Rogers' Science of Unitary Man.* New York University.

Ference, Helen. (1979). *The Relationship of Time Experience, Creativity Traits, Differentiation, and Human Field Motion.* New York University.

Gueldner, Sarah H. (1983). *A Study of the Relationship Between Imposed Motion and Human Field Motion in Elderly Individuals Living in Nursing Homes.* University of Alabama in Birmingham.

Ludomirski-Kalamin, Betty. (1984). *Relationship Between the Environmental Energy Wave Frequency Pattern Manifest in Red Light and Blue Light and Human Field Motion in Adult Individuals with Visual Sensory Perception and Those With Total Blindness.* New York University.

Macrae, Janet A. (1982). *A Comparison Between Meditating Subjects and Non-Meditating Subjects on Time Experience and Human Field Motion.* New York University.

Malinski, Violet. (1980). *The Relationship Between Hyperactivity in Children and Perception of Short Wave Length Light: An Investigation into the Conceptual System Proposed by Martha E. Rogers.* New York University.

Miller, Fay. (1984). *The Relationship of Sleep, Wakefulness, and Beyond Waking Experience: A Descriptive Study of M. Rogers' Concept of Sleep-Wake Rhythm.* New York University.

Raile, Martha M. (1982). *The Relationship of Creativity, Actualization, and Empathy in Unitary Human Development: A Descriptive Study of Rogers' Principle of Helicy.* New York University.

Rawnsley, Marilyn. (1977). *Relationships Between the Perception of the Speed of Time and the Process of Dying: An Empirical Investigation of the Holistic Theory of Nursing Proposed by Martha Rogers.* Boston University.

Reeder, Francelyn. (1984). *Nursing Research, Holism, and Philosophies of Science: Points of Congruence Between Edmund Husserl and Martha E. Rogers.* New York University.

Sarter, Barbara. (1984). *The Stream of Becoming: A Metaphysical Analysis of Rogers' Model of Unitary Man.* New York University.

Available through Dissertation Abstracts.

31

Joyce J. Fitzpatrick

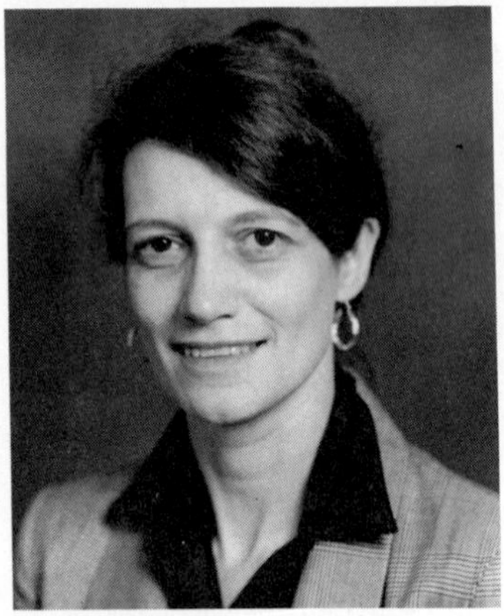

Life Perspective Model

Sarah J. Beckman, Patricia Chapman-Boyce, Sydney Coleman-Ehmke, Cheryl A. Hailway, Rhonda G. Justus, Rosalyn A. Pung, Cathy R. Smith

CREDENTIALS AND BACKGROUND OF THE THEORIST

Joyce J. Fitzpatrick was born May 4, 1944. She received her B.S.N. in 1966 from Georgetown University in Washington, D.C., and her M.S. in Psychiatric Mental Health from Ohio State University in Columbus in 1967. She took postmaster's courses in Community Health at Ohio State in 1971 to 1972, and achieved a Ph.D. in nursing from New York University in 1975. In 1987 she attended Harvard University's Institute for Educational Management.

Fitzpatrick has held many positions, including staff nurse, public health nurse, instructor, and the director of training for suicide prevention, all in Columbus, Ohio. She has served as an assistant professor at New York University and Associate Professor at Wayne State University. In addition, she has also been the chairperson for the Department of Nursing Systems and the director of the Center for Health Research at Wayne State. Fitzpatrick has been Visiting Professor at Rutgers—The State Univer-

The authors wish to express appreciation to Dr. Joyce J. Fitzpatrick for critiquing the chapter.

sity, College of Nursing. In 1982 Fitzpatrick became Professor and Dean of Nursing at Case Western Reserve University in Cleveland, Ohio, and Administrative Associate at University Hospitals of Cleveland.

Since 1974 Fitzpatrick has worked as a consultant in such areas as faculty development, research development, and development of master's and doctoral programs in nursing with several institutions, including Indiana University, Michigan State University, The Ohio State University, Rutgers University, University of Kansas, University of Virginia, Vanderbilt University, and Wright State University.

In addition, since 1984 Fitzpatrick has worked as a consultant in such areas as doctoral program development at University of South Carolina, conceptual framework development at University of Tennessee at Memphis, the development of a computerized nursing information system at Hospital Corporation of America, Nashville, Tennessee, consultant to nursing staff at a psychiatric hospital in Toronto, Ontario, and as consultant to Director of Nursing Affairs at American Medical Association.

Fitzpatrick has received honoraries and is affiliated with several organizations. Professional activities have been numerous. She has presented workshops on community health, current issues in health, stress, crisis intervention, dying and death, suicidology, theory development, and research in nursing. She has been the investigator and director for several research grants, has done numerous paper and research presentations, and has published extensively.[5]

THEORETICAL SOURCES FOR THEORY DEVELOPMENT

Fitzpatrick is a well-known, published scholar among nursing professionals. She constructed her theory model based on the ideas and work of Martha Rogers. Fitzpatrick[4;5:299-301] used rhythm patterns, which are operational modes specifying the pattern of person and environment that were explicated by Rogers. In addition, Fitzpatrick[5:310] incorporated the peak and wave pattern ideas of E. Haus and G.G. Luce. To round out the model, she drew from G. Caplan's crisis theory.[4:23-24;7:310]

USE OF EMPIRICAL EVIDENCE

Fitzpatrick's Life Perspective Model is synthesized from interpretations made from Rogers' theory work. Colleagues consider Rogers one of the most original thinkers in nursing who capitalizes on knowledge from other disciplines such as anthropology, sociology, astronomy, religion, philosophy, history, and mythology. The model's concept of environment is drawn from von Bertalanffy and others who question the failure of physical laws to explain evolution of life. According to S.M. Falco and M.L. Lobo, "There is a strong parallel between Rogers' basic assumptions and general systems theory."[2:167] Rogers also draws from Einstein in using the concept of four dimensionality.

MAJOR CONCEPTS AND DEFINITIONS

The four major concepts in this model are nursing, person, health, and environment. "The ontogenetic and phylogenetic interactions among person and health are looked upon as the essence of nursing."[7:306]

According to J.L. Pressler, in Fitzpatrick's rhythm model "nursing, as a noun, is described as the science and profession whose central concern is the meaning attached to life (health). As a verb, nursing is said to be focused on enhancing the developmental process toward health so that individuals may be led to develop their potentials as human beings."[7:313]

Person is seen as an open system, a unified whole characterized by a basic human rhythm. Health is viewed as a human dimension under continuous development—a heightened awareness of the meaningfulness of life.[7:306] According to J.L. Pressler,[7] Fitzpatrick mirrors Rogers' definition of environmental field.

MAJOR ASSUMPTIONS

Fitzpatrick repeats the five basic assumptions proposed by Rogers in her theory of unitary man:

1. Man is a unified whole possessing his own integrity and manifesting characteristics that are more than and different from the sum of his parts.
2. Man and environment are open systems, continually exchanging matter and energy with each other.
3. The life process evolves irreversibly and unidirectionally along the space time continuum.
4. Pattern and organization identify man and reflect his innovative wholeness.
5. Man is characterized by the capacity for abstraction and imagery, language and thought, sensation and emotion.[3:299-300]

According to Pressler, four implicit assumptions pertinent to understanding Fitzpatrick's model were previously identified. These are:

1. Differences in behavioral manifestations are more easily identified during the peaks of wave patterns.
2. Identified by congruency, consistency, and integrity of rhythmic patterns, health is to the manifestations of symphonic interaction of persons and their environments.
3. Emphasized through selected research on temporality, the meaning attached to life is a central concern of nursing.
4. Nursing is a philosophy, a science, and an art.[4;7:309-310]

THEORETICAL ASSERTIONS

The Life Perspective Model is a developmental model that proposes that the process of human development is characterized by rhythms. The person is treated as an open, holistic, rhythmic system that can best be described by temporal, motion, consciousness, and perceptual patterns. It is possible to identify peaks and troughs of particular human rhythms throughout the developmental process. There are patterns within a pattern or overall life patterns. Life's pattern continues toward timelessness, becoming more dominant as one's development occurs. This may best be described as patterns within a pattern or rhythms within an overall life rhythm. Health is viewed as a continuously developing characteristic of humans with the full life potential that may characterize the process of dying, as the heightened awareness of the meaningfulness of life, and as representing a more fully developed dimension of health. Health is seen as the interactions of persons with their environment. Nursing's central concern is focused on the person in relation to health, with the goal of enhancing the developmental process toward health so people may develop their potential as human beings. "The meaning attached to life, the basic understanding of human existence, is a central concern of nursing as science and profession."[3:301] The hypothesis is that "individuals experiencing crisis had difficulty integrating the present situation within their life perspective."[3:295]

A conceptual model was developed to depict the essential theoretical representation of person, environment, health, and nursing as if one were looking through a Slinky. Fitzpatrick expanded the Slinky concept to symbolize her view of man. The representation helps in picturing the relationships found in the Life Perspective Model (Figure 31-1).

LOGICAL FORM

Fitzpatrick developed the Life Perspective Model using a deductive logical approach; that is, the author uses empirical findings to support a proposed developmental model. This model indicates that human development is characteristic of temporal, motion, perceptual, and consciousness rhythms. These patterns show the continuous person-environment interaction in relation to one's personal development.

An individual's progression through life contains varying high and low intervals, but the general direction represents rapidity. While explaining the broadness in life, such progression

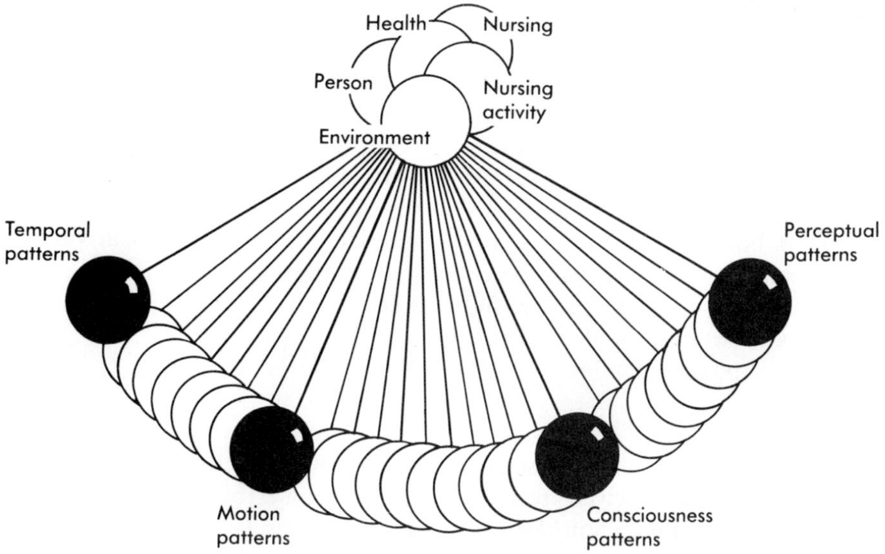

Figure 31-1. Relationships within life perspective model.
Used with permission from Pressler, J.L. (1983). Fitzpatrick's Rhythm Model: Analysis for Nursing Science. In J.J. Fitzpatrick, & A. Whall, *Conceptual models of nursing: Analysis and application*. Bowie, Md.: Robert J. Brady.

relates life and health. In this model health represents a basic human element that is a continuous development from birth to death. Understandably, the meaning one attaches to life and health or humanness is significant in this model. Accordingly, health or potentiating health is considerably influential to one's meaning in life.

Because of Fitzpatrick's extensive work and study under Rogers, Fitzpatrick bases the Life Perspective Model on Rogers' unitary man assumptions and model concepts in addition to expanding the Slinky representation in her own model. To add further merit to this model's development, Fitzpatrick drew from the biological rhythm theory and also from Caplan's crisis theory. Fitzpatrick also used her own personal interests and professional experience in crisis in the model's development. The model's hypothesis was derived based on these aspects. It states, "Individuals experiencing crisis had difficulty integrating the present situations within their life perspective."[3:295]

The next logical step is empirical testing, which is imperative in any model's development and future. Much of the testing of this model has related only to the temporal pattern with a selective population focus on the elderly in nursing homes and during hospitalization. Recent studies have dealt with terminally ill cancer patients and with suicidal individuals. Using results from the completed investigations, Fitzpatrick continues to broaden the model, such as in her meaning attached to life and death. But she acknowledges that the limitations of the empirical investigations hold back the model's developmental progress and the gathering of further logical support.

ACCEPTANCE BY THE NURSING COMMUNITY

Practice

Because her model is still in the developmental stage, Fitzpatrick encourages further study and ongoing empirical testing. With more involvement by the nursing community, progress will be made. The model is apparently not being used in practice.

Education

The majority of testing has been completed by graduate students studying with Fitzpatrick. The model has not been incorporated into any nursing curriculum, but critics feel the theory is potentially adaptable for educational purposes. Fitzpatrick has incorporated her theory and conceptualization into her graduate-level theory and nursing research courses.

Research

Fitzpatrick is active in current nursing research. From 1976 to 1984 she received research grants totaling more than $1 million. Her research projects have dealt with temporal experiences of the terminally ill cancer patients, the aging process, temporal experiences of the suicidal, the advancement of doctoral programs, and interpretations of life and death.

From 1985 to 1988 she received research grants totaling more than $1 million. Some of her projects include doctor of nursing evaluation, advanced nurse training in nurse-midwifery, the advancement of doctoral programs, the design and development of expert systems for decision-support in acute care nursing areas, and perinatal nurse major.[5] Fitzpatrick's proposals are initiating new ideas and research that is useful for the advancement of nursing science.

FURTHER DEVELOPMENT

As previously discussed, the Life Perspective Model is in a beginning developmental stage. The multiple definitions given to nursing and health in the model are problematic. The vast interrelationship between person and environment is highly complex and not easily understood. Because most of the completed research focuses on the temporal pattern, the other patterns still need to be researched. But even the completed temporal pattern research shows that operational measurement is problematic and raises other considerations for future research. Until significant investigation is completed in all rhythms, this model cannot be addressed holistically. Although the model's individual components may have merit and nursing support, the complete model still needs to be tested. Therefore, this model's future place in a creative nursing science, in nursing practice, and in nursing theory consideration is uncertain.

CRITIQUE

Clarity

Fitzpatrick consistently follows theoretical form by stating a hypothesis and listing assumptions. She continues by stating relationships of concepts and displays her theory in a four dimensional Slinky model, representing the relationship statements. Most of the empirical testing has occurred with temporal patterns, but plans are in process to develop the theory and to empirically test the conscious rhythm, perceptual rhythms, motion rhythms, and their relationships with the meaning attached to life and life perspective.

Simplicity

This model is complex in its concepts and interrelationships. Sufficiently understanding and explaining the interrelationships between health, nursing, person, environment, and nursing activity in respect to the temporal, motion, consciousness, and perceptual patterns are highly complex and involved undertakings. Such interrelationships are not easily taken from concept to operational measurement.

Generality

Most of the empirical investigations relate to the elderly, terminally ill cancer patients, and suicidal individuals and contain a heavy psychosocial orientation. Fitzpatrick acknowledges that the model needs testing in other populations such as infants, children, and adolescents.[3:315]

Empirical Precision

Fitzpatrick and her researchers have been successful in scientifically testing and evaluating several of the relationships presented in the Life Perspective Rhythm Model. But the current literature indicates that only some educators and students are in the process of empirically testing relationships in this projected model. Interested researchers and practitioners are encouraged to become involved in the efforts to further develop the Life Perspective Rhythm Model.

Derivable Consequences

The derivable consequences connect the theory with achievable nursing outcomes. Because this model is at the beginning development stage, its application and usefulness in nursing practice and science have been limited. The concepts, and some of the research, are stimulating and warrant further work and additional development. Conceivably, some concepts of the model may in the future help broaden perspectives in relation to humanness and move nursing closer to holistic nursing practice.[1:133-143]

REFERENCES

1. Chinn, P.L., & Jacobs, M.K. (1983). *Theory and nursing: A systematic approach.* St. Louis: C.V. Mosby.
2. Falco, S.M., & Lobo, M.L. (1980). Martha Rogers. In Nursing Theories Conference Group, J.B. George, Chairperson, *Nursing theories: The base for professional nursing practice.* Englewood Cliffs, N.J.: Prentice-Hall.
3. Fitzpatrick, J.J., & Whall, A.L. (1983). *Conceptual models of nursing: Analysis and application.* Bowie, Md.: Robert J. Brady.
4. Fitzpatrick, J.J. (1982). The crisis perspective: Relationship to nursing. In J.J. Fitzpatrick, et al., (Eds.), *Nursing models and their psychiatric mental health applications.* Bowie, Md.: Robert J. Brady.
5. Fitzpatrick, J.J. (1988). Curriculum vitae.
6. Goldberg, W.G., & Fitzpatrick, J.J. (1980, Nov.-Dec.). Movement therapy with the aged. *Nursing Research, 29(6)*:339-346.
7. Pressler, J.L. (1983). Fitzpatrick's rhythm model: Analysis for nursing science. In J. Fitzpatrick & A. Whall, *Conceptual models of nursing: Analysis and application.* Bowie, Md.: Robert J. Brady.

BIBLIOGRAPHY
Primary Sources
Books

Abraham, I.L., & Fitzpatrick, J.J. (In preparation). *Nursing and health research.* Philadelphia: W.B. Saunders.

Abraham, I.L., Nadzam, D.M., & Fitzpatrick, J.J. (Eds.). (In press). *Statistics and quantitative methods in nursing: Issues and strategies for research and education.* Philadelphia: W.B. Saunders.

Fitzpatrick, J.J., Johnston, A.L., & Floyd, J.A. (1982). *Nursing models and their psychiatric mental health applications.* Bowie, Md.: Robert J. Brady.

Fitzpatrick, J.J., & Taunton, R.L. (Eds.). (1987). *Annual review of nursing research* (Vol. 5). New York: Springer.

Fitzpatrick, J.J., Taunton, R.L., & Beneliol, J.Q. (1988). *Annual review of nursing research* (Vol. 6). New York: Springer.

Fitzpatrick, J.J., Taunton, R.L., & Benoliol, J.Q. (1989). *Annual Review of Nursing Research.* (Vol. 7). New York: Springer.

Fitzpatrick, J.J., & Whall, A.L. (1983). *Conceptual models of nursing: Analysis and application.* Bowie, Md.: Robert J. Brady.

Shamian, J., Cowling, W.R. III, & Fitzpatrick, J.J. *Advanced critical analysis of nursing management theories* (book prospectus, in review).

Werley, H.H., & Fitzpatrick, J.J. (Eds.). (1984). *Annual review of nursing research* (Vol. I). New York: Springer.

Werley, H.H., & Fitzpatrick, J.J. (Eds.). (1984). *Annual review of nursing research* (Vol. II). New York: Springer.

Werley, H.H., & Fitzpatrick, J.J. (Eds.). (1985). *Annual review of nursing research.* (Vol. 3). New York: Springer.

Werley, H.H., Fitzpatrick, J.J., & Taunton, R.L. (Eds.). (1986). *Annual review of nursing research* (Vol. 4). New York: Springer.

Chapters and Proceedings

Abraham, I.L., & Fitzpatrick, J.J. (1986). Expert systems for nursing practice: Developing and implementing decision-support technology in nursing. In B. DuGas, G. Hefferman, M. Light, A. O'-Connor, H. Oglivie, & E. Zwarts (Eds.),

Proceedings of the National Symposium on Computer Applications for Nursing. Ottawa, Canada: The University of Ottawa.

Abraham, I.L., & Fitzpatrick, J.J. (1986). Research environments in nursing: Rationale and requirements for computing. *Proceedings of the Ninth Annual Symposium on Computer Applications in Medical Care.* Silver Springs, Md.: IEEE Computer Society.

Abraham, I.L., & Fitzpatrick, J.J. (In press). On the scientific and technical requirements for computing resources. In V.K. Saba, K. Rieder, & D. Pocklington (Eds.). *A review of computer technology in nursing.* Berlin: Springer Verlag.

Abraham, I.L., & Fitzpatrick, J.J., & Jewell, J.A. (In press). The Artificial Intelligence in Nursing Project: Developing advanced technology for expert care. In K. Hanna (Ed.), *Clinical judgment and decision-making: The future with nursing diagnosis.* Amsterdam: North-Holland.

Abraham, I.L., Nadzam, D.M., & Fitzpatrick, J.J. (Eds.). (In press). Statistics in nursing curricula. In I.L. Abraham, D.M. Nadzam, & J.J. Fitzpatrick (Eds.), *Statistics and quantitative methods in nursing: Issues and strategies for research and education.* Philadelphia: W.B. Saunders.

Downs, F.S., & Fitzpatrick, J.J. (1984). Preliminary investigation of the reliability and validity of a tool for the assessment of body position and motor activity. In F.S. Downs (Ed.), *A Source book of nursing research* (3d ed.). Philadelphia: F.A. Davis. (Reprinted from *Nursing Research,* 1976, *25:*404-408.)

Fitzpatrick, J.J. (1976). Repatterning alcoholic behaviors: Nursing strategies. In J. Chodil (Ed.), *Proceedings of the 8th Annual Clinical Sessions.* New York: New York University.

Fitzpatrick, J.J. (1982). The crisis perspective: Relationship to nursing. In J.J. Fitzpatrick, et al., *Nursing models and their psychiatric mental health applications.* Bowie, Md.: Robert J. Brady.

Fitzpatrick, J.J. (1982). The path of nursing, the path of science? In V. Engle, *Proceedings of the Fourth Annual Research Symposium of the Michigan Sigma Theta Tau Consortium.* Indianapolis, Ind.: Sigma Theta Tau.

Fitzpatrick, J.J. (1983). Integrating the domains of nursing. In *Proceedings of the 1982 Forum on Doctoral Education in Nursing.* Cleveland, Ohio: Case Western Reserve University.

Fitzpatrick, J.J. (1983). A life perspective rhythm model. In J.J. Fitzpatrick & A.L. Whall (Eds.), *Conceptual models of nursing: Analysis and application.* Bowie, Md.: Robert J. Brady.

Fitzpatrick, J.J. (1983). Techniques of gerontological counseling. In S. Lego (Ed.), *Lippincott manual of psychiatric nursing.* Philadelphia: J.B. Lippincott.

Fitzpatrick, J.J. (1984). Gerontological counseling. In S. Lego (Ed.), *The American handbook of psychiatric nursing,* pp. 357-363. Philadelphia: J.B. Lippincott.

Fitzpatrick, J.J. (1984). Reaction to the debate: The research doctorate and the professional doctorate. In *The 1984 National Forum on Doctoral Education in Nursing Proceedings: Epistemological strategies in nursing.* Denver, Colo.: University of Colorado School of Nursing.

Fitzpatrick, J.J. (1985). Reaction to Fagin: Institutionalizing faculty practice. In *Proceedings of the Second National Conference on Faculty Practice.* Kansas City, Mo.: American Academy of Nursing.

Fitzpatrick, J.J. (1985). Research. In J.S. Jamann (Ed.), *Proceedings of doctoral programs in nursing: Consensus for quality, August, 1984.* Washington, D.C.: American Association of Colleges of Nursing.

Fitzpatrick, J.J. (1985). Response to institutionalizing practice: Historical and future perspectives. In K.E. Barnard & G.R. Smith (Eds.), *Faculty practice in action, Second Annual Symposium on Nursing Faculty Practice,* pp. 28-30. Kansas City, Mo.: American Academy of Nursing.

Fitzpatrick J.J. (1985). Response to manpower in nursing homes: Implications for research. In M.S. Harper & B. Lebowitz (Eds.), *Mental illness in nursing homes: Agenda for research,* pp. 281-305. Rockville, Md.: National Institute of Mental Health.

Fitzpatrick, J.J. (1987). Etiology: Conceptual concerns. *Proceedings of the 1986 North American Nursing Diagnosis Association (NANDA) Conference.*

Fitzpatrick, J.J. (1987). In V. Malinski (Ed.). *Explorations in Martha Rogers' science of unitary human beings.* East Norwalk, Conn.: Appleton-Century-Crofts. Chapter 1. Introduction to Rogers' science of unitary human beings. Chapter 6. Critique: Relationship between the perception of the speed of time and the process of dying (Rawnsley). Chapter 7. Critique: Relationship of time experience, creativity traits, differentiation, and human field motion (Ference). Chapter 8. Critique: Relationship between hyperactivity in children and perception of short wavelength light (Malinski). Chapter 9. Critique: Relationship between visible lightwaves and the experience of pain (McDonald). Chapter 10. Critique: Relationship of mystical experience, differentiation, and creativity in college students (Cowling). Chapter 11. Critique: Relationship of creativity, actualization, and empathy in unitary human development (Raile-Alligood). Chapter 12. Critique: Relationship between imposed motion and human field motion in elderly individuals living in nursing homes (Gueldner). Chapter 13. Critique: Investigation of the principle of helicy: The relationship of human field motion and power (Barrett).

Fitzpatrick, J.J. (1987). Nursing. In A.J. Goldstein (Ed.). *Peterson's accounting to zoology.* Princeton, N.J.: Peterson's Guides.

Fitzpatrick, J.J. (1987). Nursing education. *Peterson's Annual Guides to Graduate Study, Book 3. Graduate programs in the biological, agricultural, and health sciences 1987,* 21st ed. Princeton, N.J.: Peterson's Guides.

Fitzpatrick, J.J. (1987). Philosophical approach: Empiricism. In *Proceedings of the Fourth Nursing Science Colloquium,* pp. 19-30. Boston: Boston University.

Fitzpatrick, J.J. (1988). Toward a nursing minimum data set: Group #1 Review and summary. In H.H. Werley & N.L. Lang (Eds.), *Nursing minimum data set.* New York: Springer.

Fitzpatrick, J.J., & Abraham, I.L. (1987). Developing collegial relationships through scholarship. In W.E. Cashin & A. Noma (Eds.), *Proceedings of the Third Annual Conference on Academic Chairpersons: Unraveling the paradox, 20:*105-108. Orlando: Center for Faculty Evaluation and Development.

Fitzpatrick, J.J., Abraham, I.L., & Nadzam, D.M. (In press). Statistics and quantitative methods in nursing summarized: Issues and strategies for the future. In I.L. Abraham, D.M. Nadzam, & J.J. Fitzpatrick (Eds.), *Statistics and quantitative methods in nursing: Issues and strategies for research and education.* Philadelphia: W.B. Saunders.

Fitzpatrick, J.J., & Anderson, G.C. (1986). Group summary: Setting the agenda for the year 2000: Knowledge development in nursing. *Proceedings of the AAN Annual Meeting and Scientific Session.* Kansas City, Mo.: American Academy of Nursing.

Fitzpatrick, J.J., & Donovan, M.J. (1986). Interpretations of life and death: Relationships to health. *Proceedings of the Twelfth World Conference on Health Education.* Dublin, Ireland: International Health Educator's Association.

Fitzpatrick, J.J., & Holloran, E.J. (1985). Proactivating a collaborative service education climate. In *MAIN Proceedings Thriving or Surviving? Managing pro-active environments for nursing,* pp. 29-41. Indianapolis: Midwest Alliance in Nursing.

Fitzpatrick, J.J., & Whall, A.L. (1983). Nursing models: Summary and future projections. In J.J. Fitzpatrick & A.L. Whall (Eds.). *Conceptual models of nursing: Analysis and application.* Bowie, Md.: Robert J. Brady.

Fitzpatrick, J.J., & Whall, A.L., (1983). Overview of nursing models and nursing theories. In J.J. Fitzpatrick & A.L. Whall (Eds.), *Conceptual models of nursing: Analysis and application.* Bowie, Md.: Robert J. Brady.

Jewell, J.A., Abraham, I.L., & Fitzpatrick, J.J. (In press). The Laboratory for AI Research in Nursing: Initial equipment configuration. *Proceedings of the American Association for Medical Systems and Informatics.*

Johnston, R.L., & Fitzpatrick, J.J. (1982). Relevance of psychiatric mental health nursing theories to nursing models. In J.J. Fitzpatrick, et al., *Nursing models and their psychiatric mental health applications.* Bowie, Md.: Robert J. Brady.

Kirk, L.W., Abraham, I.L., Jane, L.-H., & Fitzpatrick, J.J. (1986). Comprehensive computerization of a school of nursing: Planning aspects and system description. In R. Salamon, B. Blum, & M. Jorgenson (Eds.), *Medinfo 86,* Vol 2, Amsterdam: North-Holland/Elsevier.

Nadzam, D.M., Fitzpatrick, J.J., & Abraham, I.L. (In press). Statistics, quantitative methods, and the discipline of nursing. In I.L. Abraham, D.M. Nadzam, & J.J. Fitzpatrick (Eds.), *Statistics and quantitative methods in nursing: Issues and strategies for research and education.* Philadelphia: W.B. Saunders.

Roy, C., et al. (1981). Theoretical framework for classification of nursing diagnosis: Panel discussion. In M.J. Kim & D. Moritz (Eds.), *Classification of nursing diagnosis: Proceedings of the third and fourth national conferences.* New York: McGraw-Hill.

Articles

Abraham, I.L., Fitzpatrick, J.J., & Jane, L.-H. (1986). Computers in critical care nursing: Yet another technology? *Dimensions of Critical Care Nursing, 5:*325-326.

Downs, F.S., & Fitzpatrick, J.J. (1976, Nov.-Dec.). Preliminary investigation of the reliability and validity of a tool for the assessment of body position and motor activity. *Nursing Research, 25:*404-408.

Fitzpatrick, J.J. (1970, Feb.). Aging and institutionalization as determinants of temporal and motor phenomena. *Image, 1:*24.

Fitzpatrick, J. (1970). Learning is . . . . *Capital, 54:*7-9.

Fitzpatrick, J. (1978). Aging and institutionalization as determinants of temporal and motor phenomena. *Image, 10:*24.

Fitzpatrick, J.J. (1980, Sept.-Oct.). Patients' perceptions of time: Current research. *International Nursing Review, 5:*143-153, 160.

Fitzpatrick, J.J. (1983, May). Suicidology and suicide prevention: Historical perspectives from the nursing literature. *Journal of Psychosocial Nursing and Mental Health Service, 5:*20-28.

Fitzpatrick, J. (1984, Sept.-Oct.) Customizing reusable stoma plates. *Journal of Enterostomal Therapy, 11:*196-198.

Fitzpatrick, J.J. (1985). Endowed chairs in nursing: State of the art. *Journal of Professional Nursing, 1(3):*145-147.

Fitzpatrick, J.J. (1985). The new breed! *Nursing Success Today, 2(3):*4-8.

Fitzpatrick, J.J. (1986). Endowed Chairs in nursing: An update. *Journal of Professional Nursing.*

Fitzpatrick, J.J. (1987). Professional doctorate as entry into clinical practice. *Perspectives in Nursing 1987-1989*. New York: National League for Nursing, pp. 53-56.

Fitzpatrick, J.J. (1987). Use of existing nursing models. *Journal of Gerontological Nursing, 13(9):*8-9.

Fitzpatrick, J.J. (1988). The clinical nurse-midwife as scientist. *Journal of Nurse Midwifery. 33(1):*37-39.

Fitzpatrick, J.J. (1988, Sept.). GN theory based on Rogers' conceptual model. *Journal of Gerontological Nursing. 14(9):*14-16.

Fitzpatrick, J.J. & Abraham, I.L. (1987). Contractual community relationships for research. *Issues in Higher Education, 25:*107-110.

Fitzpatrick, J.J., & Abraham, I.L. (1987). Toward the socialization of scholars and scientists. *Nurse Educator, 12:*23-25.

Fitzpatrick, J.J., Abraham, I.L., & Pressler, J.L. (In press). Developing scientific relationships through leadership. *Nurse Educator.*

Fitzpatrick, J.J., & Behrman, R.E. (1985). The university and the hospital: Old friends, new allies. *Nursing and Health Care, 6:*383-384.

Fitzpatrick, J.J., Boyle, K.K., & Anderson, R.M. (1986). Evaluation of the Doctor of Nursing (ND) program: Preliminary findings. *Journal of Professional Nursing 2(6):*365-372.

Fitzpatrick, J.J., & Donovan, M.J. (1978, July). Temporal experience and motor behavior among the aging. *Research in Nursing and Health, 2:* 60-68.

Fitzpatrick, J.J., & Donovan, M.J. (1979, May-June). A follow-up study of the reliability and validity of the motor activity rating scale. *Nursing Research, 3:*179-181.

Fitzpatrick, J.J., Donovan, M.J., & Johnston, R.L. (1980, June). Experience of time during the crisis of cancer. *Cancer Nursing, 3:*191-194.

Fitzpatrick, J.J., Halloran, E.J., & Algase, D.L. (1987). An experiment in nursing revisited. *Nursing Outlook. 35(1):*29-33.

Fitzpatrick, J.J., & Macaluso, J. (1985, Oct.) Shadow positioning technique: a method for postmortem identification. *Journal of Forensic Science, 30:*1226-1229.

Fitzpatrick, J.J., & Reid, P.G. (1980, Dec.). Stress in the crisis experience: Nursing interventions. *Occupational Health Nursing, 28:*19-21.

Fitzpatrick, J.J., & Whall, A.L. (1984). Points of view: Should nursing models be used in psychiatric nursing practice? *Journal of Psychosocial Nursing, 22(6):*44-45.

Fitzpatrick, J.J., & Whall, A.L. (1984, June). Should nursing models be used in psychiatric nursing practice? *Journal of Psychosocial Nursing and Mental Health Services, 222:*44-45.

Flagherty, G.G., & Fitzpatrick, J.J. (1978, Nov.-Dec.). Use of a relaxation technique to increase comfort level of postoperative patients: A preliminary study. *Nursing Research, 6:*352-355.

Goldberg, W.G., & Fitzpatrick, J.J. (1980, Nov.-Dec.). Movement therapy with the aged. *Nursing Research, 6:*339-346.

Horowitz, B., Fitzpatrick, J.J., & Flaherty, G. (1984). Relaxation techniques to relieve pain in postoperative open heart surgery patients: A clinical study. *Dimensions of Critical Care Nursing Journal. 3*(6):364-371.

Kiley, M., et al. (1983). Computerized nursing information systems (NIS). *Nursing Management, 14:*26-29.

Pacini, C.M., & Fitzpatrick, J.J. (1982, June). Sleep patterns of hospitalized aged individuals. *Journal of Gerontological Nursing, 6:*327-332.

Pressler, J.L., & Fitzpatrick, J.J. (1988). Rosemary Ellis: Contributions of Rosemary Ellis to Knowledge Development for Nursing, *Image, 20(1):*28-30.

Roberts, B.L., & Fitzpatrick, J.J. (1983, March). Improving balance. Therapy of movement. *Journal of Gerontological Nursing, 3:*150-156.

Roslaniec, A., & Fitzpatrick, J.J. (1979, Dec.). Changes in mental status in older adults with four days of hospitalization. *Research in Nursing and Health, 2:*177-187.

Study Group on Nursing Information Systems (1983). Special report computerized nursing information systems: An urgent need. *Research in Nursing and Health, 6:*101-105.

Wilson, L.M., & Fitzpatrick, J.J. (1984). Dialectic thinking as a means of understanding systems-in-development: Relevance to Rogers' principles. *Advances in Nursing Science, 6(2):*24-41.

Thesis

Fitzpatrick, J.J. (1967). *A study of staff nurses' perceptions of the importance of selected nursing activities in carrying out their nursing role.* Unpublished master's thesis. The Ohio State University.

Dissertation

Fitzpatrick, J.J. (1975). *An investigation of the relationship between temporal orientation, temporal extension, and time perception.* Unpublished doctoral dissertation. New York University.

Abstracts, Book Reviews, Editorials

Downs, F.S., & Fitzpatrick, J.J. (1977). Preliminary investigation of the reliability and validity of a tool for the assessment of body position and motor activity. *Psychological Abstracts.* Washington, D.C.: American Psychological Association (Research abstract).

Fitzpatrick, J.J. (1975). *An investigation of the relationship between temporal orientation, temporal extension, and time perception.* Unpublished doctoral dissertation, New York Univerity (Abstract).

Fitzpatrick, J. (1978). Temporal experiences among hospitalized individuals: A pilot study. In R. Williams & C. Wrotny (Eds.), *Health promotion: In health and illness: Proceedings of the First Annual Research Symposium of the Michigan Sigma Theta Tau Consortium.* Indianapolis, Ind.: Sigma Theta Tau (Abstract).

Fitzpatrick, J. (1980). Identity crisis resolved. *Center for Health Research NEWS, 2(1):*1.

Fitzpatrick, J. (1980). Review of *Nursing theory: Analysis, application, evaluation* by Barbara J. Stevens, *Nursing Research, 29:*114.

Fitzpatrick, J. (1980). Time is relevant. *Center for Health Research NEWS, 1(2):*1.

Fitzpatrick, J. (1980). Why a newsletter? *Center for Health Research NEWS, 1(1):*1.

Fitzpatrick, J. (1981). Answer 2 to research replication: Questions and answers. *Western Journal of Nursing Research, 3:*96-97.

Fitzpatrick, J. (1981). Is nursing the science of health? *Center for Health Research NEWS, 2(2):*1.

Fitzpatrick, J. (1981). Review of *The many faces of suicide: Indirect self-destructive behavior* by N.L. Farberow (Ed.). *Nursing Outlook, 29:*435.

Fitzpatrick, J. (1981). Toward the future. . . . *Center for Health Research NEWS, 2(3):*1.

Fitzpatrick, J.J. (1981 to 1985) Message from the chairperson. *CNR Council of Nurse Researchers Newsletter.* Kansas City, Mo.: American Nurses Association.

Fitzpatrick, J.J. (1982). Preface in *Creating research environments for the 1980's (MNRS).* Indianapolis: Midwest Alliance in Nursing.

Fitzpatrick, J. (1982). Review of *Readings on the research process in nursing* by D.J. Fox & I.R. Leeser (Eds.). *Nursing Research, 31:*158.

Fitzpatrick, J.J. (1983). Review of *Suicide intervention for nurses* by M. Miller (Ed.). *Journal of Psychosocial Nursing, 21(2):*39.

Fitzpatrick, J.J. (1984). Why research? *Nursing Success Today, 1(4):*3 (Editorial).

Fitzpatrick, J. J. (1987). Visions of nursing. *Nurse Educator. 12(2):*7-8.

Fitzpatrick, J.J., & Boyle, K.K. (1987). Evaluation of graduates of the Doctor of Nursing (ND) program. *Proceedings of the 11th Annual Midwest Nursing Research Society Conference* (Abstract).

Fitzpatrick, J.J., Donovan, M.J., & Johnston, R. (1979). Temporal experiences among terminally ill cancer patients: An exploratory study. *Proceedings of the Second Annual Research Symposium, Michigan Sigma Theta Tau Consortium.* Indianapolis, Ind.: Sigma Theta Tau (Abstract).

Fitzpatrick, J.J., Donovan, M.J., & Johnston, R.L. (1985). Adult devvelopmental stage, depression and the experience of time. *The Gerontologist, 25:*128-129 (Abstract).

Fitzpatrick, J.J., Johnston, R.L., & Donovan, M.J. (1980). Hospitalization as a crisis: Relation to temporal experience, in WICHE proceedings. *Communicating Nursing Research Directions for the 1980's, 13:*48 (Abstract).

Fitzpatrick, J.J., Reed, P.G., Donovan, M.J., & Zurakowski, T. (1983). Programmatic research on suicide: A nursing perspective. *Proceedings of the American Association of Suicidology Annual Meeting,* New York (Abstract).

Johnston, R.L., Fitzpatrick, J.J., & Donovan, M.J. (1982). Developmental stage: Relationship to the experience of time. *Nursing Research, 31:*120 (Abstract).

Reed, P.G., et al. (1982). Suicidal crises: Relationship to the experience of time. *Nursing Research, 31:*122 (Abstract).

See, E.M., Fitzpatrick, J.J., & Halloran, E.J. (1987). An organizational model for faculty practice. *Proceedings of the 1986 MAIN Seventh Annual Fall Workshop,* Overland Park, Kansas (Abstract).

Sills, G.M., & Fitzpatrick, J.J. (1979). Women: Psychotropic drug use and eclectic relaxation therapy. In *Nursing Research: Synopses of selected clinical studies.* Kansas City: American Nurses' Association. (Abstract).

Werley, H.H., & Fitzpatrick, J.J. (1986). Annual review of nursing research: A valuable research tool. *Proceedings of the 1986 International Nursing Research Conference,* Edmonton, Alberta, Canada (Abstract).

Correspondence

Fitzpatrick, Joyce (1984). Personal correspondence.

Interview

Fitzpatrick, J.J. (1984, March 22). Telephone interview.

Fitzpatrick, J.J. (1985). Telephone interviews.

Fitzpatrick, J.J. (1988). Telephone interviews.

Bulletins

Abraham, I.L., Nadzam, D.M., & Fitzpatrick, J.J. (1986). Statistics and quantitative methods in nursing: Overview of a recent invitational conference. *Bulletin on Teaching of Statistics in the Health Sciences,* pp. 1-4. American Statistical Association, No. 41, Winter.

Fitzpatrick, J.J. (1987). *The ND Program: Integration of past and future.* Cleveland, Ohio: Frances Payne Bolton School of Nursing.

Secondary Sources

Book Reviews

Fitzpatrick, J.J., Whall, A.L., & Johnston, R.L. (1982). *Nursing models and their psychiatric mental health applications.*
*American Journal of Nursing, 1:*102-103, January 1983.
*Nursing Outlook, 3:*148, May-June 1983.
*Research in Nursing and Health, 1:*41, March 1983.

Chapters

Beckman, S.J., Chapman-Boyce, P., Coleman-Ehmke, S., Hailway, C.A., & Pung, R.A. (1986). Joyce J. Fitzpatrick Life Perspective Model. In D.P. Carroll (Ed.). *Nursing Theorists and Their Work,* pp. 361-368. St. Louis: C.V. Mosby.

Pressler, J.L. (1983). Fitzpatrick's rhythm model: Analysis for nursing science. In J. Fitzpatrick & A. Whall, *Conceptual models of nursing: Analysis and application.* Bowie, Md.: Robert J. Brady.

Biographical Sources

Fitzpatrick, J.J. (1980, Aug.). *Directory of nurses with doctoral degrees* (Vol. 1). Kansas City: American Nurses Association.

Fitzpatrick, J.J. (1984, Jan.). *The National Faculty Directory* (Vol. 1). Detroit: Gale Research.

Other Sources

Caplan, G. (1961). *An approach to community mental health.* New York: Grune & Stratton.

Caplan, G. (1964). *Principles of preventive psychiatry.* New York: Basic Books.

Chinn, P.L., & Jacobs, M.K. (1983). *Theory and nursing: A systematic approach.* St. Louis: C.V. Mosby.

Falco, S.M., & Lobo, M.L. (1980). Martha Rogers.

In Nursing Theories Conference Group, J.B. George, Chairperson, *Nursing theories: The base for professional nursing practice*. Englewood Cliffs, N.J.: Prentice-Hall.

Haus, E. (1978). Perspectives on nursing theory. *Advances in Nursing Science, 1*:37-48.

Lachmann, F.M. (1985). On transience and the sense of temporal continuity. *Continuing Psychiatry, 21*:193.

Luce, G.G. (1970). *Biological rhythms in psychiatry and medicine*. National Institute of Mental Health. Washington, D.C.: U.S. Dept. of Health, Education, and Welfare.

Rogers, M.E. (1967). The theoretical basis of nursing. Philadelphia: F.A. Davis.

Margaret A. Newman

32

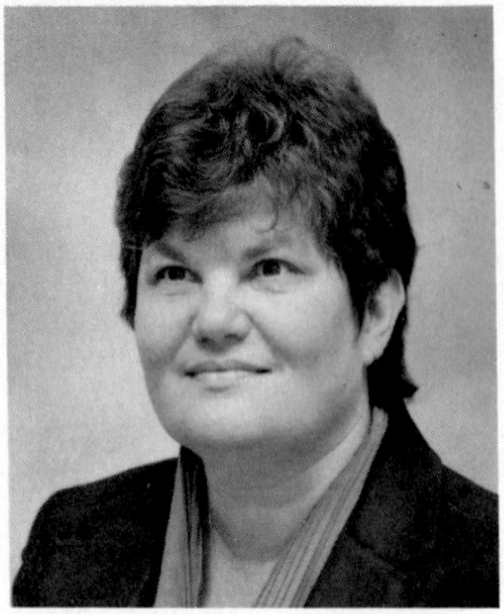

Model of Health

DeAnn M. Hensley, M. Jan Keffer, Kimberly A. Kilgore-Keever, Jill Vass Langfitt, LaPhyllis Peterson

CREDENTIALS AND BACKGROUND OF THE THEORIST

Margaret A. Newman was born October 10, 1933,[39:588] in Memphis, Tennessee. She earned her first bachelor's degree in Home Economics and English from Baylor University, in Waco, Texas, in 1954, and her second in nursing from the University of Tennessee in Memphis in 1962. She received her master's degree in medical-surgical nursing and teaching from the University of California at San Francisco in 1964 and her Ph.D. in nursing science and rehabilitation nursing from New York University in New York City in 1971.

Newman progressed through the academic ranks at the University of Tennessee, New York University, The Pennsylvania State University, and since 1984 has been a professor at the University of Minnesota in Minneapolis. In addition, she has been the director of nursing for the Clinical Research Center at the University of Tennessee, the acting director of the Ph.D. program in the Division of Nursing at New

The authors wish to express appreciation to Dr. Margaret A. Newman for critiquing the chapter.

York University, and Professor-in-Charge of the Graduate Program and Research at The Pennsylvania State University.

Newman was admitted to the American Academy of Nursing in 1976. She received the Outstanding Alumnus Award from the University of Tennessee College of Nursing in Memphis in 1975 and the Distinguished Alumnus Award from the Division of Nursing at New York University in 1984[26:1-2] She was a Latin American Teaching Fellow in 1976-1977 and an American Journal of Nursing Scholar in 1979. She was Distinguished Faculty at the Seventh International Conference on Human Functioning at Wichita, Kansas, in 1983 and is listed in *Who's Who in American Women.*[18]

In 1985, as a Traveling Research Fellow, Newman conducted workshops in four locations throughout New Zealand.[32] At the University of Tampere, Finland, in 1985 Newman was the major speaker for a week-long conference on the theory of consciousness as it related to nursing.[32] Newman has presented numerous papers on topics pertaining to her theory of health as expanding consciousness. She has published two books on the theory: *Health as Expanding Consciousness* in 1986 and *Theory Development in Nursing* in 1979. She has written numerous articles in journals and book chapters. In 1986 she did a case study analysis of practice in three sites within the Minneapolis–St. Paul area in which she discussed the background of the health care system, findings within each site, and conclusions concerning the changes necessary for hospital nursing practice.[34]

Newman has served on several editorial boards, including *Nursing Research, Western Journal of Nursing Research, Nursing and Health Care,* and *Advances in Nursing Science.* Essential to her theory and nursing diagnoses development was her participation as a member of the nurse theorist task force, since 1978, with the North American Nursing Diagnoses Association.

THEORETICAL SOURCES

Central to her assumptions was the use of the philosopher Hegel's "dialectical process of the fusion of opposites."[23:56] Newman used many fields of inquiry as sources for theory development. The rationale for drawing broad conclusions from the use of a limited number of concepts came from Capra, a physicist. Capra's position was that many phenomena can be explained in terms of a few. Newman[23:59] drew from Capra in general, and Bentov in particular, for her position on the importance of holistic health and expansion of consciousness. "Bentov has postulated that time is a measure of consciousness."[23:64] Newman[26:1] stated, "From the standpoint of nursing theorists, those who were most influential on my thinking were Dorothy Johnson, during my undergraduate studies, and Martha Rogers, in a more extensive way, during my graduate study."

Bohm's theory of implicit order helped Newman put Bentov's explanation of the evolving consciousness into perspective.[29:5] Newman stated she began to comprehend "the underlying, unseen pattern that manifests itself in varying forms, including disease, and the interconnectedness and omnipresence of all that there is."[29:5] Young's theory of human evolution pinpointed for Newman the role of pattern recognition and "was the impetus for . . . efforts to integrate the basic concepts of my theory—movement, space, time, and consciousness—into a dynamic portrayal of life and health."[29:6] Moss' experience of love as the highest level of consciousness "provided affirmation and elaboration of my intuition regarding the nature of health."[29:6]

USE OF EMPIRICAL EVIDENCE

Evidence for the theory of health emanated from Newman's early personal family experiences. Her mother's struggle with a chronic illness and her dependency upon Newman, then a young college graduate, sparked the interest in nursing. From the experience evolved the idea that "illness reflected the life patterns of the person and that what was needed was the recognition of that pattern and acceptance of it for what is meant to that person."[29:3]

Throughout Newman's writing, terms are used such as *call to nursing,*[29:2] *growing conscience-like feeling,*[29:2] *fear,*[29:3] *power,*[29:3] *meaning of life and health,*[29:4] *belief of life after death,*[29:5] *rituals of health,*[29:7] and *love.*[29:6,65,72,102] The terms provide a clue concerning Newman's endeavors to make logical a disturbing life experience. The life experience triggered her beginning maturation toward theory development in nursing. Within her philosophical framework, Newman began to develop a synthesis of disease-nondisease—health as a recognition of the total patterning of a person.

Research has been conducted on the theoretical sources used. Newman[23:23] wrote that "in order for nursing research to have meaning in terms of theory development, it must (1) have as its purpose the testing of theory, (2) make explicit the theoretical framework upon which the testing relies, and (3) reexamine the theoretical underpinnings in light of the findings." To Newman,[23:73] "The expansion of knowledge related to man's health and the development of practice based on that knowledge are the responsibility, and perhaps the 'rightful heritage,' of nursing."

MAJOR CONCEPTS AND DEFINITIONS

HEALTH. Health encompasses disease and nondisease. Health can be regarded as the explication of the underlying pattern of the person and the environment.[29:13] Health is viewed as a process of "developing awareness of self and environment together with increasing ability to perceive alternatives and respond in a variety of ways."[25:164] Health is viewed as the "pattern of the whole" of a person.[29:12]

PATTERN. Pattern is what identifies an individual as a particular person. Examples of explicit manifestations of the underlying pattern of a person would be the genetic pattern that contains information that directs our becoming, the voice pattern, the movement pattern.[29:13] Characteristics of pattern include movement, diversity, and rhythm. Pattern is "somehow intimately involved in energy exchange and transformation."[29:14]

In *Health As Expanding Consciousness,* Newman developed pattern as a major concept that was used to understand the individual as a whole being. Newman described a paradigm shift that was occurring in the field of health care. The shift was from treatment of symptoms of a disease to the search for patterns. Newman stated that the patterns of interaction of person-environment constitute health.[29:18] Embedded within the concepts of movement, time, and space is the idea that an event such as a disease occurrence is part of a larger process.

> By interacting with the event, no matter how destructive the force might seem to be, its energy augments our own and enhances our power in the situation. In order to see this, it is necessary to grasp the pattern of the whole.[29:18]

CONSCIOUSNESS. *Consciousness* is defined as the "informational capacity of the system: the ability of the system to interact with its environment."[29:33] Three correlates of consciousness (time, movement, space) serve as explanations for the changing pattern of the whole and are major concepts in the theory of health.

The life process is seen as a progression toward higher levels of consciousness.[23,25] "The expansion of consciousness is what life, and therefore health, is all about."[23:66] Newman referred to the time sense as a factor altered in the changing level of consciousness. Thus, the perception of time is an indicator of man's health status.[20:6]

Movement. "Movement is the means whereby one perceives reality and, therefore, is a means of becoming aware of self."[25:165] Newman[20:23] emphasized that "movement through space is integral to the development of a concept of time in man and is utilized by man as a measure of time." She maintained that "movement brings about change, without which there is no manifest reality."[23:61] To further explain this concept Newman[20:1] used the example of "the person restricted in his mobility by structural or psychological pathology [who] must adapt to an altered rate of movement."

Time and space. Time and space have a complementary relationship.[23:61] "The concept of space is inextricably linked to the concept of time. . . . When one's life space is decreased, as by either physical or social immobility, one's time is increased."[20:61]

Time in Newman's model includes a sense of time perspective, that is, orientation to past, present, and future, but it centers primarily on time as perceived duration. Perceived duration is defined as the ratio of the individual's awareness to content.

$$\text{Perceived duration} = \frac{\text{Awareness}}{\text{Content}}$$

Perceived duration is used synonymously with subjective time as defined by Bentov.[22:290-291] "Factors related to the awareness component include emotional state and attention to a task; factors related to content are external events, body movement, and metabolism."[24:137]

$$\text{Subjective time} = \frac{\text{Awareness}}{\text{Content}^{35:137}}$$

Newman used the theories of time perception, modified by Bentov's conceptualization of time and consciousness. "He calculates an index of consciousness by establishing a ratio of subjective time (the number of seconds judged to have elapsed) to objective time (actual clock time).[23:64]

$$\text{Index of consciousness} = \frac{\text{Subjective time}}{\text{Objective time}^{24:291}}$$

Bentov depicted the relationship of time and space as axes perpendicular to each other. He then superimposed another set of perpendicular axes representing subjective time and subjective space. Bentov hypothesized that as the subjective axes rotate, a person's index of consciousness would increase to infinity; therefore, time is converted to space.[25:167]

In *Health As Expanding Consciousness,* Newman drew heavily on the theoretical work of Young's *The Reflexive Universe: Evolution of Consciousness.* "The central theme of Young's theory is that a self, or a universe, is of the same nature. The essential nature is undefinable, but the beginning and the end are characterized by complete freedom, unrestricted choice."[29:43]

Newman established a corollary between her model of health as expanding consciousness and Young's conception of the evolution of human beings (Figure 32-1).

We come into being from a state of potential consciousness, are bound in time, find our identity in space, and through movement learn the

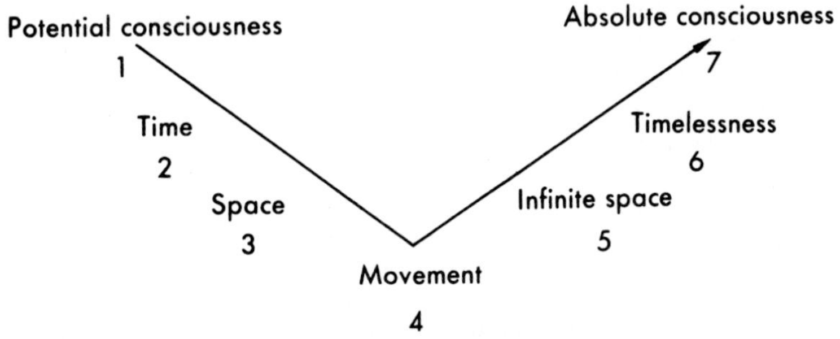

Figure 32-1. Young's process applied to expanding consciousness.
Used with permission from Newman, M. (1986). *Health As Expanding Consciousness.* St. Louis: C.V. Mosby, p. 45.

"law'" of the way things work and make choices that ultimately take us beyond space and time to a state of absolute consciousness.[29:46]

Since beginning the development of her theory, Newman moved from the "restrictions in movement-space-time" to an "awareness that extend[ed] beyond the physical self."[29:46] She assumed that the awareness corresponded to the "inward, self-generated reformation that Young [spoke] of as the turning point of the process."[29:46] "Progression to the sixth state (timelessness) involves increasing freedom from time."[29:46] Finally, the last stage is absolute consciousness, "which has been equated with love."[29:47]

MAJOR ASSUMPTIONS

The foundation for Newman's assumptions[23:56] is her definition of health, which is rationalized through the Hegelian dialectical process of thesis, antithesis, and synthesis. Another influential component is Rogers' 1970 model for nursing that focuses on wholeness, person/environment, life process, pattern/organization, and man's capacity for the higher, complex processes of the mind.[23:57] From this Newman[23:57-58] developed the following assumptions:

1. Health encompasses conditions heretofore desribed as illness, or in medical terms, pathology.
2. These "pathological" conditions can be considered a manifestation of the total pattern of the individual.
3. The pattern of the individual that eventually manifests itself as pathology is primary and exists prior to structural or functional changes.
4. Removal of the pathology in itself will not change the pattern of the individual.
5. If becoming "ill" is the only way an individual's pattern can manifest itself, then that is health for that person.

Newman developed her central premise based on these assumptions. She stated, "Health is the expansion of consciousness."[20:58] The "process of unfolding consciousness will occur regardless of what we as nurses do. We can, however, assist clients in getting in touch with what is going on, and in that way faciliate the process."[26]

Nursing's major assumptions of nursing, person, health, and environment are not addressed explicitly in the theory of health. In the following paragraphs implicit definitions from Newman's work were used to discuss the four nursing components.

NURSING. The nurse is the facilitator who helps an individual, family, or community focus on his/her pattern.[29:73] The nursing process is one of pattern recognition. Newman utilized the assessment framework developed by the nurse theorist group of the North American Nursing Diagnosis Association (NANDA) to assist the nurse in pattern identification. The dimensions of the assessment framework—exchanging, communicating, relating, valuing, choosing, moving, perceiving, feeling, and knowing—are considered to be manifestations of the unitary pattern.[29:73]

"Pattern recognition comes from within the observer."[30:38] The nurse perceives the patterns of the set of data or sequence of events and the pattern of the individual changes with the new information. The process of pattern recognition first involves an attempt to view the pattern of a person as "sequential patterns over time."[30:38] Data from interviews of "healthy" adults could be grouped into sequential patterns. A follow-up interview is then conducted to share the investigator's findings with the subjects. The nurse can use this process to identify the current pattern of an individual in order to establish a plan of care.[30]

PERSON. Throughout Newman's work the terms *client, patient, person, individual,* and *pattern* are used interchangeably. Person is defined as being consciousness.[29:33] Persons are identified as an individual by the specific pattern.

Newman addressed the concepts of implicit order and explicit order in describing the pattern of an individual. The *implicit order* was described as the underlying pattern and the *explicit order* as the things we can see, feel, and touch.[15:10]

ENVIRONMENT. Environment is not explicitly defined, but is described as being the larger whole, that which is beyond the consciousness of the individual. The pattern of consciousness that is the person interacts within the pattern of consciousness that is the family and within the pattern of community interactions.[29:32] A major assumption is that "consciousness is coextensive in the universe and resides in all matter."[29:33]

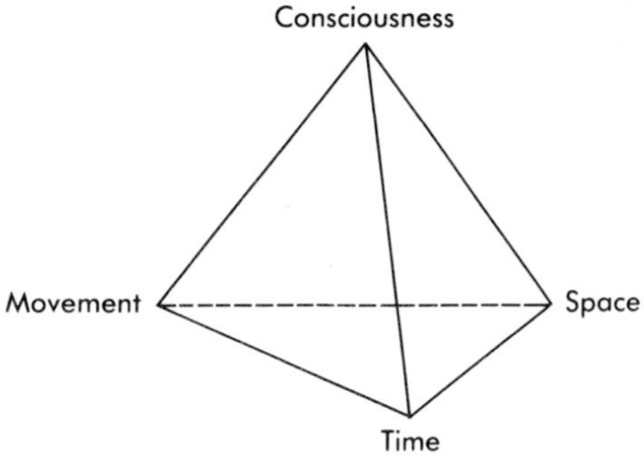

Figure 32-2. Newman's Model of Health.
Used with permission from Newman, M. (1979). *Theory Development in Nursing*. F.A. Davis, p. 60.

HEALTH. Health is the major concept of Newman's theory of expanding consciousness. A fusion of disease and nondisease creates a synthesis that is regarded as health.[23:56] Because disease and nondisease are each reflections of the larger whole a new concept is formed: pattern of the whole.[29:12] Newman stated that the "essence of the emerging paradigm of health is pattern recognition."[29:13]

THEORETICAL ASSERTIONS

In *Theory Development in Nursing,* Newman used considerable space to explain the concepts of time, space, and movement. The interrelationships of the concepts are show in Figure 32-2 and are succinctly described within her work. Newman developed five interrelationships between her major concepts.

"Time and space have a complementary relationship."[23:60;25:165] Newman gave examples of this relationship at the macrocosmic, microcosmic, and humanistic (everyday) levels. She stated that at the humanistic level "the highly mobile individual lives in a world of expanded space and compartmentalized time. When one's life space is decreased, as by either physical or social immobility, one's time is increased."[23:61]

"Movement is a means whereby space and time become a reality."[23:60;25:165] Man is in a constant state of motion and is constantly changing. This occurs both internally, at the cellular level, and externally through body movement and interaction with the environment. This movement through time and space is what gives man his own unique perception of reality. Movement brings change and enables the individual to experience the world around him.[23:61-63]

"Movement is a reflection of consciousness."[23:60;25:165] Movement not only is the means of experiencing reality, but it is also the means by which one expresses his thoughts and feelings about the reality he experiences. An individual conveys his awareness of self through the movement involved in language, posture, and body movement.[23:62] "The rhythm and pattern which are reflected in movement are an indication of the internal organization of the person and his perception of the world. Movement provides a means of communication beyond that which language can convey."[23:62]

"Time is a function of movement."[23:60;17:165] This assertion is supported by Newman's previous studies regarding the experience of time as related to movement and gait tempo. Newman's research shows that the slower one walks, the less subjective time one experiences. When compared with clock time, however, time seems to "fly." Although the individual who is moving quickly subjectively feels he is "beating the clock," he finds when checking a clock that time seems to be dragging.[23:63;20:1]

"Time is a measure of consciousness."[23:60] This assertion was first proposed in 1977 by Bentov, who measured consciousness with a ratio of subjective to objective time. Newman applied this measure of consciousness to the subjective and objective data compiled in her research. She found that the consciousness index increased with age. Some of her most recent research has also supported the finding of increasing consciousness with age.[24:293] Newman[20:64] cited this evidence as support for her position that the life process evolves toward consciousness expansion. "However, certain moods, such as depression, may be accompanied by a diminished sense of time."[35:139]

Excellent examples were used by Newman to illustrate the centrality of space-time, one of which is included here.[29:56]

> Mrs. V. made repeated attempts to *move* away from husband and to *move* into an educational program to become more independent. She felt she had no *space* for herself, and she tried to distance herself *(space)* from her husband. She felt she had no *time* for leisure (self), was overworked, and was constantly meeting other people's needs. She was submissive to the demands and criticism of her husband.

In *Health As Expanding Consciousness*, Newman used Figure 32-3 as a model of the interrelationship of the center of consciousness (person) with movement-time-space. Newman stated that the crucial task "is to be able to see the concepts of movement-space-time in relation to each other, all at once, as patterns of evolving consciousness."[29:48] The intersection represents the person as a center of consciousness and varies from "person to person, place to place, and time to time."[29:49]

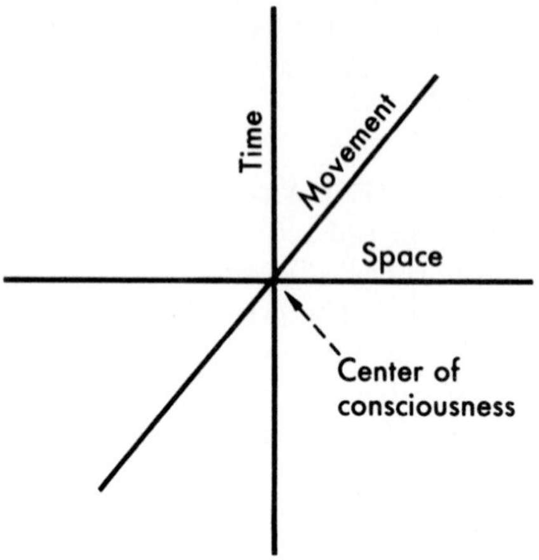

Figure 32-3. Persons as centers of consciousness with movement-time space configurations.
Used with permission from Newman, M. (1986). *Health As Expanding Consciousness*. C.V. Mosby, p. 48.

LOGICAL FORM

Newman utilized both inductive and deductive logic. Inductive logic is based on observing particular instances and then relating those instances to form a whole. Newman's theory development was derived from her earlier research on time perception and gait tempo. Time and movement, along with space and consciousness, are subsequently used as central components in her conceptual framework. These concepts help explain "the phenomena of the life process, and therefore of health."[23:59]

But Newman's theory also incorporated deductive logic.

> A holistic approach is not to be confused with, or construed to mean a multivariate approach. It is not the summing up of many factors . . . to make a whole. It is the identification of patterns which are reflective of the whole. What these parameters are will vary according to one's ability to see the whole. For some, the universe can be seen in a grain of sand. For others, characteristics which present identifiable patterns of the individual, e.g., the way a person walks or the way he talks, are a good place to start.[23:70]

ACCEPTANCE BY THE NURSING COMMUNITY
Practice

Newman's model of health is potentially useful in the practice of nursing because it contained concepts employed by the nursing profession.

Movement and time are an intrinsic part of nursing intervention, that is, range-of-motion, ambulation, turning, coughing, and deep breathing. These parameters are used each day by the nurse in practice.[9:271-272]

Doberneck, while a graduate student at The Pennsylvania State University, used Newman's model to work with caregivers of chronically ill people. She was helped by Newman's discussion of application of the model to practice in her chapter in the Clements and Roberts book *Family Health* and her further elaboration at the May 1984 Edmonton Conference. Doberneck believed Newman's model addressed issues intrinsic to caring that other theories omit, such as unconditionally being with another person and noncommitment to specific predetermined outcomes.[5]

Marchione used Newman's model to investigate and report the meanings of disabling events in families. She presented a case study in which an additional person became part of the nuclear family for an extended period of time. The addition was a disruptive event for the family and created disturbances in time, space, movement, and consciousness.[29:124-126;18:231-237] Analysis of the case study of the family suggested that Newman's work with patterns could be utilized to understand family interactions.

Newman admitted that when the current paradigm of health care is utilized (treatment of disease rather than pattern) and nursing remains bounded by hospital regulations, her nursing approach encounters difficulties.[15:11] She challenged nursing to "practice her philosophy of health in their contact with patients throughout the lifespan" whether in an acute medical crisis or not.[15:11]

The new paradigm is based on health as the "undivided wholeness of the person in interaction with the environment."[29:88] Newman believed that nursing practice should be directed toward recognition of the pattern of that interaction and acceptance of it as a process of evolving consciousness.[29:88]

Education

Roy stated,

> The function of nursing education [is] the development and sharing of knowledge concerning the theories about the phenomena of nursing and the knowledge and skills related to the theories of the practice of nursing. Since theories describe and predict nursing practice, then nursing education must develop and promote them in such a way that students become nurses who use and develop theory.[36:17]

Newman[26] did "not advocate one model as the sole basis for a curriculum. . . . Students should have the opportunity to study various approaches to health and nursing and to choose what is relevant to them in their practice and research."

Newman consulted with faculty and students from several universities, including Indiana University, Louisiana State University, Medical College of Virginia, New York University, The Pennsylvania State University, University of Akron, University of Alabama, University of California at San Francisco, University of Colorado, University of Minnesota, University of Oregon, University of Southern Florida, University of Tennessee, and Wayne State University.[20] Faculty at the University of Akron have incorporated Newman's work into the philosophical and conceptual framework of their master's program.[12] Metropolitan State University in St. Paul, Minnesota, adopted Newman's theory for use in its baccalaureate nursing program.[32] At some institutions, Newman's model is presented in classes about theoretical models in nursing, and some graduate students at various institutions conduct research based on it.

Newman's theory of pattern extended directly to the nursing process. She suggested that the task in intervention is pattern recognition accomplished by the health professional becoming "aware of the pattern of the other person by sensing into her/his *own* pattern."[33] Newman suggested that the professional should

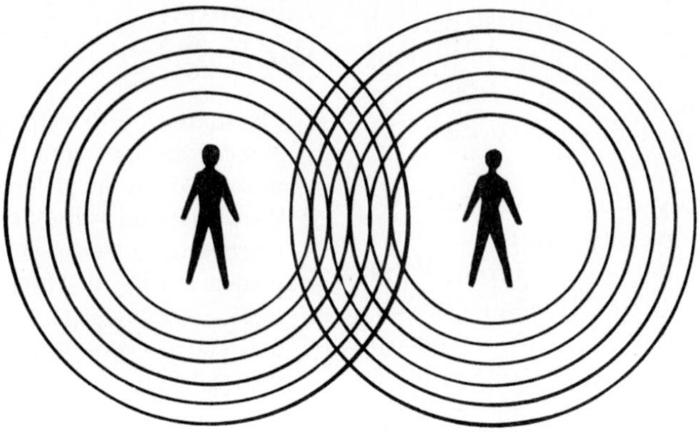

Figure 32-4. Interaction pattern of two persons: a holographic model of intervention.
Used with permission from Newman, M. (1986). *Health As Expanding Consciousness.* C.V. Mosby, p. 71.

focus on the pattern of the other person, in effect acting like the "reference beam in a hologram."[29:73] The holographic model of intervention is described by "imagining the emanating waves that appear when two pebbles are thrown into water. As the waves radiate . . . they meet and interact . . . [forming] an interference pattern"[29:70] (Figure 32-4).

Newman stated that a new role is needed for the nurse to function in the paradigm of the evolving consciousness of the whole. "Nurses need to be free to relate to patients in an ongoing partnership that is not limited to a particular place or time."[29:89] Nursing education would revolve around the "concept of pattern: pattern as substance, pattern as process, and pattern as method."[29:89] Education by this method would enable nursing to be an important resource for the continued development of health care. Newman stated that nursing is at the intersection of the focus of the health care industry; thus "nursing is in position to bring about the fluctuation within the system that will shift the system to a new higher order of functioning."[29:90]

Research

Research has a dual role: to test theory and establish a scientific knowledge base from which to practice professional nursing. In addition to Newman, several researchers have done research about time, space, or movement. They include Barnard,[1] Chapman,[2] Downs and Fitzpatrick,[6] Engle,[7;11:12] Fitzpatrick and Donovan,[13] Goldberg and Fitzpatrick,[14] Smith,[37] and Tompkins.[38] Several of these researchers, including Newman, were influenced by Rogers. By using similar methodology, a cohesive body of knowledge is being developed on the relationship between movement and time across different age groups. "Traditional methodologies may not be sufficient to examine the [relationships], because the model is future-oriented and visionary."[9:270-271]

Engle[9-11] attempted to test Newman's propositions of time, space, and movement by measuring older adults' functional health. In 1986 Engle found significant relationships between functional health and movement and between movement and time in a sample of older white women.[10]

Newman and Gaudiano focused on the occurrence of depression in the elderly. Subjective versus objective time was used as a measure of consciousness. Analysis of the study supported the hypothesis that depression was related to decreased subjective time.[35:137] In her 1987 article "Aging as Increasing Complexity," Newman discussed the Newman and Gaudiano study. A negative correlation was found between depression and subjective time, and this, in turn, could explain "findings that do not support an increasing level of consciousness with age."[31:17] The factor of depression (awareness) may be decreasing consciousness (subjective time). As awareness increases and content stays the same, subjective time increases.[31:17]

Mentzer and Schorr used Newman's model of duration of time as an index to consciousness in a study of institutionalized elderly. Findings indicated perceived duration of time was not significantly related to age or perceived control (movement or space).[19:12]

Newman stated that research should center around "participatory investigations in which subjects (clients) are our partners, our co-researchers, in our search for health patterns."[29:94] This method of inquiry is called *cooperative inquiry* or *interactive, integrative participation*. Newman has moved her research method toward this coinvestigatory method in recent research involving a community investigation.[29:95] In addition, Newman has investigated a method to describe pattern as unfolding and evolving over time. She utilized the method of interviewing a subject in different time frames to establish a pattern for that subject.[30]

FURTHER DEVELOPMENT

Newman reported that operationalization of the model of health as expanding consciousness has been approached in two ways: (1) by research methods designed to describe and test the relationships between the major concepts of movement, time, space, and consciousness and (2) by attempts to describe evolving patterns of consciousness in terms of the integration of movement-space-time.[29:48]

Several studies that address research within the Newman theoretical framework are underway. One study has examined the meaning of health in persons who have been diagnosed with breast cancer.[32] Another study investigated the experience of giving and receiving social support in elderly caregivers.[32]

Newman's current work stresses the concept of pattern recognition, of "grasping the whole in order for the parts to be meaningful."[22:36] She described her attempts to identify pattern in an individual first by using the assessment framework of the NANDA. Second, by analyzing data from interviews of "healthy" (emphasis by Newman) adults into sequential patterns, Newman identified crucial experiences in which energy flow changed and patterns were elucidated.[30] Further work in identification of patterns across the life span is recommended.

Newman's work is progressing toward a fully developed theory. She used Popper's definition that a theory is a powerful, unifying idea to guide the development of her theory. However, Newman[20:6-7] asserted that a theory must also provide for "new relationships [that] may be deduced and tested, and the data therefrom then will either strengthen or weaken the theoretical system from which the tested relationship is drawn."

Newman's concepts are being operationally defined to allow for empirical testing. The interrelationships between the concepts need to be further developed with greater focus directed toward the usefulness within applied nursing practice.

CRITIQUE

Simplicity

In Newman's *Theory Development in Nursing*, the concepts of movement, time, space, and consciousness with the five resulting relationship statements represented the evolution of the theory at that time. In *Health As Expanding Consciousness*, pattern became a major concept included for the purpose of understanding consciousness. Simplicity was sacrificed when pattern of the whole was used to describe the theory of health. Additional relationship statements are needed to incorporate pattern recognition so the theory of health can be utilized for predicting events.

Generality

The concepts in Newman's theory are broad in scope because they all relate to health. This renders her theory generalizable. The broad scope provides a focus for future theory development.

Empirical Precision

Aspects of the theory have been operationalized and tested within a traditional scientific mode. However, quantitative methods are limited in capturing the dynamic, changing nature of this model. Qualitative approaches are being developed for a full explication of its meaning and application.

The model of health has little empirical adequacy because the central concepts are not consistent in their operational definitions. Completed research has operationalized time as passage of seconds on a clock[19,21,24,33] and movement as walking cadence,[9] but the operationalized concept could also be defined in other ways. However, Newman stated that each time a study is done the concepts are operationalized. "The major concepts are meant to be summary concepts that include many more specific concepts."[33]

The concepts of health and patterns are defined as summative units.[7] The units are global and represent an entire complex phenomenon. A summative unit describes an entire entity in a few words, making definitions vague and overlapping. Any interaction between the units are not testable, limiting their utility.

Derivable Consequences

Newman's theory is useful in nursing practice because it used concepts already familiar to nursing, such as time and movement. It has received increased recognition regarding application to practice in recent publications and presentations at conferences.[5,23,32]

The domain of the model of health is the nursing process. The model would be useful for guiding nursing practice and differentiating nursing's areas of concern.

REFERENCES

1. Barnard, R. (1973). *Field-dependence/independence and selected motor abilities.* Unpublished doctoral dissertation. New York University.
2. Chapman, J. (1978). The relationship between auditory stimulation and gross motor activity of short-gestation infants. *Research in Nursing and Health, 1*:29-36.
3. Chinn, P.L. (1983). Nursing theory development: Where we have been and where we are going. In N.L. Chaska (Ed.), *The nursing profession: A time to speak.* New York: McGraw-Hill.
4. Chinn, P.L., & Jacobs, M.K. (1983). *Theory and nursing: A systematic approach.* St. Louis: C.V. Mosby.
5. Doberneck, B. (1985). Graduate student at Pennsylvania State University. Telephone interview.
6. Downs, F., & Fitzpatrick, J. (1976). Preliminary investigation of the reliability and validity of a tool for the assessment of body position and motor activity. *Nursing Research, 25*:404-408.
7. Dubin, R. (1978). *Theory building.* New York: Free Press.
8. Engle, V. (1981). *A study of the relationship between self-assessment of health, function, personal tempo and time perception in elderly women.* Unpublished doctoral dissertation. Detroit: Wayne State University.
9. Engle, V. (1983). Newman's model of health. In J.J. Fitzpatrick, & A.L. Whall (Eds.), *Conceptual models of nursing: Analysis and application.* Bowie, Md.: Robert J. Brady.
10. Engle, V.F. (1984). Newman's conceptual framework and the measurement of the older adults' health. *Advances in Nursing Science, 6*:24-36.
11. Engle, V.F. (1986). The relationship of movement and time to older adults' functional health. *Research in Nursing and Health, 9*:123-129.
12. Engle, V.F., & Graney, M.J. (1985-86). Self-assessed and functional health of older women. *International Journal of Aging and Human Development, 22(4)*:301-313.
13. Fitzpatrick, J., & Donovan, M., (1978). Temporal experience and motor behavior among the aging. *Research in Nursing and Health, 1*:60-68.
14. Goldberg, W., & Fitzpatrick, J. (1980). Movement theory and the aged. *Nursing Research, 29*:339-346.

15. Keene, L. (1985). Nursing as a partnership. *The New Zealand Nursing Journal, 78(12):*10-11.
16. Kim, H.S. (1983). *The nature of theoretical thinking in nursing.* Norwalk, Conn.: Appleton-Century-Crofts.
17. Marchione, J. (1985). Associate professor at the University of Akron, Telephone interview.
18. Marchione, J.M. (1986). Pattern as methodology for assessing family health: Newman's theory of health. In P. Winstead-Fry (Ed.), *Case Studies in Nursing Theory.* New York: NLN.
19. Mentzer, C.A., & Schorr, J.A. (1986). Perceived situational control and perceived duration of time: Expressions of life patterns. *Advances in Nursing Science, 9(1):*12-20.
20. Newman, M.A. (1971). *An investigation of the relationship between gait tempo and time perception.* Unpublished doctoral dissertation. New York University.
21. Newman, M.A. (1972). Time estimation in relation to gait tempo. *Perceptual and Motor Skills, 34:*359-366.
22. Newman, M.A. (1978). *Second Annual Nurse Educator's Conference.* Held in New York City, December 4-6, 1978. (Audiotape).
23. Newman, M.A. (1979). *Theory development in nursing.* Philadelphia: F.A. Davis.
24. Newman, M.A. (1982, Sept.-Oct.). Time as an index of expanding consciousness with age. *Nursing Research, 31:*290-293.
25. Newman, M.A. (1983). Newman's health theory. In I.W. Clements, & F.B. Roberts, *Family health: A theoretical approach to nursing care.* New York: John Wiley & Sons.
26. Newman, M.A. (1984). Personal correspondence.
27. Newman, M.A. (1985). Personal correspondence.
28. Newman, M.A. (1985) Telephone interview.
29. Newman, M.A. (1986). *Health as expanding consciousness.* St. Louis: C.V. Mosby.
30. Newman, M.A. (1987). Patterning. In M. Duffy & N.J. Pender (Eds.), *Conceptual issues in health promotion, a report of proceedings of a Wingspread conference,* Racine, Wisc., April 13-15, 1987. Indianapolis: Sigma Theta Tau.
31. Newman, M.A. (1987). Aging as increasing complexity. *Journal of Gerontological Nursing, 13(9):*16-18.
32. Newman, M.A. (February 1988). Personal correspondence.
33. Newman, M.A. (March 1988). Personal correspondence.
34. Newman, M.A., & Autio, S. (1986). *Nursing in a Prospective Payment System Health Care Environment.* Minneapolis, MN: Univ. of Minn.
35. Newman, M.A., & Gaudiano, J.F. (1984, May-June). Depression as an explanation for decreased subjective time in the elderly. *Nursing Research, 33:*137-139.
36. Roy, C. (1979, March-April). Relating nursing theory to education: A new era. *Nurse Educator, 29:*16-21.
37. Smith, M. (1979). Duration experience for bed-confined subjects: A replication and refinement. *Nursing Research, 28:*139-144.
38. Tompkins, E. (1980). Effect of restricted mobility and dominance in perceived duration. *Nursing Research, 29:*333-338.
39. *Who's Who of American Women.* (1983-1984). Chicago: Marquis.

BIBLIOGRAPHY

Primary Sources

Books

Downs, F.S., & Newman, M.A. (Eds.). (1977). *A source book of nursing research.* Philadelphia: F.A. Davis.

Newman, M.A. (1980). *Theory development in nursing.* Philadelphia: F.A. Davis.

Newman, M.A. (1986). *Health as Expanding Consciousness.* St. Louis: C.V. Mosby.

Newman, M.A., & Autio, S. (1986). *Nursing in a Prospective Payment System Health Care Environment.* Minneapolis: University of Minnesota.

Book Chapters

Feild, L., & Newman, M. (1982). Clinical application of the unitary man framework: Case study analysis. In M.J. Kim & D.A. Morita (Eds.), *Classification of nursing diagnosis.* New York: McGraw-Hill.

Newman, M.A. (1973). Identifying patient needs in short-span nurse-patient relationships. In M.E. Auld, & L.H. Birum (Eds.), *The challenge of nursing.* St. Louis: C.V. Mosby.

Newman, M.A. (1981). The meaning of health. In G.E. Laskar (Ed.), *Applied systems research and cy-*

bernetics: Vol. 4. *Systems research in health care, biocybernetics and ecology.* New York: Pergamon.

Newman, M.A. (1983). The continuing revolution: A history of nursing science. In N.L. Chaska (Ed.), *The nursing profession: A time to speak.* New York: McGraw-Hill.

Newman, M.A. (1983). Nursing's theoretical evolution. In T.A. Duespohol (Ed.), *Nursing in transition.* Rockville, Md.: Aspen Systems.

Newman, M.A. (1983). Newman's health theory. In I. Clements & F. Roberts (Eds.), *Family health: A theoretical approach to nursing care.* New York: John Wiley & Sons.

Newman, M.A. (1983). Health as expanding consciousness. In *Proceedings of Seventh International Conference on Human Functioning.* Wichita, Kan.: Biomedical Synergistics Institute.

Newman, M.A. (In press). Nursing paradigms and realities. In N.L. Chaska (Ed.), *The nursing profession: Turning points.* New York: McGraw-Hill.

Newman, M.A. (In press). Professionalism: Myth or reality. In N.L. Chaska (Ed.), *The nursing profession: Turning points.* New York: McGraw-Hill.

Newman, M.A. (1987). Nursing's emerging paradigm: The diagnosis of pattern. In A.M. McLane (Ed.) *Classification of nursing diagnoses,* Proceedings of the Seventh Conference, North American Nursing Diagnosis Association. St. Louis: C.V. Mosby.

Newman, M.A. (1987). Patterning. In M. Duffy, & N.J. Pender (Eds.), *Conceptual issues in health promotion, a report of proceedings of a Wingspread conference.* Racine, Wisc.: Indianapolis: Sigma Theta Tau.

Roy, C., et al. (1982). Nursing diagnosis and nursing theory. In M.J. Kim, & D.A. Moritz (Eds.), *Classification of nursing diagnosis.* New York: McGraw-Hill.

Articles

Butrin, J., & Newman, M.A. (1986). Health promotion in Zaire: Time perspective and cerebral hemispheric dominance as relevant factors. *Public Health Nursing, 3*(3):183-191.

Newman, M.A. (1966). Identifying and meeting patient's needs in short-span nurse-patient relationships. *Nursing Forum, 5:*76-86.

Newman, M.A. (1972). Time estimation in relation to gait tempo. *Perceptual and Motor Skills, 34:*359-366.

Newman, M.A. (1972, July). Nursing's theoretical evolution. *Nursing Outlook, 20:*449-453.

Newman, M.A. (1975, Nov.). The professional doctorate in nursing: A position paper. *Nursing Outlook, 23:*704-706.

Newman, M.A. (1976, Aug.). Movement, tempo and the experience of time. *Nursing Research, 25:*273-279.

Newman, M.A. (1982, Sept.-Oct.). Time as an index of expanding consciousness with age. *Nursing Research, 31:*290-293.

Newman, M.A. (1982, Oct.). What differentiates clinical research? *Image, 14:*86-88.

Newman, M.A. (1983). Editorial. *Advances in Nursing Science, 5:*x-xi.

Newman, M.A. (1984, Dec.). Nursing diagnosis: Looking at the whole. *American Journal of Nursing, 84(12):*1496-1499.

Newman, M.A. (1987). Aging as increasing complexity. *Journal of Gerontological Nursing, 13(9):*16-18.

Newman, M.A. (1987). Commentary: Perception of time among Japanese inpatients. *Western Journal of Nursing Research, 9(3):*299-300.

Newman, M.A., & Gaudiano, J.K. (1984, May-June). Depression as an explanation for decreased subjective time in the elderly. *Nursing Research, 33:*137-139.

Newman, M.A., & O'Brien, R.A. (1978, Feb.). Experiencing the research process via computer simulation. *Image, 10:*5-9.

Portonova, M., Young E., & Newman, M.A. (1984). Elderly women's attitudes toward sexual activity among their peers. *Health Care for Women, International, 5(5/6):*289-298.

Dissertation

Newman, M.A. (1971). An investigation of the relationship between gait tempo and time perception. Unpublished doctoral dissertation. New York University, School of Education.

Reports

Newman, M.A. (1977). Nursing course content in doctoral education. *Proceedings of National Conference on Doctoral Education in Nursing.* Philadelphia: University of Pennsylvania.

Newman, M.A. (1982). What differentiates clinical research? *Proceedings of the Second Phyllis J. Verhonick Nursing Research Course.* Washington, D.C.:

Nursing Research Service, Walter Reed Army Medical Center.

Newman, M.A., et al. (1980). Movement, time, and consciousness: Parameters of health. (Symposium). Proceedings of Western Society for Research. *Nursing Research, 13:*45-49.

Newman, M.A., & Gaudiano, J.K. (1983). Depression as an explanation for decreased subjective time in the elderly. In M.C. Smith (Ed.). *Proceedings of the Second Annual Research Conference of the Southern Council on Collegiate Education in Nursing.*

Audiotapes

Newman, M.A. (1978, Dec. 4-6). Paper presented at Second Annual Conference, New York City. Tapes available from Teach 'em Inc., 160 E. Illinois Street, Chicago, Ill. 60611.

Newman, M.A., (1984, May). Paper presented at Nursing Theory Conference, Boyle, Letourneau Conference, Edmonton, Canada. Tapes available from Ed Kennedy, Kennedy Recording, R.R. 5, Edmonton, Alberta, Canada T5P4B7 (403-470-0013).

Correspondence

Newman, M.A. (1984). Personal correspondence.

Newman, M.A. (1985). Personal correspondence.

Interview

Newman, M.A. (1985). Telephone interview.

Secondary Sources

Book Reviews

Newman, M.A. (1980). *Theory development in nursing.*
*Continuing Education in Nursing, 2:*8†, Nov.-Dec. 1979.
*Nursing Administration Quarterly, 4:*81-82, Spring, 1980
*Nursing Leadership, 3:*38, March, 1980
*Nursing Research, 29:*311, Sept.-Oct., 1980
*Western Journal of Nursing Research, 2:*250-251, Spring, 1980

Books

Chinn, P.L., & Jacobs, M.K. (1983). Theory in nursing: A current overview In P.L. Chinn & M.K. Jacobs (Eds.), *Theory and nursing.* St. Louis: C.V. Mosby.

Kim, H.S. (1983). *The nature of theoretical thinking in nursing.* Norwalk, Conn.: Appleton-Century-Crofts.

Rogers, M.E. (1970). *An introduction to the theoretical basis of nursing.* Philadelphia: F.A. Davis.

Who's Who of American Women (1983-1985). Chicago: Marquis Who's Who.

Book Chapters

Burd, C. (1985). Appendix D. Newman's Nursing Theory of Health. In B.W. Duldt & K. Geffin, *Theoretical Perspectives for Nursing.* Boston: Little, Brown.

Chinn, P.L. (1983). Nursing theory development: Where we have been and where we are going. In N.L. Chaska (Ed.), *The nursing profession: A time to speak.* New York: McGraw-Hill.

Engle, V. (1983). Newman's model of health. In J.J. Fitzpatrick & A.L. Whall (Eds.), *Conceptual models of nursing: Analysis and application.* Bowie, Md.: Robert J. Brady.

Marchione, J.M. (1986). Pattern as methodology for assessing family health: Newman's theory of health. In P. Winstead-Fry (Ed.), *Case Studies in Nursing Theory,* New York, NLN.

Articles

Batra, C. (1987). Nursing theory for undergraduates. *Nursing Outlook, 35(4):*189-192.

Cull-Wilby, B.L., & Pepin, J.I. (1987). Towards a coexistence of paradigms in nursing knowledge development. *Journal of Advanced Nursing, 12:*515-521.

DeGrott, H.A., Ferketich, S.L., & Larson, P.J. (1987). Theory development in a non-university service setting. *Journal of Nursing Administration, 17(4):*38-44.

Doherty, W.J. (1985). Family interventions in health care. *Family Relations, 34:*129-137.

Engle, V.F. (1984, Oct.). Newman's conceptual framework and the measurement of older adults' health. *Advances in Nursing Science, 7(1):*24-36.

Engle, V.F. (1986). The relationship of movement and time to older adults' functional health. *Research in Nursing and Health, 9:*123-129.

Engle, V.F., & Graney, M.J. (1985-86). Self-assessed and functional health of older women. *International Journal of Aging and Human Development, 22(4):*301-313.

Gupta, S., & Cummings, L.L. (1986). Perceived

speed of time and task affect. *Perceptual and Motor Skills, 63:*971-980.

Jennings, B.M. (1987). Nursing theory development: Successes and challenges. *Journal of Advanced Nursing, 12:*63-69.

Keene, L. (1985). Nursing as a partnership. *The New Zealand Nursing Journal, 78(12):*10-11.

Mentzer, C.A., & Schorr, J.A. (1986). Perceived situational control and perceived duration of time: Expressions of life patterns. *Advances in Nursing Science, 9(1):*12-20.

Moccia, P. (1985). A further investigation of "dialectical thinking as a means of understanding systems-in-development: Relevance to Roger's principles." *Advances in Nursing Science, 7(4):*33-38.

Peplau, H.E. (1988). The art and science of nursing: Similarities, differences, and relations. *Nursing Science Quarterly, 1(1):*8-15.

Pridham, K.F., & Hansen, M.F. (1985). Nursing and medicine: Complementary modes of thought and action. *Public Health Nursing, 2(4):*195-201.

Reed, P.G. (1986). Developmental resources and depression in the elderly. *Nursing Research, 35(6):*368-374.

Rosenbaum, J.N. (1986). Comparison of two theorists on care: Orem and Leininger. *Journal of Advanced Nursing, 11:*409-419.

Roy, C. (1979, March-April). Relating nursing theory to education: A new era. *Nurse Educator, 29:*16-21.

Sanders, S.A. (1986). Development of a tool to measure subjective time experience. *Nursing Research, 35(3):*178-182.

Sarter, B. (1987). Evolutionary idealism: A philosophical foundation for holistic nursing theory. *Advances in Nursing Science, 9(2):*1-9.

Shah, S.K., Harasymiw, S.J., & Stahl, P.L. (1986). Stroke rehabilitation: Outcome based on Brunnstrom recovery stages. *The Occupational Therapy Journal of Research, 6(6):*365-376.

Silva, M.C. (1986). Research testing nursing theory: State of the art. *Advances in Nursing Science, 9(1):*1-11.

Silva, M.C., & Rothbart, D. (1984). An analysis of changing trends in philosophies of science on nursing theory development and testing. *Advances in Nursing Science, 6:*1-13.

Smith, M.J. (1984). Temporal experience and bed rest: Replication and refinement. *Nursing Research, 33(5):*298-302.

Tompkins, E. (1980, Nov.-Dec.). Effect of restricted mobility and dominance in perceived duration. *Nursing Research, 29(6):*333-338.

Whall, A.L. (1986). The family as the unit of care in nursing: A historical review. *Public Health Nursing, 3(4):*240-249.

News Releases

Brown, N.M. (1983, Nov.). The body is not a machine. *Research/Penn State 4(4):*19-20.

M.A. Newman appointed as full tenured professor at University of Minnesota School of Nursing. (1984, March). *Nursing Outlook, 32:*2.

Abstracts

Newman, M.A. (1981). Relationship of age to perceived duration. *Abstracts of ANF funded research 1979-1980.* Kansas City: American Nurses' Foundation.

Dissertation Proposal

Page, G. (1985). *An exploration of the relationship between a person's daily patterning and weight loss; Maintenance or non-maintenance.* Dissertation proposal. Wayne State University.

Master's Theses

Butren, J. (1983). *Differences in time perspective and hemisphericity between educated and noneducated Zairians.* Masters thesis. Pennsylvania State University.

Griscavage, D. (1982). *Relationships among state anxiety time estimation, body movement, and repression-sensitization in preoperative patients.* Master's thesis. Pennsylvania State University.

Pollard, M. (1981). *Emotional expressiveness in cancer and noncancer patients.* Master's thesis. Pennsylvania State University.

Pollock, D. (1983). *The relationship of sleep deprivation to cerebral hemisphericity and temporal orientation.* Master's thesis. Pennsylvania State University.

Zack, C. (1983). *Hospitalized patients' personal space preferences in relation to female and male nurses.* Master's thesis. Pennsylvania State University.

Other

Acton, H.B. (1967). George Wilhelm Friedrich Hegel 1770-1831. In *The encyclopedia of philosophy* (Vols. 3 & 4). New York: Macmillan & Free Press.

Barnard, R. (1973). *Field-dependence-independence and selected motor abilities.* Unpublished doctoral dissertation. New York University.

Bentov, I. (1977). *Stalking the wild pendulum.* New York: E.P. Dutton.

Bentov, I. (1978, Nov. 17-20). *The mechanics of consciousness.* Paper presented at the symposium on New Dimensions of Consciousness, sponsored by Sufi Order in the West. New York.

Capra, F. (1975). *The tao of physics.* Boulder, Col.: Thambhala Publications.

Chapman, J. (1978). The relationship between auditory stimulation and gross motor activity of short-gestation infants. *Research in Nursing and Health, 1:*29-36.

Downs, F., & Fitzpatrick, J. (1976). Preliminary investigation of the reliability and validity of a tool for the assessment of body position and motor activity. *Nursing Research, 25:*404-408.

Engle, V. (1981). *A study of the relationship between self-assessment of health, function, personal tempo and time perception in elderly women.* Unpublished doctoral dissertation. Wayne State University.

Fitzpatrick, J., & Donovan, M. (1978). Temporal experience and motor behavior among the aging. *Research in Nursing and Health, 1:*60-68.

Goldberg, W., & Fitzpatrick, J. (1980). Movement therapy and the aged. *Nursing Research, 29:*339-346.

Marcuse, H. (1954). *Reason and revolution: Hegel and the rise of social theory* (2d ed.). New York: Beacon.

Rogers, M.E. (1980). Nursing, a science of unitary man. In J.P. Reihl & C. Roy, *Conceptual models for nursing practice.* New York: Appleton-Century-Crofts.

Smith, M. (1979). Duration experience for bed-confined subjects: A replication and refinement. *Nursing Research, 28:*139-144.

Tompkins, E. (1980). Effect of restricted mobility and dominance in perceived duration. *Nursing Research, 29:*333-338.

Interviews

Doberneck, B. (1985). Graduate student at Pennsylvania State University. Telephone interview.

Marchione, J. (1985). Associate professor at the University of Akron. Telephone interview.

Index

Page numbers in *italics* indicate illustrations.
Page numbers followed by *t* indicate tables.